PRIMER ON MR IMAGING OF THE ABDOMEN AND PELVIS

DIEGO R. MARTIN, M.D., Ph.D.
Division of Abdominal Radiology
Emory University Hospital
Atlanta, Georgia

MICHÈLE A. BROWN, M.D.
Department of Radiology
University of California, San Diego Medical Center
San Diego, California

RICHARD C. SEMELKA, M.D.
Department of Radiology
University of North Carolina School of Medicine
Chapel Hill, North Carolina

 **WILEY-LISS**

A JOHN WILEY & SONS, INC., PUBLICATION

Published by John Wiley & Sons, Inc., Hoboken, New Jersey.
Published simultaneously in Canada.

For general information on our other products and services please contact our Customer Care Department within the U.S. at 877-762-2974, outside the U.S. at 317-572-3993 or fax 317-572-4002.

Wiley also publishes its books in a variety of electronic formats. Some content that appears in print, however, may not be available in electronic format.

Library of Congress Cataloging-in-Publication Data:

Martin, Diego R.
    Primer on MR imaging of the abdomen and pelvis / Diego R. Martin, Michèle
A. Brown, Richard C. Semelka.
        p. ; cm.
    Includes bibliographical references and index.
    ISBN 0-471-37340-0 (pbk.)
    1. Abdomen—Magnetic resonance imaging.   2. Pelvis—Magnetic resonance imaging.
    [DNLM: 1. Abdomen—physiopathology.   2. Digestive System Diseases—diagnosis.   3. Magnetic Resonance
Imaging—methods.   4. Pelvis—physiopathology.   5. Urologic Diseases—diagnosis. WI 900 M379p 2005]
    I. Brown, Michèle A.   II. Semelka, Richard C.   III. Title.

RC944.M375   2005
617.5′507548—dc22   2004013847

Printed in the United States of America.

10 9 8 7 6 5 4 3 2

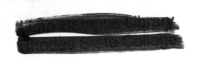

PRIMER ON MR IMAGING OF THE ABDOMEN AND PELVIS

CONTENTS

PREFACE

The inspiration for this book derives from the observation that there exists a gap between the utility and the utilization of MRI as applied for diagnostic evaluation of abdominal and pelvic diseases. The objective of this book is to provide readers with a reference that facilitates an understanding of MR imaging techniques and the appearance of the diseases as depicted with these techniques, with the hope that it will encourage others to help close this gap. We have organized the diseases by organ system, and the information is displayed as lists of key points, with a short explanation of the disease, followed by key imaging features. Emphasis has been placed on images showing each of the disease entities. While MR continues to develop in ways that will make imaging easier to perform reliably and with shorter exam times, it is important to note that current techniques can reliably yield diagnostic images that can be used in place of CT for most important diseases of the abdomen and pelvis, and with results that have been shown to provide more information about these diseases. There has been increasing concern regarding the risks of CT in relation to radiation and iodinated contrast exposure. As utilization of cross-sectional imaging in our population continues to increase, there is a greater pressure for radiologists to be able to offer alternatives. Becoming more conversant with MR imaging is a key element to success in this process. Aiming towards maximizing efficiency, many of the images shown in this publication can be found in another textbook, "*Abdominal-Pelvic MRI*" by Richard Semelka, published by Wiley & Sons. Where the prior textbook represents an exhaustive comprehensive detailed reference, the current Primer is targeted towards radiology residents, fellows, and practicing radiologists who may find this book useful to provide a rapid reference to help with both acquisition and analysis of images.

ACKNOWLEDGMENT

The authors would like to thank Tiffany Snyder for her tireless efforts helping in the preparation of this primer.

CHAPTER 1

INTRODUCTION

FUNDAMENTALS OF MR IMAGING TECHNIQUES APPLIED TO THE ABDOMEN AND THE PELVIS

Image quality, reproducibility of image quality, and good conspicuity of disease require the use of sequences that are robust and reliable and that avoid artifacts. Maximizing these principles to achieve high-quality diagnostic MR images usually requires the use of fast scanning techniques, with the overall intention of generating images with consistent image quality that demonstrate consistent display of disease processes. The important goal of shorter examination time may be achieved with the same principles that maximize diagnostic quality. With the decrease of imaging times for individual sequences, a greater variety of sequences may be employed without increasing the total examination time. This approach contributes to one of the major strengths of MRI, which is comprehensive information on disease processes.

Respiration, bowel peristalsis, and vascular pulsations may result in major artifacts that lessen the reproducibility of MRI. Breathing-independent sequences and breath-hold sequences form the foundation of high-quality MRI studies of the abdomen. Breathing artifact is less problematic in the pelvis, and high spatial and contrast resolution imaging have been the mainstay for maximizing image quality for pelvic studies.

Disease conspicuity depends on the principle of maximizing the difference in signal intensities between diseased tissues and background tissue. For disease processes situated within or adjacent to fat, this is readily performed by manipulating the signal intensity of fat, which can range from low to high on both T1-weighted (T1W) and T2-weighted (T2W) images. For example, diseases that are low in signal intensity on T1W images, such as peritoneal fluid or retroperitoneal fibrosis, are most conspicuous on T1W sequences in which fat is high in signal intensity (i.e., sequences without fat suppression). Conversely, diseases that are high in signal intensity, such as subacute blood or proteinaceous fluid, are more conspicuous if fat is rendered low in signal intensity with the use of fat-suppression techniques. On T2W images, diseases that are low in signal intensity, such as fibrous tissue, are most conspicuous on sequences in which background fat is high in signal intensity, such as echo-train spin-echo sequences. Diseases that are moderate to high in signal intensity, such as lymphadenopathy or

Primer on MR Imaging of the Abdomen and Pelvis, edited by Diego R. Martin, Michele A. Brown, and Richard C. Semelka ISBN 0-471-37340-0 Copyright © 2005 Wiley-Liss, Inc.

ascites, are most conspicuous on sequences in which fat signal intensity is low, such as fat-suppressed sequences.

Gadolinium chelate enhancement may be routinely useful because it provides at least two further imaging properties that facilitate detection and characterization of disease, specifically the pattern of blood delivery (i.e., capillary enhancement) and the size and/or rapidity of drainage of the interstitial space (i.e., interstitial enhancement). Capillary phase image acquisition is achieved by using a short-duration sequence initiated immediately after gadolinium injection. Spoiled gradient-echo (GRE or SGE) sequence performed as multisection two- or three-dimensional acquisition is an ideal sequence to use for capillary phase imaging.

The majority of focal mass lesions are best evaluated in the capillary phase of enhancement, particularly lesions that do not distort the margins of the organs in which they are located (e.g., focal liver, spleen, or pancreatic lesions). Images acquired 1.5–10 min after contrast administration are in the interstitial phase of enhancement, with the optimal window being 2–5 min postcontrast. Diseases that are superficial, spreading, or inflammatory in nature are generally well shown on interstitial phase images. The concomitant use of fat suppression serves to increase the conspicuity of disease processes characterized by increased enhancement on interstitial phase images including peritoneal metastases, cholangiocarcinoma, ascending cholangitis, inflammatory bowel disease, and abscesses.

The great majority of diseases can be characterized by defining their appearance on T1, T2, and early and late postgadolinium images. Throughout this text the combination of these four parameters for the evaluation of abdomino-pelvic disease is stressed.

T1-WEIGHTED SEQUENCES

T1W sequences are routinely useful for investigating diseases of the abdomen, and they supplement T2W images for investigating diseases of the pelvis. The primary information that pre-contrast T1W images provide includes (1) information on abnormally increased fluid content or fibrous tissue content that appears low in signal intensity on T1W images and (2) information on the presence of subacute blood or concentrated protein, which are both high in signal intensity. T1W sequences obtained without fat suppression also demonstrate the presence of fat as high-signal intensity tissue. The routine use of an additional fat attenuating technique facilitates reliable characterization of fatty lesions.

Spoiled Gradient-Echo (GRE or SGE) Sequences

SGE sequences are the most important and versatile sequences for studying abdominal disease. These sequences provide T1W imaging and may be used with phased-array multicoil imaging, to replace longer-duration sequences such as the T1W spin-echo (SE) sequence. Image parameters for SGE are (1) relatively long repetition time (TR) (approximately 150 ms) to maximize signal-to-noise ratio and the number of sections that can be acquired in one multisection acquisition and (2) the shortest in-phase echo time (TE) (approximately 6.0 ms at 1.0 T and 4.2–4.5 ms at 1.5 T) to maximize signal-to-noise ratio and the number of sections per acquisition. Hydrogen protons in a voxel containing 100% fat will precess approximately 220–230 Hz slower than in a voxel comprised of 100% water at 1.5 T. Thus, every 4.4 ms the fat protons will lag behind by 360° and regain in-phase orientation relative to water protons, while at 2.2 ms the fat and water protons will be 180° out-of-phase.

Current generation MR control software has incorporated dual-echo breath-hold SGE sequences that can acquire two sets of k-space filled to obtain two sets of images, one set in-phase, the other out-of-phase, with spatially matched slices. For routine T1W images, in-phase TE may be preferable to the shorter out-of-phase echo times (4.0 ms at 1.0 T and 2.2–2.4 ms at 1.5 T) to avoid both phase cancellation artifact around the borders of organs and fat-water phase cancellation in tissues containing both fat and water protons. The flip angle should be approximately 70–90° to maximize the T1W signal. With the use of the larger built-in body coil, the signal-to-noise ratio of SGE sequences is usually suboptimal with section thickness less than 8 mm, whereas with the phased-array surface coils, section thickness of 5 mm results in diagnostically adequate images. On new MRI machines more than 22 sections may be acquired in a 20 s breath-hold, or 44 paired sections, when using the dual-echo technique.

Application of Out-of-Phase SGE Sequences

Out-of-phase (opposed-phase) SGE images are useful for demonstrating diseased tissue in which mixtures of fat and water protons are present within the same voxel. A voxel containing predominantly fat or water will not demonstrate diminished signal on out-of-phase images. A TE of 2.2 ms is advisable at 1.5 T, and 4.4 ms is advisable at 1.0 T. A TE of 6.6 ms is also out-of-phase at 1.5 T, but the shorter TE of 2 ms is preferable because there are decreased susceptibility effects (i.e., the shorter echo time reduces the time for dephasing effects to accumulate, as is caused by metals or gas), more sections can be acquired per sequence acquisition, the signal is higher, the sequence is more T1W, and in combination with a T2W sequence it is easier to distinguish fat and iron in the liver.

At 1.5 T, both fat and iron cause liver signal decrease on out-of-phase images using a TE of 6.6 ms, relative to the in-phase images acquired with a TE of 4.4 ms, whereas on 2.2 ms out-of-phase TE images fat is darker and iron is brighter relative to a TE of 4.4 ms (fig. 1.1). Relative sensitivity to magnetic susceptibility effects, which increase with an increase in TE, can also be used to distinguish iron-containing paramagnetic structures (e.g., surgical clips, or foci of iron deposition in the spleen or liver) from nonmagnetic signal void structures (e.g., calcium). To illustrate this point, the signal void susceptibility artifact from surgical clips

increases in size as the TE increases from 2.2 to 4.4 ms, whereas the signal void from calcium remains unchanged. However, the most common indications for out-of-phase imaging are the detection of abnormal fat accumulation within the liver and the detection of lipid within adrenal masses, a feature used to characterize benign adrenal adenomas. As discussed previously, current MRI systems can acquire both in- and out-of-phase images during a single breath-hold SGE acquisition, and this feature is useful on routine imaging of the abdomen.

Intravascular Gadolinium-Chelate Contrast-Enhanced SGE Sequences

In addition to its use as precontrast T1W images, SGE should be used routinely for multiphase image acquisition after gadolinium administration for investigation of the liver, spleen, pancreas, and kidneys. An important feature of the multisection acquisition of SGE is that the central phase-encoding steps are generally used to fill central k-space, which determines image contrast. This contrast component of the data set is acquired over a 4–5 s period for the entire data set and is essentially shared by each individual section. Thus, the data acquisition is sufficiently short for the entire data set to isolate a distinct phase of enhancement (e.g., hepatic arterial dominant phase). Furthermore, this ensures that images of organs, such as the liver, are shown uniformly in the same phase of contrast enhancement throughout the volume of the tissue.

Fat-Suppressed SGE Sequences

Fat-suppressed (FS) SGE sequences are routinely used as precontrast images for evaluating the pancreas and for the detection of subacute blood. Fat suppression is generally achieved on SGE images by selectively stimulating slower precessing hydrogen protons associated with fat using a tuned radio-frequency (rf) pulse, followed by spoiler gradients, prior to performing the gradient echo imaging components of the sequence. This process is termed excitation – spoiling fat suppression. Image parameters are similar to those for standard SGE. It may be advantageous to employ a lower out-of-phase echo time (2.2–2.5 ms at 1.5 T), which benefits from additional fat-attenuating effects and increases signal-to-noise ratio and the number of sections per acquisition.

On current MRI machines fat-suppressed SGE may acquire 22 sections in a 20 s breath-hold with reproducible uniform fat suppression. One method used by modern systems to reduce the amount of time that fat suppression adds to the SGE sequence and to acquire a greater number of slices per breath-hold is to perform an FS step only after several phase-encoding steps instead of after every phase encode. Another approach called water excitation selectively tunes the stimulation rf pulse to activate protons in water but not in fat, thus eliminating the need to add fat-saturation pulses.

Fat-suppressed SGE images are used to improve the contrast between intra-abdominal fat and diseased tissues and blood vessels on interstitial phase gadolinium-enhanced images. Gadolinium enhancement generally increases the signal intensity of blood vessels and disease tissue, and fat suppression diminishes the competing high signal intensity of background fat.

Three-Dimensional Gradient-Echo (3D GRE or 3D SGE) Sequences

3D SGE imaging has been used extensively for MR angiography (MRA) but has evolved only recently into an accepted technique for soft-tissue imaging in the abdomen and pelvis. This development has partly been achieved simply by reducing the flip angle from 70–90° used for angiography to 12–15°. Advantages include the ability to acquire a volumetric data set that can be sectioned into thinner parts than typically used for 2D images, generally in the range of 2.5–3.0 mm per slice with contiguous slices and with images that can be postprocessed into other imaging planes.

Although there are differences between some of the sequence features among various vendor MR systems, generically they are all 3D GRE sequences. Vendor-specific acronyms are different (e.g., 3D-VIBE, 3D-THRIVE, and T1-FAME). Fat suppression on 3D GRE tends to be superior with greater uniformity as compared to 2D SGE. On some MR systems, it is also possible to image a larger volume of tissue than with 2D SGE during the same breath-hold period. A potential limitation of 3D SGE imaging has been diminished contrast to noise. This has led to concern regarding use of this technique other than for gadolinium-enhanced fat-suppressed interstitial phase imaging, where the gadolinium effectively improves the contrast-to-noise ratio.

Motion-Insensitive SGE

One limitation of 2D and 3D SGE images is relative motion sensitivity and thus requirements for patient cooperation in following breathing instructions. In uncooperative patients, SGE may be modified as a single-shot technique using the minimum TR to achieve breathing-independent images. Such sequences have included magnetization-prepared rapid acquisition gradient echo (MP-RAGE) and turbo-fast low-angle shot (Turbo FLASH). This single-shot technique has been achieved using magnetization-prepared GRE, where an inversion prepulse leads to the ability to improve T1W contrast during a single-slice short acquisition. As the protons recover magnetization, a single-slice short TR GRE imaging sequence is performed. An inversion time of around 0.5 s provides optimal T1W contrast, and sufficient time to allow the protons to recover between slices leads to an effective slice-to-slice TR of no less than 1.5 s. This technique can be performed to yield through-plane bright or dark flowing blood by making the prepulse either slice selective or nonselective, respectively. Limitations of this technique have included the inability to obtain the same high or predictable T1W contrast as with standard SGE. Another limitation is that the magnetization-prepared gradient-echo slice-by-slice technique performs suboptimally for dynamic gadolinium-enhanced imaging of the liver, particularly during the hepatic arterial dominant phase. As each slice requires an acquisition time of around 1.5 s, the time difference accumulated between the top and bottom liver slices results in variation in the phase of enhancement through the entire liver.

With MP-RAGE sequences, it is advisable to use the slice-selection inversion pulse, since it permits acquisition of the individual sections without a time delay between them. The non-slice-selective technique results in superior image quality but requires a 2–3 s delay between each individual image slice to maintain image quality and to avoid disturbing variations in tissue signal and contrast resulting from variable tissue relaxation. In contrast, the standard SGE sequences, although motion sensitive, offer much superior time resolution for the entire volume of tissue imaged, with the critical contrast data acquired in less than 5 s and with these data time averaged throughout the entire set of slices, facilitating capture of the entire liver in the same phase of contrast enhancement.

Another strategy dealing with motion is based on motion correction. Older methods using slow spin-echo sequences require several minutes per acquisition using bellows around the patient's lower chest to detect the respiratory cycle and trigger acquisition of data only during end expiration. Although similar in strategy, a more accurate method has been developed in conjunction with rapid imaging sequences where a continuous series of sagittal images are acquired at a rate of greater than one image per second across the right hemidiaphragm using an MP-RAGE–type sequence. The liver-lung interface produces a high-contrast border that can be automatically detected by the specialized software and used to trigger image acquisition at the same phase of the respiratory cycle. Another approach uses phase accumulation during motion of the tissue in order to calculate a correction factor, with application of spatial correction factors in order to restore the detected signal to the location from where it would have originated had there not been any movement. These methods are still considered developmental.

A third approach, which may result in the best solution for patients unable to suspend respirations, is parallel imaging techniques. Development of these techniques is ongoing. With this approach, individual elements of a multielement phased-array receiver surface coil are used to separately collect the signal. The separated signal provides the usual collected information regarding signal frequencies and intensities but also uses the coils to provide additional positional information. The data obtained in this fashion can allow k-space undersampling and can lead to time savings with relatively conserved signal-to-noise ratios (using a variety of techniques beyond the scope of this text). The theoretical reduction in acquisition time is dependent on the number of coil elements used, with reduction in time on the order of 2–4-fold with current generation systems. For example, reduction in time of acquisition for an SGE sequence from 20 s to 10 s or less will be sufficient to facilitate consistent image quality for a majority of patients.

T2-WEIGHTED SEQUENCES

The predominant information provided by T2W sequences is (1) the presence of increased fluid in diseased tissue, which results in high signal intensity, (2) the presence of chronic fibrotic tissue, which results in low signal intensity, and (3) the presence of iron deposition, which results in very low signal intensity.

Standard Spin-Echo and Fast Spin-Echo Sequences

Standard T2W SE is a relatively long method requiring several minutes to acquire slices through the abdomen or pelvis. Advantages include good contrast to noise. With abdominal imaging, breathing-related motion precludes use of this sequence, unless used in conjunction with a motion correction method such as respiratory gating or multiple averaging. This approach adds to the total scan time, and the motion compensation is not reliable or accurate, resulting in at least mild edge blurring, effectively deteriorating resolution. Typical scan times are between 5 and 12 min, depending on the respiratory rate and pattern. It is not unusual for the acquisition to be of poor quality due to motion artifact, thus necessitating repetition.

Pelvic imaging can be performed without breath-holding in most patients, with little image deterioration as breathing-related motion is less severe than in the upper abdomen. Motion due to contracting bowel can cause image deterioration and can be reduced using intravenous or intramuscular glucagon. Latest-generation echo-train spin-echo techniques, including turbo spin-echo and fast spin-echo sequences, are based on intermediate-length echo trains. Acquisition time can be reduced to as low as 2.5 min for the pelvis.

Echo-Train Spin-Echo Sequences

Echo-train spin-echo (ETSE) sequences are classified as single-shot echo-train fast spin-echo (SS-ETSE), single-shot turbo spin-echo, or rapid acquisition with relaxation enhancement (RARE) sequences. The principle of echo-train spin-echo sequences is to summate multiple echoes within the same repetition time interval to decrease examination time, increase spatial resolution, or both. The single-shot techniques are slice-by-slice approaches, where a single slice-selective excitation pulse is followed by a series of echoes, typically using between eighty and one hundred 180° pulses, each separated by approximately 3 ms, to fill in k-space for the entire slice. The T2W contrast is achieved by using the echoes obtained around 80–90 ms for filling central k-space, where central k-space is responsible for image contrast. Although the theoretical TR is infinite, each slice requires around 1.2–1.5 s before continuing to the next slice. However, the motion-sensitive component represents only a smaller fraction of the entire acquisition period, making this technique relatively insensitive to breathing artifacts. Single-shot echo-train spin-

echo has achieved widespread use because of these advantages.

In contrast, conventional T2 spin-echo or longer-duration echo-train sequences are lengthy and suffer from patient motion and increased examination time. The major disadvantage of echo-train sequences is that T2 differences between tissues are decreased. This generally is not problematic in the pelvis because of the substantial differences in the T2 values between diseased and normal tissue. In the liver, however, the T2 difference between diseased and background normal liver may be small, and the T2 averaging effects of summated multiple echoes blur this T2 difference. This results in relatively diminished lesion conspicuity for lesions with mildly elevated T2W signal intensity, such as hepatocellular carcinoma, as compared to standard spin-echo sequences. Fortunately, diseases with T2 values similar to those of the liver generally have longer T1 values than the liver, so lesions poorly visualized on echo-train spin-echo are generally well visualized on SGE or immediate postgadolinium SGE images as low-signal lesions.

ETSE and T2W sequences in general are important for evaluating the abdomen and pelvis. In liver masses, T2W images are especially necessary for lesion characterization, while T1W images are important for both lesion detection sensitivity and characterization. T2W images are also critical for assessment of diffuse liver disease, including iron deposition, edema related to active liver disease, and fibrosis. Echo-train T2W sequences are important for assessment of fluid-filled structures, including the bile duct, gallbladder, and pancreatic duct, the stomach, and the bowel, as well as cysts or cystic masses, abscesses or collections, or free fluid in the abdomen or pelvis.

The relative resistance of echo-train images to motion degradation generally yields better resolution of structures internal to cystic masses, such as the septations within a pancreatic serous or mucinous tumor. MR cholangiopancreatography (MRCP) is based on modified echo-train sequences, where the effective TE is made longer, on the order of 250–500 ms.

Lengthening the TE results in heavily T2W high-contrast images that yield most soft tissues dark and make the fluid in bile ducts, the gallbladder, and the pancreatic duct very bright. MRCP can be performed in thin sections of 3–4 mm for higher resolution, or by using a single thick slab of 3–4 cm to include the majority of the pancreatic and bile ducts in a single image. Echo-train imaging is well suited to image the bowel, due to insensitivity to both respiratory motion and bowel peristalsis as well as relative resistance to distorting paramagnetic effects of intraluminal bowel gas as a result of repeated refocusing echo pulses.

On T2W sequences, fat is high in signal intensity on echo-train spin-echo sequences in comparison to conventional spin-echo sequences, in which fat is intermediate in signal intensity. The MR imaging determination of recurrent malignant disease versus fibrosis for pelvic malignancies illustrates this difference. Recurrent malignant disease in the pelvis (e.g., cervical, endometrial, bladder, or rectal cancer) generally appears high in signal intensity on conventional spin-echo sequences because of the higher signal intensity of the diseased tissue relative to the intermediate signal intensity of fat. In contrast, fat is high in signal intensity on echo-train spin-echo images, and recurrent disease will commonly appear relatively lower in signal intensity. The observation that abnormal tissue is not high in signal intensity on echo-train T2W images relative to fat is not specific for neoplasm, as fibrosis can have a similar appearance. This is particularly problematic in posttherapy patients.

Fat may also be problematic in the liver because fatty liver will be high in signal intensity on echo-train spin-echo sequences, thereby diminishing contrast with the majority of liver lesions, which are generally high in signal intensity on T2W images. It may be essential to use fat suppression on T2W echo-train spin-echo sequences for liver imaging. Fat suppression should generally be applied on at least one set of T2W images of the abdomen or pelvis, to ensure optimal contrast between high-signal abnormalities such as fluid collections or cystic masses and adjacent intra-abdominal or pelvic fat.

MRI EXAMINATION: GENERAL APPROACH

A fundamental approach for successful use of MRI to image the abdomen and pelvis is to employ set protocols for various organ systems that do not require routine on-the-spot adjustment by supervising physicians. Our approach is to employ a set series of sequences that are performed by the technologist. In this fashion, MRI is performed similarly to CT.

MRI is currently considered an expensive and time-intensive imaging modality, which has hampered its appropriate utilization. A balance must always be achieved between acquiring a variety of sequences that provide sufficiently comprehensive information and a short enough study time to accommodate patients' ability to cooperate and a busy MR schedule. We generally aim for abdominal studies of approximately 30 min duration (ideally 15 min) and total abdominal and pelvis studies of 45 min or less. Even shorter studies can be performed in the setting of follow-up examinations. Depending on the amount of information needed, a follow-up study that employs coronal single-shot echo-train spin-echo, transverse precontrast SGE, arterial and venous phase postgadolinium SGE, and 2 min interstitial phase postgadolinium fat-suppressed SGE provides relatively comprehensive information in a 15 min time frame. An even more curtailed examination can be performed if only change in lesion size is being assessed. An adrenal mass or lymphadenopathy may be adequately followed by precontrast SGE alone, and, in the case of an adrenal adenoma, using dual echo out-of-phase and in-phase SGE.

Uncooperative Patients

It is crucial to recognize that separate protocols are required for uncooperative patients. In general, uncooperative patients fall into two categories: (1) those who cannot suspend respiration but breathe in a regular fashion and (2) those who cannot suspend respiration and cannot breathe in a regular fashion. The most common patient population that fits into the first group are sedated pediatric patients. Agitated patients are the most commonly encountered population that fits into the second group. Imaging strategies differ for each.

In sedated patients, substitution of breathhold images (e.g., SGE) can be made readily with breathing-averaged spin-echo images, the image quality of which is improved by using fat suppression. With sedation, breathing is in a more regular pattern than that observed for all other patients. Additionally, breathing-independent T2W single-shot echo-train spin-echo is useful, as is T1W MP-RAGE, if dynamic gadolinium-enhanced images are required

In patients who are agitated, only single-shot techniques should be used, including breathing-independent T2W single-shot echo-train spin-echo and T1W MP-RAGE pre- and postgadolinium administration. Parallel imaging approaches, which provide superior image quality, may supplant single-section techniques to image uncooperative patients.

CHAPTER 2

LIVER

NORMAL LIVER

Figure 2.1 shows a normal liver exam. T2W images are used to aid in the characterization of focal masses. High-signal lesions have high water content and most commonly represent benign lesions including cysts, benign bile duct hamartomas, and hemangiomas. Malignant masses often show an elevated T2 signal but are usually heterogeneous and not as high-signal as cysts, hemangiomas, or bile duct hamartomas on single-shot echo-train spin-echo. The higher-signal malignancies generally represent more vascular or cystic tumors. Sensitivity for metastases is lower on single-shot T2W images compared to standard spin-echo, but this is the trade-off for higher-speed studies that are robust and insensitive to respiratory motion. T2W images should be relied on for characterization of tumors, assessment of diffuse disease (edema, fat or iron deposition), and examination of other related fluid-filled structures such as bile ducts and the gallbladder.

T1W images are obtained with pre- and postgadolinium acquisitions. Pregadolinium images are obtained as in-phase and out-of-phase techniques individually or as dual-echo in/out-of-phase techniques to examine for fatty infiltration. Pregadolinium in-phase sequences should be used to detect masses. Most metastatic malignancies will be low-signal and conspicuous. Postgadolinium images can increase focal lesion conspicuity and provide the most critical data for lesion characterization supported by T2W image findings. All T1W imaging should be obtained using the spoiled gradient-echo technique acquired during a breath-hold. This imaging is motion sensitive. Use of 3D gradient-echo is definitely recommended for the postgadolinium equilibrium phase with fat suppression and is useful for higher-resolution anatomical imaging of normal structures and pathology of all abdominal organs, including the GI tract, vessels, retroperitoneum, and peritoneum. Use of 3D gradient-echo for arterial and venous phase soft-tissue imaging is less certain, as 2D imaging still produces improved contrast, which may yield critical additional information, particularly for detecting small lesions and characterizing liver masses and subtle perfusion abnormalities that can be seen in the liver.

Primer on MR Imaging of the Abdomen and Pelvis, edited by Diego R. Martin, Michele A. Brown, and Richard C. Semelka ISBN 0-471-37340-0 Copyright © 2005 Wiley-Liss, Inc.

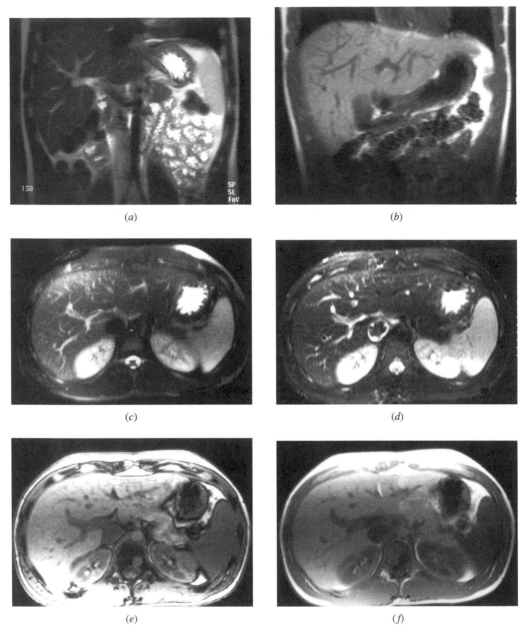

FIGURE 2.1   Liver and pelvis protocol. Coronal T2W single-shot echo-train spin-echo (*a*), coronal T1W SGE (*b*), axial T2W fat-suppressed single-shot echo-train spin-echo (*c*), T2W breath-hold STIR (short tau inversion recovery) (*d*), T1W out-of-phase (*e*),

LIVER MASSES

The superiority of MR over CT for the detection of lesions is most apparent for hypervascular lesions such as small hemangiomas and focal nodular hyperplasias (FNHs), small hepatocellular carcinomas (HCCs), and small hypervascular metastases. A major advantage of MR over CT imaging is lesion characterization, particularly in lesions less than 1–2 cm

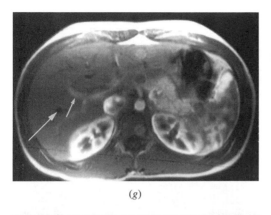

(g)

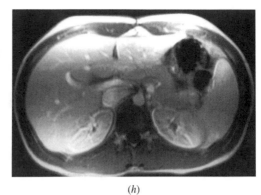

(h)

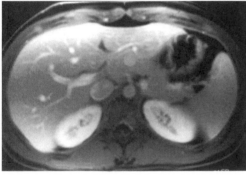

(i)

FIGURE 2.1   (*Continued*) T1W in-phase SGE (*f*), hepatic arterial dominant phase SGE (*g*), 1 min postgadolinium SGE (*h*), 1.5 min postgadolinium fat-suppressed SGE (*i*).

in diameter. A common problem occurs in patients with known malignancy, where the liver is found to have multiple small lesions, often with one or more of these lesions found to be too small to characterize on CT. Around a quarter to half of liver lesions in patients with a primary malignancy are benign. MR imaging is excellent in these cases, with characterization specificity of approximately 95%. Percutaneous needle biopsy has an inadequate yield in a third of cases, making MR the method of choice for liver lesion characterization. In patients with malignancy, the ability to characterize a liver lesion as benign or malignant can be as important as identifying metastases. For example, small liver cysts or bile duct hamartomas are common in adult patients and can be too small for accurate density measurement on CT, but they can be resolved even down to 1 mm cysts on MR due to a very high signal produced on T2W imaging. Generally, the advantages of MR over CT arise from the greater contrast resolution

and the variety of different soft-tissue contrast achieved through implementation of multiple sequences.

Table 2.1 summarizes MRI findings for the most common liver masses.

Cysts

Background
- Commonly found in adults
- Etiology unclear, but may result from different mechanisms, including developmental and acquired causes
- Pathology generally shows single-layer lining with cuboidal to columnar epithelial cells
- Categorization
  - Nonparasitic
  - Parasitic
    - Echinococcus
  - Hemorrhagic
    - Spontaneous/posttraumatic
  - Polycystic diseases

TABLE 2.1 MRI Findings for the Majority of Encountered Liver Masses

	T1	T2	Early Gd (Arterial)	Late Gd (Venous and Equilibrium)	Other Features
Benign					
Cyst	↓↓	↑↑	O	O	Well-defined borders
Hamartoma	↓↓	↑↑	Thin rim	Thin rim	<1 cm
Hemangioma	↓↓	↑↑	Peripheral nodules	Nodules coalesce, retain	<1.5 cm lesion may enhance
FNH	↓-∅	∅-↑	Homogeneous intense, nonenhancing scar	Homogeneous washout, late scar enhancement	Central scar liver is commonly fatty
Adenoma	↓-↑	∅-↑	Homogeneous intense	Homogeneous washout	Uniform signal loss on out-of-phase T1, larger lesions may bleed
Bacterial abscess	↓↓	↑-↑↑	Perilesional enhancement, capsule enhances	Perilesional enhancement fades, capsule remains enhanced	Resemble metastases but not progressive lesion enhancement
Regenerative nodules	↓-∅	↓-∅	Negligible	Negligible	Lesions generally <1.5 cm and homogeneous
Malignant OR Premalignant Primary Neoplasm					
Mildly dysplastic nodule	↓-↑	—	Minimal	Minimal	Lesions generally <cm and homogeneous
Severely dysplastic nodule	↓-↑	—	Homogeneous intense	Fade to isointense with liver	Lesions generally <1.5 cm, homogeneous, and no capsule

	T1	T2	Enhancement	Dynamic	Comments
HCC—small (<3 cm) HCC—large (>3–5 cm)	↓-↑↓-↑	Ø-↑Ø-↑	Diffuse Heterogeneous	Rapid washout Heterogeneous +/− foci showing washout	Larger lesions may appear infiltrative, poorly marginated, and demonstrate portal vein invasion
Fibrolamellar carcinoma	↓	↑-↑↑	Diffuse radiating bands	Slow washout	Usually >5 cm
Cholangiocarcinoma	Ø-↓	Ø-↑	Negligible	Progressive heterogeneous	Associated liver atrophy intrahepatic duct dilatation
Lymphoma (primary)	↓	↑	Diffuse heterogeneous	Progressive with heterogeneous washout	Resemble HCC, rarely may resemble cholangiocarcinoma
Secondary Neoplasms					
Metastasis	↓	↑	+/− ring, +/− perilesional	Heterogeneous	Mucinous adenoma have ↑↑T2 and more perilesional enhancement
Hypervascular metastases	↓	↑ - ↑↑	Heterogeneous	Variable washout	
Lymphoma (secondary)	↓	↑	Ring	Progressive mild enhancement	Resemble metastases

↓↓ Moderately to markedly decreased signal intensity
↓ Mildly decreased signal intensity
Ø Isointense
↑ Mildly increased signal intensity
↑↑ Moderately to markedly increased signal intensity
O No enhancement

- Autosomal-dominant polycystic kidney disease (APCKD)
  - Liver cysts common, 70%
- Von Hippel–Lindau disease
  - Liver cysts in 20%, pancreatic cysts uncommon
  - High incidence of renal, pancreatic, and adrenal neoplasms
  - Brain and/or cord multiple hemangioblastomas

Imaging (fig. 2.2)
- Uniformly smooth and round, ovoid, or slightly lobulated margins
- High T2, similar to cerebral spinal fluid around spinal cord
  - Can resolve down to 1 mm due to high contrast
- Low T1
- Postgadolinium imaging shows no enhancement

Variants
- May be slightly complicated with septations, lobulation
- Multiple adjacent cysts may appear to represent a cyst with septations
- Elevated T1 signal may be due to protein or blood products, consistent with hemorrhagic cyst (uncommon) (fig. 2.3)
- If associated with a thin enhancing rim, likely represents a bile duct hamartoma (see next section)
- Ciliates hepatic foregut cysts arise along convex outer surface of liver, typically intersegmental in Location, bulge liver contour, possess thin enhancing rim, and may be high signal intensity on T1W images (mucin).

Mimickers
- Cystic neoplasms
  - Mucinous/serous ovarian carcinoma
    - Usually superficial and bulge liver surface contour
  - Mucinous cystadenocarcinoma

- These tumors show postgadolinium enhancement, often perilesional

Benign Bile Duct Hamartoma

Background
- Biliary hamartomas are benign and common, occurring in 3% of the population
- Histopathologically comprised of small, irregular branching bile ducts that may be dilated and embedded in a fibrous stroma

Imaging (fig. 2.4)
- Often peripheral and <1 cm
- High T2 and low T1 signal, indistinguishable from simple cysts
- Postgadolinium imaging shows a thin peripheral enhancing rim that persists unchanged between early and late postcontrast images

Mimickers
- Other lesions that have high T2 signal intensity and rim enhancement on postgadolinium images
  - Metastases with high T2 signal may show peripheral rim enhancement, but also most often have progressive central filling on delayed images
  - Mucinous cystic carcinomas will have high T2 signal, but will show distinctive perilesional enhancement with variable central enhancement on delayed images
  - Hypervascular metastases can have high T2 signal, but will show a greater amount of stromal enhancement on arterial phase images

Hemangiomas

Background
- Common benign liver neoplasm, occuring in up to 20% of the general population
- Seen commonly in young adult females
- Multiple in at least half of the patients with hemangiomas

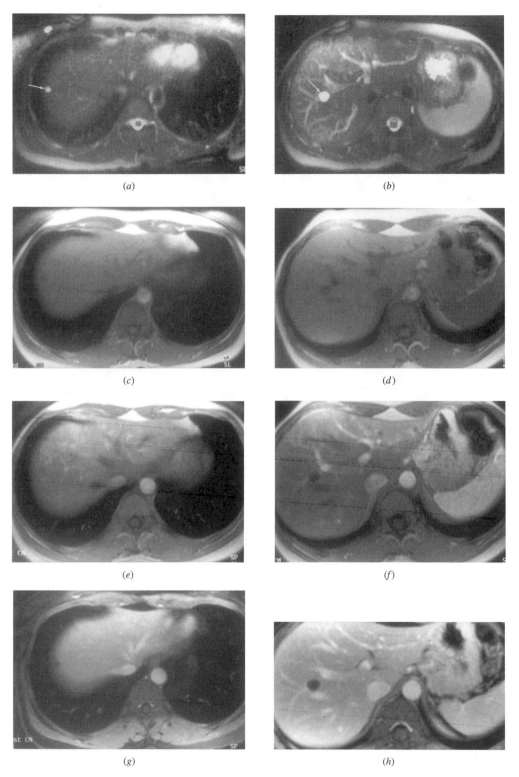

FIGURE 2.2 Simple cyst. Transverse T2W fat-suppressed SS ETSE (*a*, *b*), SGE (*c*, *d*), immediate postgadolinium (*e*, *f*) and 90 s postgadolinium fat-suppressed SGE (*g*, *h*) images. There are two homogeneous, well-defined lesions (arrow, *a*, *b*) that are high signal on T2 (*a*, *b*) and low signal on T1W images (*c*, *d*), which do not enchance after administration of gadolinium on early (*e*, *f*) and late (*g*, *h*) postcontrast images, consistent with simple liver cysts.

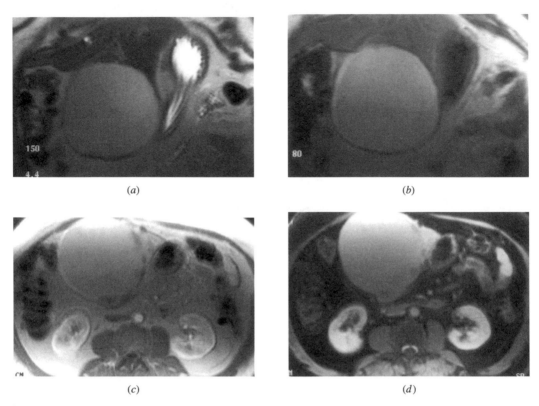

(a) (b)

(c) (d)

FIGURE 2.3 Hemorrhagic cyst. Coronal T2W SS ETSE (a), Coronal SGE (b), transverse immediate postgadolinium SGE (c), and 90 s postgadolinium fat-suppressed SGE (d) images. A large cystic mass with a thickened and irregular wall arises from the lateral segment and demonstrates increased signal on T2W (a) and T1W (b) images and no enhancement on early (c) and late (d) postcontrast images. A blood-filled cyst was proven by histopathology.

- Comprised of vascular lakes and channels, some of which can develop thrombosis and fibrosis

Imaging (fig. 2.5)
- Small lesions are round, and lesions <2 cm are round or lobular and sharply marginated with liver
- Elevated T2 signal intensity
  - Moderately elevated on single-shot echo-train spin-echo (i.e., typically slightly lower signal than cysts)
  - Large hemangiomas (many <2 cm and all >5 cm) show central strands of low-signal stroma and foci of high signal
  - Show increasing signal intensity as TE increased from 90 to over 120 ms on standard spin-echo
    - This approach is no longer recommended due to inadequate specificity and excessive length of exam
- Low T1 signal intensity
- Postgadolinium imaging highly specific diagnostically
  - Hepatic arterial phase shows interrupted peripheral nodules, with enlargement and coalescence of nodules and variable central filling on subsequent venous and delayed images
  - Typing has been made based on how quickly the hemangioma fills centrally
    - Smaller lesions generally fill more quickly
    - Larger lesions are more likely to show slower central filling and more likely to have thrombosis and fibrosis, seen as central persistent nonfilling

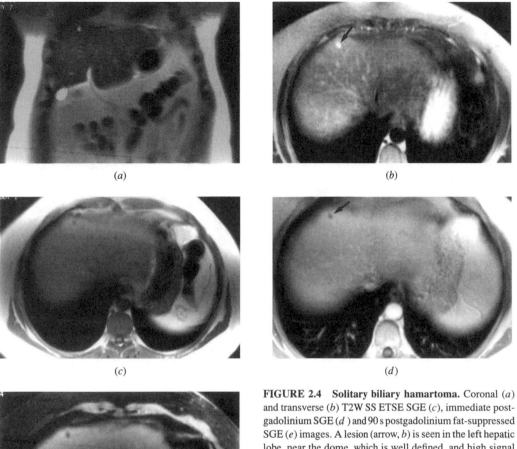

(a)

(b)

(c)

(d)

(e)

FIGURE 2.4   Solitary biliary hamartoma. Coronal (*a*) and transverse (*b*) T2W SS ETSE SGE (*c*), immediate post-gadolinium SGE (*d*) and 90 s postgadolinium fat-suppressed SGE (*e*) images. A lesion (arrow, *b*) is seen in the left hepatic lobe, near the dome, which is well defined, and high signal on the T2W (*a*, *b*) and low signal on the T1W (*c*) images. On the immediate postgadolinium image (*d*), the lesion does not enhance with gadolinium, but a thin perilesional rim of enhancement is appreciated (arrow, *d*). (Reproduced with permission from Semelka RC, Hussain SM, Marcos HB, Woosley JT. Biliary hamartomas: Solitary and multiple lesions shown on current MR techniques including gadolinium enhancement. *J Magn Reson Imaging* 10: 196–201, 1999.)

- Variants
  - Rapid enhancement may simulate enhancement of more aggressive lesions
  - Giant hemangiomas can occupy up to entire hepatic lobe and may expand liver contour
  - Rarely hemorrhage
  - Occasionally exhibit perilesional enhancement (fig. 2.6)
- Mimickers
  - Chemotherapy-treated metastases
    - May show slowly progressive central enhancement
    - Do not show interrupted peripheral nodules that coalesce
- Notes to Emphasize
  - Well-timed arterial phase is important to see peripheral nodular enhancement, particularly in smaller (<1.5 cm) hemangiomas that may fill in rapidly

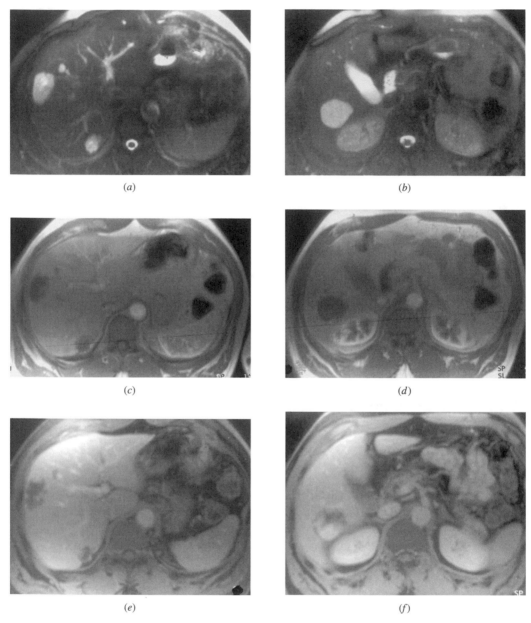

FIGURE 2.5   Multiple hemangiomas. T2W fat-suppressed SS ETSE (a, b), immediate postgadolinium SGE (c, d), and 90 s postgadolinium fat-suppressed SGE (e, f) images. Multiple hemangiomas are appreciated throughout the liver. All of these lesions show increased T2 signal intensity (a, b), peripheral nodular enhancement after contrast administration (c, d), and enlargement and coalescence of nodules on delayed postcontrast images (e, f), consistent with hemangiomas.

Focal Nodular Hyperplasia (FNH)

- Background
  - Etiology unclear, but pathology may be related to underlying developmental abnormality, with hyperplastic response of liver parenchyma, and disorganized growth pattern of hepatocytes and ducts
  - Forms an unencapsulated mass, with central stellate fibrovascular core with malformed vessels and bile duct proliferation

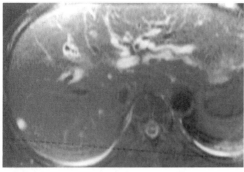

(a)

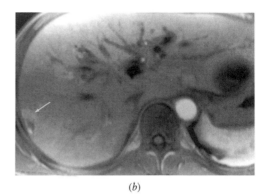

(b)

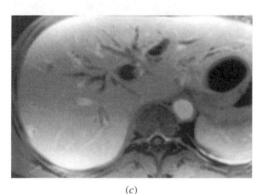

(c)

FIGURE 2.6   Hemangioma with perilesional enhancement. T2W SS ETSE (*a*), immediate postgadolinium SGE (*b*), and 90 s postgadolinium fat-suppressed SGE (*c*) images. This patient, who has an inflammatory pseudotumor arising in the common hepatic duct that causes dilatation of the biliary tree, also demonstrates a round, well-defined lesion, which is hyperintense on T2 (*a*) and shows peripheral nodular enhancement on the immediate postcontrast image (*b*) with nearly complete fill-in of the lesion on the delayed image (*c*). Note the transient ill-defined increased perilesional enhancement (arrow, *b*) on the immediate postcontrast image (*b*) that reflects high flow in vessels related to the hemangioma.

- ○ Common in young adult females. Likely related to hormonal stimulation, regresses with age
- ○ Can be multiple
- ○ No malignant potential
- ○ Hemorrhage is exceedingly rare
- Imaging (fig. 2.7)
  - ○ On single-shot echo-train T2
    - ▪ Isointense to very mildly elevated signal intensity mass
    - ▪ Central core may have higher signal than surrounding mass in around 50% of cases, representing central scar
  - ○ T1 spoiled gradient echo
    - ▪ Iso- to mildly hypointense, central core may be very low signal
    - ▪ Background liver commonly fatty
  - ○ Postgadolinium
    - ▪ Arterial phase shows uniform enhancement, usually very intensely
    - ▪ If isointense on precontrast images, may only be observed on arterial phase images; more often noted in small (<1.5 cm) lesions
    - ▪ Rapidly fades in venous to interstitial phases to become isointense or slightly hyperintense to liver
    - ▪ Central core does not enhance in arterial phase, but becomes progressively enhanced in venous and interstitial phases in around 70% of cases
      - • Central core is small and has angular margins
      - • Thin radial septations may be visible
      - • Difficult to see in smaller (<1.5 cm) lesions
      - • Central core may only partially fill in with contrast in larger (>5 cm) lesions
  - ○ Other contrast agents
    - ▪ Gd-EOB-DTPA: early arterial phase blush and late hepatocellular uptake
    - ▪ Mn-DPDP: similar uptake as normal liver
    - ▪ SPIO: similar uptake as normal liver
- Mimickers
  - ○ Adenoma
    - ▪ May be near isointense on precontrast images and also show arterial phase transient uniform enhancement

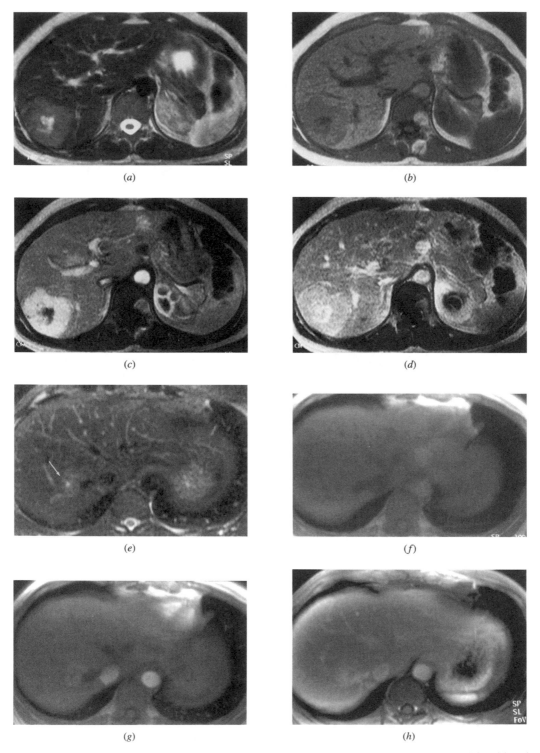

FIGURE 2.7 Medium-sized focal nodular hyperplasia. T2W ETSE (*a*), SGE (*b*), immediate postgadolinium (*c*), and 5 min postgadolinium SGE (*d*) images. A 5.5 cm mass is present in the right lobe of the liver. The tumor is mildly hyperintense on T2 (*a*) and mildly hypointense on T1 (*b*).

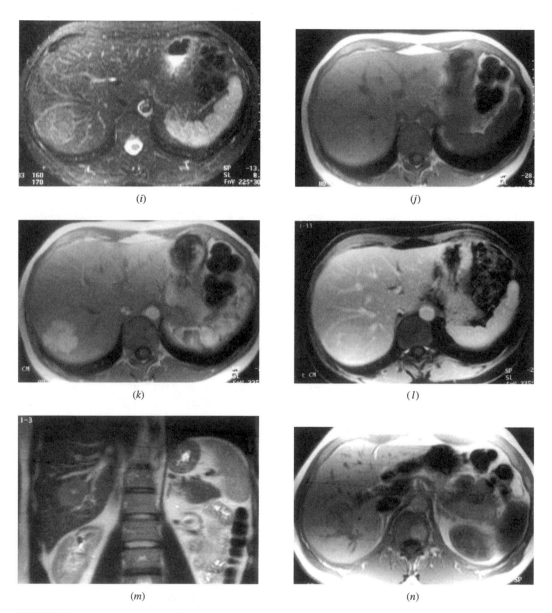

(i) *(j)* *(k)* *(l)* *(m)* *(n)*

FIGURE 2.7 *(Continued)* A central scar is present that is low in signal intensity on T1 (*b*) and high in signal intensity on T2 (*a*). On the immediate postgadolinium image (*c*), the tumor enhances with a uniform capillary blush, whereas the central scar remains low in signal intensity. On the late postgadolinium image (*d*), the tumor fades to near isointensity with background liver, whereas the central scar shows delayed enhancement. This lesion is a classic focal nodular hyperplasia. (Courtesy of Susan M. Ascher, MD, Department of Radiology, Georgetown University Medical Center.)

Echo-train STIR (*e*), SGE (*f*), immediate postgadolinium SGE (*g*), and 90 s postgadolinium SGE (*h*) images in a second patient. There is a lesion in the right hepatic lobe (arrow, *e*) that demonstrates minimally high signal on the T2W image (*e*) and isointensity on the T1W image (*f*), enhances with a uniform blush on the immediate postgadolinium image (*g*), and fades to near isointensity on the delayed image (*h*). Note the small central scar that is high signal intensity on T2 (*e*) and low signal intensity on T1 (*f*) and immediate postgadolinium (*g*) images and enhances to hyperintensity over time (*h*).

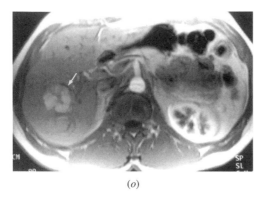

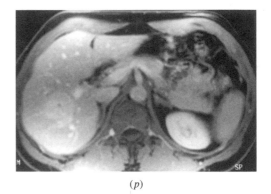

(o)   (p)

FIGURE 2.7   (*Continued*) Echo-train STIR (*i*), SGE (*j*), immediate postgadolinium SGE (*k*), and 90 s postgadolinium fat-suppressed SGE (*l*) images in a third patient. There is a lobular lesion in the right hepatic lobe that has minimally increased signal on T2 (*i*), near isointensity on T1 (*j*), demonstrates intense uniform enhancement on the immediate postgadolinium image (*k*), and fades to near isointensity on late image (*l*). There is a small central scar best seen as a low-signal linear structure on the immediate postcontrast image (*k*).

Coronal T2W SS ETSE (*m*), SGE (*n*), immediate postgadolinium SGE (*o*) and 90 s postgadolinium fat-suppressed SGE (*p*) images in a fourth patient. The 3.5 cm FNH has a partial pseudocapsule (arrow, *o*). The pseudocapsule and central scar show partial enhancement on the delayed image (*p*). The lesion otherwise has a typical MRI appearance for an FNH.

- Adenoma has these features:
  - Presence of capsule (variable)
  - Fatty infiltration of the mass shown on out-of-phase images
  - A central core with high T2 signal and late enhancement is not seen
  - Pregadolinium T1W images may show heterogeneous high-signal blood products, or mildly hyperintense and homogeneous due to fat content
- ○ HCC or hypervascular metastases
  - HCC develops in background of cirrhosis or chronic liver disease
  - Has a capsule, seen as high-signal peripheral rim enhancement on venous or equilibrium phase images
  - A central scar with late enhancement may be seen in HCC
  - HCC, that mimics FNH with central scar, shows irregular enhancement that usually persists into equilibrium phase, while FNH shows uniform enhancement that typically becomes near isointense on equilibrium phase images
  - Out-of-phase images may show fat in HCC, but globular and not confined to a central scar, if present
  - Also look for portal venous tumor thrombus in HCC
- ○ Fibrolamellar carcinoma
  - Typically large (>10 cm) lesions with larger central scar
  - Central scar is lower and more heterogeneous in signal on T2W images and enhances early and heterogeneously on postgadolinium images
  - Arterial phase enhancement of the mass is more irregular and develops radiating bands of enhancement
  - Equilibrium phase central scar enhancement is more irregular
- Notes to Emphasize
  - ○ Utilize complete abdominal imaging technique, including single-shot T2W images, spoiled gradient-echo T1W images (in-phase/out-of-phase), and optimally timed arterial, venous, and equilibrium phase postgadolinium imaging to maximize sensitivity and specificity, especially for small FNHs that may be seen only on arterial phase images, or for discriminating between FNH and mimickers

Hepatic Adenoma

- Background
  - Benign epithelial neoplasm
  - Majority of lesions occur in young females on oral contraceptives
    - Lesion will involute if oral contraceptives discontinued
    - Other rare associations include
      - Exogenous anabolic steroids
      - Galactosemia
      - Glycogen storage disease type Ia
  - Patient can present with abdominal pain related to spontaneous intralesional hemorrhage (rare)
    - Can rarely bleed excessively into peritoneum and require emergency intervention
  - Pathology shows two- to three-layer sheets of normal hepatocytes separated by sinusoids and thin veins with areas of microhemorrhage
    - No bile ducts
    - Forms a pseudocapsule due to compressed adjacent liver
- Imaging (fig. 2.8)
  - T2W imaging shows iso- to moderate hyperintensity
  - T1W imaging ranges from mildly hypo- to mildly hyperintense, depending on presence of fat or blood products
    - If fat is present—commonly seen uniformly throughout lesion
      - T1W in-phase images may be mildly hyperintense
      - T1W out-of-phase images show drop in signal or low signal on fat-suppressed T1W images
    - If acute blood products are present
      - Irregular foci of high signal on T1W and T2W images that do not drop on out-of-phase or fat-suppressed T1W images
  - Postgadolinium
    - Arterial phase blush
    - Rapid fading, usually to hypo- or isointensity to liver

- Adenomas are the only benign lesions that may commonly show washout (i.e., lower signal than liver parenchyma)
- Often develops pseudocapsule rim enhancement on delayed images
- If blood products present, enhancement may appear irregular
- May demonstrate an enhancing scar
- Mimickers
  - FNH
    - Has a small central scar
    - No capsule enhancement
    - No diffuse fat or hemorrhage within lesion
  - HCC
    - History of cirrhosis or hepatitis
    - Background of cirrhosis or chronic liver disease
    - Only very rarely shows internal fat on out-of-phase or fat-suppressed T1W images
    - May see portal vein tumor thrombus
  - Liver adenomatosis
    - Represents a rare and distinct entitity
      - Equal incidence in males and females with no steroid correlation
      - Associated with abnormal elevated liver enzymes
      - Higher risk of hemorrhage and of malignant transformation
    - Multiple (>10) lesions
    - Irregular enhancement
    - Difficult to distinguish from HCC

Infectious and Inflammatory Masses

- Background
  - Infectious
    - Pyogenic abscess (fig. 2.9)
      - Most common causes are bacteria entering portal venous system, seeding liver from a bowel source related to diverticulitis, appendicitis, or Crohn's disease
      - Central purulent necrosis forms a relatively hypo- or avascular core, a surrounding rind of vascularized granulation tissue is generally present,

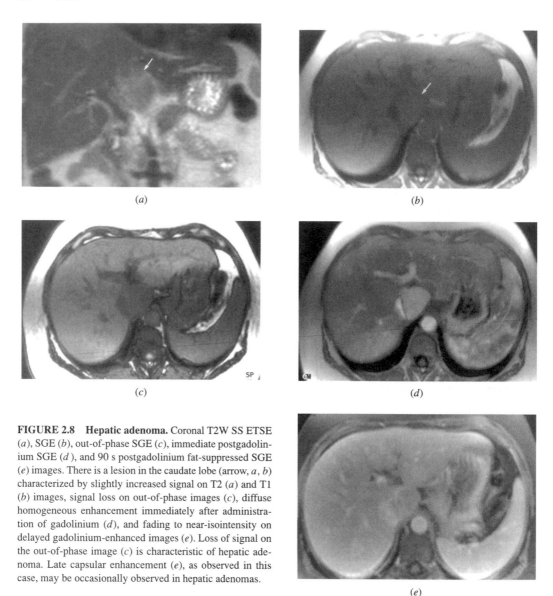

(a)

(b)

(c)

(d)

FIGURE 2.8 Hepatic adenoma. Coronal T2W SS ETSE (*a*), SGE (*b*), out-of-phase SGE (*c*), immediate postgadolinium SGE (*d*), and 90 s postgadolinium fat-suppressed SGE (*e*) images. There is a lesion in the caudate lobe (arrow, *a*, *b*) characterized by slightly increased signal on T2 (*a*) and T1 (*b*) images, signal loss on out-of-phase images (*c*), diffuse homogeneous enhancement immediately after administration of gadolinium (*d*), and fading to near-isointensity on delayed gadolinium-enhanced images (*e*). Loss of signal on the out-of-phase image (*c*) is characteristic of hepatic adenoma. Late capsular enhancement (*e*), as observed in this case, may be occasionally observed in hepatic adenomas.

(e)

occurring early, and the rind develops increasing fibrous tissue with time
- Imaging
  - Solitary or multiple lesions
  - Central low T1, intermediate heterogeneous T2 signal
  - Postgadolinium-enhancing rind with arterial enhancement that persists into equilibrium phase, becoming more pronounced with maturity of the abscess

- No progressive internal stromal enhancement over time
- Perilesional enhancement due to hyperemic inflammatory effects on adjacent liver
○ Nonpyogenic abscess
  ▪ Amoebic (fig. 2.10)
    • Related to *Entamoeba histolytica*, rare in industrialized countries and usually related to travel in the tropics

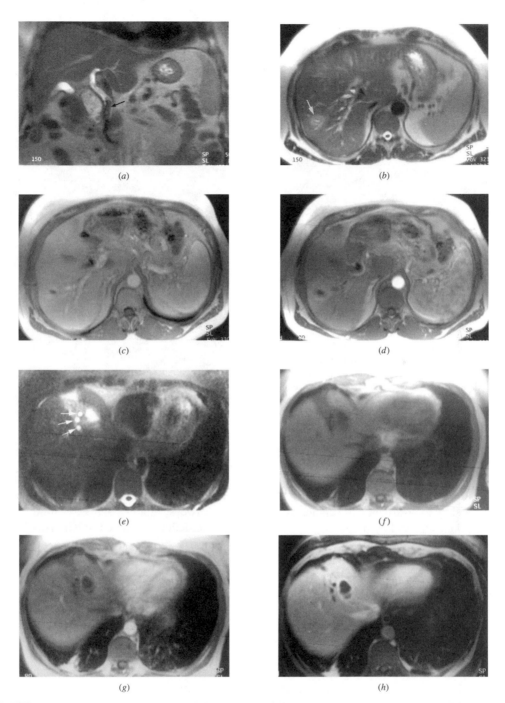

FIGURE 2.9 Liver abscesses secondary to infective cholangitis. Coronal (*a*) and transverse (*b*) T2W SS ETSE, and immediate (*c*) and 45 s (*d*) postgadolinium SGE images. There is a lesion in the right hepatic lobe (arrow, *b*) that demonstrates increased signal intensity on T2 (*b*), decreased signal on T1 (not shown), and circumferential ill-defined perilesional and capsular enhancement on immediate postgadolinium images (*c*), with fading of the perilesional enhancement and persistent capsular enhancement on 45 s images (*d*). There is no enhancement of internal stroma or fill-in of the lesion with time. Note the biliary stent (arrow, *a*) situated in the common bile duct (*a*). T2W SS ETSE (*e*), SGE (*f*), immediate postgadolinium SGE (*g*) and 90 s postgadolinium fat-suppressed SGE (*h*) images in a second patient. There is an irregular region of increased signal on T2 (*e*) and decreased signal on T1 (*f*) in the dome of the liver. Adjacent to this area, there are multiple rounded structures (arrows, *e*) that demonstrate increased signal on T2 (*e*) and decreased signal on T1 (*f*), which represent dilated ducts. After gadolinium administration (*g*, *h*), a cystic mass with a thickened enhancing wall and internal septations is identified, consistent with an abscess secondary to segmental infective cholangitis.

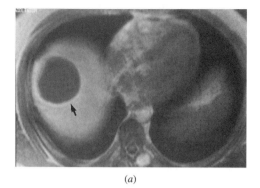

(a)

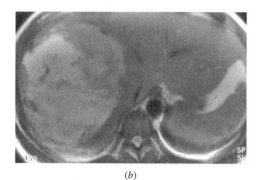

(b)

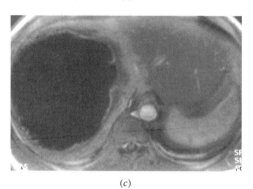

(c)

FIGURE 2.10 **Amoebic abscess.** Immediate postgadolinium SGE (a) image demonstrates a 7 cm cystic lesion located superiorly in the right lobe of the liver. The amoebic abscess has a prominent enhancing wall (arrow, a) distinguishing it from a simple cyst.

T2W SS ETSE (b) and immediate postgadolinium magnetization-prepared gradient-echo (c) images in a second patient. A large cystic lesion is seen in the right hepatic lobe, near the dome of the diaphragm, with a thick irregular wall, and perilesional and capsular enhancement after gadolinium administration, consistent with abscess.

- Clinically the patient has a septic picture, including nausea, vomiting, and weight loss
- Results from hepatocyte necrosis secondary to obstruction of venules by the trophosites and by-products
- Imaging
  - Usually solitary, most frequently in right lobe
  - Central low T1 and moderate T2 (this lesion can appear as a cyst on CT)
  - Thick (5–10 mm) enhancing capsule discriminates amoebic abscess from cyst
  - May involve diaphragm, pleura, and lung with empyema and consolidation, best seen with combination of single-shot T2W and breath-hold postgadolinium 3D GRE T1W images for assessment of pleura and lung
  - Echinococcal (fig. 2.11)
    - E. granulosis
- Causes hydatid cyst and is found in North America, Europe, and Asia, with sheep as primary host and humans as accidental carriers
- Cysts are spherical and form a fibrous rim
- Typically there is little tissue reaction, unless cyst ruptures and leaks fluid, which can induce a marked inflammatory reaction
- Imaging
  - May become large (>10 cm) with well-defined margins
  - Mixed, usually high T2, and mixed low T1 signal, due to internal proteinaceous fluid
  - May see internal daughter cyst septae internally, or occasionally externally, best seen on single-shot T2W images
  - Calcifications occur in 10–15%, seen on CT, but appear as nonspecific dark bands or thickening on MR
  - Thin enhancing wall seen on gadolinium-enhanced GRE
  - E. alveolaris
    - Rare parasitic disease, with fox as main host

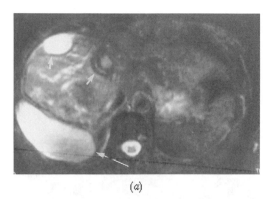 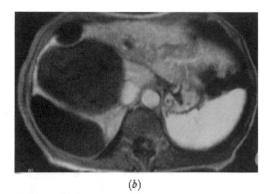

(*a*)   (*b*)

FIGURE 2.11   Hydatid cyst. T2W fat-suppressed SE (*a*), and immediate postgadolinium SGE (*b*) images. A multicystic lesion is present, with the large cyst appearing heterogeneous and moderate in signal intensity on T2 (*a*), and contains peripherally arranged daughter cysts (arrows, *a*). A satellite cyst is also present (long arrow, *a*). The hydatid cyst walls enhance after gadolinium administration (*b*). This appearance is typical for a hydatid cyst.

- Multilocular or confluent disease with necrotic cavities and irregular nonencapsulated margins. Appears as mixed high-T2 signal large lesions with extensive heterogeneous enhancement on postgadolinium images. Portal vein can be thrombosed
- Mycobacterial
  - *M. tuberculosis*
    - Globally the most common cause of infectious hepatic granulomas
    - Increased incidence in AIDS
    - Imaging
      - Multiple small lesions that have similar appearance to fungal abscesses (see below)
      - Additionally, disease involves portal triad with periportal high T2 signal and increased enhancement appreciated on equilibrium phase postgadolinium T1W images
      - Enlarged portal and retroperitoneal lymph nodes
  - *Mycobacterium avium*-intracellulare (MAI) (fig. 2.12)
    - Most common hepatic infection in AIDS, found in 50% of autopsy specimens
    - Imaging
      - Periportal and porta hepatis high T2 signal and enhancement on equilibrium phase T1W images

- Lymphadenopathy in retroperitoneum and mesentery
- Fungal (fig. 2.13)
  - Patients are typically immunocompromised
  - *Candida albicans* is most common
  - Often concomitant involvement of spleen and occasionally kidneys
  - Imaging
    - Acute fungal infection seen as multiple peripheral <1 cm lesions with high T2 signal
      - Conspicuity may be increased in patients who have undergone blood transfusions and possess low-signal livers due to the paramagnetic effect of blood breakdown products (transfusional hemosiderosis)
    - Appear as low-signal foci on gadolinium-enhanced T1W images, usually without enhancing abscess wall
      - Absence of granulation tissue capsule likely related to neutropenic immunocompromised state
    - Fungal abscess features change with response to treatment
      - Develop central focus of high T2 signal

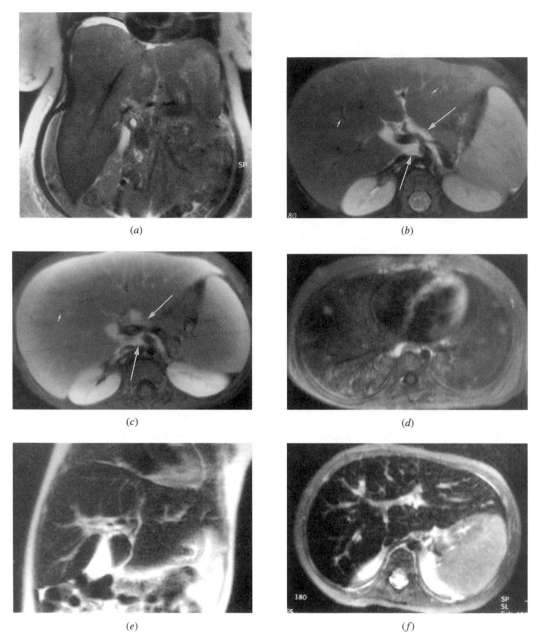

(a)

(b)

(c)

(d)

(e)

(f)

FIGURE 2.12   *Mycobacterium avium*-intracellulare (MAI) hepatic infection. Coronal T2W SS ETSE (*a*), transverse T2W fat-suppressed ETSE (*b*), and interstitial phase gadolinium-enhanced T1W fat-suppressed SE (*c*) images. The coronal image (*a*) demonstrates hepatomegaly. On the fat-suppressed T2W image (*b*), high-signal-intensity soft tissue is present in the porta hepatis (long arrows, *b*) that extends along periportal tracks (short arrows, *b*). After gadolinium administration (*c*), enhancing porta hepatis tissue is clearly shown on the fat-suppressed image (long arrows, *c*), and enhancement is also noted of the periportal tissue (short arrow, *c*). Periportal distribution is a common pattern of involvement with MAI. Gadolinium-enhanced, gated T2W fat-suppressed SE image (*d*) of the lungs demonstrates a ground-glass appearance with irregularly marginated 1 cm enhancing nodules consistent with MAI lung infection.

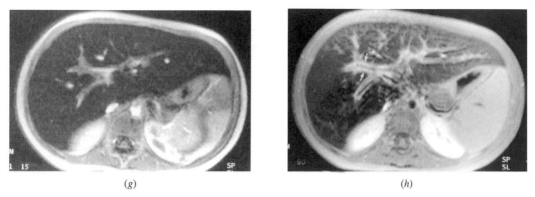

(g)   (h)

FIGURE 2.12   (*Continued*) Coronal T2W SS ETSE (*e*), T2W fat-suppressed SS ETSE (*f*), immediate postgadolinium SGE (*g*), and 90 s postgadolinium fat-suppressed SGE (*h*) images in a second patient, who has a history of hereditary blood dyscrasia and currently has MAI infection, demonstrate tissue in the porta hepatis and periportal tracks that is high signal on T2 (*e*, *f*), and enhances on late gadolinium-enhanced fat-suppressed T1W images (arrows, *h*). Note also the iron deposition in the liver from transfusional siderosis.

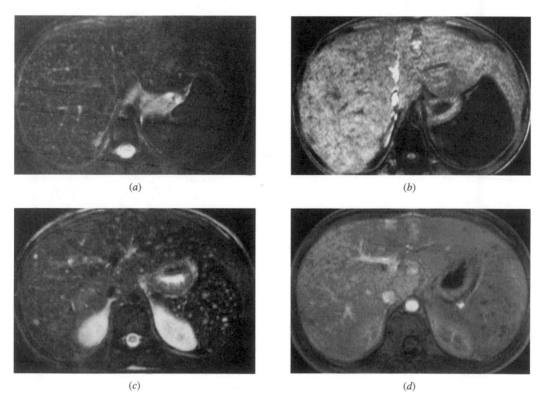

(a)   (b)

(c)   (d)

FIGURE 2.13   Acute hepatosplenic candidiasis. T2W fat-suppressed ETSE (*a*) and immediate postgadolinium SGE (*b*) images. On the T2W images (*a*), multiple well-defined <1 cm high-signal-intensity foci are scattered throughout the hepatic parenchyma with a smaller number of similar lesions apparent in the spleen. On the immediate postgadolinium image (*b*), the liver lesions are near signal void and do not show ring or perilesional enhancement.

T2W fat-suppressed SS ETSE (*c*) and immediate postgadolinium SGE (*d*) images in a second patient. Multiple well-defined <1 cm high-signal-intensity lesions are scattered throughout the liver and spleen on the T2W image (*c*). Lesions are near signal void and do not show ring or perilesional enhancement on the immediate postgadolinium image (*d*).

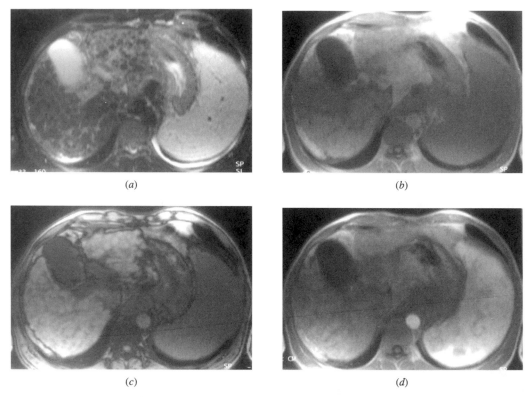

(a)

(b)

(c)

(d)

FIGURE 2.14   Cirrhosis with regenerative nodules. Echo-train STIR (*a*), SGE (*b*), out-of-phase SGE (*c*), immediate postgadolinium SGE (*d*), and 90 s postgadolinium fat-suppressed SGE (*e*) images. The liver is small with an extensive nodular pattern. A reticular pattern of fibrosis is present, which is well shown on out-of-phase images (*c*) as low-signal-intensity linear tissue and demonstrates negligible enhancement on immediate postgadolinium images (*d*) with progressive enhancement on late images (*e*).

- Central focus enhances on post-gadolinium T1
- A rind of dark signal is present in liver surrounding the central ring, seen on pre- and postcontrast TIW images, correlating to the paramagnetic effect of iron-laden macrophages that are found at histopathology
- Mimickers
  - Lymphoma
    - Lower signal on T2W images
    - Show greater enhancement on early and late postgadolinium images
  - Metastases
    - Show progressive internal stromal enhancement on delayed postgadolinium images, not seen with abscesses

Regenerative Nodules (RNs) (fig. 2.14)

- Background
  - Associated with chronic liver disease and cirrhosis
- Imaging
  - See section on cirrhosis

Dysplastic Nodules (DNs) (fig. 2.15)

- Background
  - Associated with chronic liver disease and cirrhosis
  - Represent premalignant lesions, ranging from low- to high-grade dysplasia
  - HCC can develop within DN, within 4 months
  - Usually >1 cm, larger than most RNs

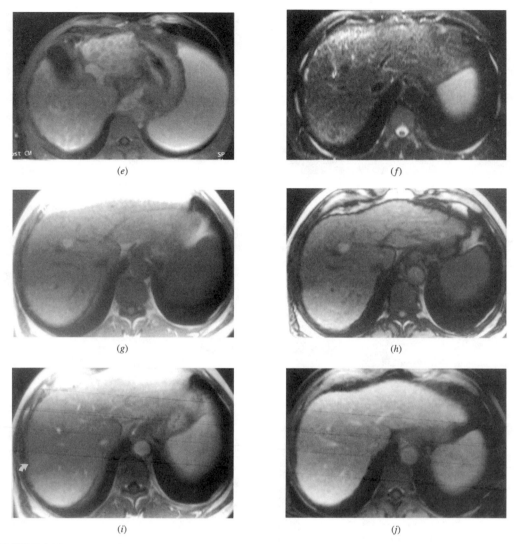

(e)

(f)

(g)

(h)

(i)

(j)

FIGURE 2.14 *(Continued)* Multiple regenerative nodules appear as rounded <1 cm masses best seen as high-signal lesions on out-of-phase images (*c*). Ascites, splenomegaly, and paraesophageal varices are present. Echo-train STIR (*f*), SGE (*g*), out-of-phase SGE (*h*), 45 s postgadolinium SGE (*i*), and 90 s postgadolinium fat-suppressed SGE (*j*) images in a second patient. There are multiple scattered, rounded foci throughout the liver that show decreased signal on T2W (*f*) and increased signal on noncontrast T1W (*g*) and out-of-phase (*h*) images. Lesions are not apparent on early (*i*) or late (*j*) postgadolinium images, consistent with regenerative or mildly dysplastic nodules. Note also the fine reticular pattern on postgadolinium images (*i, j*) with progressive enhancement, consistent with fibrotic change associated with cirrhosis. A small transiently enhancing focus (curved arrow, *i*) is present in *segment 8,* which reflects a vascular phenomenon.

- ○ Most DNs fed by portal veins
- ○ Can receive supply from hepatic artery, which may be related to grade of dysplasia
- • Imaging
  - ○ Variable characteristics, at least partly depending on degree of dysplasia, and partly a result of variables including degree of intracellular iron accumulation and protein content
  - ○ Low-grade DNs generally isointense on T2, mildly hyperintense on T1, and show comparable enhancement to background liver on early and late postgadolinium images

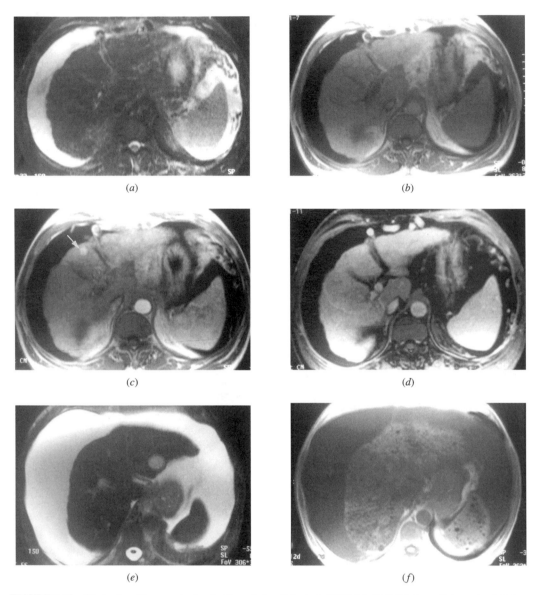

FIGURE 2.15 Cirrhosis with severely dysplastic nodules. Echo-train STIR (*a*), SGE (*b*), immediate postgadolinium SGE (*c*), and 90 s postgadolinium fat-suppressed SGE (*d*) images. The liver is small and nodular, compatible with cirrhosis. There is a 1 cm lesion (arrow, *c*) in *segment 4* that is not evident on T2W (*a*) or T1W (*b*) images but displays intense enhancement on the immediate postgadolinium image (*c*) and fades to isointensity on the late image (*d*), consistent with a severely dysplastic nodule. Note also the presence of ascites and collateral vessels. T2W fat-suppressed SS ETSE (*e*), SGE (*f*), immediate postgadolinium SGE (*g, h*), and 90 s postgadolinium fat-suppressed SGE (*i*) images in a second patient. The liver is very small, nodular, and irregular in contour, consistent with cirrhosis.

○ High-grade DNs generally show isointense on T2, hypo- to isointense on T1, intense early enhancement with fading to background liver

○ Washout of lesion to lower signal than background liver and late capsular enhancement are features of HCC

○ It is crucial to serially reimage patients with lesions that show intense early enhancement at 3-month intervals. Observation of change in size from 1 cm to 2 cm requires rf ablation.

○ Lesions that measure 2 cm in size and show early capillary enhancement with rapid

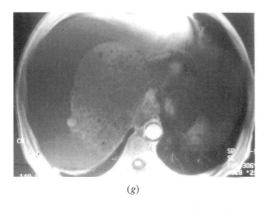

(g)

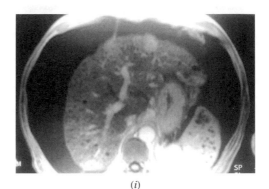

(h)

(i)

FIGURE 2.15 *(Continued)* Multiple nodules are identified in the liver and demonstrate isointense to moderate high signal intensity on T2 (*e*), low signal intensity on T1 (*f*), and intense enhancement immediately after administration of contrast (*g, h*) that persist on late images (*i*), compatible with severe dysplastic nodules. Note the Gamna-Gandy bodies in the spleen and large-volume ascites.

fading and isointense to mildly increased signal on T2W images require rf ablation or other curative therapy

Hepatocellular Carcinoma (HCC) (Fig. 2.16)

- Background
  - Most common primary hepatic malignancy
  - Generally develops in livers with underlying chronic liver disease
  - Most common underlying liver disease is alcoholic cirrhosis in developed Western countries; related to viral hepatitis globally, with relative highest frequency in East Asia. Viral hepatitis is increasing in frequency in Western countries and may surpass alcohol as the underlying etiology in the near future.
  - Hepatic arterial supply
  - Hepatic and portal veins also proliferate around HCC, possibly related to propensity of HCC to invade these vessels
- Imaging
  - Associated with greater surrounding liver distortion from alcoholic cirrhosis
  - Viral hepatitis leads to less liver distortion,

and any mass has high likelihood of representing HCC
  - Solitary in 50% of cases
  - Multifocal in 40% of cases
  - Diffuse in 10% of cases
  - Overlapping features with high-grade DN
  - Variable T2 and T1 signals
  - Most common is mildly elevated T2, mildly low T1, and heterogeneous arterial phase enhancement
    - If <1.5 cm, most commonly isointense on both T1W and T2W images and only seen on immediate (arterial phase) postgadolinium T1W images
  - Typical postgadolinium T1W imaging
    - Arterial phase irregular enhancement
    - Rapid venous and interstitial phase washout with development of persistent pseudocapsule enhancement
  - Diffuse HCC shows irregular T2 and T1, with irregular enhancement that has regions that wash out while other regions may persist
    - Almost invariably seen in association with portal vein tumor thrombosis

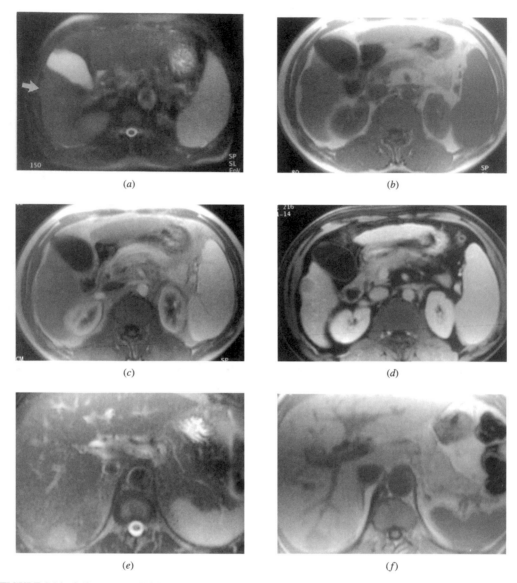

FIGURE 2.16   Solitary small HCC. T2W fat-suppressed SS ETSE (*a*), SGE (*b*), immediate postgadolinium SGE (*c*), and 90 s postgadolinium fat-suppressed SGE (*d*) images. There is a 2 cm mass that bulges the liver contour slightly in the right lobe of the liver. The mass is minimally hyperintense on T2 (*a*) and mildly hypointense on T1 (*b*), demonstrates intense uniform enhancement on the immediate postgadolinium image (*c*), and fades to hypointensity by 90 s (*d*) with late enhancement of a pseudocapsule. Intense hepatic arterial dominant phase enhancement is the most sensitive technique for the detection of small HCCs. Washout to hypointensity with late capsular enhancement is the most specific.

- Alpha-fetoprotein elevated in the majority of patients, but a sizable minority (20%) may have normal alpha-fetoprotein
- Mimickers
  - High-grade DN may show arterial phase enhancement, fade but do not wash out, and do not develop an enhancing pseudocapsule on delayed images
  - Metastases usually show peripheral lesion enhancement, rarely diffuse heterogeneous enhancement as seen with HCC

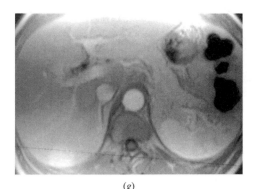

(g)

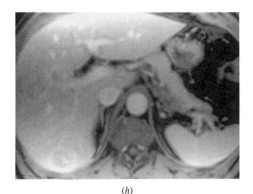

(h)

FIGURE 2.16   *(Continued)* T2W fat-suppressed SS ETSE (*e*), SGE (*f*), immediate postgadolinium SGE (*g*), and 90 s postgadolinium fat-suppressed SGE (*h*) images in a second patient exhibit similar features for a 2.5 cm tumor.

○ Diffuse HCC may resemble active hepatitis, but is usually also associated with portal vein involvement and marked elevation of alpha-fetoprotein (fig. 2.17), which are not features of active hepatitis.

Fibrolamellar Carcinoma (fig. 2.18)

- Background
  - Distinct subtype of HCC
  - Usually occurs in younger patients, predominantly females, but can be seen in any age
  - Underlying liver is normal without chronic liver disease
  - Indolent tumor with good prognosis, in contrast to HCC
  - Pathologically find cellular lobules with fibrous septa with a central stellate scar formed by collagenous network surrounding large polygonal eosinophilic cells
- Imaging
  - Large mass, often > 10 cm, occupying and expanding an entire liver segment
  - T2 imaging
    - Moderately high, heterogeneous signal mass, with a large central radiating heterogeneous stromal pattern
    - Central scar is lower in signal than surrounding mass and is heterogeneous
  - T1 imaging
    - Lower signal than liver
  - Postgadolinium

- Irregular transient arterial phase enhancement, forming coarse bands radiating from center
- Irregular central scar enhances progressively and heterogeneously in the equilibrium phase
- Mimickers
  - See section on FNH

Cholangiocarcinoma (fig. 2.19)

- Background
  - Second most common primary malignant tumor affecting liver, after HCC
  - Subtypes
    - Classifications
      - By anatomical location as intrahepatic, at bifurcation of right and left hepatic ducts (Klatskin's), and distal common bile duct (CBD)
      - Morphologically as superficial spreading or mass-like
    - Superficial spreading
      - Spread along wall of bile ducts, generally contiguously, and involving intra- or extrahepatic ducts, or both
    - Klatskin's tumor is a superficial spreading tumor occurring at the hepatic duct bifurcation, causing right and left branch obstruction
    - Intrahepatic disease most commonly appears as solitary or multifocal intrahepatic masses

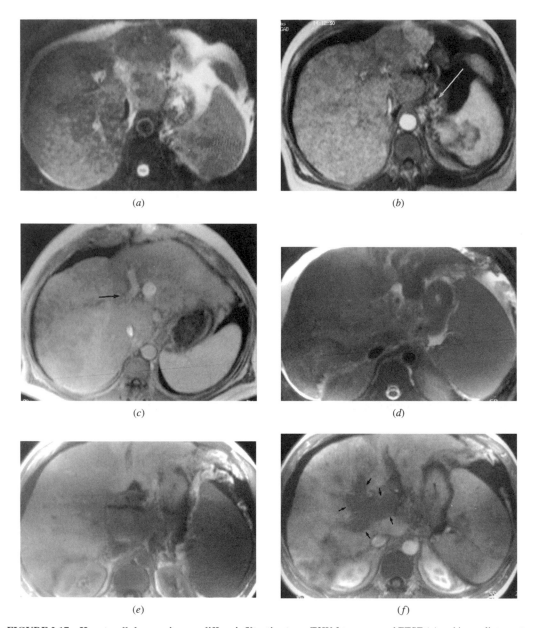

(a)

(b)

(c)

(d)

(e)

(f)

FIGURE 2.17   Hepatocellular carcinoma, diffuse infiltrative type. T2W fat-suppressed ETSE (*a*) and immediate post-gadolinium SGE (*b*) images. Mottled diffuse high signal intensity is present throughout the liver on the T2W image (*a*). Diffuse mottled heterogeneous enhancement is appreciated on the immediate postgadolinium image (*b*). This finding represents diffuse infiltrative HCC. Mottled signal intensity is the most common MRI appearance for diffuse infiltrative HCC. Occasionally, diffuse infiltrative HCC will appear as low in signal intensity on T2W images and very low in signal intensity on postgadolinium images. Prominent varices are present along the lesser curvature of the stomach (arrow, *b*).

Transverse 45 s postgadolinium SGE (*c*) in a second patient. There is a large heterogeneous region of mottled enhancement throughout the right lobe of the liver consistent with an infiltrating HCC. Note the irregularity of liver contour. Tumor thrombus of the right portal vein (arrow, *c*) is present.

Transverse T2W fat-suppressed SS ETSE (*d*), SGE (*e*), and immediate postgadolinium SGE (*f*) images in a third patient. The liver is diffusely heterogeneous in appearance with diffuse heterogeneous enhancement consistent with infiltrative HCC. The main, right, and left portal veins are distended with tumor thrombus (arrows, *f*). Note ascites and splenomegaly.

These cases illustrate the mottled heterogeneity of infiltrative HCC and that tumor thrombus in veins is almost invariably present. A third important feature is that alpha-fetoprotein is almost always extremely high.

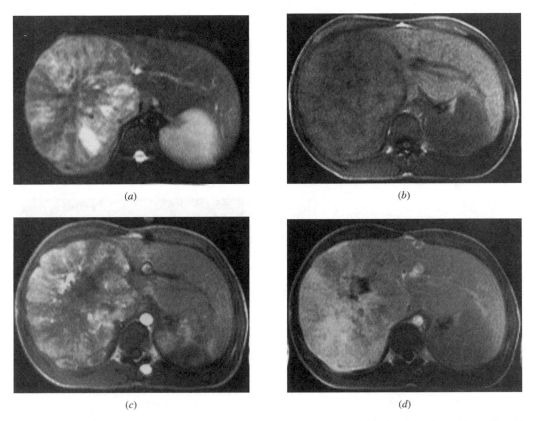

(a)   *(b)*

(c)   *(d)*

FIGURE 2.18   Fibrolamellar hepatocellular carcinoma. T2W fat-suppressed ETSE (*a*), SGE (*b*), and immediate (*c*) and 10 min (*d*) postgadolinium SGE images. A 14 cm fibrolamellar hepatocellular carcinoma is present in this adolescent male with no history of liver disease and 1 yr duration of gynecomastia. The tumor is hypointense on the T1W image with a low-signal-intensity central scar (*b*) and heterogeneously hyperintense on the T2W image (*a*) with the central radiating scar largely low in signal intensity. On the immediate postgadolinium SGE image (*c*), the tumor exhibits diffuse heterogeneous enhancement with negligible enhancement of the radiating scar. On the 10 min image (*d*), the bulk of the tumor has become isointense with background liver. Portions of the central scar are higher in signal intensity than surrounding tissue, whereas other parts remain low in signal. In contrast to FNH, the scar in fibrolamellar HCC is much larger and exhibits more heterogeneous signal on T2 and early and late postgadolinium images.

- ○ Generally tumors have a high fibrous tissue content
- ○ Typically slow growing
- ○ Risk factors include choledochal cyst, Caroli's disease, sclerosing cholangitis, recurrent pyogenic oriental cholangitis
- Imaging
  - ○ Superficial spreading tumors are assessed using a combination of T2W MRCP single-shot images to visualize bile duct lumen and fat-suppressed gadolinium-enhanced interstitial phase images to visualize bile duct walls

- ○ Irregular narrowing of involved ducts with peripheral duct obstruction and dilatation
  - ▪ Can range from short segmental involvement to extensive multiple branch pattern
  - ▪ Duct thickening >5 mm observed on postgadolinium equilibrium phase fat-suppressed GRE combined with progressive enhancement is suggestive of diagnosis, but not specific
  - ▪ Klatskin's tumor frequently causes relatively minor thickening (3 mm) of the bile duct wall, but is associated with

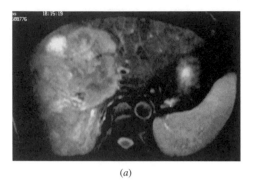

(a)

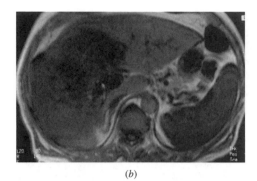

(b)

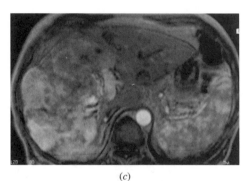

(c)

FIGURE 2.19 Intrahepatic cholangiocarcinoma. T2W fat-suppressed ETSE (*a*), SGE (*b*), and immediate postgadolinium SGE (*c*) images. A 14 cm tumor is present in the right lobe of the liver that is moderately high in signal intensity on the T2W image (*a*) and moderately low in signal intensity on the T1W image (*b*) and enhances in an intense diffuse heterogeneous fashion on the immediate postgadolinium SGE image (*c*). The appearance resembles that of an HCC.

high-grade bile duct dilatation despite apparent minimal disease
- Surrounding thin stranding and small lymph nodes often seen on interstitial phase gadolinium-enhanced fat-suppressed images is consistent with tumor involvement
○ Focal mass subtype shows low T1, moderate irregular increased T2, with irregular progressive equilibrium phase enhancement, with peripheral bile duct dilatation
- Less common (~10%)
○ Combination of features highly suggestive of superficial spreading cholangiocarcinoma include
- Segmental atrophy without evidence of mass
- Diffuse fibrosis, seen as progressive late enhancement
- Segmental peripheral duct dilatation and irregular narrowing centrally
- On single-shot T2 and MRCP images, the intrahepatic central bile ducts appear drawn into a vortex at the level of the common hepatic duct (CHD)

○ Involvement of central common bile duct can obstruct pancreatic duct
○ Not associated with cirrhosis
• Mimickers
○ Sclerosing cholangitis
- May be difficult to discriminate
- Intrahepatic bile ducts generally not as dilated
○ HCC
- In diffuse HCC, portal vein invasion is typical, but is not seen with cholangiocarcinoma
- In focal HCC, enhancement is arterial and transient
○ Sclerosing primary hepatic lymphoma
- Rare mimicker, may be indistinguishable, causing segmental hepatic atrophy and fibrosis
○ Central tumors dilating both the common bile duct and the pancreatic duct have: the following differential diagnosis:
- Pancreatic adenocarcinoma
- Ampullary or duodenal adenocarcinoma
  - Central tumors may have histopathological overlap

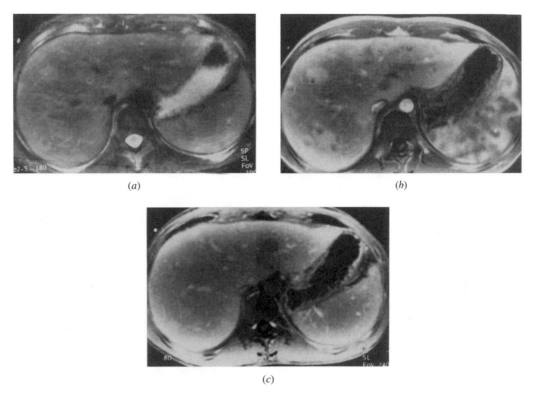

(a)   (b)

(c)

FIGURE 2.20   Hodgkin's lymphoma. T2W fat-suppressed ETSE (*a*), immediate postgadolinium SGE (*b*), and 90 s postgadolinium fat-suppressed SGE (*c*) images. Multiple focal mass lesions smaller than 2 cm are present throughout the liver, many of which show mildly hyperintense tumor periphery on T2 (*a*) and demonstrate ring enhancement with ill-defined perilesional enhancement on immediate postgadolinium images (*b*). Arciform enhancement of the spleen is present on the immediate postgadolinium image, with no evidence of focal low-signal-intensity masses (*b*). By 90 s postgadolinium (*c*), many of the hepatic masses have become isointense with liver.

- Notes to Emphasize
  - Many features of cholangiocarcinoma can be ameliorated (e.g., severe intrahepatic bile duct dilatation) or mimicked (e.g., increased duct wall enhancement) by the placement of a biliary drain. Imaging prior to bile duct intervention is recommended to avoid these diagnostic confounding variables.

Lymphoma (fig. 2.20)

- Background
  - Stage IV Hodgkin's or non-Hodgkin's lymphoma commonly involves liver
  - Extensive retroperitoneal, mesenteric lymph node enlargement in combination with splenomegaly is common. Lymph nodes are generally homogeneous in signal on all sequences.

- Imaging
  - Focal masses, typically low on T1, ranging from low to moderately high on T2
    - High-T2 lesions more likely to show greater arterial phase enhancement
    - Enhancement is predominantly peripheral, as seen generally with metastases
    - May develop transient perilesional enhancement
  - Can have infiltrative pattern with vascular encasement observed as tissue thickening in porta hepatis tracking along portal triads
    - Best seen with fat-suppressed T2 as moderately increased signal intensity tissue

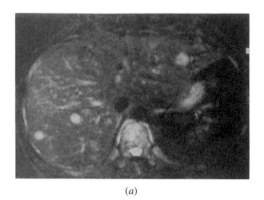

(a)

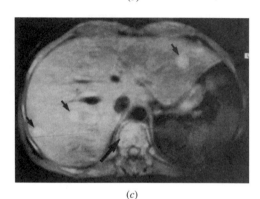

(b)

(c)

FIGURE 2.21 Multiple myeloma. T2W fat-suppressed ETSE (*a*), SGE (*b*), and T1W fat-suppressed spin-echo (*c*) images. Multiple focal masses smaller than 1.5 cm are present in the liver that are moderately hyperintense on T2 (*a*), nearly isointense on T1W image (*b*), and moderately hyperintense on the T1W fat-suppressed spin-echo image (black arrows, *c*). High signal intensity on T1W and T2W images is also present in vertebral bodies (large arrow, *c*) because of myelomatous involvement.

- ○ Very rare form of primary lymphoma can appear as segmental atrophy with progressive persistent diffuse enhancement in equilibrium phase, similar to cholangiocarcinoma
- ○ Very rarely multiple myeloma can involve liver and result in multiple, usually small (~1 cm) lesions, with mildly elevated T2 and isointense or hyperintense T1 signal (fig. 2.21)
  - The distinctive mildly hyperintense T1 signal is likely due to abundant intracellular protein
- Mimickers
  - ○ Metastases of other cell types

Metastases

- Background
  - ○ Most common malignant hepatic tumor
  - ○ Solitary or multiple masses, with multiple masses occasionally confluent, rarely appears as infiltrative tumor

- ○ Primary blood supply is hepatic arterial
- ○ Metastases can be further classified as hypovascular, hypervascular, or near isovascular
- ○ Hypovascular
  - Colon adenocarcinoma is most common
  - Hypovascularity corresponds to a lower tumor vessel count histologically
- ○ Hypervascular
  - Most consistently hypervascular and possibly most common are neuroendocrine tumors, including carcinoid and islet cell tumors
  - Other tumors include renal cell carcinoma, melanoma, pancreatic ductal adenocarcinoma, thyroid cancer, and breast cancer
  - Hypervascularity corresponds to a higher tumor vessel count histologically
- ○ Near isovascular
  - Most commonly seen in chemotherapy-treated metastases

▪ May be well visualized on noncontrast images
- Imaging
  ○ Hypovascular (fig. 2.22)
    ▪ Variable T2 signal
    ▪ Typically most conspicuous on T1W SGE breath-hold pre- and postgadolinium images—these images provide maximal sensitivity and specificity for detection and diagnosis
    ▪ Rim enhancement is the hallmark of metastases, reflecting increased enhancement of the peripheral, most vascularized portion of the tumor
    ▪ Even in hypovascular tumors, rim enhancement may be well seen on hepatic arterial phase images; occasionally lesions are sufficiently hypovascular that the rim is better appreciated on later phases
    ▪ Postgadolinium images show progressive venous interstitial phase enhancement, predominantly filling in from the outer margins
    ▪ Colon cancer metastases usually have a pseudocapsule peripheral rim enhancement seen on all phases of enhancement, contributing to a cauliflower appearance
    ▪ Perilesional enhancement of adjacent liver is frequently seen with adenocarcinoma, most commonly mucinous type from colon, stomach, or pancreas, and is usually best seen on arterial phase
  ○ Hypervascular (fig. 2.23)
    ▪ Variable T2 signal, but frequently moderate to moderately intense heterogeneous signal
    ▪ Low T1 signal
    ▪ Melanoma is an exception and can present with iso- to hyperintense T1 signal, but this is seen in only a minority (15%) of cases (fig. 2.24)
    ▪ Postgadolinium enhancement generally well or best appreciated in hepatic arterial phase and may be homogeneous (most often seen in small, <1.5 cm, tumors), ring (most common pattern, seen in all sizes),

or irregular (rare, difficult to distinguish from HCC)

Diffuse Liver Diseases

- Background
  ○ Acute Liver Disease
    ▪ Acute hepatitis
      - Viral
      - Alcoholic
      - Nonalcoholic steatotic hepatitis (NASH)
      - Drug related
      - Autoimmune
      - Idiopathic
    ▪ HELLP syndrome of acute toxemia of pregnancy
    ▪ If cause for acute hepatitis is persistent or recurrent, disease can progress to cirrhosis
  ○ Chronic Liver Disease
    ▪ Pathology classifications
      - Chronic persistent hepatitis
      - Chronic active hepatitis
      - Cirrhosis
- Etiologies include
  ○ Congenital
    ▪ Wilson's disease
    ▪ Primary biliary cirrhosis
    ▪ Primary sclerosing cholangitis
  ○ Acquired
    ▪ Viral hepatitis
    ▪ Alcohol hepatitis
  ○ Depositional diseases
    ▪ Hepatic steatosis, or fatty liver
    ▪ Hemochromatosis
      - Primary
      - Secondary
- Cirrhosis
  ○ End stage of chronic liver disease, with fibrosis

Acute Hepatitis (fig. 2.25)
- Generally cannot discriminate between etiologies
- Liver is generally enlarged
- Normal liver enhancement is uniform in intensity in all phases

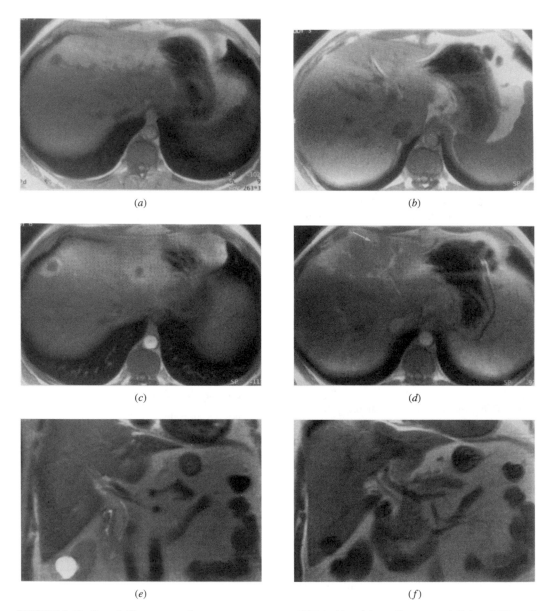

(a)

(b)

(c)

(d)

(e)

(f)

FIGURE 2.22 Low-fluid-content colon cancer metastases. SGE (a, b) and immediate postgadolinium SGE (c, d) images. Lesions, especially small lesions, are difficult to discern on noncontrast T2W (not shown) and T1W images (a, b). On immediate postgadolinium images (c, d), lesions are rendered conspicuous because of ring enhancement. Lesions <1 cm in size may be detected and characterized with this technique.

Coronal T2W SS-ETSE (e), coronal SGE (f), transverse T2W SS ETSE (g), and transverse immediate postgadolinium SGE (h) images in a second patient. There are multiple metastases in the liver that are near isointense on T2W (e, g), hypointense on T1W images (f), and demonstrate ring enhancement on postgadolinium images (h).

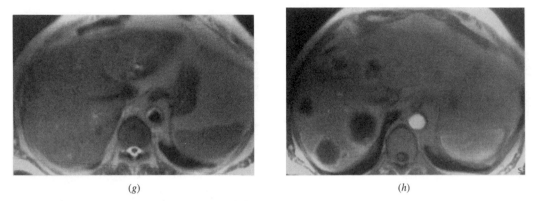

(g)   (h)

FIGURE 2.22 (*Continued*) These liver metastases are poorly seen on T2 (*e*, *g*), well seen on T1 (*f*), and very well shown on immediate postgadolinium images (*h*).

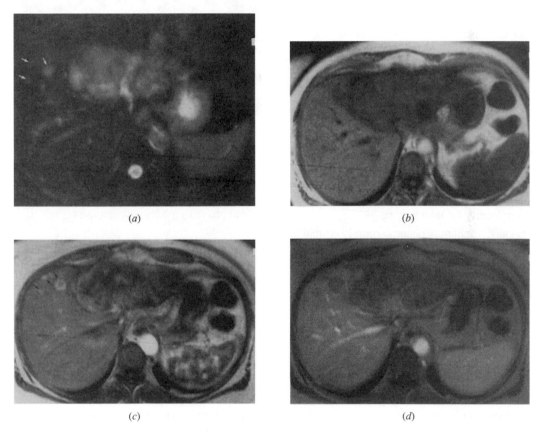

(a)   (b)

(c)   (d)

FIGURE 2.23 **Hypervascular liver metastases.** T2W fat-suppressed ETSE (*a*), SGE (*b*), immediate postgadolinium SGE (*c*), and 90 s postgadolinium SGE (*d*) images. A 7 cm metastasis is identified in the left lobe of the liver (*a–d*). Several metastases smaller than 1 cm are present in the medial and anterior segments. These small metastases are moderately high in signal intensity on T2 (arrows, *a*) and not visible on T1 (*b*), enhance intensely on immediate postgadolinium images (arrows, *c*), and wash out to lower signal intensity than liver on 90 s postgadolinium images (*d*). On the immediate postgadolinium image (*c*), the smallest lesions enhance homogeneously, whereas the 1 cm metastasis has ring enhancement.

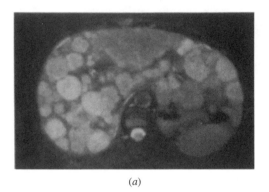

(a)

(b)

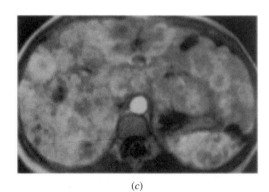

FIGURE 2.24 Melanoma metastasis. T2W fat-suppressed ETSE (*a*), SGE (*b*), and immediate postgadolinium SGE (*c*) images. Melanoma metastases are a mixed population of low- to high-signal-intensity lesions on T2W (*a*) and T1W (*b*) images. This reflects the paramagnetic properties of melanin. Intense ring enhancement is present on the immediate postgadolinium image (*c*), demonstrating the hypervascularity of these metastases.

(c)

- Hepatitis results in heterogeneous enhancement best appreciated on hepatic arterial dominant phase, which may equilibriate to isointensity on later phases
- Enhancement may become entirely normal in venous and equilibrium phases
- Nonuniform enhancement can be seen in venous and equilibrium phases in
  - Severe acute hepatitis
  - Additional background chronic liver disease
- T2 signal intensity can be elevated nonuniformly and is generally related to greater severity of disease. Increased T2 signal reflects hepatic edema with possibly concomitant steatohepatitis.

Chronic Hepatitis (fig. 2.26)
- MRI is sensitive to fibrosis related to chronic liver disease and cirrhosis
- Fibrosis often best seen on short TE (2.2 ms) out-of-phase images

- Fibrosis will enhance progressively and persistently into equilibrium phase, from negligible enhancement on hepatic arterial dominant phase to moderately intense on interstitial phase
- Generally see patterns of either fine reticular or coarse curvilinear late enhancement
- Reticular pattern conforms to and surrounds regenerative nodules, seen as innumerable subcentimeter soft-tissue nodules that enhance progressively into the venous phase, then slowly through the equilibrium phase (i.e., similar to normal liver) (refer to the section on dysplastic nodules, fig. 2.27)
- Enhancement may be heterogeneous in arterial and venous phases in advanced cirrhosis or in the setting of active superimposed acute on chronic liver disease
- Fibrosis is generally poorly appreciated on T2 images and may be lower or moderately high signal, reflecting fluid content and often age of the fibrous tissue

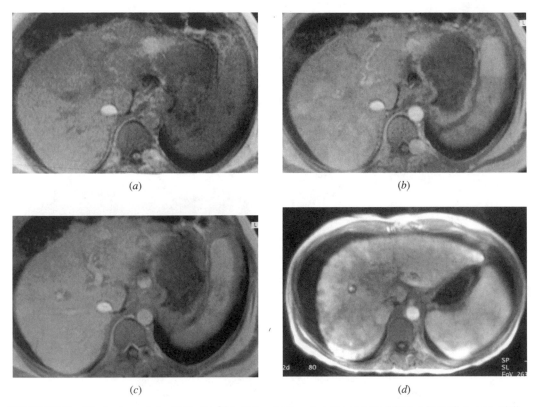

(a)　*(b)*

(c)　*(d)*

FIGURE 2.25   Cirrhosis, acute hepatitis resulting in transient early enhancement. SGE (*a*), immediate postgadolinium SGE (*b*), and 45 s postgadolinium SGE (*c*) images. Normal signal intensity of the liver is present on the T1W image (*a*). Ill-defined, <2 cm regions of blotchy enhancement are present on the immediate postgadolinium image (*b*), which resolve by 45 s (*c*). The presence of enhancing tissue immediately after contrast raises the concern of HCC in a cirrhotic patient. Diffuse HCC usually results in a mottled enhancement pattern with smaller foci of enhancing tissue. Diffuse HCC also is associated with venous tumor thrombus. The underlying cause for this enhancement abnormality in this patient is superimposed acute hepatitis on chronic hepatitis.

Immediate postgadolinium SGE image (*d*) in a second patient demonstrates patchy transient increased enhancement throughout the liver.

- Patchy, nonuniform increased T2 signal may be seen in chronic hepatitis with superimposed active acute hepatitis

Hepatic Steatosis (fig. 2.28)
- Background
  - Fatty infiltration can be diffuse or focal
  - MR is more sensitive and specific than CT or ultrasound
  - More commonly seen in obese patients
- Imaging
  - Seen on GRE in-phase and opposed phase as individual sequences or dual-echo imaging
    - In-phase 4.4 ms
      - Liver brighter than spleen
    - Opposed-phase 2.2 ms
      - Liver diminishes in signal intensity relative to spleen
      - Spleen never accumulates fat and therefore remains constant in signal intensity regardless of echo sampling time
- Can be seen in association with findings of acute or chronic hepatitis (see previous section)

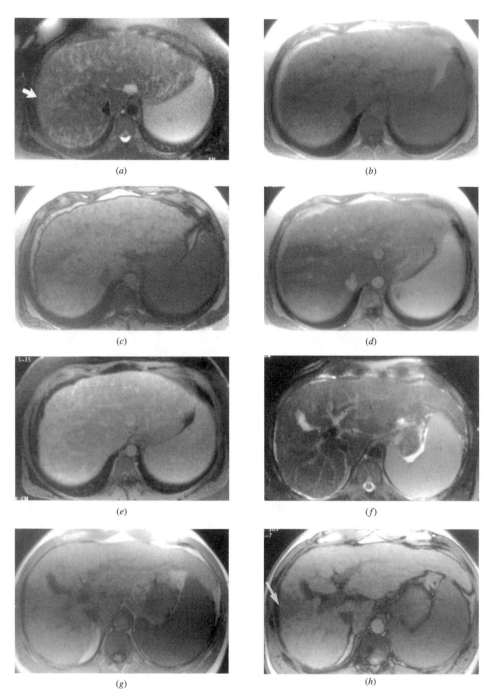

FIGURE 2.26 Cirrhosis with confluent fibrosis. Echo-train STIR (*a*), SGE (*b*), out-of-phase SGE (*c*), immediate postgadolinium SGE (*d*), and 90 s postgadolinium fat-suppressed SGE (*e*) images. There is a linear pattern of fibrosis throughout the liver with a focal region of confluent fibrosis (arrow, *a*) that is mildly high in signal on T2W (*a*) and mildly low in signal on T1W images (*b*) and demonstrates negligible enhancement on early postcontrast (*d*) and late mild enhancement (*e*). Note that the fine pattern of fibrosis present throughout the liver is particularly well shown on the short TE out-of-phase image (*c*) as low-signal linear structures and on late postgadolinium as linear-enhancing structures (*e*). T2W fat-suppressed SSETSE (*f*), SGE (*g*), out-of-phase SGE (*h*), immediate postgadolinium SGE (*i*), and 90 s postgadolinium fat-suppressed SGE (*j*) images in a second patient. The liver is small and nodular in contour and demonstrates a reticular heterogeneous enhancement pattern consistent with cirrhosis. A confluent region of fibrosis is evident in *segment 8* peripherally (arrow, *h*). No focal lesion is identified within the liver. Note the presence of splenomegaly.

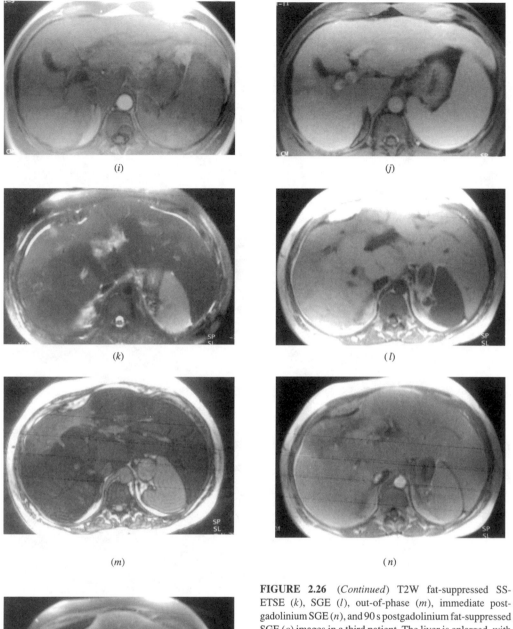

(i)

(j)

(k)

(l)

(m)

(n)

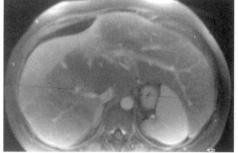

(o)

FIGURE 2.26 (*Continued*) T2W fat-suppressed SS-ETSE (k), SGE (l), out-of-phase (m), immediate post-gadolinium SGE (n), and 90 s postgadolinium fat-suppressed SGE (o) images in a third patient. The liver is enlarged, with the left lobe extending lateral to the spleen. On the out-of-phase image (m) there is a drop in signal of the hepatic parenchyma with focal sparing of the superficial parenchyma in *segments 4* and *5*. This is consistent with diffuse fatty infiltration of the liver, with lack of fatty infiltration in the region of fibrosis. Note the presence atrophy in association with the fibrosis. The region of confluent fibrosis shows negligible early enhancement (n) with late increased enhancement (o).

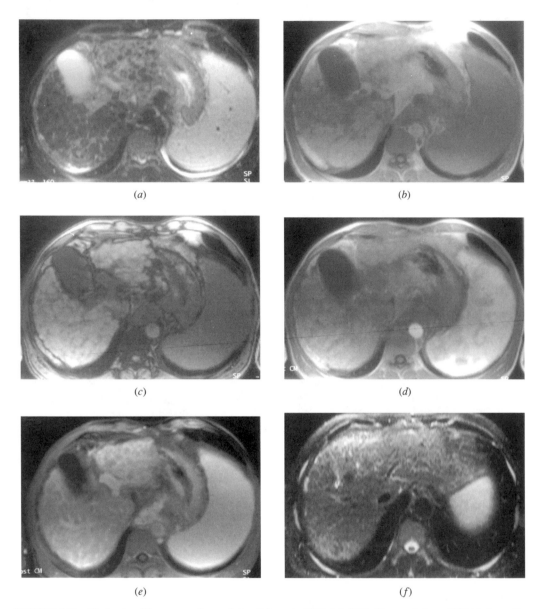

(a)

(b)

(c)

(d)

(e)

(f)

FIGURE 2.27   Cirrhosis with regenerative nodules. Echo-train STIR (*a*), SGE (*b*), out-of-phase SGE (*c*), immediate postgadolinium SGE (*d*), and 90 s postgadolinium fat-suppressed SGE (*e*) images. The liver is small with an extensive nodular pattern. A reticular pattern of fibrosis is present, which is well shown on out-of-phase images (*c*) as low-signal intensity linear tissue and demonstrates negligible enhancement on immediate postgadolinium images (*d*) with progressive enhancement on late images (*e*). Multiple regenerative nodules appear as rounded <1 cm masses best seen as high-signal lesions on out-of-phase images (*c*). Ascites, splenomegaly, and paraesophageal varices are present. Echo-train STIR (*f*), SGE (*g*), out-of-phase SGE (*h*), 45 s postgadolinium SGE (*i*), and 90 s postgadolinium fat-suppressed SGE (*j*) images in a second patient. There are multiple scattered, rounded foci throughout the liver that show decreased signal on T2 (*f*) and increased signal on noncontrast T1W (*g*) and out-of-phase (*h*) images.

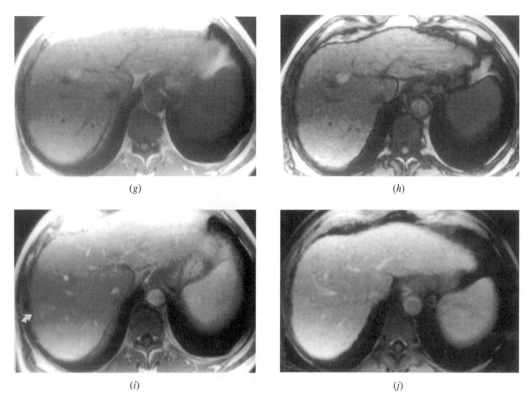

(g)

(h)

(i)

(j)

FIGURE 2.27 (*Continued*) Lesions are not apparent on early (*i*) or late (*j*) postgadolinium images, consistent with regenerative or mildly dysplastic nodules. Note also the fine reticular pattern on postgadolinium images (*i*, *j*) with progressive enhancement, consistent with fibrotic change associated with cirrhosis. A small transiently enhancing focus (curved arrow, *i*) is present in *segment 8* that reflects a vascular phenomenon.

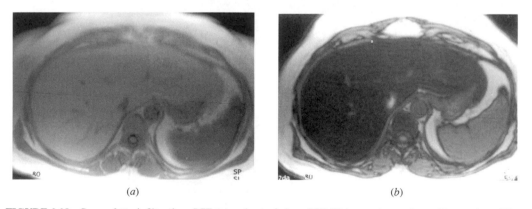

(a)

(b)

FIGURE 2.28   Severe fatty infiltration. SGE (*a*) and out-of-phase SGE (*b*) images in a patient with an enlarged liver and marked fatty infiltration.

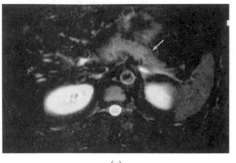

(a)

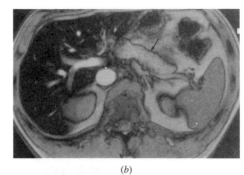

(b)

FIGURE 2.29 Idiopathic hemochromatosis, early disease. T2W fat-suppressed ETSE (*a*), out-of-phase SGE (*b*), and immediate postgadolinium SGE (*c*) images. The liver is low in signal intensity on noncontrast T2W (*a*) and T1W (*b*) images consistent with substantial iron deposition. The spleen is relatively normal in signal intensity on these sequences, reflecting that iron is not in the RES but in hepatocytes. The pancreas (arrow, *a*, *b*) is normal in signal intensity on noncontrast images and enhances normally with gadolinium. Iron deposition limited to the liver is consistent with early precirrhotic disease.

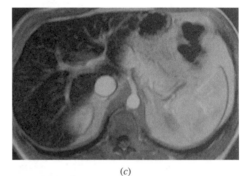

(c)

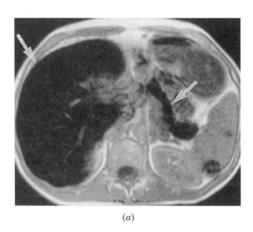

(a)

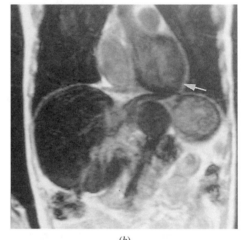

(b)

FIGURE 2.30 Idiopathic hemochromatosis, advanced disease. Transverse (*a*) and coronal SGE (*b*), and coronal 45 s postgadolinium SGE (*c*) images. The precontrast T1W image (*a*) demonstrates signal void liver and pancreas (arrows, *a*). The coronal SGE image (*b*) also demonstrates low-signal-intensity left ventricular myocardium (arrow, *b*). On the 45 s postgadolinium image (*c*), multiple enhanced varices are shown (arrows, *c*) that reflect portal hypertension secondary to cirrhosis.

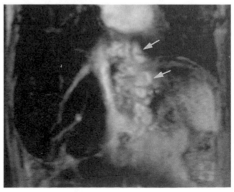

(c)

Hemochromatosis (figs. 2.29 and 2.30)
- Background
  - Results from abnormal iron deposition in soft tissues
  - Two major causes of disease, are increased GI absorption and increased erythrocyte turnover
    - Abnormal iron uptake from the GI tract
      - Genetic hemochromatosis is most important form
      - Gene mutation prevalence around 1:10; homozygous in 1:250
      - Variable penetrance
      - Iron can also deposit as hemosiderin within hepatocytes
      - Other tissues accumulating iron include
        - Pancreas
          - Develop diabetes
        - Myocardium
          - Develop congestive heart failure and arrhythmias
      - Excess iron leads to free oxidative radicals that can cause protein and DNA damage, leading to chronic liver disease and tumor formation
    - Abnormal increased erythrocyte turnover
      - Blood transfusion is most common cause
      - Intrinsic increased red cell turnover is an alternative or contributing etiology
      - Iron deposits in liver Kupffer cells, phagocytic cells that take up senescing red cells
      - Part of the reticuloendothelial system
      - Also deposits in spleen and bone marrow
- Imaging
  - Cellular iron is paramagnetic and causes field inhomogeneity in the microenvironment, leading to increased $T2^*$ decay
  - Can be seen as low signal on single-shot ETSE T2W imaging, comparing liver and spleen to psoas muscle, more easily appreciated on coronal images
  - Skeletal muscle is relatively spared in hemochromatosis and is used as a control
  - Can be seen on standard T1 GRE images as darkened signal in more severe disease

- A measure of liver $T2^*$ can be obtained using multiecho GRE images, setting TE to progressively longer in-phase values. This has been proposed as a more sensitive and semiquantitative method. On routine out/in-phase images (TE = 2.2/4.4 at 1.5 T), abnormal elevated iron level in liver will lead to a decreased signal on the in-phase images due to $T2^*$ effects of longer echo time
  - In addition to the liver, the spleen, pancreas, and heart can also be involved
  - Complications in the form of cirrhosis and hepatocellular carcinoma can be identified by routine MR imaging

Budd-Chiari Syndrome
- Background
  - Although originally described for acute, usually fatal, thrombotic occlusion of the hepatic veins, the definition of Budd-Chiari syndrome has been broadened to include subacute and chronic occlusive syndromes
  - Obstruction of venous outflow from the liver results in portal hypertension, ascites, and progressive hepatic failure
  - This condition is more common in females, and an underlying thrombotic tendency is present in up to half of patients
  - Predisposing conditions include pregnancy, postpartum state, and intra-abdominal cancer, especially HCC
  - Although the disease most commonly involves major hepatic veins, demonstration of patent central hepatic veins may be observed as small, or intermediate-sized veins may be occluded in isolation
  - In the chronic setting, regions with completely obstructed hepatic venous outflow will develop shunting of blood from hepatic arteries to portal veins. The involved liver parenchyma is thereby deprived of portal vein supply.
  - Hepatic regeneration, hypertrophy, and atrophy depend in part on the degree of portal perfusion
  - The syndrome most often results in atrophy of peripheral liver, which experiences

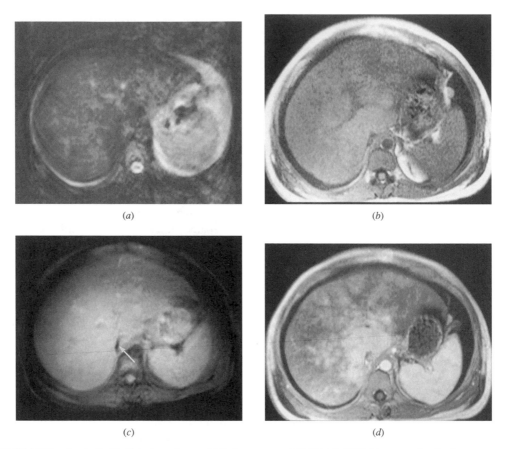

(a) (b)

(c) (d)

FIGURE 2.31   Acute Budd-Chiari syndrome. T2W fat-suppressed ETSE (a), SGE (b), proton-density fat-suppressed spin-echo (c), and immediate postgadolinium SGE (d) images. The T2W image (a) shows normal signal intensity of the caudate lobe and central liver and heterogeneous higher signal intensity of the peripheral liver. On the precontrast T1W image (b), the caudate lobe and central portion of the liver are normal in signal intensity, whereas the peripheral liver is low in signal intensity. The proton-density image (c), acquired at the expected level of the hepatic veins, demonstrates absence of hepatic veins and a compressed IVC (arrow, c). On the immediate postgadolinium SGE image (d), the caudate lobe and central liver enhance intensely, whereas peripheral liver is low in signal intensity. (Reproduced with permission from Noone T, Semelka RC, Woosley JT, Pisano ED: Ultrasound and MR findings in acute Budd-Chiari syndrome with histopathologic correlation. *J Comput Assist Tomogr* 20: 819–822, 1996).

severe venous obstruction, and hypertrophy of the caudate lobe and central liver, which are relatively spared
- Imaging
  - Enhancement patterns differ for acute, subacute, and chronic Budd-Chiari, with combinations of enhancement patterns present when acute is superimposed on subacute disease
  - In acute-onset Budd-Chiari syndrome, the peripheral liver enhances less than the central liver, presumably due to acute increased

tissue pressure with resultant diminished blood supply from both hepatic arterial and portal venous systems
- The liver demonstrates a dramatic appearance of increased central enhancement compared to decreased enhancement of the peripheral liver that persists on later postcontrast images. This is associated with low signal on T1W, and moderately high signal on T2W images of peripheral liver reflecting associated edema (figs. 2.31 and 2.32).

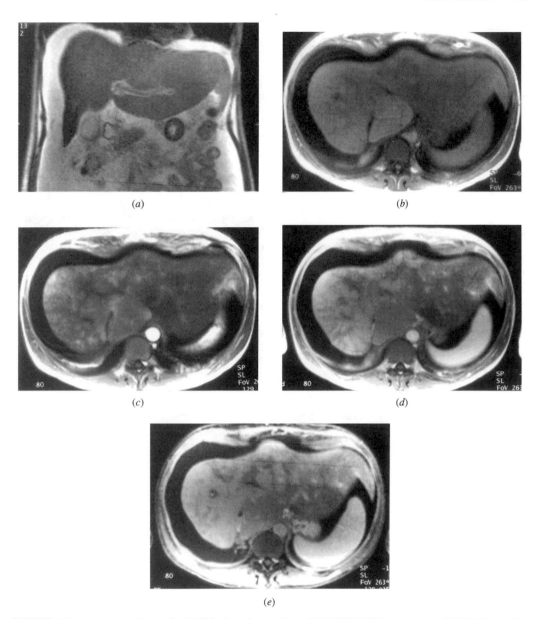

FIGURE 2.32   Acute on subacute Budd-Chiari syndrome. Coronal T2W SS ETSE (*a*), transverse SGE (*b*), immediate (*c*) and 45 s (*d*) postgadolinium SGE, and 90 s postgadolinium fat-suppressed SGE (*e*) images. The coronal T2W image (*a*) shows high signal of the lateral segment relative to the right lobe. On the T1W image (*b*), moderately diminished signal is identified in the enlarged lateral segment of the left lobe, with mild diminished signal of the right lobe. The enlarged caudate lobe possesses a more normal signal intensity. The immediate postgadolinium image (*c*) reveals markedly diminished enhancement of the lateral segment, consistent with acute changes of Budd-Chiari, and mildly heterogeneous and increase signal of the right lobe, consistent with subacute changes of Budd-Chiari. The caudate lobe has a mild heterogeneity with signal intensity intermediate between the acutely affected lateral segment and subacutely affected right lobe. Enchancement abnormalities diminish but persist on late postcontrast images (*d*, *e*).

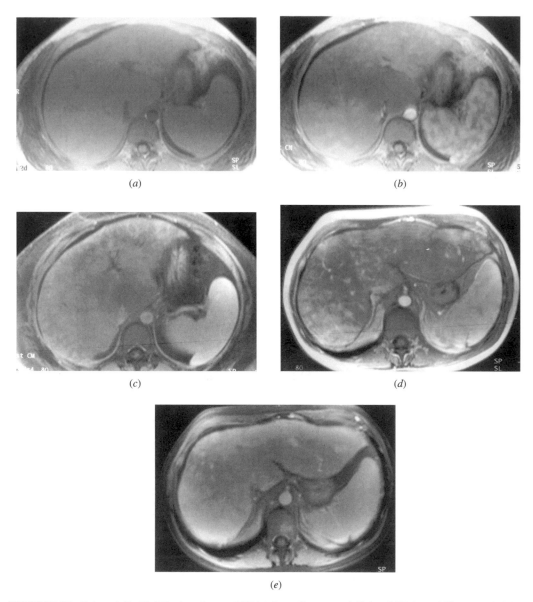

(a)

(b)

(c)

(d)

(e)

FIGURE 2.33   Subacute Budd-Chiari syndrome. SGE (*a*), immediate postgadolinium SGE (*b*), and 90 s postgadolinium fat-suppressed SGE (*c*) images. Peripheral liver is diminished in signal on T1W image (*a*) and demonstrates a diffuse, heterogeneous, mildly increased enhancement on immediate postgadolinium image (*b*) that persists on later image (*c*), consistent with hepatic vascular compensation to venous thrombosis as observed in subacute Budd-Chiari syndrome. (Reproduced with permission from Noone TC, Semelka RC, Siegelman ES, Balci NC, Hussain SM, Kim PN, Mitchell DG. Budd-Chiari Syndrome: Spectrum of appearances of acute, subacute, and chronic disease with magnetic resonance imaging. *J Magn Reson Imaging* 11: 44–50, 2000.)

Immediate postgadolinium SGE (*d*) and 90 s postgadolinium fat-suppressed SGE (*e*) images in a second patient. The liver is enlarged with an irregular contour. There is mild hypertrophy of the caudate lobe. After administration of contrast (*d*), the liver enhances in a diffusely heterogeneous pattern and becomes more homogeneous on the later image (*e*).

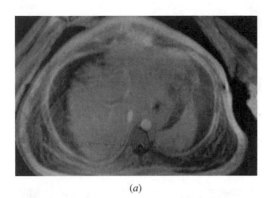

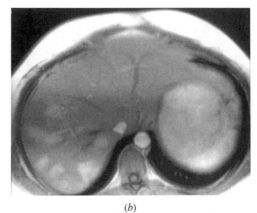

(a)   (b)

FIGURE 2.34   HELLP syndrome. Transverse 45 s postgadolinium SGE image (*a*) demonstrates an abnormal serrated margin of the liver and massive ascites. Liver changes reflect ischemic injury.

Immediate postgadolinium image (*b*) in a second patient with HELLP syndrome shows an early patchy enhancement of the liver.

○ In subacute Budd-Chiari syndrome, reversal of flow in portal veins and development of small intra- and extrahepatic venovenous collaterals occur
  ▪ Many of the collaterals are capsule based, and dynamic gadolinium-enhanced MR images show mildly increased and heterogeneous enhancement in the peripheral liver relative to the central liver on hepatic arterial dominant phase images, which on later postgadolinium images become more homogeneous with the remainder of the liver. Signal of the peripheral liver is mildly low on T1 and mildly increased on T2, similar to acute Budd-Chiari syndrome. Caudate lobe hypertrophy is mild to moderate, and collateral vessels are not prominent in the subacute setting (fig. 2.33).
○ In chronic Budd-Chiari syndrome, hepatic edema is not a prominent feature, and fibrosis develops
  ▪ Fibrosis results in decreased signal of peripheral liver on T1W and T2W images. Enhancement differences between peripheral and central liver on serial postgadolinium images become more subtler.
  ▪ Venous thrombosis, appreciated in acute and subacute disease, is usually not observed in chronic disease

  ▪ Massive caudate lobe hypertrophy, enlarged bridging intrahepatic collaterals, extrahepatic collaterals, and mildly dysplastic and regenerative nodules are all features observed in chronic Budd-Chiari syndrome

Toxemia of Pregnancy/Preeclampsia-Eclampsia/HELLP Syndrome
• Background
  ○ Hepatic disease is common in preeclampsia and may result in hemolytic anemia, elevated liver enzymes, and low platelet count (HELLP) syndrome
  ○ Liver is affected by peripheral vascular occlusions, infarcts, and hemorrhage, which can range from microscopic to macroscopic in degree
• Imaging
  ○ MR images show peripheral wedge-like enhancement defects (fig. 2.34)
    ▪ Regions of decreased enhancement on postgadolinium images and heterogeneous high-signal intensity on T2W images may result from edema and, in more severe disease, infarction
    ▪ Hematoma appears as a peripheral fluid collection with signal intensity depending on the age of the blood products, usually

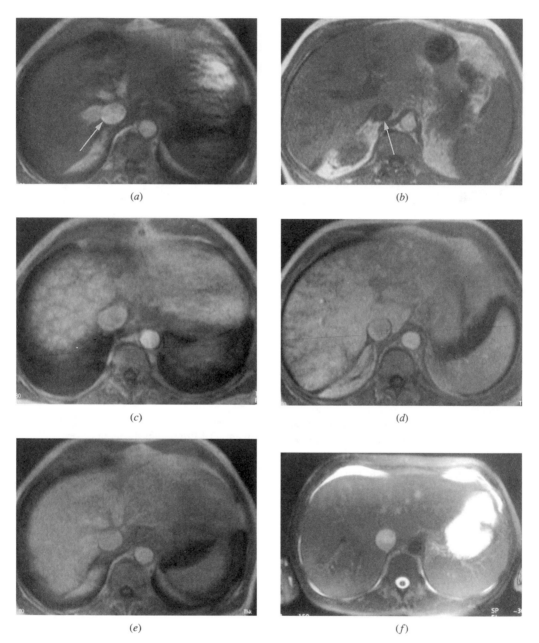

(a)   *(b)*

(c)   *(d)*

(e)   *(f)*

FIGURE 2.35   Mosaic enhancement secondary to congestive heart failure. Immediate (*a*, *b*), 45 s postgadolinium (*c*, *d*) and 90 s postgadolinium SGE (*e*) images. The immediate postgadolinium images (*a*, *b*) demonstrate the presence of gadolinium in the superior IVC early in the arterial phase of enhancement with no enhancement of the abdominal organs, because of the low cardiac output state of the patient. Reflux of gadolinium into the dilated suprahepatic IVC and hepatic veins is present (arrow, *a*) with no contrast present in the infrahepatic IVC (arrow, *b*). On the 45 s postgadolinium images (*c*, *d*), a mosaic enhancement pattern is present throughout the liver, reflecting hepatic congestion. This mosaic enhancement resolves on the 90 s postgadolinium image (*e*).

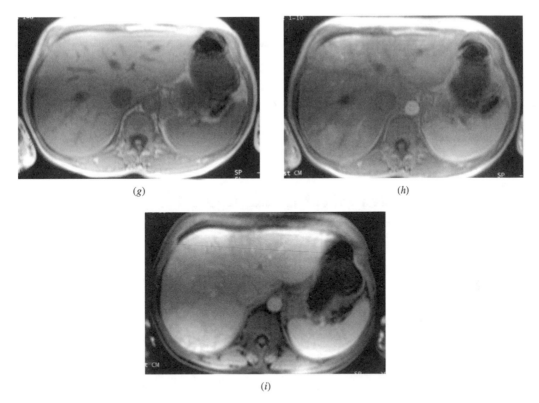

(g) (h)

(i)

FIGURE 2.35 (*Continued*) T2W fat-suppressed SS ETSE (*f*), SGE (*g*), immediate postgadolinium SGE (*h*), and 90 s postgadolinium fat-suppressed SGE (*i*) images in a patient with systemic amyloidosis and restrictive cardiomyopathy. The liver is enlarged with a mosaic enhancement pattern immediately after gadolinium administration (*h*) that diminishes on late images (*i*). Note dilatation of the inferior vena cava and small volume of ascites.

deoxyhemoglobin or intracellular methe-moglobin reflecting the acute nature of the disease process

Congestive Heart Failure
- Background
  - Patients with congestive heart failure may present with hepatomegaly and hepatic enzyme elevations
  - Pathology corresponds to nutmeg liver, and if chronic, can lead to cirrhosis
- Imaging
  - The suprahepatic inferior vena cava (IVC) is frequently enlarged with enlargement of the hepatic veins. Contrast injected in a brachial vein may appear earlier in the hepatic veins and suprahepatic IVC than in the portal veins and infrahepatic IVC, reflecting reflux of contrast from the heart (fig. 2.35).
  - On early dynamic contrast-enhanced MR images, the liver may enhance in a mosaic fashion with a reticulated pattern of low-signal-intensity linear markings
  - By 1 min postcontrast, the liver becomes more homogeneous
  - Chronic changes of cirrhosis may superimpose (see section on cirrhosis)

CHAPTER 3

GALLBLADDER AND BILE DUCTS

GALLBLADDER

BACKGROUND

MR provides unparalleled imaging for comprehensive examination of the gallbladder, in combination with the liver parenchyma and intra/extrahepatic bile ducts, pancreas, and pancreatic duct. This is important, as disease can frequently involve more than one of these systems, and evaluation of all these organ systems can help direct patient management. While gallbladder can be assessed well using motion-insensitive T2W MRCP techniques, it is suggested that a comprehensive examination, including pre/postgadolinium-enhanced T1W GRE, following a standard protocol for examination of the liver and other abdominal organs, is warranted. With such an approach, a relatively quick examination can be performed extracting the full utility of MR for evaluation of all possible associated disease processes. In addition to T2W imaging for the gallbladder and ducts, T1W imaging in combination with contrast agents excreted by the liver into bile has been proposed.

Normal Gallbladder (GB)
• Imaging (fig. 3.1)
  ○ On T2W images

• Bile is bright and uniform
• GB wall mildly hypointense and thin (<3 mm)
• GB lumen is less than 4 cm in diameter
• Single-shot echo-train imaging can be performed even in patients who are unable to breath-hold, by performing acquisition during quiet breathing
• Combination of axial and coronal images provide complementary views of the gallbladder and related bile duct anatomy
  ○ On T1W SGE
• Bile is dark (concentrated bile may be high signal)
• GB wall is mildly hypointense
• Gadolinium enhancement of the wall is intermediate in intensity
  ○ Variations include
• Phrygian-cap configuration
• Ectopic location (intrahepatic, retrohepatic, or beneath the left lobe)

Nonneoplastic Diseases

Gallstones and Sludge
• Imaging (fig. 3.2)
  ○ On T2W images
    • Gallstones are dark and conspicuous against bright bile fluid

Primer on MR Imaging of the Abdomen and Pelvis, edited by Diego R. Martin, Michele A. Brown, and Richard C. Semelka ISBN 0-471-37340-0 Copyright © 2005 Wiley-Liss, Inc.

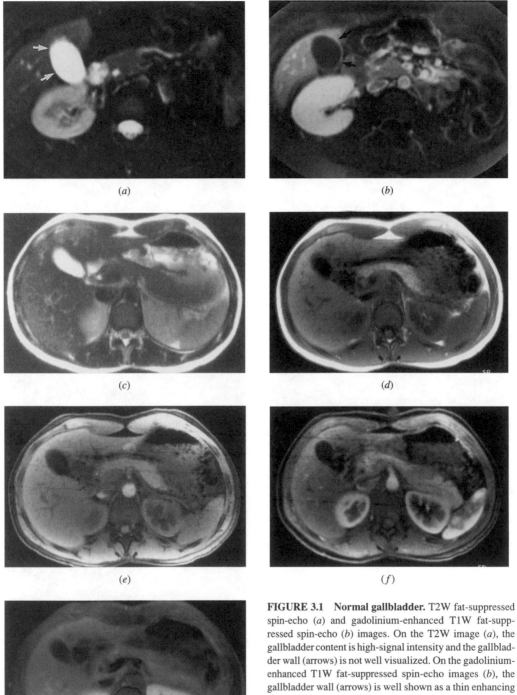

(a)

(b)

(c)

(d)

(e)

(f)

(g)

FIGURE 3.1   Normal gallbladder. T2W fat-suppressed spin-echo (*a*) and gadolinium-enhanced T1W fat-suppressed spin-echo (*b*) images. On the T2W image (*a*), the gallbladder content is high-signal intensity and the gallbladder wall (arrows) is not well visualized. On the gadolinium-enhanced T1W fat-suppressed spin-echo images (*b*), the gallbladder wall (arrows) is well shown as a thin enhancing structure. The gallbladder wall adjacent to the liver is not clearly defined because the enhancement of the gallbladder wall and the liver are similar. T2W spin-echo (*c*), T1W SGE (*d*), fat-suppressed SGE (*e*), immediate postgadolinium fat-suppressed SGE (*f*), and 2 min postgadolinium fat-suppressed spin-echo (*g*) images in a second patient with normal gallbladder. The bile is high in signal on the T2W images (*c*) and low in signal on the T1W images (*d–g*). The normal gallbladder wall is barely perceptible as a thin line, best shown on the immediate postgadolinium image (*f*).

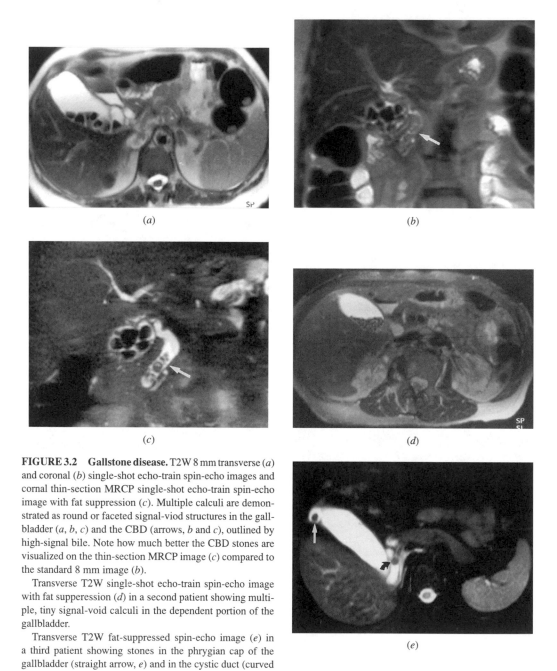

(a)

(b)

(c)

(d)

FIGURE 3.2   Gallstone disease. T2W 8 mm transverse (*a*) and coronal (*b*) single-shot echo-train spin-echo images and cornal thin-section MRCP single-shot echo-train spin-echo image with fat suppression (*c*). Multiple calculi are demonstrated as round or faceted signal-viod structures in the gallbladder (*a*, *b*, *c*) and the CBD (arrows, *b* and *c*), outlined by high-signal bile. Note how much better the CBD stones are visualized on the thin-section MRCP image (*c*) compared to the standard 8 mm image (*b*).

Transverse T2W single-shot echo-train spin-echo image with fat supperession (*d*) in a second patient showing multiple, tiny signal-void calculi in the dependent portion of the gallbladder.

Transverse T2W fat-suppressed spin-echo image (*e*) in a third patient showing stones in the phrygian cap of the gallbladder (straight arrow, *e*) and in the cystic duct (curved arrow, *e*).

(e)

- Sludge appears as a dark layer of sediment usually collecting along the dependent aspect of the gallbladder
  ○ On T1W images
    - Gallstones are generally not perceptible, but may occasionally possess high signal (fig. 3.3)
    - Sludge may appear as mildly to moderately elevated signal layering within the dependent aspect of the gallbladder

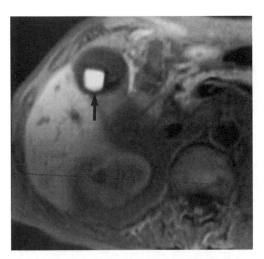

FIGURE 3.3 Hyperintense gallstone. T1W fat-suppressed spin-echo image showing a gallstone (arrow) of uniform high-signal intensity of its central portion with a signal-void peripheral rim. (Courtesy of Caroline Reinhold, MD, Dept. of Radiology, McGill University.)

Wall Thickening (defined as >3 mm)
- Etiologies include
  - Acute cholecystitis
  - Chronic cholecystitis
  - Adenomyomatosis
  - Edema
  - Hemorrhage
- Acute Cholecystitis (fig. 3.4)

Imaging
- On T2W images
  - Gallbladder lumen dilated over 4 cm
  - Wall thickening conspicuous
  - May appear as thickened homogeneous low-signal wall
  - Alternatively, the wall may be moderately high signal and may be up to several millimeters thick, likely due to wall edema
  - Associated pericholecystic high-signal fluid within the gallbladder fossa
  - May see patchy increased signal in liver parenchyma immediately adjacent to the gallbladder fossa
  - Usually can identify calculi within the gallbladder lumen, or in cystic or common bile duct
  - In acalculus acute cholecystitis, above

findings are present, but without evidence of gallstones
- On T1W images
  - Precontrast images may show high signal, reflecting, hemorrhage
  - Postgadolinium enhancement, equilibrium phase images show enhancing thickened gallbladder
  - Liver adjacent to gallbladder fossa may show abnormal increased enhancement in the arterial phase, fading by the venous phase, due to hyperemic response to gallbladder inflammation
- Chronic Cholecystitis (fig. 3.5)
  - On T2W images
    - Gallbladder is often contracted
    - Wall thickening, uniform dark signal
    - Pericholecystic fluid unusual
    - May see stones and/or sludge
  - On T1W images
    - Postgadolinium images show enhancing thickened wall
    - Liver usually does not show perfusion hyperemic changes adjacent to the gallbladder fossa
    - Suspect tumor of the gallbladder wall, if the wall is thickened irregularly and focally
  - Additional notes
    - Xanthogranulomatous cholecystitis (fibroxanthogranulomatous inflammation) is a rare, focal or diffuse, destructive inflammatory disease of the gallbladder that is considered a variant of chronic cholecystitis
    - Pathogenesis is thought to be occlusion of mucosal outpouchings (Rokitansky-Aschoff sinuses) with subsequent rupture and intramural extravasation of inspissated bile and mucin, which causes an inflammatory reaction with multiple intramural xanthogranulomatous nodules
    - Imaging
      - On T2W images
        - High-signal foci in the wall associated with small intramural abscesses

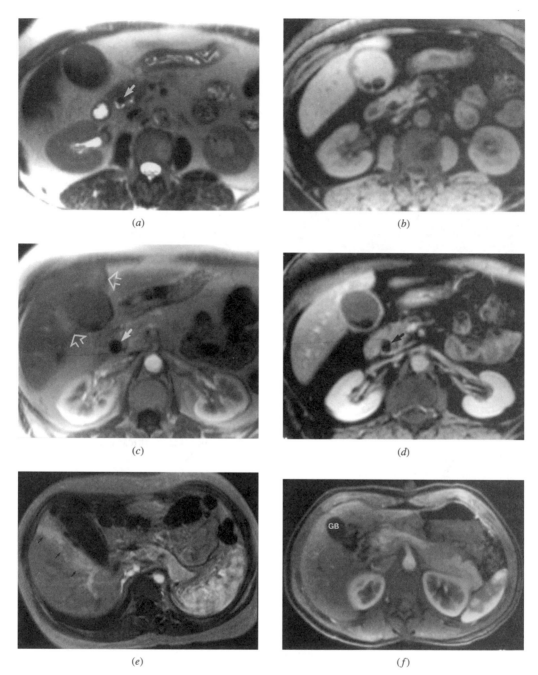

FIGURE 3.4 **Acute cholecystitis with gallstones.** T2W single-shot echo-train spin-echo (*a*), T1W fat-suppressed SGE (*b*), immediate postgadolinium SGE (*c*), and 2 min postgadolinium fat-suppressed SGE (*d*) images. The bile in the gallbladder is highly concentrated, showing low signal on the T2W image (*a*) and high signal on the T1W image (*b*). Several low-signal gallstones are visualized in the gallbladder and the CBD (arrows, *a*, *c*, *d*). The gallbladder wall is thickened. On the immediate postgadolinium image (*c*), the adjacent liver parenchyma demonstrates transient increased enhancement (open arrows, *c*). Immediate postgadolinium SGE image (*e*) in another patient demonstrating transient hyperemic enhancement of the liver (arrows, *e*) adjacent to the gallbladder.

Immediate postgadolinium fat-suppressed SGE image (*f*) in a normal subject for comparison, demonstrating homogeneous enhancement of the liver. GB, gallbladder.

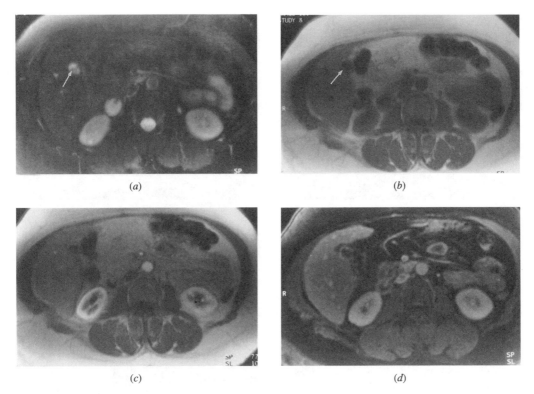

FIGURE 3.5   Chronic cholecystitis. T2W fat-suppressed spin-echo (*a*), T1W SGE (*b*), immediate postgadolinium SGE (*c*), and 90 s postgadolinium fat-suppressed SGE (*d*) images. On the T2W image (*a*), the gallbladder is shrunken and irregular in shape with poorly defined walls and a low-signal gallstone (arrow, *a*). On the precontrast T1W image (*b*), the gallbladder wall is partly hyperintense (arrow, *b*). It enhances mildly on the immediate postgadolinium image (*c*), but no increased enhancement is noted in the adjacent liver parenchyma. On the 90 s postgadolinium fat-suppressed image (*d*), the gallbladder wall shows progressive enhancement. T2W single-shot echo-train spin-echo (*e*), T1W fat-suppressed SGE (*f*), and 2 min postgadolinium fat-suppressed SGE (*g*) images in a second patient with chronic cholecystitis. The gallbladder is shrunken and irregular in shape and shows pronounced wall thickening. On the T2W image (*e*), small hyperintense foci (short arrows, *e*) represent intramural fluid collections. The gallbladder shows enhancement on the 2 min postgadolinium image (*g*).

- On T1W images
  - Low-signal intramural abscesses
- Adenomyomatosis (fig. 3.6)
  - Found in approximately 5% of the population
  - Histologically find hyperplasia of epithelial and muscular elements with mucosal outpouching of epithelium-lined cystic spaces into a thickened muscularis layer
  - Imaging
    - On T2W images
      - Focal gallbladder wall thickening and possible narrowing of lumen
      - Most common site is the fundus: when located in the gallbladder body, this may create the appearance of a waist-like narrowing—"hour-glass gallbladder" configuration
    - On T1W images
      - No specific features
      - May enhance similarly to adjacent normal-appearing gallbladder wall
  - Edema
    - Examples of secondary causes include ascites with fluid overload (hydrops) and hepatitis with secondary inflammation or cirrhosis

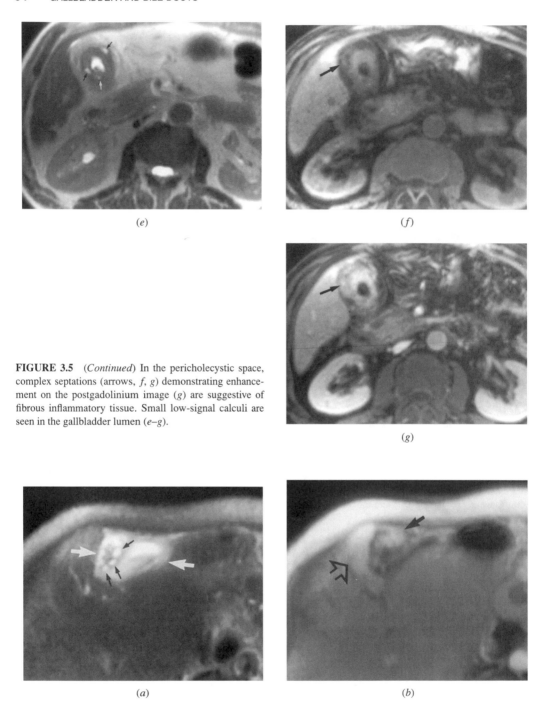

(e)

(f)

(g)

FIGURE 3.5 (*Continued*) In the pericholecystic space, complex septations (arrows, *f*, *g*) demonstrating enhancement on the postgadolinium image (*g*) are suggestive of fibrous inflammatory tissue. Small low-signal calculi are seen in the gallbladder lumen (*e–g*).

(a)

(b)

FIGURE 3.6   Gallbladder adenomyomatosis. T2W fat-suppressed single-shot echo-train spin-echo (*a*) and immediate postgadolinium T1W SGE (*b*) images. The gallbladder (large arrows, *a*) has a phrygian cap configuration, is shrunken, and shows partial severe wall thickening. Layering of low-signal concentrated bile in the dependent portion is demonstrated on the T2W image (*a*). Rokitansky-Aschoff sinuses (small arrows, *a*) are visualized as high-signal foci in the gallbladder wall on the T2W image (*a*). On the postgadolinium image (*b*), the gallbladder (arrows, *b*) and the adjacent liver parenchyma (open arrow, *b*) show increased enhancement, reflecting inflammation. In this patient who also has primary sclerosing cholangitis, the liver is cirrhotic with nodular enlargement of the caudate lobe.

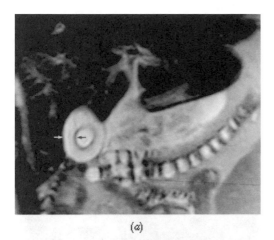

(a)

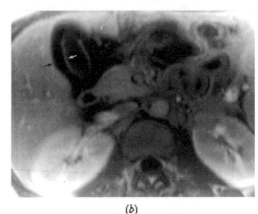

(b)

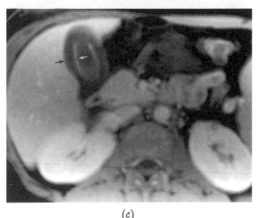

(c)

FIGURE 3.7 Gallbladder wall edema. Coronal T2W fat-suppressed single-shot echo-train spin-echo (*a*), T1W immediate postgadolinium SGE (*b*), and 2 min postgadolinium fat-suppressed SGE (*c*) images. In this patient after bone marrow transplantation, the gallbladder wall is markedly edematous and thickened (arrows, *a–c*). Because of the high fluid content of the wall, the signal intensity is high on the T2W image (*a*) and low on the T1W images (*b*, *c*). The gallbladder mucosa shows moderate early and late enhancement (*b*, *c*). The adjacent liver parenchyma is normal.

- Imaging (fig. 3.7)
  - On T2W images
    - Thickened wall has bright signal arising from within the wall
    - Challenging to differentiate between wall edema and inflammation—extent of enhancement is important
    - Gallbladder lumen within normal limits, <4 cm
  - On T1W images
    - Precontrast images generally show low signal
    - High signal reflects hemorrhage in the wall (see below)
    - Gadolinium enhancement allows for assessment of inflammation (see above)

  - Hemorrhagic Cholecystitis
    - Hemorrhagic cholecystitis is more prevalent in patients with acalculous cholecystitis than in patients with calculous cholecystitis
    - Blood breakdown products in the gallbladder wall and lumen can be clearly identified with precontrast MRI sequences
    - Imaging (fig. 3.8)
    - On T2W images
      - May see high to low signal in the thickened gallbladder wall or lumen depending on the age and composition of the blood products (fig. 3.8)
    - On T1W images
      - Variable low to high signal

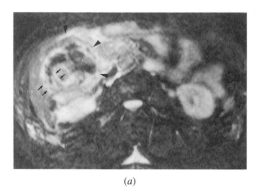

(a)

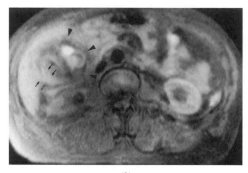

(b)

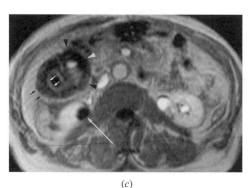

(c)

FIGURE 3.8 Hemorrhagic cholecystitis. T2W fat-suppressed echo-train spin-echo (a), T1W fat-suppressed spin-echo (b), and immediate postgadolinium SGE (c) images. On the T2W image (a), the thickened gallbladder wall (small arrows, a) shows areas of high and low signal. A pericholecystic area of predominantly low signal (arrowheads, a) is located anteromedially. On the T1W image (b), areas of high-signal intensity consistent with hemorrhage are noted within the substantially thickened gallbladder wall (small arrows, b). The large complex anteromedial area (arrowheads, b) is predominantly of high signal, which in combination with the low signal on the T2W image is consistent with intracellular methemoglobin in an area of hemorrhage. The delayed postgadolinium SGE image (c) shows to better advantage the thick gallbladder wall (small arrows, c) and the hemorrhagic pericholecystic fluid collection (arrowheads, c). A calculus (long arrow, c) is incidentally shown in the right renal collecting system.

Neoplastic Diseases

Benign Neoplasm

- Polyps
  - If less than 10 mm, may not require follow-up, or can be followed up by MR imaging at 3, 6, and 12 months, and if stable, diagnostic certainty for a benign polyp would be high
  - Imaging
    - On T2W images
    - Dark signal, equal to gallbladder wall, conforming to a polypoid filling defect, <1 cm in diameter, protruding into the lumen
    - On T1W images
      - Postgadolinium arterial and venous phases optimally show enhancement of a typically vascularized polyp
      - Enhancement serves to discriminate between polyp and stone
  - Mimickers
    - Stone
      - Stones do not enhance and generally aggregate on the dependent aspect of the gallbladder
    - Adenomyomatosis
      - This entity may be difficult to discriminate if focal and small
      - Look for typical patterns of this disease with focal involvement of the fundus or midwaist of the gallbladder

Malignant Neoplasm

- Gallbladder Adenocarcinoma
  - Although an association with gallstones and cholecystitis is noted, there appears to be less than a 1% associated risk
    - Risk is greater in the presence of large symptomatic stones
  - 5-year survival of around 6%

- Usually presents with local invasion and unresectable disease
- Imaging (fig. 3.9)
  - On T2W images
    - Dark signal mass similar to normal gallbladder wall
    - Fungating mass >1 cm, with irregular borders, discriminates from benign polyp
    - Earlier-stage local disease confined to intraluminal and superficial mucosal growth
    - Higher-stage disease shows extension of soft tissue beyond the smooth outer border of the gallbladder wall
    - May invade into adjacent liver, seen as higher signal than normal liver
    - Direct extension to involve CBD or pancreatic head can lead to CBD/pancreatic duct obstruction and dilatation, also seen on MRCP
      - Malignant cutoff sign of duct seen as abrupt irregular truncation, as opposed to benign pattern smoothly tapered duct
  - On T1W images
    - Pregadolinium images generally contribute little for primary disease localized to gallbladder, but show extension of lower-signal tumor into higher-signal liver and fat adjacent to free wall
    - Postgadolinium shows irregular heterogeneously enhancing mass that differs substantially from normal wall, with direct liver extension well shown on venous and interstitial phase images as heterogeneously lower-signal tissue extending into normal liver
    - Hematogeneous metastases well shown on hepatic arterial/capillary images
- Metastases
  - Most commonly from
    - Breast
    - Melanoma
    - Lymphoma
  - Imaging
    - Lymphoma more commonly appears as diffuse thickening (fig. 3.10)

- On T2W images
  - Abnormal focal and diffuse thickening may be apparent, corresponding to the metastatic mass with low to intermediate signal
- On T1W images
  - Low signal with enhancement increasing on the interstitial phase gadolinium-enhanced images (fig. 3.10)

BILE DUCTS
OVERVIEW

- One of the main indications for MRCP and/or conventional MRI of the biliary system is to reveal the cause for biliary obstruction and to characterize the lesion process as benign or malignant
- Common causes for benign obstruction are gallstone disease or strictures resulting from prior inflammation (usually a result of passing stones or secondary to pancreatitis) or from surgery (as may occur from complicated cholecystectomy)
- Malignant causes include
  - Pancreatic neoplasm in the head of the pancreas
  - Compression from porta hepatis mass, usually enlarged lymph nodes
  - Ampullary tumors
  - Primary bile duct tumors
- To date, standard dedicated MRCP images are T2W single-shot echo-train sequences with a very long echo time of 150–450 ms
  - This achieves very high contrast, rendering bile fluid very bright while all surrounding tissues are very dark
  - Single-shot 2D acquisition makes these sequences motion insensitive, and thin sections of 3–4 mm yield good resolution of the ducts
  - Pitfalls include
    - Flow void effects, which can produce artifactual dark signal in the center of the duct on axial images, simulating a filling defect

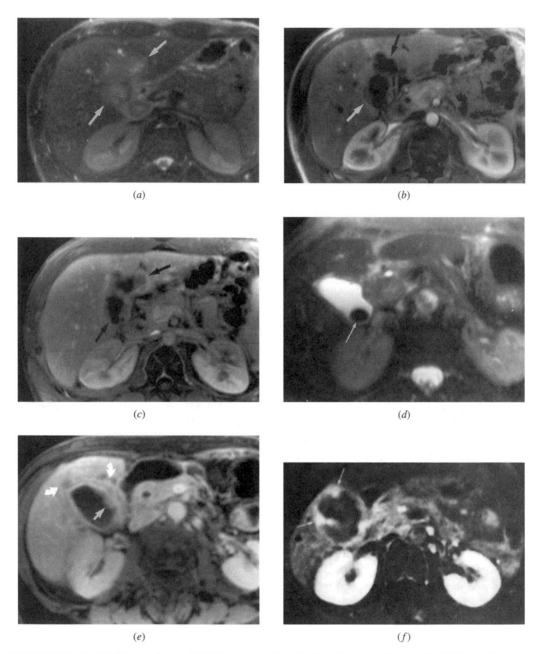

FIGURE 3.9 Gallbladder carcinoma. T2W fat-suppressed single-shot echo-train spin-echo (*a*), T1W immediate post-gadolinium SGE (*b*), and 2 min postgadolinium fat-suppressed SGE (*c*) images. The gallbladder (arrows, *a–c*) has a masslike appearance and shows an irregular and markedly thickened wall (arrows) that is moderately hyperintense on the T2W image (*a*). Intense, slightly heterogeneous enhancement is demonstrated on the immediate and 2 min postgadolinium images (*b, c*), showing poor delineation from liver parenchyma. T2W fat-suppressed single-shot echo-train spin-echo (*d*) and T1W 2 min postgadolinium fat-suppressed SGE (*e*) images in a second patient with adenocarcinoma of the gallbladder. A signal-void stone is shown on the T2W image (*d*). The gallbladder wall demonstrates partial irregular thickening (arrow, *e*) best visualized on the postgadolinium image (*e*). Small hypoenhancing areas in the adjacent liver parenchyma (curved arrows, *e*) are suggestive of metastases to the liver.

Transverse T1W 2 min postgadolinium fat-suppressed SGE image (*f*) in a third patient with gallbladder cancer demonstrates irregular nodular thickening of the gallbladder wall (arrows, *f*).

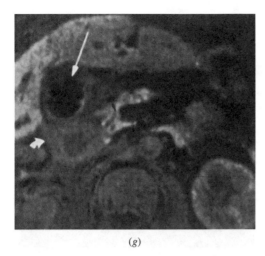

(g)

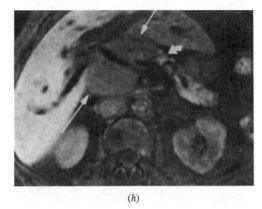

(h)

FIGURE 3.9 (*Continued*) T1W fat-suppressed spin-echo images (*g*, *h*) in a fourth patient demonstrating gallbladder cancer, which is intermediate in signal intensity and infiltrates along the duodenal wall (curved arrow, *g*) and head of the pancreas encasing the gastroduodenal artery (short arrow, *g*). Signal-void calculi are present within the gallbladder (long arrow, *g*). On a more superior image at the level of the porta hepatis (*h*), a large tumor (straight arrows, *h*) is demonstrated. Good contrast is observed between intermediate-signal tumor and high-signal pancreas (curved arrow, *h*).

- These sequences are prone to cross-talk and require that the images are acquired noncontiguously, intercalating alternating slices (e.g., slice numbers 1, 3, 5, 7, ... are acquired first, followed by slice numbers 2, 4, 6, 8, ...)
  - If there is any respiratory movement, this results in marked spatial misregistration with potential to miss imaging areas of interest

  - Option: respiratory-triggered or navigator-triggered acquisition, however these techniques result in longer total acquisition time
- Vessel crossing the extrahepatic duct (e.g., hepatic artery) may mimic a filling defect
  - To overcome some of these potential pitfalls, it is useful to perform two planes of acquisition, one in the axial and a second

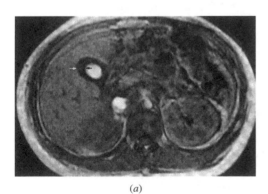

(a)

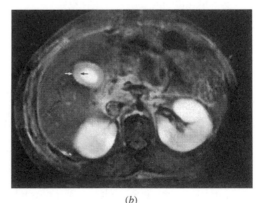

(b)

FIGURE 3.10 **Burkitt's lymphoma of the gallbladder.** T1W SGE (*a*) and 2 min postgadolinium fat-suppressed spin-echo (*b*) images. The gallbladder wall (arrows, *a*, *b*) is diffusely thickened because of infiltration by lymphoma. Note the uniform moderate enhancement of the wall after contrast administration (*b*), which is less than that observed for acute cholecystitis.

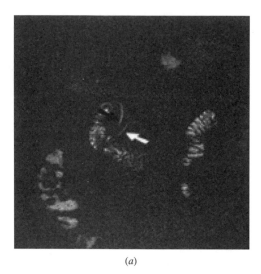 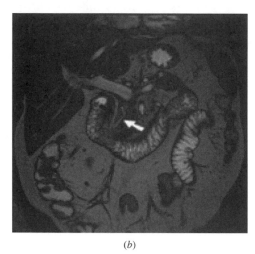

(a)   (b)

FIGURE 3.11   Comparison of MRCP imaging sequences. Coronal conventional MRCP (*a*) and coronal True-FISP images (*b*) show normal common bile duct (black arrow) and pancreatic duct (white arrow) converging in the pancreatic head at the level of the duodenal sweep. Note that the True-FISP image provides equally good depiction of the ducts, but also provides excellent representation of the relation of the ducts to the surrounding soft tissues and blood vessels.

in the coronal plane, both acquired with 3–4 mm thick sections
- This allows verification of any abnormality seen on one plane of imaging—for example, a flow void artifact seen on axial images of the CBD may not be apparent on the coronal images
- These images are best reviewed on a computer workstation scrolling through the stacked images
- Optional maximum intensity projection images (MIPs) can be constructed with software readily available on all current MR console software to provide 3D rendering of the images
○ Optional imaging includes a thick slab—for example, 40 mm thick—acquired in the coronal plane, typically as a 5–8 acquisition, which can produce an overview of the pancreatic and the intra- and extrahepatic bile duct configuration
- Pitfall of relying exclusively on thick slabs is that small abnormalities such as an intraductal stone partially filling the lumen may become obscurel due to volume averaging with bright signal bile fluid surrounding the stone

○ Alternative bile duct imaging includes use of 2D Free Induction Steady-State Precession (True-FISP) sequences that have T2W properties, making fluid-filled structures very conspicuous, including bile ducts, gallbladder, pancreatic duct, stomach, and duodenum (fig. 3.11)
- These are also slice-by-slice acquisitions that can take less than 1 s per slice and are remarkable for motion insensitivity
- Advantages over standard MRCP include
  • Insensitive to through-plane signal flow void, avoiding artifacts that mimic disease
  • Resistant to cross-talk, allowing contiguous slice acquisitions that reduce spatial misregistration between slices
  • Maintains a full gray scale for visualization of the surrounding soft tissues, useful for anatomic referencing to both normal and abnormal soft tissues, including vessels
    ○ Vessels remain high signal internally with dark walls and are easily visualized and separated from the bile ducts
○ As a general observation, dedicated MRCP imaging is not recommended in isolation

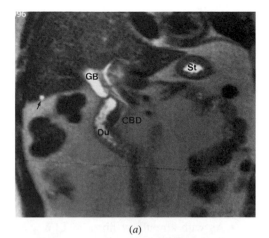

(*a*)

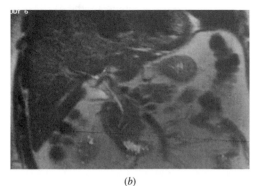

(*b*)

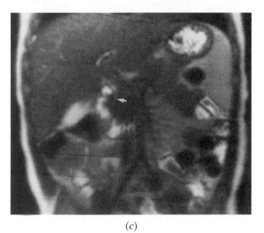

(*c*)

FIGURE 3.12 Normal biliary tree. Coronal T2W single-shot echo-train spin-echo images (*a, b, c*) in three patients. In the first patient (*a*), the biliary tree is visualized with high signal, allowing clear depiction of normal anatomy. The second part of the duodenum (Du) is outlined by a small amount of physiologic fluid in this fasting patient (*a*) (CBD, common bile duct; GB, gallbladder; St, stomach). A small liver cyst (arrow, *a*) is present in the right lobe. In a second adult patient (*b*), the right and left hepatic, common hepatic, and common bile duct are demonstrated. A short portion of the pancreatic duct is also seen. In a 1-year-old child (*c*), the CBD (arrow) is well visualized despite the lack of patient cooperation.

and should be performed in addition to standard comprehensive abdominal imaging pre- and postgadolinium administration with the full complement of T2W and T1W acquisitions

- This facilitates superior sensitivity and specificity for disease affecting the ducts, including inflammation and mass effect mediated by other soft-tissue structures such as tumors, as is shown in the following sections
  ◦ The normal CBD as visualized with MRCP (measured on coronal source images) is considered 7 mm in patients with gallbladder in place and 10 mm in patients after cholecystectomy
- Duct diameter can increase with age, and duct diameter may increase by 1 mm per decade above 60 years of age

- Normal intrahepatic bile ducts show smooth contours that taper gradually and uniformly toward the periphery of the liver, and the CBD should taper smoothly toward the ampulla (fig. 3.12)
- Notes to Emphasize
  ◦ Stent placement can significantly impair diagnostic sensitivity, specificity, and accuracy of imaging studies (including ultrasound and CT)
  ◦ Unless considered a medical emergency, it is highly advisable to coordinate imaging studies with the gastroenterology interventionalist to ensure that the MRI is performed first as the presence of a biliary start results in inflammatory changes in the duct wall, which can be difficult to distinguish from intrinsic disease.

Benign Disease

Choledocholithiasis
- Calculi in the biliary ducts are the most common cause of extrahepatic obstructive jaundice
- MRI is significantly more sensitive and specific than ultrasound and CT
- Although endoscopic retrograde cholangiopancreatography (ERCP) is generally viewed as a gold standard, it should be reserved for therapeutic intervention, with MRCP performed when the underlying disease process is uncertain
  - For example, ERCP drawbacks include
    - Invasive procedure requiring patient sedation
    - Difficulty visualizing above the level of obstruction
    - Inability to visualize any of the soft-tissue structures surrounding the ducts
    - Associated risk of inducing pancreatitis, which has a high morbidity
    - Failure rates of ERCP are between 5% and 20%
- Imaging
  - MRCP can reliably identify obstructing and nonobstructing duct and gallbladder calculi (fig. 3.13)

Ampullary Stenosis
- The clinical symptoms of ampullary stenosis include recurrent, intermittent upper abdominal pain, abnormal liver tests, and dilatation of the common bile duct
- Two benign causes include ampullary fibrosis and papillary dysfunction
- Ampullary fibrosis
  - Is the most common cause
  - Most likely a result of prior stone passage with induced inflammation followed by fibrosis and stricture
  - Imaging
    - MRCP images show a dilated CBD that tapers smoothly toward the ampulla, having a benign configuration and without any obstructing filling defects (fig. 3.14)

- T1W gadolinium-enhanced multiphase imaging is important to fully evaluate the pancreatic head and exclude the possibility of tumor
- Papillary dysfunction
  - Functional stenosis of the sphincter of Oddi includes spasm or uncoordinated contractions of the sphincter of Oddi, resulting in delayed drainage of the CBD
  - Imaging
    - MRI can demonstrate the presence of abnormal CBD dilatation with benign configuration on MRCP (fig. 3.15)
    - As with ampullary fibrosis, T1W gadolinium-enhanced imaging should be performed to exclude pancreatic head disease including tumor (fig. 3.15)
    - Administration of secretin to induce gallbladder bile discharge to possibly exacerbate duct dilatation secondary to dysfunction has been proposed

Sclerosing Cholangitis
- Characterized by inflammation and obliterative fibrosis of intrahepatic and extrahepatic bile ducts
- Progressive periductal fibrosis eventually leads to disappearance of small ducts and strictures of larger ducts
- Disease can be focal, multifocal, or diffuse
- Primary sclerosing cholangitis
  - Approximately 70% of patients with primary sclerosing cholangitis (PSC) also have inflammatory bowel disease
  - 87% of these patients have ulcerative colitis and 13% have Crohn's disease
  - PSC results in cholestasis with progression to secondary biliary cirrhosis and hepatic failure
  - Progression rate of disease is highly variable and can be rapid or indolent
  - Prognosis is poor
  - Associated increased risk of cholangiocarcinoma
- Imaging
  - MRCP shows multifocal, irregular strictures and dilatations of segments of the intra- and extrahepatic ducts (fig. 3.16)

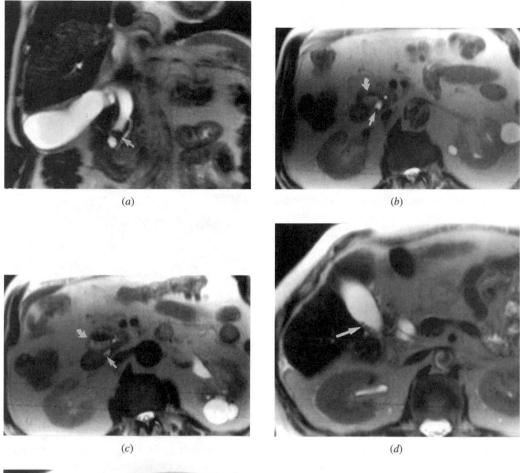

(a)

(b)

(c)

(d)

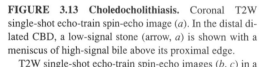

(e)

FIGURE 3.13 Choledocholithiasis. Coronal T2W single-shot echo-train spin-echo image (*a*). In the distal dilated CBD, a low-signal stone (arrow, *a*) is shown with a meniscus of high-signal bile above its proximal edge.

T2W single-shot echo-train spin-echo images (*b*, *c*) in a second patient revealing a 2 mm low-signal choledocholith (arrow, *b*) in the mildly dilated distal CBD and another tiny calculus more caudally (*c*) in the preampullary CBD (arrow, *c*). A duodenal diverticulum (curved arrows, *b*, *c*) is shown with high-signal fluid content in the dependent and a signal-void air bubble in the nondependent portions. High-signal cortical renal cysts are present in the left kidney.

Transverse T2W single-shot echo-train spin-echo images (*d*, *e*) in a third patient demonstrating several low-signal 2 mm calculi in the gallbladder (arrow, *d*) and in the preampullary CBD (arrow, *e*).

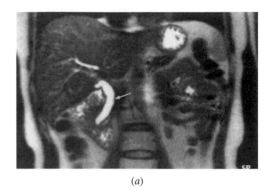

(a)

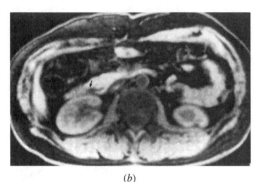

(b)

FIGURE 3.14   Ampullary fibrosis. Coronal T2W thin-section MRCP single-shot echo-train spin-echo image (*a*) shows the entire dilated CBD (arrow, *a*), excluding ductal calculi.

Transverse T1W fat-suppressed SGE (*b*) and immediate postgadolinium SGE (*c*) images in a second patient with ampullary fibrosis. The pancreas and ampulla appear normal on the fat-suppressed SGE image (*b*) at the level of the ampulla (arrow, *b*), with no evidence of a mass. This is confirmed on the immediate postgadolinium image (*c*), which shows homogeneous enhancement of the pancreas at the level of the ampulla (arrow, *c*), excluding tumor.

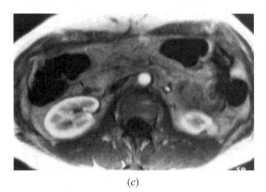

(c)

- ○ The strictures are usually short and annular, alternating with normal or slightly dilated segments, producing a beaded appearance (fig. 3.16)
- ○ Due to fibrosis of higher-order intrahepatic bile ducts, the biliary tree has the appearance of cutoff peripheral ducts, described as pruning
- ○ The disease may involve intrahepatic ducts or extrahepatic ducts alone or both, with the cystic duct usually spared
- ○ Slowly progressive disease may lead to chronic intrahepatic segmental obstruction and result in segmental liver atrophy
- ○ Cirrhosis eventually develops with PSC often having a distinctive appearance of extensive fibrosis associates with central large regenerative nodules and peripheral atrophy (see cirrhosis section in chap. 2) (fig. 3.17)
- • Mimickers
  - ○ Cholangiocarcinoma
    - ▪ Duct-infiltrating type of this disease may have a comparable appearance to PSC;

obstruction and vascular changes more severe with cholangiocarcinoma
    - ▪ ERCP with brushings has low yield and frequently fails to provide a diagnosis
    - ▪ Additionally, PSC can lead to development of cholangiocarcinoma
  - ○ Cirrhosis with secondary sclerosing cholangitis

Infectious Cholangitis
- • Infectious bacterial ascending cholangitis is a clinically defined syndrome caused by complete or partial biliary obstruction with associated ascending infection from the duodenum
  - ○ Classical clinical description includes Charcot's triad
    - ▪ Jaundice, abdominal pain, and fever with elevated white cells indicative of sepsis
    - ▪ Present in approximately 70% of patients
- • Disease severity ranges from mild to life-threatening
- • Prerequisite conditions are the presence of microorganisms in the bile and the presence of partial or complete biliary obstruction

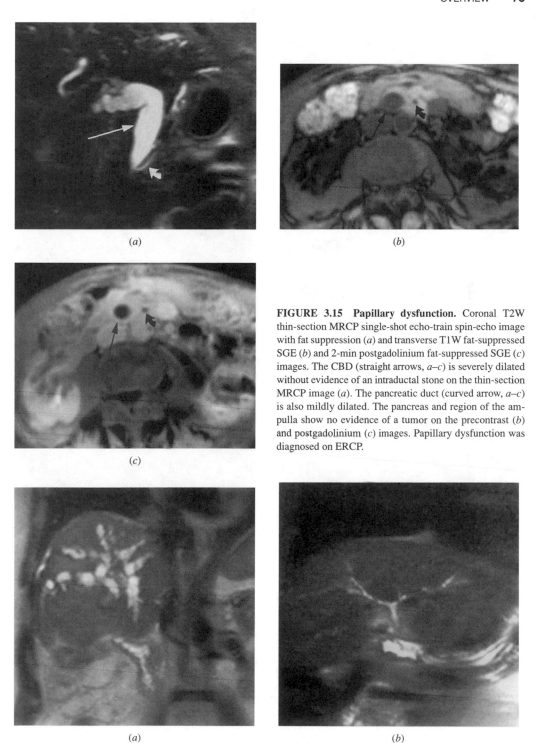

(a)

(b)

(c)

FIGURE 3.15 Papillary dysfunction. Coronal T2W thin-section MRCP single-shot echo-train spin-echo image with fat suppression (a) and transverse T1W fat-suppressed SGE (b) and 2-min postgadolinium fat-suppressed SGE (c) images. The CBD (straight arrows, a–c) is severely dilated without evidence of an intraductal stone on the thin-section MRCP image (a). The pancreatic duct (curved arrow, a–c) is also mildly dilated. The pancreas and region of the ampulla show no evidence of a tumor on the precontrast (b) and postgadolinium (c) images. Papillary dysfunction was diagnosed on ERCP.

(a)

(b)

FIGURE 3.16 Primary sclerosing cholangitis (PSC), beading. Coronal T2W single-shot echo-train spin-echo images without (a) and with fat suppression (b) in two different patients (a, b, respectively). The high-signal intrahepatic bile ducts demonstrate beading caused by short strictures alternating with dilated (a) or normal-caliber (b) segments.

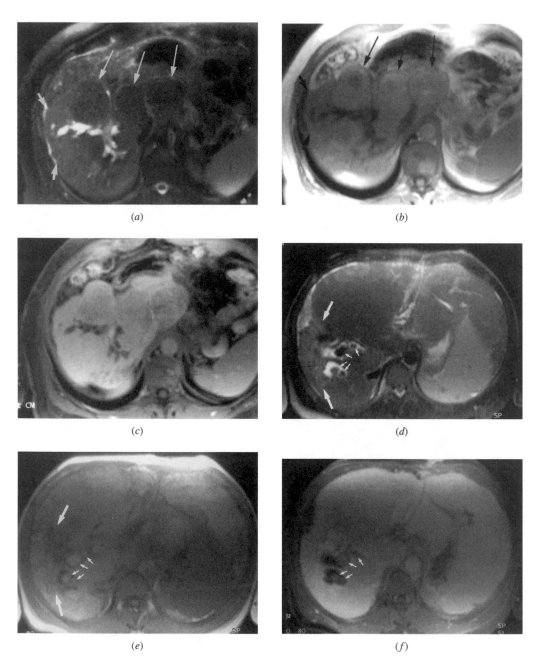

FIGURE 3.17 Primary sclerosing cholangitis (PSC), cirrhosis. T2W fat-suppressed single-shot echo-train spin-echo (*a*), T1W SGE (*b*), and 2 min postgadolinium fat-suppressed SGE (*c*) images. The intrahepatic bile ducts are dilated and demonstrate beading. The liver is nodular and cirrhotic in this patient with late-stage PSC. Three large macroregenerative nodules (long arrows, *a*, *b*) located in the central portion of the liver appear to obstruct the bile ducts centrally. The nodules are slightly hypoenhancing on the 2 min postgadolinium image (*c*). A subsegmental distal area of atrophic liver parenchyma (short arrows, *a*, *b*) appears slightly hyperintense on the T2W image (*a*) and hypointense on the T1W image (*b*). T2W fat-suppressed single-shot echo-train spin-echo (*d*), T1W SGE (*e*), and 2 min postgadolinium fat-suppressed SGE (*f*) images in a second patient. The liver shows multiple large macroregenerative nodules. The bile ducts in the right lobe of the liver are severely dilated and contain several calculi (small arrows, *d–f*) that are high signal on the T1W image (*e*). A wedge-shaped peripheral area of liver parenchyma (arrows, *d, e*) is atrophic, showing high signal on the T2W image (*d*) and low signal on the T1W image (*e*) with late enhancement on the 2 min postgadolinium image (*f*).

T1W 2 min postgadolinium SGE image with fat suppression (*g*) in a third patient demonstrating a beaded appearance of the intrahepatic bile ducts (arrows, *g*).

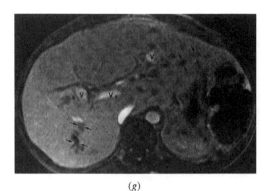

(g)

FIGURE 3.17 (*Continued*) The branches of the portal vein (V, *g*) are enhanced, facilitating differentiation from low-signal dilated intrahepatic bile ducts. The liver demonstrates a mildly irregular surface and enlargement of the left lobe.

- Oriental cholangiohepatitis
  - A particular form of infectious cholangitis possibly caused by infestation of the biliary tract by *Clonorchis sinensis* or other parasites
    - This infection is regionally ubiquitous among certain Asians, but the disease manifests in only a subset
    - Characterized by inflammatory infiltration of bile ducts, proliferative fibrosis, periductal abscesses, intrahepatic duct-layering sludge and calculi (pigment stones)
    - May develop multiple intrahepatic abscesses
- AIDS cholangiopathy
  - In HIV-positive patients, involvement of the pancreatico-biliary tract may be an early feature of AIDS
  - Inflammation and edema of the biliary mucosa, resulting in mucosal thickening and irregularity, is the hallmark of AIDS cholangiopathy
  - This may lead to strictures, dilatations, and pruning, resembling sclerosing cholangitis
  - When the ampulla of Vater is involved, ampullary stenosis with common bile duct dilatation may result
  - The gallbladder may also be involved and show acalculous cholecystitis with similar imaging features to acute cholecystitis

  - Patients can develop superimposed infectious cholangitis often by unusual pathogens, including cytomegalovirus, cryptosporidium, mycobacteriae, and *Candida albicans*
- Imaging
  - Bile duct walls are commonly mild to moderately thickened and show increased enhancement, which can be best appreciated on fat-suppressed T1W interstitial phase gadolinium-enhanced images (fig. 3.18)
  - On T2W images streaky increased signal can be present in the periportal area and wedge-shaped hyperintense regions in the liver parenchyma (fig. 3.18)
  - On pregadolinium T1W images, these wedge-shaped regions in the liver are usually hypointense, but may also show increased signal intensity
  - On immediate postgadolinium images, increased focal parenchymal enhancement may frequently be observed, consistent with inflammation (fig. 3.18)
  - Liver abscesses may complicate infectious cholangitis and are best visualized on T2W and T1W dynamic gadolinium-enhanced images
  - Thrombosis of the portal vein may occur and is easily visualized on gadolinium-enhanced T1W images
    - A distinguishing feature from sclerosing cholangitis, in which portal vein thrombosis is rare

Cystic Diseases of Bile Ducts
- Congenital biliary cysts comprise choledochal cysts, diverticula originating from extrahepatic ducts, choledochocele, Caroli's disease, and segmental cysts, depending on the location of the dilatation of the biliary tract
- MRCP can display the anatomical distribution, extent, and size of these lesions and diagnose associated findings such as stone disease, and, in combination with gadolinium-enhanced T1W images, evaluate for malignancy

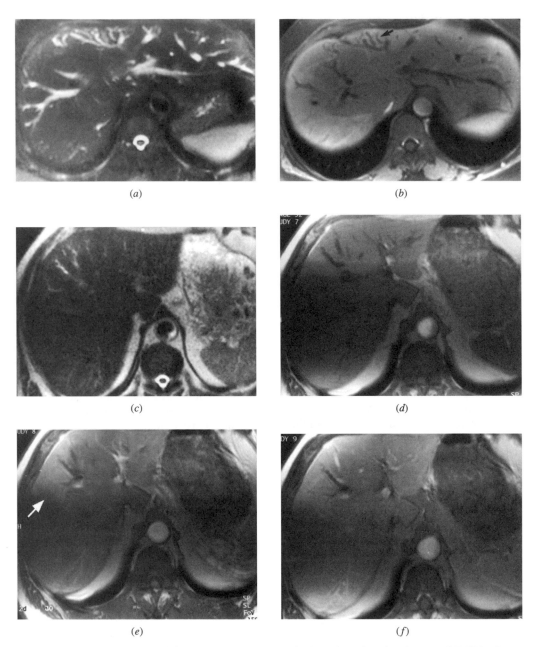

(a)

(b)

(c)

(d)

(e)

(f)

FIGURE 3.18 Infectious cholangitis. T2W fat-suppressed single-shot echo-train spin-echo (a) and T1W 2 min post-gadolinium fat-suppressed SGE (b) images. The entire intrahepatic biliary tree is severely dilated, visualized as high signal on the T2W image (a). On the T1W image (b), the low-signal ducts are well differentiated from gadolinium-enhanced vessels. The walls of the bile ducts show increased enhancement that is most pronounced in *segment 4* of the liver (arrow, b).

T2W single-shot echo-train spin-echo (c), T1W SGE (d), immediate postgadolinium SGE (e), and 2 min postgadolinium fat-suppressed SGE (f) images in a second patient. A periferal wedge-shaped area of liver parenchyma between *segments 4* and *8* shows moderate biliary ductal dilatation. The liver parenchyma in this area demonstrates increased signal on both the T2W (c) and T1W (d) images, consistent with inspissated bile. Increased enhancement of this area (arrow, e) is demonstrated on the postgadolinium images (e, f), reflecting local inflammation and hyperemia in the liver parenchyma. The bile duct walls show increased enhancement, best visualized on the 2 min postgadolinium image (f).

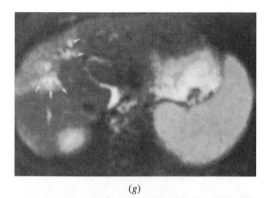

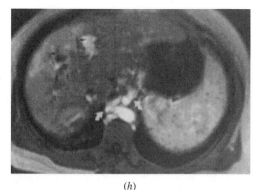

(g)

(h)

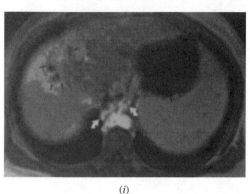

(i)

FIGURE 3.18 (*Continued*) T2W fat-suppressed spin-echo (*g*) and T1W immediate (*h*), and 90 s (*i*) postgadolinium SGE images in a third patient with liver cirrhosis and infectious cholangitis. A peripheral wedge-shaped area of liver parenchyma in the right lobe is hyperintense on the T2W image (*g*) and demonstrates increased enhancement on the postgadolinium images (*h*, *i*), reflecting acute inflammation. The bile ducts (arrows, *g–i*) in this area are dilated and show increased mural enhancement, best demonstrated on the 90 s postgadolinium image (*i*). The spleen is enlarged, showing multiple small low-signal foci (Gamna-Gandy bodies) (*g–i*). Esophageal varices (curved arrows, *h*, *i*) are shown on the postgadolinium images (*h*, *i*).

- Todani classification system is widely used and useful for presurgical planning
  - Type I, choledochal cyst
  - Type II, diverticulum of extrahepatic ducts
  - Type III choledochocele
  - Type IV, multiple segmental cysts
  - Type V, Caroli's disease
- Choledochal Cyst
- The most common cystic dilatation (77–87%)
- Presents before age 10 in approximately 50% of cases
- Associated with an increased incidence of other biliary anomalies, gallstone disease, pancreatitis, and cholangiocarcinoma
- The etiology may result from anomalous junction of the CBD and the pancreatic duct proximal to the major papilla, where there is no ductal sphincter
  - Allows reflux of pancreatic enzymes into the biliary system, weakening the walls of the bile ducts

- Imaging
  - Choledochal cysts are segmental aneurysmal dilatations of the CBD alone or of the CBD and CHD (fig. 3.19)
- Choledochocele
- Imaging
  - Choledochoceles are cystic dilatations of the distal CBD that herniate into the lumen of the duodenum and create a "cobra-head" appearance on MRCP images (fig. 3.20).
- Caroli's Disease
  - An uncommon form of congenital dilatations of intrahepatic bile ducts with normal extrahepatic ducts
  - Demonstration that these multiple cystic spaces communicate with the biliary tree is mandatory for the differentiation from cystic disease of the liver
  - Imaging
    - Optimally demonstrated with thin-section T2W or T1W images where

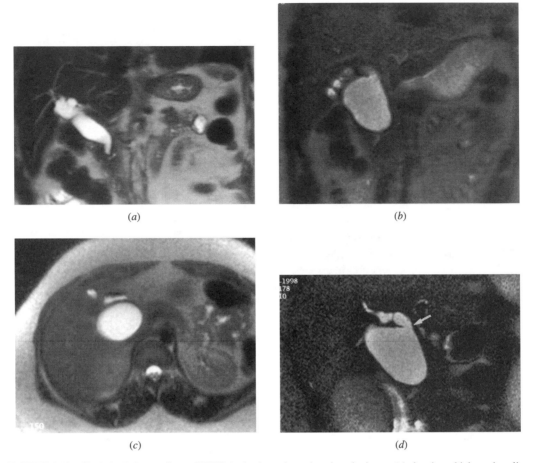

(a)

(b)

(c)

(d)

FIGURE 3.19   Choledochal cyst. Coronal T2W single-shot echo-train spin-echo image (a) showing a high-grade cylindrical dilatation of the CHD and CBD. The intrahepatic bile ducts are normal.

T2W coronal (b) and transverse (c) single-shot echo-train spin-echo images and coronal thin-section MRCP single-shot echo-train spin-echo image with fat suppression (d) in a child demonstrating a saccular choledochal cyst arising from the CHD. The MRCP image (d) shows the origin of the choledochal cyst (arrow, d).

Caroli's disease presents with rounded cystic dilatations with signal intensity of bile (bright on T2W and low on T1W images), in direct communication with bile ducts (fig. 3.21)

Postsurgical Biliary Complications
- Benign biliary strictures usually arise secondary to surgical injury (laparoscopic cholecystectomy, gastric and hepatic resection, biliary-enteric anastomosis, biliary reconstruction following liver transplantation)
- The remainder are secondary to penetrating or blunt trauma, inflammation associated with

gallstone disease, chronic pancreatitis, ampullary fibrosis, toxic or ischemic lesions of the hepatic artery, or primary infection
- The advent of minimally invasive therapeutic procedures performed by interventional radiology or endoscopy have greatly increased the need for preoperative diagnosis and imaging in order to plan the optimal therapeutic approach
- The major advantage of MRCP is the ability to visualize the biliary tree above and below a high-grade stricture or complete obstruction
- The bile ducts distal to a stenosis, however, may be collapsed and miniscule on

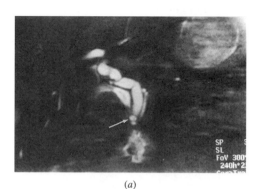

(a)

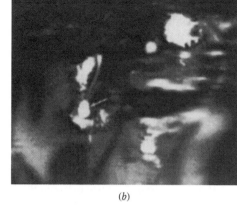

(b)

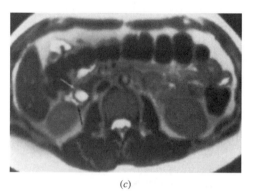

(c)

FIGURE 3.20 Choledochocele. Coronal this-section MRCP single-shot echo-train spin-echo image with fat suppression (a). The ampullary section of the CBD shows a small cystic dilatation (arrow, a) that protrudes into the lumen of the duodenum. The rest of the CBD is also dilated.

T2W single-shot echo-train spin-echo images in the coronal plane with fat suppression (b) and the transverse plane without fat suppression (c) in a second patient. The CBD shows a cystic expansion (white arrows, b, c) of its ampullary section. The transverse image (c) demonstrates that the choledochocele (white arrows, c) bulges into the duodenum (black arrow, c), which contains high-signal-intensity intraluminal fluid.

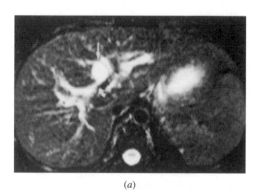

(a)

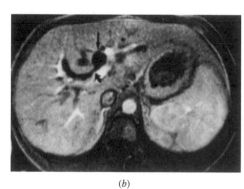

(b)

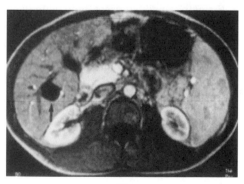

(c)

FIGURE 3.21 Caroli's disease. T2W fat-suppressed spin-echo (a) and immediate postgadolinium SGE (b, c) images. Cystic intrahepatic biliary dilatation (straight arrows, a–c) is present in the left (a, b) and right (c) lobes of the liver. Differentiation from liver cysts is made by demonstration of continuity with a mildly dilated bile duct (curved arrow, a, b). Differentiation of bile ducts from portal vein branches is facilitated on the postgadolinium images (b, c), where the latter demonstrate enhancement.

MIP-reconstructed images, leading to overestimation of the stricture length

- Thin-section source images must be used to evaluate the extent of high-grade stenosis
- Other biliary complications of cholecystectomy are retained bile duct stones, biliary leak, and biliary fistula
- High-grade biliary stricture and transsection of bile ducts can both present as abrupt termination of a dilated duct, and consequently MRCP may fail to distinguish between these entities. Contrast agents eliminated through the biliary system are useful in this setting to make the distinction, with leak into surrounding tissues evident with bile duct laceration or transsection.
- In patients with biliary-enteric anastomoses, ERCP often cannot be performed
- Imaging
  - MRCP may be used to visualize the anatomy of the anastomosis, strictures of the anastomosis or of intrahepatic ducts, and biliary tract stones proximal to the anastomosis in most patients
  - Metallic surgical clips and pneumobilia can also produce artifacts that should not be mistaken for stones or strictures

Neoplastic Lesions

Benign Masses

- May cause obstruction and result in sequelae of chronic obstruction, including duct dilatation and atrophy of the affected hepatic segments
- Benign tumors of the biliary ducts are rare histological types including
  - Giant cell tumor
  - Imaging (fig. 3.22)
    - tumors are generally small and well defined.
  - Papillary adenomas
    - Rare benign epithelial tumors that have an increased risk for malignant transformation
    - Multiple small papillomas scattered

throughout the biliary tree are characteristic of biliary papillomatosis
- Associated with an irregular pattern of intrahepatic bile duct dilatation due to obstruction by the papillomas
  - Imaging
    - These small tumors are best visualized on fat-suppressed T1W interstitial phase gadolinium-enhanced GRE images as tiny enhancing mass lesions (fig. 3.23)

Malignant Diseases

Cholangiocarcinoma

- Primary duct malignancy far outweighs the incidence of metastases, which include primary disease from breast, melanoma, lung, and lymphoma
- Cholangiocarcinomas are well-differentiated sclerosing adenocarcinomas in two-thirds of cases; the remainder are anaplastic, squamous cell, or cystadenocarcinomas
- The most common predisposing diseases in Western countries are ulcerative colitis and sclerosing cholangitis
- In Far Eastern countries, recurrent pyogenic Oriental cholangitis is the most common cause
- Other predisposing factors include Caroli's disease, choledochal cysts, alpha-1-antitrypsin deficiency, and autosomal-dominant polycystic kidney disease
- Cholangiocarcinoma is typically a malignancy of older patients (>50 years)
- Patients usually present with jaundice and weight loss
- Tumor growth may be focal or diffuse infiltration of the duct walls (appearing similar to sclerosing cholangitis), or may develop an intrahepatic mass
- Three types of cholangiocarcinomas may be classified according to their anatomical location
  - Peripheral (or intrahepatic) type arising from peripheral bile ducts in the liver

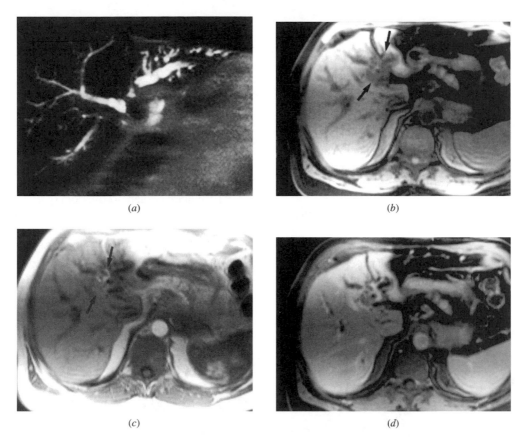

FIGURE 3.22   **Giant cell tumor of the bile duct.** Coronal thin-section MRCP single-shot echo-train spin-echo image with fat suppression (*a*), transverse T1W fat-suppressed SGE (*b*), immediate postgadolinium SGE (*c*), and 2 min postgadolinium fat-suppressed SGE (*d*) images. An obstruction at the confluence of the right and left main hepatic ducts is visualized on the MRCP image (*a*) with dilatation of the right and left intrahepatic biliary system. The tumor (arrow, *b*) appears moderately low signal intensity on the T1W image (*b*). On the immediate postgadolinium image (*c*), the tumor demonstrates increased enhancement (arrow, *c*), with persistent enhancement on the 2 min postgadolinium image (*d*). The liver parenchyma distal to the tumor shows delayed increased enhancement (*d*). The tumor mimics the MRI appearance of Klatskin's tumor but was diagnosed giant cell tumor of the left hepatic duct at histopathology.

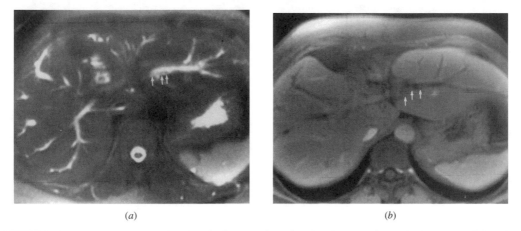

FIGURE 3.23   **Biliary papillomatosis.** T2W single-shot echo-train spin-echo (*a*) and T1W 2 min postgadolinium fat-suppressed SGE (*b*) images. Several small, biliary intraductal, papillary tumors (arrows, *a*, *b*) show enhancement on the postgadolinium image (*b*). The entire biliary tree is moderately dilated because of a obstruction by papillomas in the CHD and CBD.

○ Hilar type (Klatskin's tumor), which originates at the confluence of the right and left hepatic ducts

○ Extrahepatic type, arising from the main hepatic ducts, CHD or CBD

• The peripheral type constitutes approximately 10% of all cholangiocarcinomas and is the second most common primary liver tumor after hepatocellular carcinoma (HCC)

○ Usually present as mass-like lesions that do not obstruct the central bile ducts

○ As a result, these can obtain a large size and show intrahepatic metastases before they cause clinical symptoms

• Klatskin's tumors are usually small and superficial spreading tumors that result in early biliary obstruction and dilatation of proximal ducts

• Extrahepatic cholangiocarcinomas usually grow in a circumferential pattern similar to Klatskin's tumors and arise in the CBD, resulting in high-grade duct obstruction

○ Imaging

▪ Peripheral cholangiocarcinoma

• Typical appearance is a mass lesion that is mildly heterogeneous with moderately low signal intensity on T1W images and mildly to moderately hyperintense signal on T2W images (fig. 3.24)

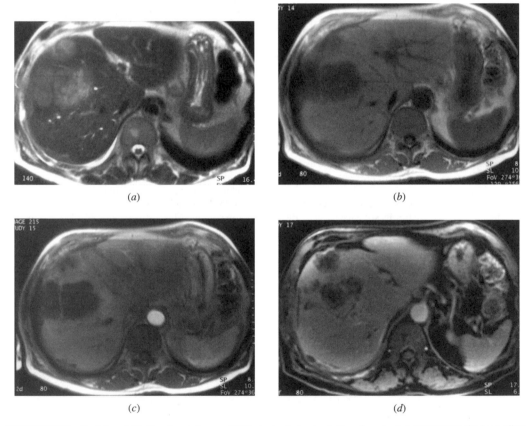

(a) (b)

(c) (d)

FIGURE 3.24 **Peripheral cholangiocarcinoma.** T2W single-shot echo-train spin-echo (a), T1W SGE (b), immediate postgadolinium SGE (c), and 2 min postgadolinium fat-suppressed SGE (d) images. A large tumor with intrahepatic metastases is observed in the right lobe of the liver. The signal is moderately hyperintense on the T2W image (a) and hypointense on the T1W image (b). On the immediate postgadolinium image (c) the tumors are hypoenhancing and demonstrate mild perilesional enhancement. Progressive heterogeneous enhancement of the tumors is observed on the 2 min postgadolinium image (d).

- Immediate postgadolinium images usually show mild to moderate enhancement that is usually diffuse and heterogeneous in pattern
- Progressive enhancement may be observed on late fat-suppressed images, reflecting a high content of fibrous tissue (fig. 3.24)
- Mimickers
  ◦ HCC
    ▪ Typically shows arterial enhancement with rapid washout
    ▪ Typically shows portal venous invasion, which is rare for cholangiocarcinomas
- Klatskin's tumor
  - Tumors typically present early due to obstruction, and thickness of tumor may be 3–4 mm at initial presentation
  - At initial presentation, intrahepatic bile duct dilatation is severe and apparently out of proportion to the volume of tissue
  - Usually see duct stricture at the hepatic duct confluence with intrahepatic duct dilatation (fig. 3.25)

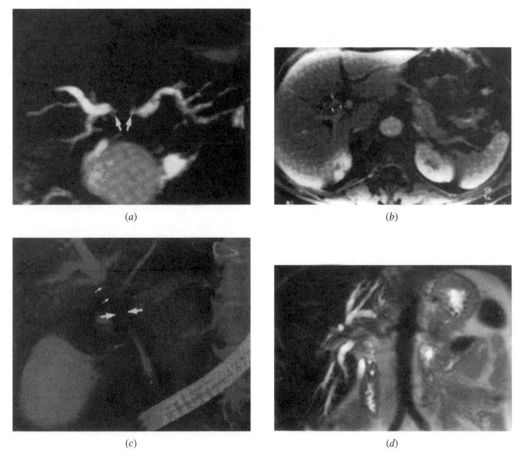

(a)

(b)

(c)

(d)

FIGURE 3.25   Klatskin's tumor. Coronal MRCP MIP reconstruction (*a*), transverse T1W 2 min postgadolinium fat-suppressed SGE (*b*), and ERCP (*c*) images. Obstruction of the right and left main hepatic ducts (arrows, *a*) at the level of the porta hepatis with dilatation of peripheral ducts is visualized on the MRCP image (*a*). A small enhancing tumor (small arrows, *b*), measuring 4 mm in diametre, extends from the CHD into the right main hepatic duct, as shown on the postgadolinium image (*b*). ERCP (*c*) also shows the obstruction (arrows, *c*) at the level of the porta hepatis and the extension of the tumor into the right main hepatic duct (small arrows, *c*). Note the poor visualization of the left biliary ductal sytem on the ERCP image (*c*) because of underfilling.

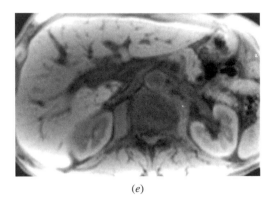
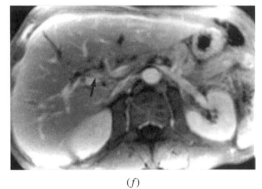

(e)   (f)

FIGURE 3.25 (*Continued*) Coronal T2W single-shot echo-train spin-echo (*d*), transverse T1W fat-suppressed SGE (*e*), and 2 min postgadolinium fat-suppressed SGE (*f*) images in a second patient. Dilatation of the right and left intrahepatic biliary tree is observed on the T2W image (*d*). The tumor shows poor conspicuity on the precontrast SGE image (*e*). On the 2 min postgadolinium image (*f*), the small Klatskin's tumor (arrow, *f*) in the porta hepatis demonstrates enhancement and can be well differentiated from surrounding structures.

- Tumor best seen on 2 min postgadolinium fat-suppressed T1W GRE images as mildly increased enhancement tissue
- Small regional lymph nodes or reticular stranding is common and consistent with direct tumor extension
- Segmental liver atrophy may occur associated with intrahepatic duct dilatation
- Compression of adjacent portal vein results in transient arterial phase increased enhancement of the affected liver parenchyma due to compensatory increased hepatic arterial inflow
- Extrahepatic cholangiocarcinomas on MRCP images show dilatation of the proximal biliary tree with stricture or abrupt termination at the tumor, typically showing a shoulder sign (fig. 3.26)
  - Irregularity of the ductal wall is indicative of infiltration and raises a high suspicion of malignancy
  - Occasionally, tumors show intraluminal papillary growth, presenting as a filling defect on MRCP images
  - Appearance comparable to Klatskin's tumor

- ERCP results in poor opacification of ducts above the lower level of obstruction, underestimating disease, and does not evaluate the liver parenchyma for tumor invasion or metastases
- Findings indicating unresectability include
  - Vascular encasement
  - Direct invasion of liver parenchyma
  - Metastases

Periampullary and Ampullary Carcinoma
- Carcinomas arising from the ampulla of Vater, periampullary duodenum, or distal CBD are grouped together and termed periampullary carcinomas
- Presentation is similar to that of pancreatic head ductal adenocarcinoma including obstruction of both the CBD and pancreatic duct
- The prognosis of periampullary carcinoma is significantly better than that of pancreatic carcinoma, with a 5-year survival rate up to 85%
  - Ampullary adenocarcinoma misdiagnosed as pancreatic duct adenocarcinoma may account for some of the favorable posttherapy outcomes for small pancreatic head masses

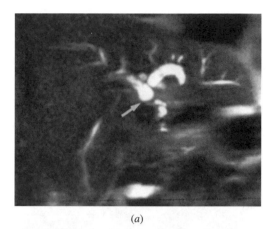

(*a*)

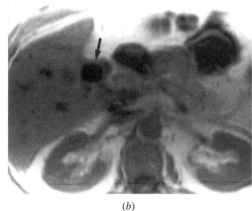

(*b*)

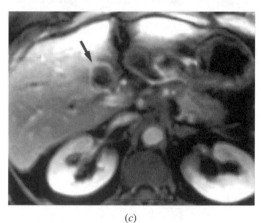

(*c*)

FIGURE 3.26 Extrahepatic cholangiocarcinoma. Coronal T2W this-section MRCP single-shot echo-train spin-echo image with fat suppression (*a*), transverse T1W SGE (*b*) and 2 min postgadolinium fat-suppressed SGE (*c*) images. Obstruction of the proximal CBD (arrow, *a*) is present, showing an abrupt cutoff ("shoulder sign") on the MRCP image (*a*). The intrahepatic biliary tree is markedly dilated (*a*). The extrahepatic cholangiocarcinoma shows circumferential growth along the dilated proximal CBD (arrows, *b*, *c*). On the late postgadolinium image (*c*), the tumor shows intense enhancement (arrows, *c*) and can be differentiated from adjacent liver parenchyma.

- Periampullary carcinomas can cause ampullary obstruction and become clinically symptomatic even when they are only a few millimeters in size
- Signs and symptoms of dilatation of the biliary tree and the pancreatic duct are observed relatively early in the course of these tumors
- Choledochoceles can be associated with an increased risk for periampullary carcinoma
- Imaging
  - MRCP images demonstrate abrupt or irregular obstruction at the level of the ampulla
  - On T1W fat-suppressed images, periampullary carcinomas typically appear as low-signal-intensity masses that enhance to a lesser degree than the adjacent normal pancreas (fig. 3.27)
  - On interstitial T1W delayed phase postgadolinium fat-suppressed images, a thin rim of peripheral enhancement may be observed, presumably representing the tumor border or compressed adjacent pancreatic tissue
  - Pancreatic duct obstruction may lead to pancreatitis with chronic changes
    - Chronic pancreatitis can lead to abnormal pancreatic perfusion with delayed increasing enhancement of the parenchyma adjacent to the ampullary tumor

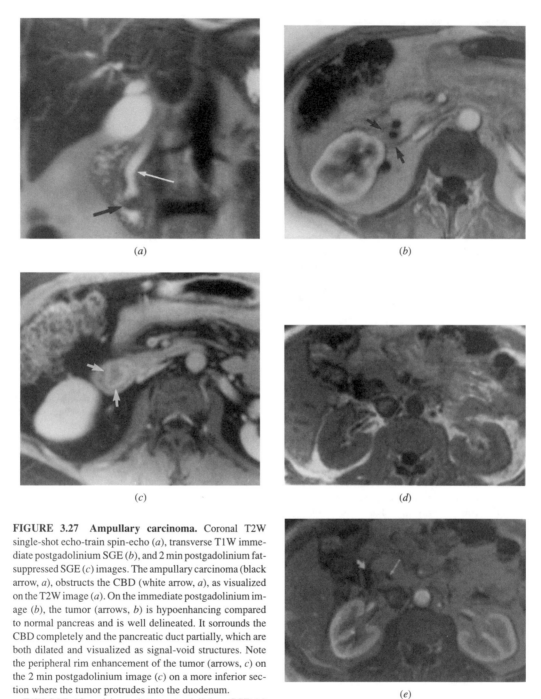

(a)

(b)

(c)

(d)

(e)

FIGURE 3.27 Ampullary carcinoma. Coronal T2W single-shot echo-train spin-echo (a), transverse T1W immediate postgadolinium SGE (b), and 2 min postgadolinium fat-suppressed SGE (c) images. The ampullary carcinoma (black arrow, a), obstructs the CBD (white arrow, a), as visualized on the T2W image (a). On the immediate postgadolinium image (b), the tumor (arrows, b) is hypoenhancing compared to normal pancreas and is well delineated. It sorrounds the CBD completely and the pancreatic duct partially, which are both dilated and visualized as signal-void structures. Note the peripheral rim enhancement of the tumor (arrows, c) on the 2 min postgadolinium image (c) on a more inferior section where the tumor protrudes into the duodenum.

T1W SGE (d) and immediate postgadolinium SGE (e) images in a second patient demonstrating a 2.5 cm ampullary carcinoma of low signal intensity that shows good contrast against high-signal pancreas on the precontrast image (d). The tumor is hypoenhancing compared to pancreatic parenchyma (e), surrounds the distal CBD (straight arrow, e), and protrudes into the duodenum (curved arrow, e).

CHAPTER 4

PANCREAS

Normal Pancreas (fig. 4.1)

- Breath-hold T1W GRE
  - Pancreas is relatively bright and higher in signal than normal liver
  - This contrast is increased on fat-suppressed T1W imaging, where the high signal from peripancreatic fat is suppressed and signal intensity of the protein in the normal pancreas is accentuated
  - Immediate postgadolinium is the most informative sequence for the demonstration of pancreatic disease
- T2W single-shot echo-train breath-hold
  - Pancreas is slightly brighter than normal liver and darker than normal spleen
  - T2W imaging allows assessment for pancreatic duct configuration
  - Fat suppression facilitates assessment of the peripancreatic retroperitoneal and peritoneal spaces for edema or abnormal fluid collections
- MRCP
  - This is essentially a variation of single-shot echo-train T2 breath-hold, with longer TE creating higher-contrast images (fig. 4.2)

Developmental Variants and Abnormalities

- Pancreas Divisum (fig. 4.2)
  - Most common and clinically important variant, seen in up to 7% of the population
  - Embryologic dorsal pancreas forms tail, but duct fails to fuse with ventral pancreatic duct and drains separately from secondary duct (also called minor duct or duct of Santorini) into second part of duodenum, more superiorly than the normal ampulla
  - Embryologic ventral pancreas forms pancreatic uncinate process, and draining duct (major duct or duct of Wirsung) drains normally from ampulla into distal second part of duodenum, attaching to the posterior distal segment of the common bile duct
  - Abnormalities
    - Poor drainage of the secondary duct can develop
      - Imaging shows secondary duct dilation
      - Findings related to pancreatitis (see section on pancreatitis)
- Uncommon Variants
  - Annular pancreas (fig. 4.3)

Primer on MR Imaging of the Abdomen and Pelvis, edited by Diego R. Martin, Michele A. Brown, and Richard C. Semelka ISBN 0-471-37340-0 Copyright © 2005 Wiley-Liss, Inc.

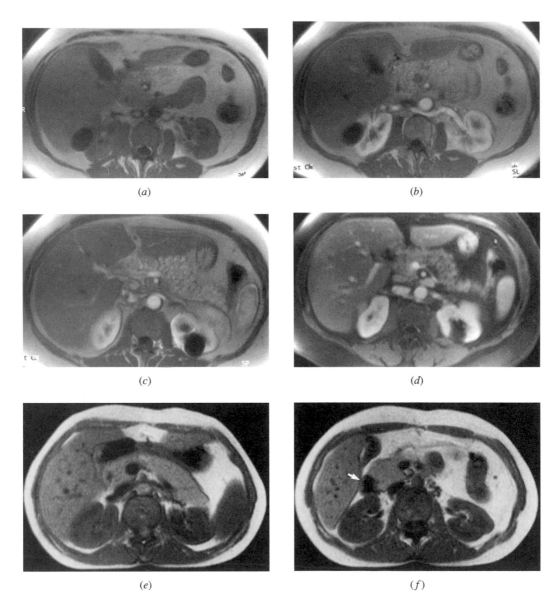

FIGURE 4.1 **Normal pancreas.** T1W SGE (*a*), immediate postgadolinium T1W SGE (*b*, *c*), and 90 s postgadolinium fat-suppressed SGE (*d*) images. The pancreas has a marbled appearance, which is a normal finding associated with aging.

T1W SGE (*e*, *f*), T1W fat-suppressed spin-echo (*g*, *h*), and immediate postgadolinium T1W SGE images (*i*, *j*) in a second patient. Images of the pancreatic body (*e*, *g*, *i*) and head (*f*, *h*, *j*) illustrate the appearance of normal pancreas. Lack of breathing artifact renders the pancreas well shown on T1W SGE images (*e*, *f*). The normal pancreas is high in signal intensity on T1W fat-suppressed images (*g*, *h*) because of the presence of aqueous protein in the acini of the pancreas. A uniform capillary blush is apparent on the immediate postgadolinium images (*i*, *j*). The head of the pancreas is clearly distinguishable from the duodenum (arrow, *f*, *h*, *j*). The small bowel has a feathery appearance and is moderate in signal intensity on T1W fat-suppressed images (long arrow, *h*), which is clearly different from the homogeneous or marbled high-signal intensity of the pancreas.

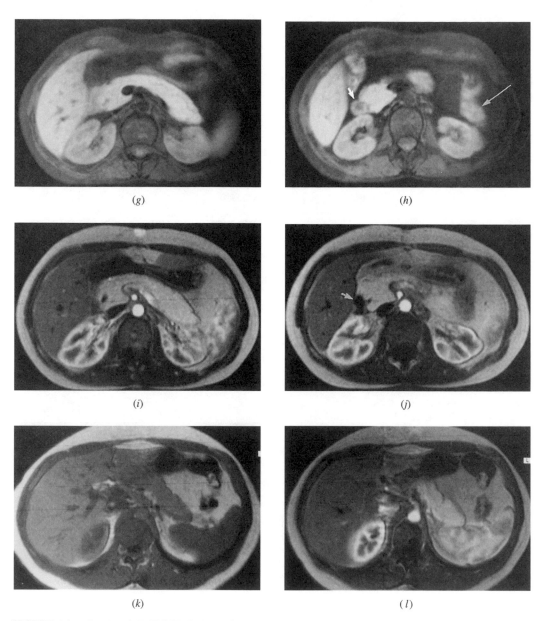

(g)

(h)

(i)

(j)

(k)

(l)

FIGURE 4.1   (*Continued*) T1W SGE (*k*), immediate postgadolinium T1W SGE (*l*), and 45 s postgadolinium T1W SGE (*m*) images in a third patient. Normal pancreas has lower signal intensity than background fat on T1W images (*k*), enhances with a uniform capillary blush resulting in a signal intensity greater than background fat on immediate postgadolinium images (*l*), and fades in signal intensity to isointense with background fat by 45 s (*m*).

Immediate postgadolinium images through the mid- (*n*) and inferior (*o*) pancreatic head in a fourth patient. Enhancement of the pancreas is more intense than that of normal bowel on immediate postgadolinium images. The inferior aspect of the pancreatic head (small arrow, *o*) can be distinguished from lesser-enhancing adjacent duodenum (long arrows, *o*).

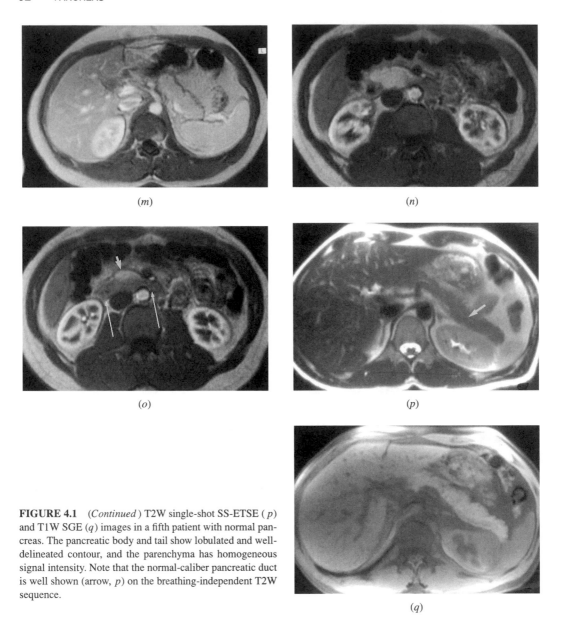

(m)   *(n)*

(o)   *(p)*

(q)

FIGURE 4.1 *(Continued)* T2W single-shot SS-ETSE (*p*) and T1W SGE (*q*) images in a fifth patient with normal pancreas. The pancreatic body and tail show lobulated and well-delineated contour, and the parenchyma has homogeneous signal intensity. Note that the normal-caliber pancreatic duct is well shown (arrow, *p*) on the breathing-independent T2W sequence.

- Pancreas encircles second part of duodenum and can be associated with duodenal atresia or stenosis, presenting with duodenal obstruction
  ○ Short pancreas in polysplenia (fig. 4.4)
    - Associated with congenital bilateral left-sidedness, with multiple small scattered splenules in the right upper quadrant

Nonneoplastic Diseases

Acute Pancreatitis
- Most common acquired associations include excessive alcohol consumption, passage of gallstones or bile sludge, hypertriglyceridemia, and hypercalcemia
- Most common congenital association is pancreas divisum

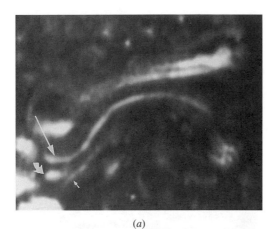

(a)

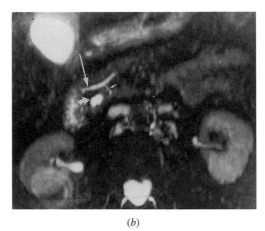

(b)

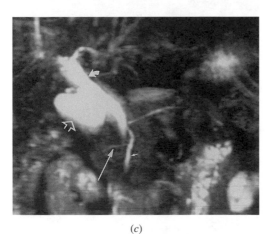

(c)

FIGURE 4.2 Pancreas divisum. MRCP image (a) formatted in an oblique tranverse plane demonstrates separate entry of the ducts of Santorini (long arrow, a) and Wirsung (short arrow, a) into the duodenum with no communication between the ductal systems. MRCP image (b) in a second patient with dominant dorsal duct syndrome shows a large duct of Santorini (long arrow, b) and a small communication with a diminutive duct of Wirsung (short arrow, b). The common bile duct (curved arrow, a, b) is identified between the ducts of Santorini and Wirsung. Oblique coronal MRCP (c) in a patient with normal ductal anatomy shows a small duct of Santorini (long arrow, c) and a larger duct of Wirsung (short arrow, c). The common bile duct (curved arrow, c) and gallbladder (hollow arrow, c) are also shown. MR pancreatography has the advantage of being a noninvasive diagnostic method for pancreas divisum. (Courtesy of Caroline Reinhold, MD, Dept. of Radiology, McGill University.)

- Results from leakage of activated proteolytic enzymes
- Mild form leads to pancreatic edema, with progressively severe forms involving greater degrees of pancreatic ischemia and hemmorhagic fat necrosis in the pancreas and peripancreatic retroperitoneal fat
- Fluid may accumulate in or around the pancreas as fluid-filled spaces, which can evolve to form pseudocysts over a period of weeks
- Treatment remains supportive, with severe pancreatitis frequently leading to severe morbidity and mortality
- Findings
  - Mild Acute Pancreatitis
    - Edema

- High signal on fat-suppressed T2W single-shot echo-train SE within and insinuating around the pancreas (fig. 4.5)
- On precontrast fat-suppressed T1W images normal pancreatic high signal is preserved
  - Moderate Acute Pancreatitis
    - Diminished perfusion
      - Impaired arterial-capillary phase enhancement without evidence of persistence or increased enhancement into the interstitial phase
      - On precontrast fat-suppressed T1W images normal high signal of the pancreas may still be preserved
      - These findings are seen in addition to edema

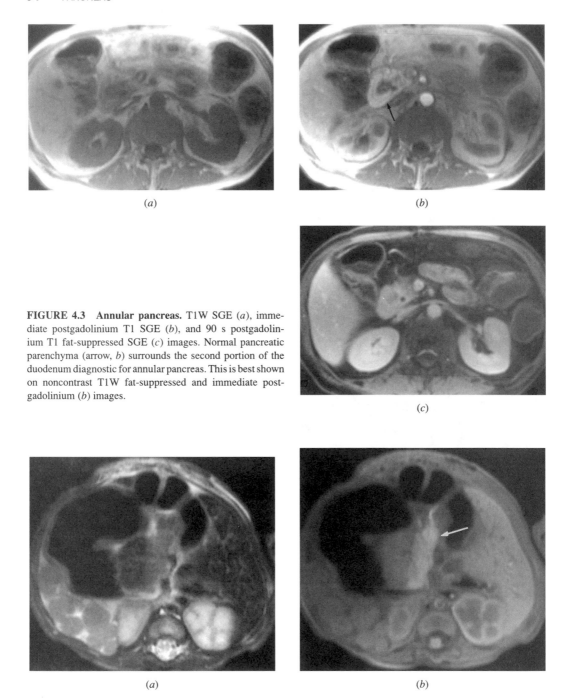

(a)

(b)

(c)

FIGURE 4.3 Annular pancreas. T1W SGE (a), immediate postgadolinium T1 SGE (b), and 90 s postgadolinium T1 fat-suppressed SGE (c) images. Normal pancreatic parenchyma (arrow, b) surrounds the second portion of the duodenum diagnostic for annular pancreas. This is best shown on noncontrast T1W fat-suppressed and immediate postgadolinium (b) images.

(a)

(b)

FIGURE 4.4 Short pancreas in the polysplenia syndrome. T2W fat-suppressed SS-ETSE (a) and T1W fat-suppressed spin-echo (b) images in a 9-week-old boy with polysplenia syndrome. The pancreas has an abnormal anterior posterior orientation and appears short (arrow, b), but the parenchyma signal intensity is normal. The most common pancreatic finding in polysplenia syndrome is short pancreas. Note situs inversus and multiple small spleens.

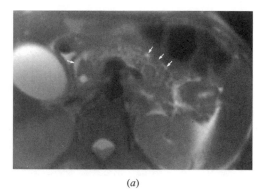 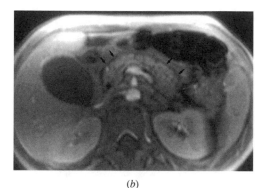

(a)   (b)

FIGURE 4.5   T2W fat-suppressed SS-ETSE (a) and early postgadolinium single-shot magnetization-prepared gradient-echo (b) images demonstrate mild diffuse enhancement of the pancreas and a thin film of peripancreatic fluid surrounding the pancreas (small arrows) and throughout the interstices of the marbled pancreatic parenchyma. Fat-suppressed breathing-independent single-shot T2W sequences are very effective at showing small volumes of fluid, as surrounding fat and pancreas are both low signal and only fluid will be high signal (a). This case is also noteworthy in that image quality is reasonable despite the fact that the patient was very ill and a noncooperative MR imaging protocol was employed, which uses only breathing-independent single-shot images.

- Severe Acute Pancreatitis
  - Edema and diminished heterogeneous arterial-capillary phase perfusion and heterogeneous signal on noncontrast fat-suppressed T1W images
  - Pancreatic and peripancreatic high signal on fat-saturated T1 GRE
    - Degree of abnormal signal correlates with severity and with prognosis for poor outcome
  - Other Findings
    - Pseudocyst formation (figs. 4.6 and 4.7)

Chronic Pancreatitis
- Results from recurrent inflammation and development of irreversible changes, including fibrosis
- Most common related factor is alcohol abuse, with other causes of acute pancreatitis rarely associated with chronic pancreatitis
- A hereditory form of chromic pancreatitis exists with disease manifesting itself offer in the tenage years.
  - Irregular pancreatic duct dilation is usually present, likely due to repeated acute pancreatitis and focal duct scarring with stenosis

- Findings (fig. 4.8)
  - Diminished signal on precontrast fat-suppressed T1W GRE images
  - Diminished heterogeneous arterial-capillary phase enhancement with development of delayed increased enhancement on interstitial phase images
  - Duct dilatation
    - Can be seen on standard T2W single-shot echo-train, MRCP, as well as T1W GRE imaging
  - Focal pancreatitis may appear mass-like (fig. 4.9)

Pancreatic Transplants
- Transplanted pancreas is typically placed in the lower right abdominal quadrant with duct anastomosis to the corresponding side of the dome of the urinary bladder
- Vascular supply is derived from grafted vessels anastomosed to the iliac artery and vein on the corresponding side
- Complications include rejection, pancreatitis, vascular compromise, and pancreatic duct obstruction
- Dynamic gadolinium-enhanced MRI may be used to assess rejection of pancreatic transplants

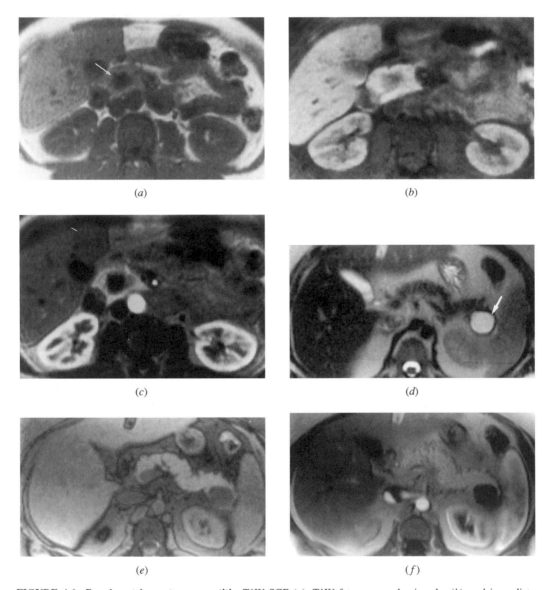

(a) (b)

(c) (d)

(e) (f)

FIGURE 4.6 Pseudocyst in acute pancreatitis. T1W SGE (*a*), T1W fat-suppressed spin-echo (*b*), and immediate postgadolinium T1W SGE (*c*) images. A low-signal-intensity pseudocyst (arrow, *a*) is present in the head of the pancreas (*a–c*). The pancreas has normal high signal intensity on the T1W fat-suppressed image (*b*), and there is normal uniform enhancement of the pancreas on the immediate postgadolinium image (*c*). These imaging features are consistent with a pseudocyst in the setting of acute pancreatitis because the background pancreas has normal signal intensity features. The lesion did not change in size and shape on delayed images, excluding a poorly vascularized tumor. T2W SS-ETSE (*d*), T1W fat-suppressed SGE (*e*), immediate postgadolinium T1W SGE (*f*), and 90 s postgadolinium fat-suppressed SGE (*g*) images in a second patient. A 3 cm pseudocyst (arrow, *d*) arises in the pancreatic tail. The pancreas is normal in signal on noncontrast T1W fat-suppressed images (*e*) and enhances normally on early (*f*) and late (*g*) images, consistent with no substantial parenchymal disease. There is progressive enhancement of the wall of the pseudocyst (*g*), which is typically for fibrous tissue. The pancreas and liver are hypointense on T2W images (*d*) secondary to iron deposition from multiple blood transfusion.

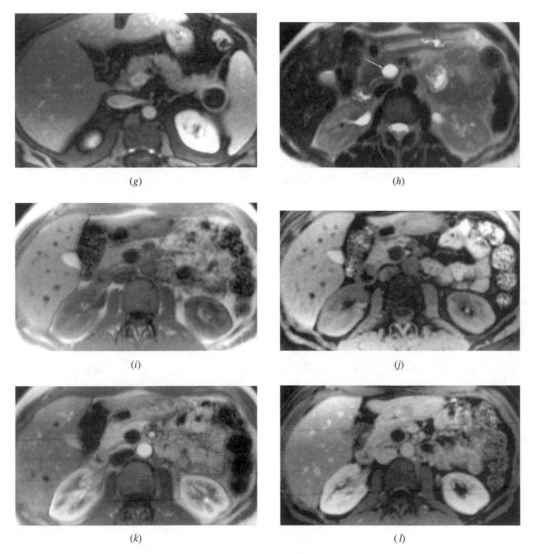

FIGURE 4.6   (*Continued*) T2W SS-ETSE (*h*), T1W SGE (*i*), T1W fat-suppressed SGE (*j*), immediate postgadolinium T1W SGE (*k*), and 90 s postgadolinium fat-suppressed SGE (*l*) images demonstrate a 2 cm pseudocyst (arrow, *h*) in the uncinate process of the pancreas. The normal signal intensity of the pancreas, especially on noncontrast T1W fat-suppressed (*j*) and immediate postgadolinium SGE (*k*) images, shows that background pancreas is not substantially diseased.

- ◦ Percentage of enhancement in normal grafts is higher (100% increase in signal) than in dysfunctional grafts (42% increase in signal)
- • MR angiography may be employed to detect acute vascular compromise (fig. 4.10)
  - ◦ Complications such as venous thrombosis are well shown on gadolinium-enhanced GRE or 3D gradient echo imaging

- • Imaging features of acute and chronic pancreatitis may be evaluated as described earlier in this chapter
- • T2W single-shot echo-train and True-FISP imaging may be utilized to assess the diameter of the pancreatic duct
  - ◦ Increased dilatation may occur in the setting of stricture, usually at the site of anastomosis

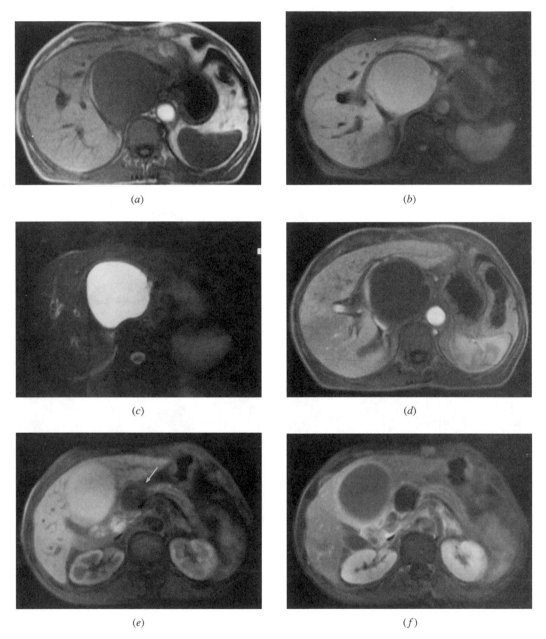

(a)

(b)

(c)

(d)

(e)

(f)

FIGURE 4.7   Pseudocysts—large. T1W SGE (*a*), T1W fat-suppressed spin-echo (*b*), T2W fat-suppressed SS-ETSE (*c*), and immediate postgadolinium T1W SGE (*d*) images obtained superior to the pancreas, T1W fat-suppressed spin-echo (*e*) and gadolinium-enhanced T1W fat-suppressed spin-echo (*f*) images at the level of the body of the pancreas, coronal gadolinium-enhanced T1W SGE images from midhepatic (*g*) and more anterior (*h*) locations, and sagittal plane (*i*) T1W SGE images. An 8 cm pseudocyst is present in the region of the porta hepatis that is mildly high in signal intensity on T1W images (*a*, *b*) and high in signal intensity on the T2W image (*c*).The mild, high signal intensity on T1W images is more conspicuous with fat suppression (*b*) and consistent with dilute blood or protein. The homogeneous signal intensity on T2W images suggests that the fluid, although proteinaceous, is not complicated by infection or cellular debris. A 3 cm pseudocyst (arrow, *e*) is identified within the body of the pancreas (*e*, *f*). Fluid in the pseudocyst is low in signal intensity on the precontrast T1W image (*e*). Capsular enhancement of the pseudocysts is shown on the fat-suppressed gadolinium-enhanced image (*f*).

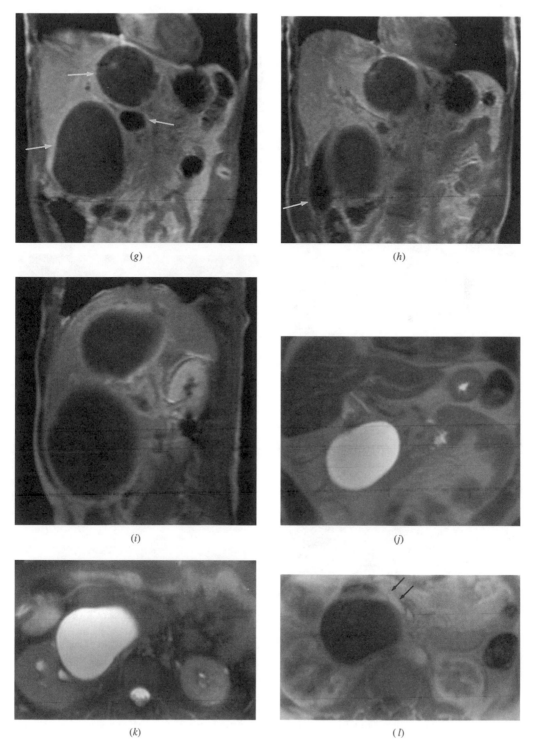

FIGURE 4.7 (*Continued*) Coronal plane gadolinium-enhanced T1W SGE images (*g*, *h*) demonstrate the relationship of the pseudocysts to surrounding structures. Three pseudocysts (arrows, *g*) are shown in the coronal plane (*g*). Gallbladder (arrow, *h*) is displaced laterally by the large pseudocyst in the porta hepatis. The sagittal plane image (*i*) demonstrates the anteroposterior orientation of the pseudocysts to other structures.

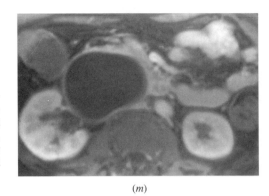

(*m*)

FIGURE 4.7 (*Continued*) Coronal SS-ETSE (*j*), transverse fat-suppressed SS-ETSE (*k*), immediate postgadolinium T1W SGE (*l*), and 90 s postgadolinium fat-suppressed SGE (*m*) images in a second patient. A large (8 × 7 cm), pancreatic pseudocyst is situated between the right kidney and second portion of the duodenum. The pancreatic head is displaced anteriorly (arrows, *l*).

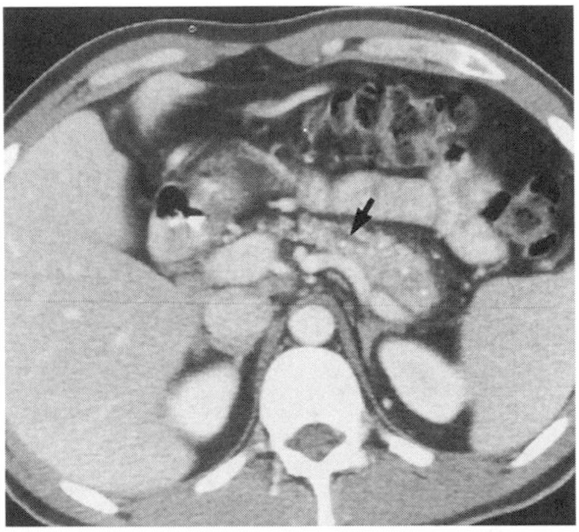

(*a*)

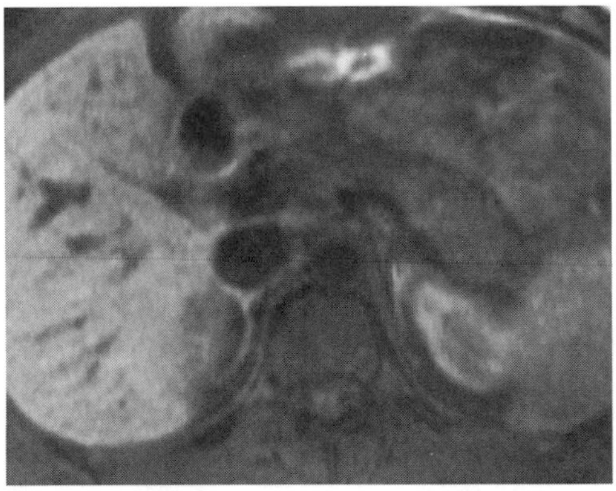

(*b*)

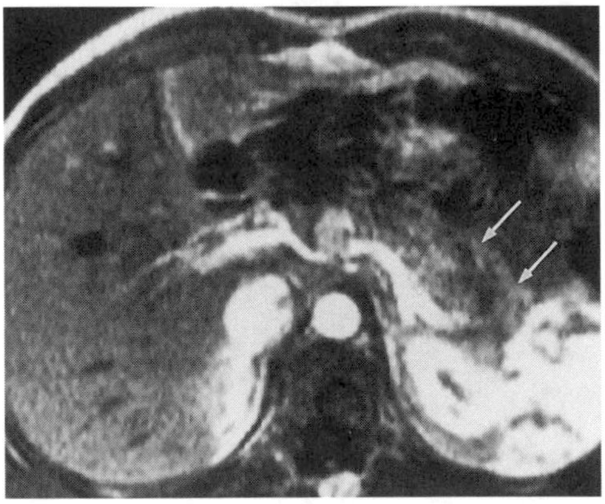

(*c*)

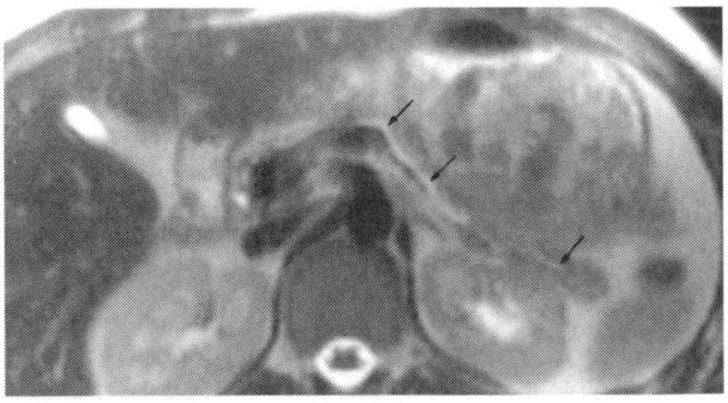

(*d*)

FIGURE 4.8   Chronic pancreatitis. Contrast-enhanced CT (*a*) T1W fat-suppressed spin-echo (*b*) and immediate postgadolinium T1W SGE (*c*) images. The CT image demonstrates pancreatic calcifications, which is diagnostic for chronic pancreatitis. Mild pancreatic ductal dilatation (arrow, *a*) and mild pancreatic enlargement are also present. The pancreas is low in signal intensity on the T1W fat-suppressed image, which is consistent with loss of aqueous protein in the acini.

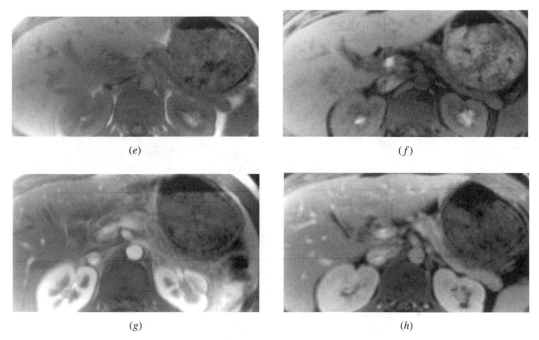

FIGURE 4.8   (*Continued*) The immediate postgadolinium T1W SGE image demonstrates heterogeneous diminished enhancement of the pancreas (arrows, *c*), reflecting replacement of the normal capillary bed with lesser vascularized fibrotic tissue. (Reproduced with permission from Semelka RC, Kroeker MA, Shoenut JP, Kroeker R, Yaffe CS, Micflikier AB: Pancreatic disease: Prospective comparison of CT, ERCP, and 1.5 T MR imaging with dynamic gadolinium enhancement and fat suppression. *Radiology* 181: 785–791, 1991.)

T2W SS-ETSE (*d*), T1W SGE (*e*), noncontrast T1W fat-suppressed SGE (*f*), immediate postgadolinium T1W SGE (*g*), and 90 s postgadolinium fat-suppressed SGE (*h*) images in a second patient. Moderate dilatation of the pancreatic duct is present (arrows, *d*). There is moderate atrophy of the pancreatic parenchyma, which is low signal on T1W fat-suppressed SGE (*f*) and demonstrates minimal enhancement on immediate postgadolinium images (*g*) with progressive enhancement on 90 s postcontrast images (*h*). These are classic features for chronic pancreatitis.

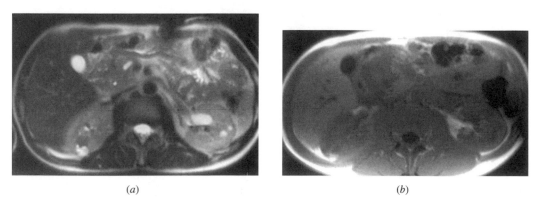

FIGURE 4.9   **Chronic pancreatitis simulating pancreatic cancer.** Coronal (*a*) and transverse (*b*) T2W SS-ETSE, immediate postgadolinium T1W SGE (*c*), and 90 s postgadolinium fat-suppressed SGE (*d*) images. The CBD (arrow, *a*) and pancreatic (arrow, *b*) ducts are severely dilated, with atrophy of the pancreatic body (*b*) creating the double duct sign.

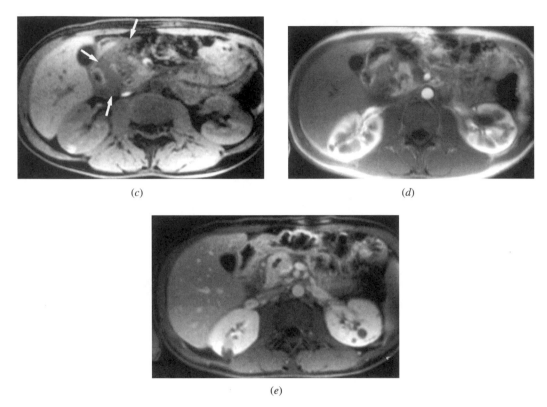

(c)

(d)

(e)

FIGURE 4.9 (*Continued*) On early (*c*) and late (*d*) postgadolinium images, no demarcated pancreatic mass is observed in the head of the pancreas. Instead, the enlarged pancreas shows a marbled texture (arrows, *c*) comparable in appearance to the remainder of the pancreas.

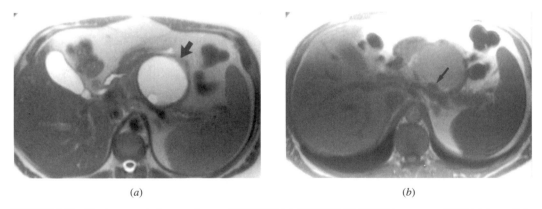

(a)

(b)

FIGURE 4.10 **Mucinous cystadenocarcinoma.** T2W ETSE (*a*), T1W SGE (*b*), T1W fat-suppressed SGE (*c*), immediate postgadolinium T1W SGE (*d*), and 90 s postgadolinium fat-suppressed SGE (*e*) images. There is a large cystic mass (arrow, *a*) arising from the pancreatic body, which has a thickened and slightly irregular wall, demonstrating increased enhancement (arrow, *e*) on interstitial phase gadolinium-enhanced fat-suppressed images.

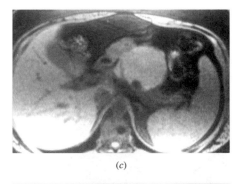

(c)

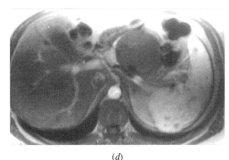

(d)

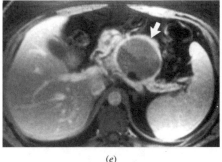

(e)

FIGURE 4.10 (*Continued*) The cyst is high in signal on T1W images (*b*, *c*), reflecting the presence of high protein content from mucin. The cyst contains a smaller cystic structure (arrow, *b*).

- Acute complications of surgery can be easily evaluated including abnormal peripancreatic fluid collections and abscess formation
  - Edema and fluid may be shown on T2W single-shot echo-train images, most clearly appreciated with concomitant fat suppression
  - Inflammatory reaction with abscess formation can be shown on gadolinium-enhanced fat-suppressed T1W images and appears as a thick rim of moderately enhancing tissue surrounding a lower-signal nonenhancing central core. T2W images may show a central core with mildly elevated signal, representing a liquid environment containing cellular debris, which can exhibit a fluid debris layer along the dependent aspect of the abscess cavity.

Neoplastic Diseases

Pancreatic Duct Adenocarcinoma
- Originates from pancreatic exocrine duct
- Represents 95% of pancreatic malignancies, and fourth most common cause of cancer-related mortality with 5-year survival rate of 5%
- Two-thirds occur in pancreatic head, with remainder in body, followed by tail in frequency
- Pancreatic head masses tend to obstruct the common bile duct and therefore present smaller in size with painless jaundice; tail masses present later with larger tumors that may be associated with pain secondary to local extension
- Findings
  - Masses have lesser perfusion compared with normal pancreas and enhance more slowly
  - Small masses are most conspicuous on arterial phase images (fig. 4.11)
  - Pancreatic head masses obstruct the pancreatic and common bile ducts (fig. 4.12)
  - Pancreatic tail masses typically present as larger masses with local infiltration and typically may involve the splenic vein, spleen, and posterior gastric fundus or body (fig. 4.13)

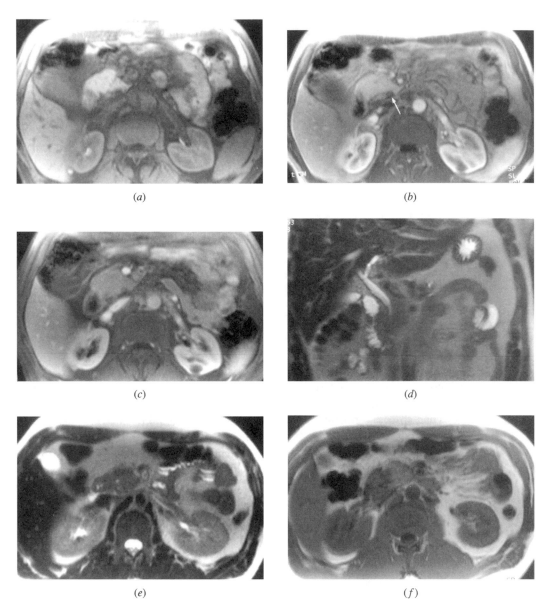

FIGURE 4.11   Small pancreatic cancer arising in the head. T1W fat-suppressed SGE (*a*), immediate postgadolinium T1W SGE (*b*), and 90 s postgadolinium fat-suppressed SGE (*c*) images. A 6 mm tumor (arrow, *b*) is present in the uncinate process of the pancreas, which does not result in ductal obstruction because of its small size and location. Note that the mass is most clearly shown on the immediate postgadolinium image (*b*) as a small hypoenhancing lesion. Coronal (*d*) and transverse (*e*) T2W SS-ETSE, T1W SGE (*f*), T1W fat-suppressed SGE (*g*), and immediate (*h*) and 45 s (*i*) postgadolinium T1W SGE and 90 s postgadolinium fat-suppressed SGE (*j*) images in a second patient with moderately differentiated adenocarcinoma. There is a 1.5 cm mass arising in the lateral aspect of the pancreatic head, which invades the duodenal wall and causes biliary ductal dilatation.

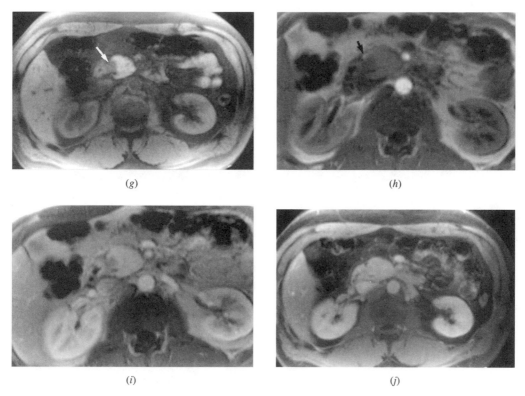

(g)   (h)

(i)   (j)

FIGURE 4.11 (*Continued*) On the T2W images (*d*, *e*), CBD obstruction is well shown, but the tumor itself is almost imperceptible. The tumor (arrow, *g*) is most clearly appreciated on the noncontrast T1W fat suppressed SGE image (*g*) and the immediate postgadolinium SGE image (*h*). Progressive tumor enhancement and pancreatic parenchyma washout over time (*i*, *j*) diminish the tumor-pancreas contrast, which is most problematic with small tumors. The gastroduodenal artery (arrow, *h*) is well shown on the immediate postgadolinium image as an enhancing structure. The tumor is shown to abut this vessel. Approximately one-quarter of all pancreas head cancers exhibit some degree of duodenal wall invasion.

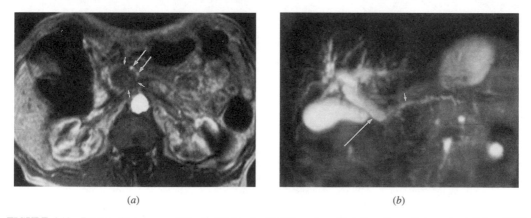

(a)   (b)

FIGURE 4.12 **Pancreatic cancer arising in the head with biliary tree dilatation.** Immediate postgadolinium T1W SGE (*a*) and non-breath-hold 3D MIP MRCP (*b*) images. A 3.5 cm cancer arises from the head of the pancreas. On the immediate postcontrast image (*a*), the tumor is well shown as a low-signal-intensity mass (small arrows, *a*) that is closely applied to the superior mesenteric vein and superior mesenteric artery (arrows, *a*). The MRCP image (*b*) demonstrates obstruction of the CBD (long arrow, *b*) and pancreatic duct (small arrow, *b*), creating the "double duct" sign.

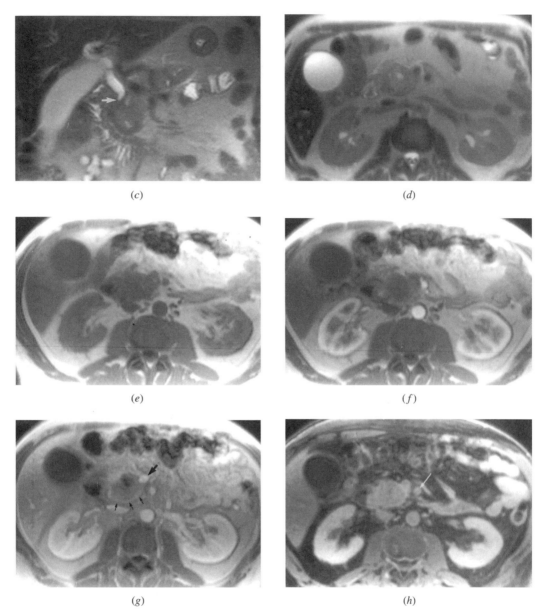

(c) *(d)*

(e) *(f)*

(g) *(h)*

FIGURE 4.12 *(Continued)* Coronal (*c*) and transverse (*d*) T2W SS-ETSE, T1W SGE (*e*), immediate (*f*) and 45 s (*g*) postgadolinium T1W SGE, and transverse (*h*) and coronal (*i*) interstitial phase gadolinium-enhanced fat-suppressed SGE images in a second patient with a poorly differentiated pancreatic adenocarcinoma arising in the head. Obstruction of the CBD (arrow, *e*) by the pancreatic head cancer is clearly shown on the coronal image (*c*). The pancreatic mass is mildly heterogeneous and hyperintense on T2W (*c*, *d*) images with minimal enhancement on early postcontrast images (*f*) and progressive enhancement on later images (*h*). The tumor partially encases the superior mesenteric vein (arrow, *h*), and a definable margin with a thin rim of adjacent pancreas (small arrows, *g*) is appreciated. Duskiness of the fat around the superior mesenteric artery (arrow, *h*) is shown on the interstitial phase gadolinium-enhanced fat-suppressed image (*h*). The coronal gadolinium-enhanced fat-suppressed image shows a patent portal vein (arrow, *i*) and its relationship with the cancer.

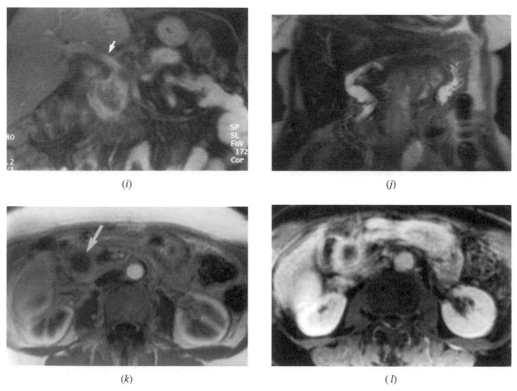

(i)   *(j)*

(k)   *(l)*

FIGURE 4.12 *(Continued)* Coronal T2W SS-ETSE (*j*), immediate postgadolinium T1W SGE (*k*), and 90 s postgadolinium fat-suppressed SGE (*l*) images in a third patient with pancreatic cancer. Obstruction of the CBD is present. A hypoenhancing tumor (arrow, *k*) with definable margins with adjacent pancreas is clearly shown on the immediate postgadolinium image (*k*), which has central necrotic areas and causes biliary tree dilatation.

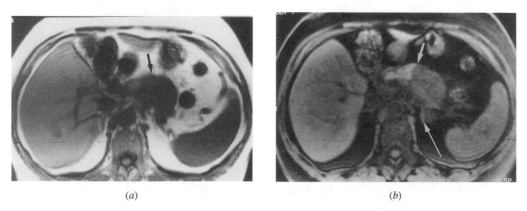

(a)   *(b)*

FIGURE 4.13 **Pancreatic cancer arising from the tail.** T1W SGE (*a*), fat-suppressed T1W SGE (*b*), and interstitial phase gadolinium-enhanced T1W SGE (*c*) images. A large pancreatic tail cancer is present that has encased the splenic vein. The tumor is low in signal intensity on the T1W image (arrow, *a*). Demarcation of tumor from uninvolved pancreas (arrow, *b*) is clearly shown on the precontrast T1W fat-suppressed image (*b*). The left adrenal is involved (long arrow, *b*). Heterogeneous enhancement with central low signal intensity is apparent on the interstitial phase image (*c*).

Interstitial phase gadolinium-enhanced T1W SGE image (*d*) in a second patient demonstrates a pancreatic tail cancer (arrows, *d*) that invades the splenic hilum.

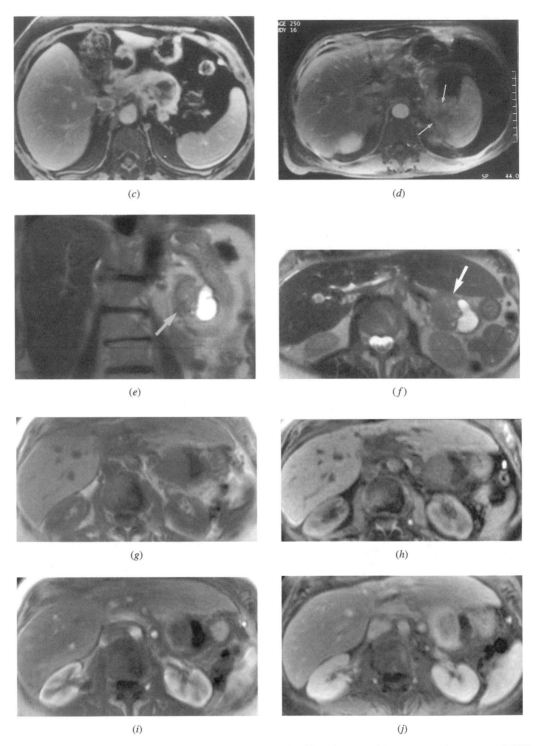

(c)

(d)

(e)

(f)

(g)

(h)

(i)

(j)

FIGURE 4.13 *(Continued)* Coronal (*e*) and transverse (*f*) T2W SS-ETSE, T1W SGE (*g*), T1W fat-suppressed SGE (*h*), immediate postgadolinium T1W SGE (*i*), and 90 s postgadolinium fat-suppressed SGE (*j*) images in a third patient. A 5-cm cancer (arrow, *e*, *f*) arises from the tail of the pancreas and contains a cystic component. The tumor displaces the lesser gastric curvature laterally, best appreciated on the coronal image (*e*).

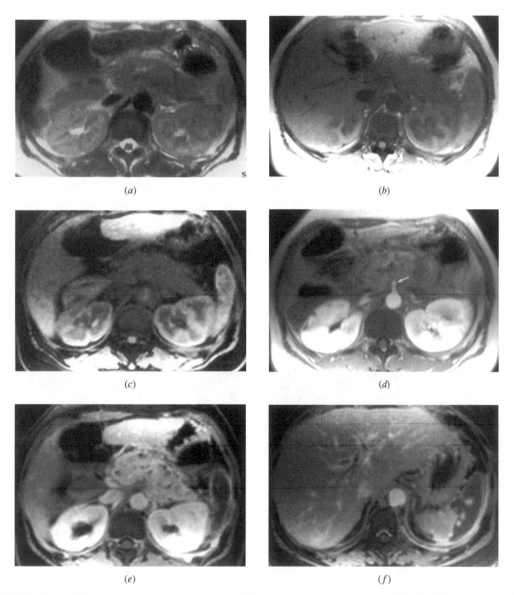

FIGURE 4.14 Diffuse pancreatic adenocarcinoma. T2W echo-train spin-echo (*a*), T1W SGE (*b*), T1W fat-suppressed SGE (*c*), immediate postgadolinium T1W SGE (*d*), and 90 s postgadolinium fat-suppressed SGE (*e*, *f*) images. The pancreas is diffusely enlarged and hypointense on T2W (*a*) and T1W (*b*) images, with diminished and heterogeneous enhancement on early (*d*) and late (*e*) gadolinium-enhanced images. The tumor encases the superior mesenteric artery (arrow, *d*) and occludes the superior mesenteric vein and splenic vein. Extensive infarction of the spleen (*f*) reflects the vascular occlusion of splenic vessels.

- Pancreatic adenocarcinoma can present with diffuse pancreatic infiltration (fig. 4.14)
- Local staging is best performed with gadolinium-enhanced interstitial phase fat-suppressed T1 GRE or 3D GRE imaging to assess local retroperitoneal lymph nodes, vessels (SMA, SMV, portal, and splenic veins), spleen, and stomach

○ In at least one-third of patients with liver metastases, the metastases are less than 1 cm in size, hypervascular, subcapsular, and may be visible only on arterial-capillary phase images

Islet Cell Tumors
• Uncommon tumors of neuroendocrine cell origin

• Can be nonfunctional (fig. 4.15) or can secrete specific hormone and present with clinical symptoms associated with hormonal hypersecretion
  ○ Most common types are
    ▪ Insulinoma (fig. 4.16): hypoglycemia; obesity
    ▪ Gastrinoma (figs. 4.17 to 4.20): Zollinger-Ellinson syndrome

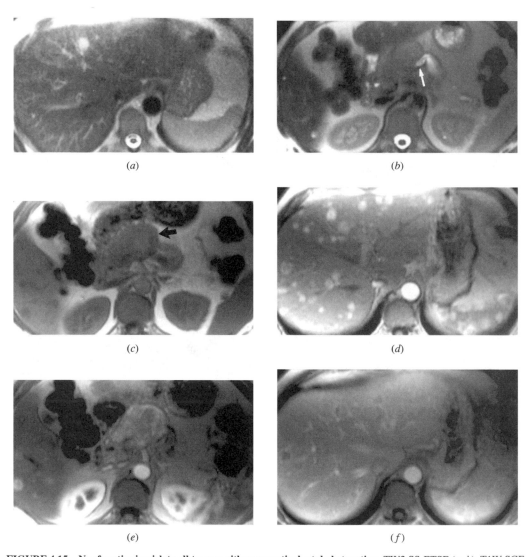

(a)   (b)   (c)   (d)   (e)   (f)

FIGURE 4.15   Nonfunctioning islet cell tumor with pancreatic ductal obstruction. TW2 SS-ETSE (*a, b*), T1W SGE (*c*), immediate (*d, e*) and 45 s (*f*) postgadolinium T1W SGE, and 90 s postgadolinium fat-suppressed SGE (*g*) images. There is a 5 cm lobulated tumor (arrow, *c*) arising from the neck/proximal body of the pancreas. The tumor is mildly hyperintense on T2 (*b*) and mildly hypointense on T1 (*c*) and shows diffuse moderately intense enhancement on immediate postgadolinium SGE (*e*) with moderate washout on interstitial phase images (*g*).

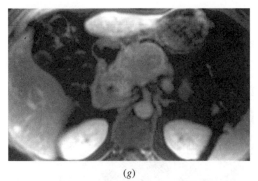

(g)

FIGURE 4.15 (*Continued*) The pancreatic duct (arrow, *b*) is obstructed by the tumor with associated distal atrophy of the pancreas. Multiple extensive liver metastases are present measuring up to 1.5 cm in diameter. These metastatic lesions are best seen as hyperintense uniform or ring-enhancing lesions on immediate postgadolinium images (*d*). Rapid washout of the metastasis occurs by 45 after injection (*f*).

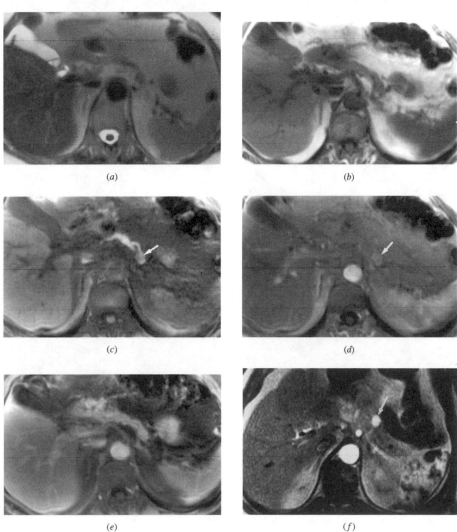

(a)

(b)

(c)

(d)

(e)

(f)

FIGURE 4.16 Insulinoma. T2W ETSE (*a*), T1W SGE (*b*), T1W fat-suppressed SGE (*c*), immediate postgadolinium T1W SGE (*d*), and 90 s postgadolinium fat-suppressed SGE (*e*) images. A 1 cm tumor (arrow, *c*) arising in the superior aspect of the midbody of the pancreas is isointense on T2W (*a*) and T1W (*b*) images and low signal on T1W fat-suppressed image (*c*) and enhances intensely and homogeneously (arrow, *d*) on the immediate postgadolinium image. The lesion fades to isointensity with background pancreas (*e*).

Immediate postgadolinium T1 SGE image (*f*) demonstrates a 1.2 cm uniformly enhancing insulinoma (arrow) arising from the body of the pancreas.

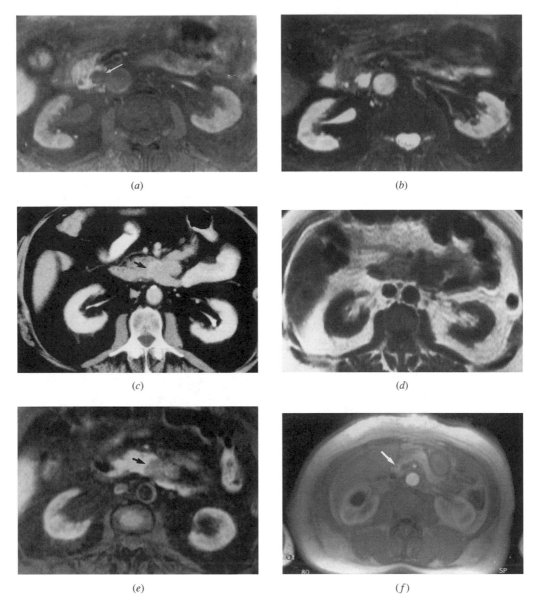

FIGURE 4.17 Islet cell tumor—gastrinoma. T1W fat-suppressed spin-echo (*a*) and T2W fat-suppressed spin-echo (*b*) images. Islet cell tumors (arrow, *a*) are usually low in signal intensity in a background of high-signal intensity pancreas on T1W fat-suppressed images (*a*) and high in signal intensity on T2W images (*b*). The uncinate process is a common location for gastrinomas, because it is located in the "gastrinoma triangle."

Dynamic contrast-enhanced CT (*c*), T1W SGE (*d*), and T1W fat-suppressed spin-echo (*e*) images in a second patient. A 2 cm gastrinoma arises from the uncinate process of the pancreas (*c*–*e*). The tumor is most conspicuous on the T1W fat-suppressed spin-echo image with a "beak" sign apparent (arrow, *e*) and was not identified on the CT examination prospectively. An enhancing rim (arrow, *c*) is apparent on the CT image.

Immediate postgadolinium SGE image (*f*) in a third patient demonstrates an 8 mm ring-enhancing tumor (arrow, *f*) in the neck of the pancreas diagnostic for a gastrinoma on the appropriate clinical setting. Gastrinomas most commonly possess uniform ring enhancement in both the primary tumor and liver metastases. This patient had two recent CT examinations that were both negative for gastrinoma.

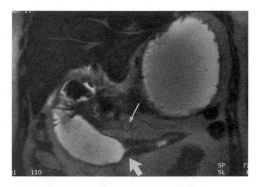

FIGURE 4.18 Coronal SS-ETSE.

- Nonfunctioning
- Glucagonoma
- Somatostatinoma
- VIPoma (fig. 4.21): watery diarrhea
- Findings
  ◦ Usually high signal on T2W images
  ◦ Low signal intensity on T1 breath-hold GRE images, with improved conspicuity seen on fat-suppressed T1W GRE images
  ◦ Typically enhance moderately intensely in arterial phase, and enhancement may persist into equilibrium phase
  ◦ Enhancement may appear as peripheral rim or diffuse throughout mass
  ◦ Insulinomas are often benign
  ◦ Metastases usually occur in the liver and occasionally in local lymph nodes
  ◦ Distinguishing features of islet cell tumors compared to pancreatic duct adenocarcinoma include

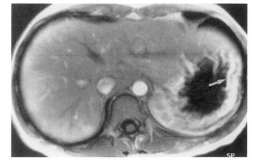

FIGURE 4.19 Gastric wall hyperplasia. Immediate postgadolinium T1W SGE image demonstrates intense enhancement of the prominent gastric rugal folds (arrow) in a patient with gastrinoma.

- Discrete margination
- Surrounding pancreas normal, making tumor more conspicuous
- Moderately high T2 signal, unlike ductal adenocarcinoma, which usually has low T2 signal
- Only rarely encase retroperitoneal vessels or thrombose splenic vein, which commonly occur in ductal adenocarcinoma
- Primary tumor is often hypervascular
- Liver metastases are hypervascular for all sizes of metastases

Cystic Neoplasms
- Serous (Microcystic) Cystadenoma
  ◦ Benign mass (rare reports of malignant variant)
  ◦ Occurs most frequently in older age
  ◦ Pathologically comprised of multiple fluid-filled small cysts (<1 cm) packed into a mass typically ranging from 1 to 12 cm in overall size
  ◦ May have a central scar
  ◦ Findings (fig. 4.22)
    ▪ Best evaluated using T2W single-shot echo-train images in combination with gadolinium-enhanced GRE images
    ▪ T2W images show high-signal-intensity fluid within closely packed cystic spaces
    ▪ Contrast-enhanced images show enhancing septations and may show central scar that can have progressive enhancement on delayed images
    ▪ Outer mass wall may be smooth or lobulated, but is well demarcated, without evidence of infiltrative growth into surrounding tissues
    ▪ Pancreatic duct obstruction is very rare
- Mucinous (Macrocystic) Cystadenoma/Cystadenocarcinoma
  ◦ May present as benign or malignant neoplasm
  ◦ Most commonly observed in females over 40 years of age; located more commonly in the pancreatic body or tail

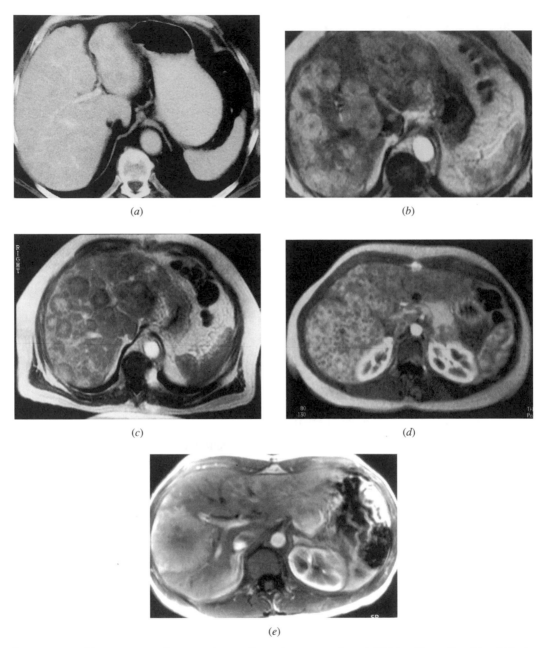

(a)

(b)

(c)

(d)

(e)

FIGURE 4.20 Liver metastases from gastrinomas. Dynamic contrast-enhanced CT (a) and immediate (b) and 10 min (c) postgadolinium T1W SGE images. Metastases are poorly visualized on the CT image (a). On the immediate post-gadolinium T1W SGE image (b), multiple metastases of similar size are identified with uniform intense rim enhancement. Peripheral washout is well shown on the 10 min postcontrast image (c).

Immediate postgadolinium SGE images (d) in a second patient show extensive <1.5 cm liver metastases throughout the liver with uniform ring enhancement.

Immediate postgadolinium SGE image (e) in a third patient shows an unusual pattern for gastrinoma liver metastases with varying size lesions with intense, almost uniform enhancement of a 5 cm metastasis. Often these large hypervascular islet cell metastases that enhance nearly uniformly on immediate postgadolinium images possess a radiating spoke-wheel pattern of bands of lesser-enhancing stroma.

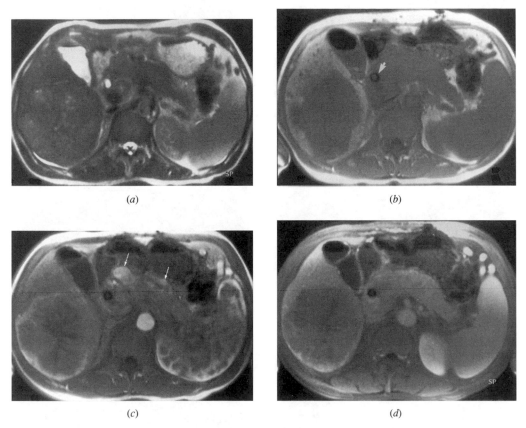

(a)   (b)

(c)   (d)

FIGURE 4.21   VIPoma. T1W fat-suppressed SGE (*a*), coronal T2W SS-ETSE (*b*), and immediate postgadolinium T1W SGE (*c*) images in a patient with VIPoma. A 1.5 cm tumor arises from the tail of the pancreas (arrow, *a*) that appears low in signal intensity on the T1W image. Multiple metastases are present that are moderately low signal intensity on the T1W image (*a*) and moderately high signal intensity on the T2W image (*b*) and enhance in a moderately intense peripheral spoke-wheel-type radial fashion on the immediate postgadolinium T1W SGE image (*c*).

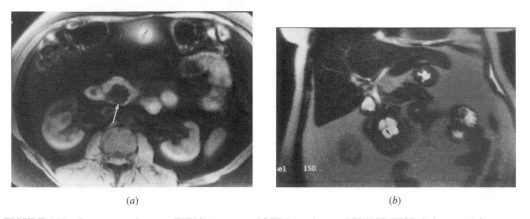

(a)   (b)

FIGURE 4.22   Serous cystadenoma. T1W fat-suppressed SGE (*a*) and coronal T2W SS-ETSE (*b*) images. A 3 cm mass lesion is present in the head of the pancreas. The lesion is well defined and low in signal intensity (arrow, *a*) in a background of high-signal-intensity pancreas on the fat-suppressed T1W SGE image (*a*). On the breathing-independent T2W image (*b*), definition of fine septations (small arrow, *b*) within the cystic mass shows that the cysts are microcysts measuring <1 cm in diameter. The serous cystadenoma is high in signal intensity on the T2W image because of the high fluid content.

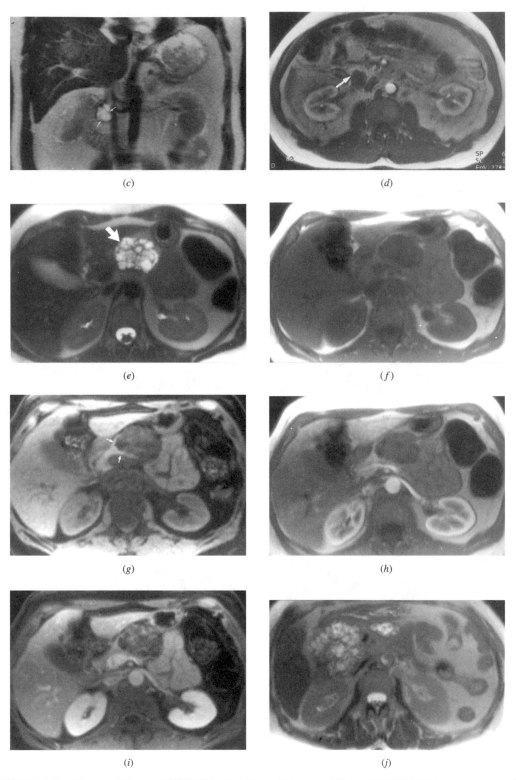

(c)

(d)

(e)

(f)

(g)

(h)

(i)

(j)

FIGURE 4.22 (*Continued*) Coronal T2W ETSE (*c*) and immediate postgadolinium T1W SGE (*d*) images in a second patient demonstrate a 3 cm serous cystadenoma in the head of the pancreas. Fine septations are apparent on the T2W image (arrows, *c*), and the tumor is sharply demarcated from normal-enhancing pancreas on the immediate postgadolinium image (arrow, *d*).

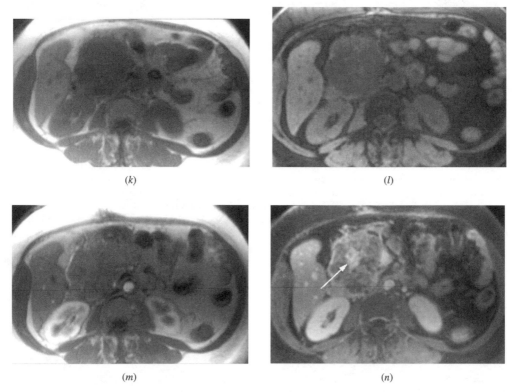

(k)   *(l)*

(m)   *(n)*

FIGURE 4.22   *(Continued)* T2W SS-ETSE (*e*), T1W SGE (*f*), T1W fat-suppressed SGE (*g*), immediate postgadolinium T1W SGE (*h*), and 90 s postgadolinium fat-suppressed SGE (*i*) images in a third patient. There is a 6 cm multicystic mass (arrows, *e*) arising in the pancreatic body with thin septations creating <2 cm cysts. The single-shot T2W sequence performs very well at defining the septations in cystic masses. A "beak sign" is demonstrated in the pancreas (arrow, *g*), which is best shown on the noncontrast T1W fat-suppressed (*g*) and immediate postgadolinium SGE (*h*) images, confirming that the mass originates from this organ. The septations enhance minimally on immediate postgadolinium images (*h*) with progressive enhancement on late images (*i*).

T2W ETSE (*j*), T1W fat-suppressed SGE (*k*), immediate postgadolinium T1W SGE (*l*), and 90 s postgadolinium fat-suppressed SGE (*m*) images in a fourth patient.

An 8 cm serous cystadenoma is present in the head of the pancreas, best shown on the single-shot T2W sequence. There is a central scar typical for serous cystadenoma that enhances on late images (arrow), which is consistent with fibrosis.

Serous cystadenomas occur predominantly in women as seen in these cases. The importance of the MR study is to differentiate this benign entity from mucinous cystadenomas, which are potentially malignant.

- ○ Pathologically comprised of mucin-filled cysts with lining cells showing at least moderate epithelial dysplasia
- ○ Cystadenomas should be treated by complete surgical resection
- ○ Complete surgical resection of cystadenocarcinoma may be curative if there is no evidence of metastases
- ○ Even in cases with metastases, surgery plus chemotherapy may yield 5-year survival rate up to 65%

- ○ Findings (figs. 4.23, 4.24, and 4.25)
  - ▪ Large encapsulated cysts greater than 2 cm in diameter (fig. 4.23)
  - ▪ Likelihood of adenocarcinoma increases as cysts become more numerous, show greater wall irregularity, or demonstrate intracystic papillary excrescence with more solid-appearing soft-tissue components (fig. 4.24)
  - ▪ Cyst fluid is typically high in signal on T2W single-shot echo-train images

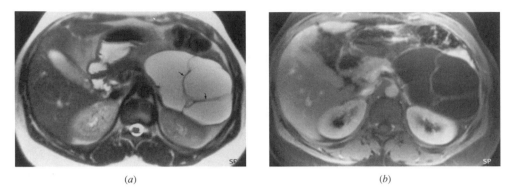

(a)   (b)

FIGURE 4.23 Mucinous (macrocystic) cystadenoma. T2W SS-ETSE (*a*) and 90 s postgadolinium fat-suppressed T1W SGE (*b*) images. A well-defined cystic mass arises from the body and tail of the pancreas that is low in signal intensity on the T1W image (not shown) and high in signal intensity on the T2W image (*a*) and demonstrates enhancement of septations on the postgadolinium T1W SGE image (*b*). No evidence of tumor nodules, invasion of adjacent tissue, or liver metastases is appreciated. The uniform thickness of the septations is clearly defined on the breathing-independent SS-ETSE image (arrows, *a*). Mucinous cystadenoma is potentially a low-grade malignant neoplasm.

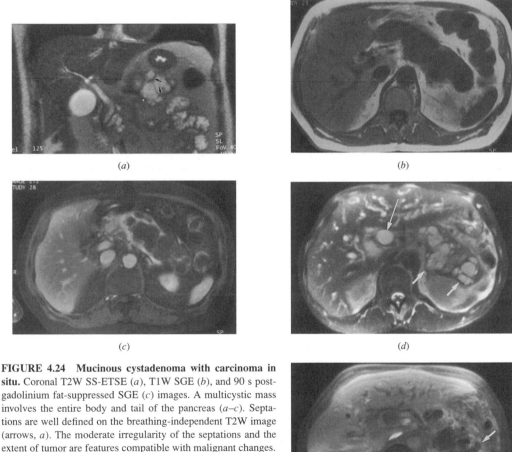

(a)   (b)

(c)   (d)

FIGURE 4.24 Mucinous cystadenoma with carcinoma in situ. Coronal T2W SS-ETSE (*a*), T1W SGE (*b*), and 90 s postgadolinium fat-suppressed SGE (*c*) images. A multicystic mass involves the entire body and tail of the pancreas (*a–c*). Septations are well defined on the breathing-independent T2W image (arrows, *a*). The moderate irregularity of the septations and the extent of tumor are features compatible with malignant changes.

T2W SS-ETSE (*d*) and 90 s postgadolinium fat-suppressed T1W SGE (*e*) images in a second patient demonstrate a mucinous cystadenocarcinoma in the body and tail (arrows, *d, e*). Dilatation of the CBD (long arrow, *d*) and intrahepatic biliary tree are also present.

(e)

- Pancreatic duct usually normal in caliber
- Cyst fluid can be low or high signal on T1W GRE: images. High signal results from T1 shortening effects of glycoprotein in mucin
- Capsule and cyst walls show moderate enhancement on gadolinium-enhanced T1W GRE images
- Local tumor extension may be seen as infiltrative soft tissue
- Metastases typically involve liver
- Liver metastases are frequently cystic and appear high signal on T2W images (fig. 4.25), and occassionally high signal on T1W images reflecting the presence of mucin

- Liver metastases may show peripheral and perilesional enhancement
- Papillary Cystic Epithelial Neoplasm
  - Rare tumor that is most commonly seen in young females
  - Pathologically appears related to ovarian stromal tissue and may be related to embryologic rest cells within the pancreas that progress into neoplasm
  - Low malignant potential
  - Growth may be stimulated and tumor may present during pregnancy
  - Management relies on complete surgical resection
  - Findings (fig. 4.26)
    - Can look indistinguishable from a mucinous macrocystic tumor

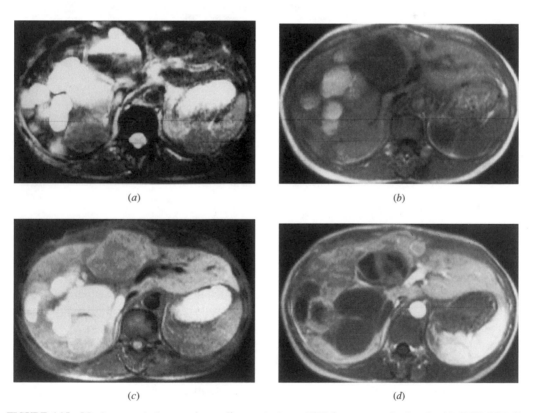

(a)   (b)

(c)   (d)

FIGURE 4.25 Mucinous cystadenocarcinoma liver metastases. T2W fat-suppressed spin-echo (a), T1W SGE (b), T1W fat-suppressed spin-echo (c), and immediate postgadolinium T1W SGE (d) images. Multiple metastases are present throughout the liver that are mixed low- and high-signal intensity on T1W (b, c) and T2W (a) images. This appearance is consistent with the presence of mucin in these tumors. On the immediate postgadolinium image (d), enhancement of the walls of the cysts is appreciated.

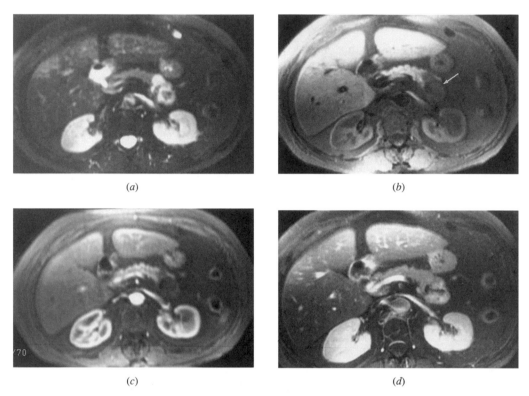

(a)   (b)

(c)   (d)

FIGURE 4.26   Solid and papillary epithelial neoplasm. T2W fat-suppressed spin-echo (*a*), T1W fat-suppressed SGE (*b*), immediate postgadolinium T1W fat-suppressed SGE (*c*), and 90 s postgadolinium fat-suppressed SGE (*d*) images. A 4 cm tumor mass arises from the tail of the pancreas that is low in signal intensity on the T1W image (arrow, *b*) and heterogeneous on the T2W image (*a*), enhances negligibly on the immediate postgadolinium T1W SGE image (*c*), and shows heterogeneous enhancement on the interstitial phase image (*d*). This rare low-grade malignant tumor is more frequent in young females and is typically located in the tail of the pancreas. MRI may be useful in these lesions by showing cystic degeneration and hemorrhagic necrosis, which are characteristic of this entity. (Courtesy of Caroline Reinhold, MD, Dept. of Radiology, McGill University.)

- Intraductal Papillary Mucinous Tumor (IPMT)
  - ○ Pathologically classified as a mucin-producing variant of duct adenocarcinoma with lower-grade malignancy potential
  - ○ Two forms are described: one arises from the main pancreatic duct and the other from side branches
  - ○ May demonstrate papillary growth
  - ○ Therapy depends on ability to completely resect surgically
  - ○ Findings (fig. 4.27)
    - ▪ T2W single-shot or longer-echo T2 MRCP images show marked dilatation of the main duct, usually involving the pancreatic head duct, with high or intermediate T2 signal, reflecting protein content
    - ▪ Papillary components within dilated duct well seen on T2W single-shot echo-train SE
    - ▪ Gadolinium-enhanced GRE images may show enhancement along the margins of the pancreatic duct and enhancement of papillary excrescences
    - ▪ Side branch disease appears as cyst-like expansion of branches extending from the main duct
    - ▪ Side branch disease may have a benign course, unlike main branch disease

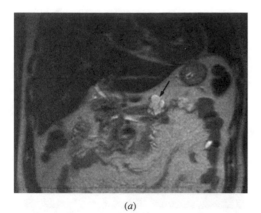

(a)

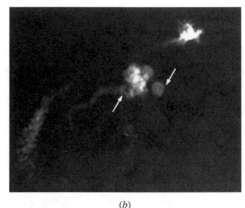

(b)

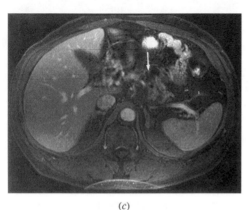

(c)

FIGURE 4.27 Intraductal papillary mucin-secreting tumor—main duct type. T2W echo-train spin-echo (*a*), thick-slab MRCP (*b*), immediate postgadolinium fat-suppressed SGE (*c*), and interstitial phase gadolinium-enhanced fat-suppressed SGE (*d*) images. There is massive dilatation of the entire main pancreatic duct (arrows, *b*), which is well shown on the T2W sequence (*a*) and MRCP (*b*). Enhancing tumor stroma is appreciated on the postcontrast images (*c, d*), with progressive enhancement on the later interstitial phase images (*d*). (Courtesy of Masayuki Kanematsu, M.D., Gifu University School of Medicine, Japan.)

Lymphoma

- Non-Hodgkin's lymphoma may directly infiltrate pancreatic parenchyma and involve peripancreatic lymph nodes
- Findings
  - Lymphoma appears as low-signal infiltrative tissue extending into high signal normal pancreas on noncontrast fat-suppressed T1 GRE images (fig. 4.28)
  - Typically appears as a mildly hetergeneous mass even when large, with mildly heterogeneous enhancement, showing low propensity for necrosis, in distinction to carcinomas or sarcomas

Metastases

- Most common hematogeneous metastases arise from renal cell carcinoma (RCC), lung cancer, breast cancer, or melanoma

- Direct invasion most commonly arises from transverse colon, which extends along transverse mesocolon or stomach, with extension from posterior wall through lesser sac
- RCC represents the most common metastases and can appear as hypervascular tumors, either solitary or multiple
- Findings (fig. 4.29)
  - Lower signal than adjacent normal high-signal pancreas on T1W GRE images, most conspicuous on fat-suppressed T1W GRE images
  - Hypervascular RCC may show intense enhancement persisting into venous and equilibrium phases. Metastases tend to appear uniformly enhancing when small and show peripheral enhancement when larger (>1 cm).
  - Other metastases may appear hypovascular, seen as minimal enhancement on

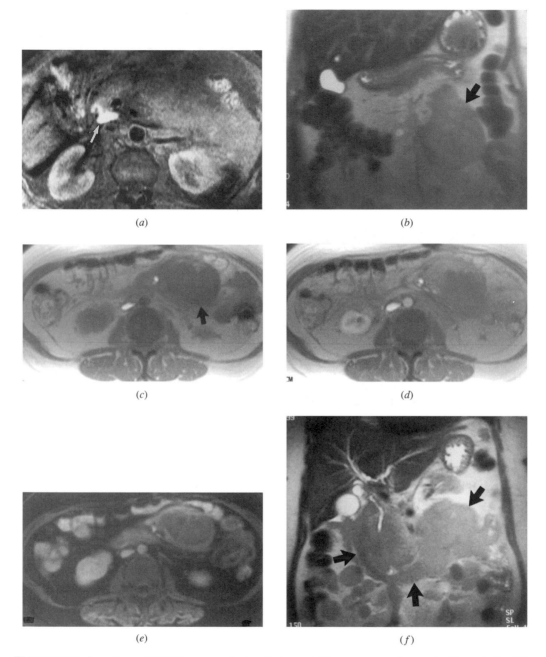

(a)

(b)

(c)

(d)

(e)

(f)

FIGURE 4.28 Lymphoma. T1W fat-suppressed spin-echo image (a) demonstrates replacement of the majority of the pancreas with intermediate-signal ill-defined lymphomatous tissue. The ventral portion of the pancreatic head is spared (arrow, a). (Reproduced with permission from Semelka RC, Shoenut JP, Kroeker MA, Micflikier AB. The Pancreas. In: Semelka RC, Shoenut JP. *MRI of the Abdomen with CT Correlation*. New York: Raven Press, pp. 59–76, 1993.)

Coronal T2W SS-ETSE (b), T1W SGE (c), immediate postgadolinium T1W SGE (d), and 90 s postgadolinium fat-suppressed SGE (e) images in a second patient who has Burkitt's lymphoma. A 10 cm mass (arrow, b, c) involves the pancreatic body and tail, which is mildly hypointense in signal intensity on both T1W (c) and T2W (b) images and enhances minimally on early (d) and late (e) postgadolinium images.

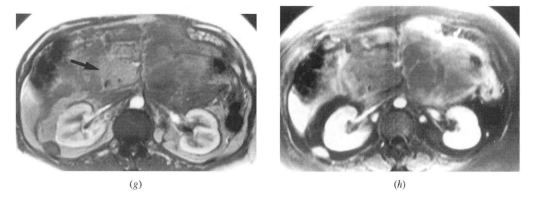

(g)   (h)

FIGURE 4.28   (*Continued*) Coronal T2W SS-ETSE (*f*), immediate postgadolinium SGE (*g*), and 90 s postgadolinium fat-suppressed SGE (*h*) images in a third patient who has non-Hodgkin's lymphoma. A large mass is present in the mesentery, which involves the pancreas as well. Mild enhancement of the mesenteric tumor and tumor involving the pancreatic head (arrow, *g*) is present on early (*g*) and late (*h*) postgadolinium images. As these cases illustrate, lymphoma typically exhibits mild enhancement on early and late postcontrast images.

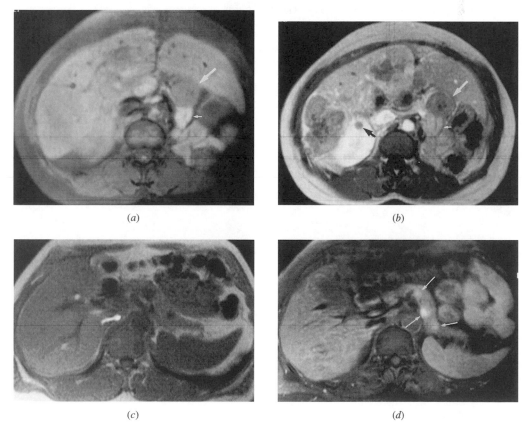

(a)   (b)

(c)   (d)

FIGURE 4.29   Pancreatic metastases from renal cancer. T1W fat-suppressed spin-echo (*a*) and immediate postgadolinium T1W SGE (*b*) images demonstrate a 3 cm mass in the distal body of the pancreas (arrow, *a*, *b*). The uninvolved tail of the pancreas has a normal high-signal intensity (small arrow, *a*, *b*). Multiple liver metastases are present that demonstrate predominant rim enhancement on the immediate postgadolinium image (*b*). Multiple renal cancers are present (black arrow, *b*).

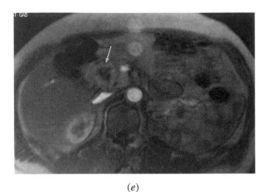 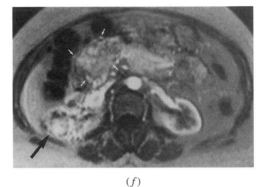

(e)   (f)

FIGURE 4.29 (*Continued*) T1W SGE (*c*) and interstitial phase gadolinium-enhanced T1W fat-suppressed spin-echo (*d*) images of the body of the pancreas and immediate postgadolinium T1W SGE image (*e*) in a second patient. Three metastases are present in the body of the pancreas (arrows, *d*) that are low in signal intensity on the precontrast T1W SGE image (*c*) and enhance uniformly and with moderate intensity on the interstitial phase gadolinium-enhanced image (*d*). A larger (3 cm) metastasis is present in the head of the pancreas that demonstrates rim enhancement on the immediate postgadolinium image (arrow, *e*).

Immediate postgadolinium T1W SGE image (*f*) in a third patient demonstrates multiple micronodular metastases to the pancreas <5 mm, which enhance uniformly and intensely on the immediate postgadolinium image (small arrows, *f*). The renal cancer is also shown (arrow, *f*). (Reproduced with permission from Kelekis NL, Semelka RC, Siegelman ES: MRI of pancreatic metastasis from renal cell cancer. *J Comput Assist Tomogr* 20: 249–253, 1996.)

Renal cell cancer is among the most common metastatic lesions to the pancreas.

arterial phase, with variable enhancement on venous and delayed phases
- T2W single-shot echo-train and MRCP usually show normal-size pancreatic duct, and tumor may have heterogeneous intermediate to high signal compared to adjacent pancreas

- Mimickers
  - Neuroendocrine tumors of the pancreas
  - Distinction from pancreatic ductal adenocarcinoma is that metastases rarely obstruct pancreatic ducts

CHAPTER 5

SPLEEN

Normal Spleen

MR Technique

- Basic abdominal MR imaging (see chap. 1) can fully assess the spleen
- Includes breath-hold T2W single-shot, breath-hold pregadolinium T1W GRE in/out-of-phase and postgadolinium T1W images
- Spleen is high signal on T2W images, higher signal intensity than muscle and normal liver (fig. 5.1) in the adult
  - Newborn spleen lacks white pulp and is iso- to hypointense relative to liver
- T1W images show signal lower than normal liver (fig. 5.1)
- Contrast enhancement is typically serpiginous in the arterial phase (20 s delay), becoming uniform by the venous phase (60–80 s)
  - Represents differential perfusion kinetics of white/red pulp, or fast-channel/low-channel red pulp
  - May become uniformly enhancing more quickly in patients with inflammatory or neoplastic conditions, possibly due to immune system stimulation (fig. 5.2)

Accessory Spleens

- Seen in 40% of patients
  - Clinical relevance
    - Differentiation from tumors
      - MR features on T1W, T2W, and gadolinium enhancement are identical to spleen and usually easily distinguishable from metastatic perisplenic deposits
    - Must be identified in patients undergoing therapeutic splenectomy for hypersplenia, where the accessory splenule may grow if not removed

Asplenia

- Congenital
  - Asplenia syndrome, Ivemark's syndrome
  - Right isomerism with high degree of associated thoraco-abdominal abnormalities and congenital heart disorders with high infant mortality of 80% by 1 year
- Acquired
  - Autosplenectomy can result from progressive severe splenic atrophy, with patient subsequently at increased risk of sepsis
  - Associated with sickle cell disease due to repeated splenic infarcts

Primer on MR Imaging of the Abdomen and Pelvis, edited by Diego R. Martin, Michele A. Brown, and Richard C. Semelka ISBN 0-471-37340-0 Copyright © 2005 Wiley-Liss, Inc.

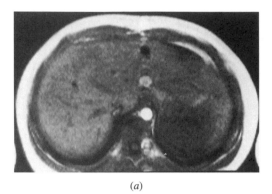
(a)

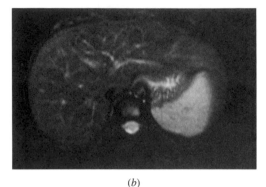
(b)

FIGURE 5.1   Normal spleen. T1W SGE (a) and T2W fat-suppressed spin-echo (b) images. Normal spleen is low in signal intensity on T1W image (a) and high in signal intensity on T2W image (b). Liver is higher in signal intensity on T1W images and lower in signal intensity on T2W images than spleen, which results in a clear distinction between the elongated lateral segment of the liver and the adjacent spleen in this patient.

○ Postsurgical, posttraumatic; the underlying cause has associated tissue changes, surgical clips, and appropriate history
• Polysplenia
  ○ Congenital syndrome associated with other abnormalities including left isomerism and cardiac malformations, but lower mortality than seen in asplenia syndrome
  ○ Other abnormalities seen on abdominal MRI include

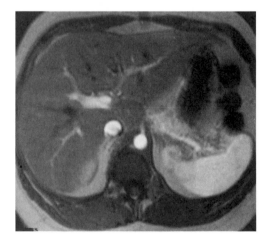

FIGURE 5.2   Homogeneous intense splenic enhancement. The spleen is noted to enhance intensely and uniformly in the capillary phase of enhancement. Contrast in hepatic arteries and portal veins and no contrast in hepatic veins demonstrate that the image was acquired in the capillary phase of enhancement.

  ▪ Situs inversus with gut malrotation, azygous continuation of the inferior vena cava, short pancreas
  ○ Imaging shows between 2 and 16 small splenules along the greater curvature of the stomach (fig. 5.3), and splenules may demonstrate infarcts and hemorrhage

Focal Disease

• MR imaging patterns of the most common focal splenic lesions are shown in table 5.1

Benign Masses

Cyst
Background
• Cysts are the most common of the benign splenic lesions
• Three types
  ○ Pseudocysts = posttraumatic
    ▪ No epithelial lining
  ○ Epidermoid
    ▪ Epithelial lining and may have trabeculations/septations
  ○ Hydatid (echinococcal)
    ▪ Relatively rare cause of splenic cysts
    ▪ Hydatid cysts are characterized by extensive wall calcification, but this is only seen in approximately 25% of cases
    ▪ May have daughter cysts internally

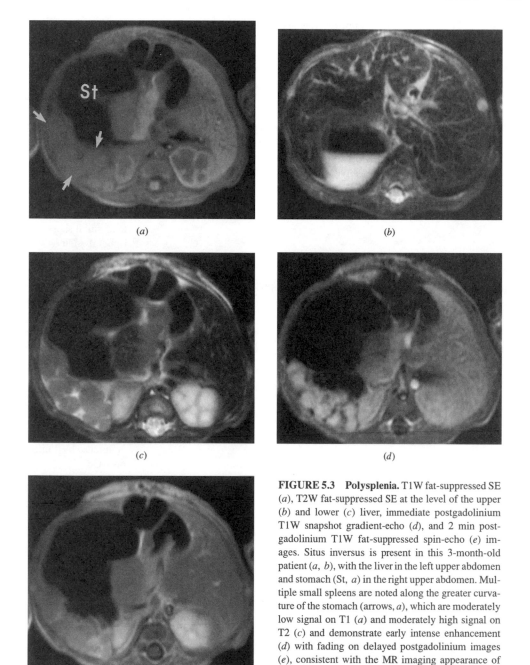

(a)

(b)

(c)

(d)

(e)

FIGURE 5.3   Polysplenia. T1W fat-suppressed SE (*a*), T2W fat-suppressed SE at the level of the upper (*b*) and lower (*c*) liver, immediate postgadolinium T1W snapshot gradient-echo (*d*), and 2 min postgadolinium T1W fat-suppressed spin-echo (*e*) images. Situs inversus is present in this 3-month-old patient (*a, b*), with the liver in the left upper abdomen and stomach (St, *a*) in the right upper abdomen. Multiple small spleens are noted along the greater curvature of the stomach (arrows, *a*), which are moderately low signal on T1 (*a*) and moderately high signal on T2 (*c*) and demonstrate early intense enhancement (*d*) with fading on delayed postgadolinium images (*e*), consistent with the MR imaging appearance of multiple spleens.

Imaging

• Cysts have sharp lesion margination, low signal intensity on T1W images, and very high and uniform signal intensity on T2W images (fig. 5.4)

• Cysts complicated by proteinaceous fluid or hemorrhage are usually posttraumatic and may have regions of high signal intensity on T1W images and regions of mixed-signal intensity on T2W images (fig. 5.5)

TABLE 5.1 Pattern Recognition of the Most Common Splenic Lesions

	T1	T2	Early Gd	Late Gd	Other Features
Cyst	↓ - Ø	↑↑	none	none	Well defined
Hamartoma	Ø	Ø - ↑	Heterogeneous intense	Homogeneous isointense	Usually >4 cm and arises from the medial surface of the midspleen
Hemangioma	↓ - Ø	↑	Peripheral nodules or homogeneous	Centripetal enhancement; retain contrast	Usually <2 cm
					Lesion more commonly enhances homogeneously on immediate post-Gd images compared to liver hemangiomas, reflecting their small size
					Peripheral nodules are not as clearly defined as liver hemangiomas
Metastases	↓ - Ø	Ø -↑	Focal lesions with minimal enhancement	Isointense	Metastases commonly become isointense by 1 min post-Gd
Lymphoma focal	↓ - Ø	↓ - ↑	Focal lesions with minimal enhancement	Isointense	Other sites of nodal disease. Lymphomatous lesions commonly become isointense by 1 min post-Gd
Lymphoma diffuse	↓ - Ø	↓ - ↑	Irregular regions with minimal enhancement	Isointense	Other sites of nodal disease. Lymphomatous lesions commonly become isointense by 1 min post-Gd

↓↓ Moderately to markedly decreased
↓ Mildly Decreased
Ø Isointense
↑ Mildly Increased
↑↑ Moderately to mildly Increased

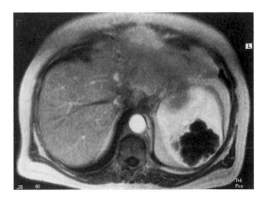

FIGURE 5.4 Epidermoid cyst. Immediate postgadolinium T1W SGE image demonstrates a signal-void cystic lesion with peripheral septations.

- Cysts do not enhance on postgadolinium images

Hemangioma
Background
- Hemangiomas are the most common of the benign splenic tumors
- Lesions may be single or multiple

Imaging
- Mildly to moderately hyperintense on T2W images, similar to hepatic hemangiomas in absolute signal intensity
  - Spleen is normally slightly hyperintense to liver on T2W images, which results in

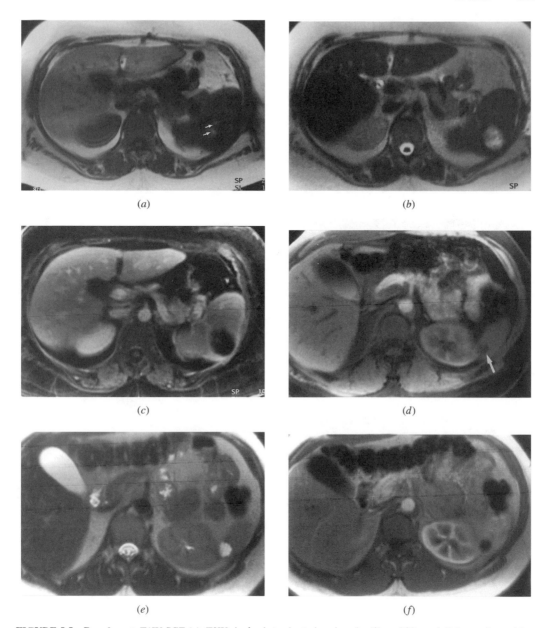

FIGURE 5.5   Pseudocyst. T1W SGE (*a*), T2W single-shot echo-train spin-echo (*b*), and 90 s gadolinium-enhanced fat-suppressed SGE (*c*) images. High-signal-intensity foci are identified in the cyst on the precontrast SGE image (arrows, *a*), a finding consistent with hemorrhage. Slight heterogeneity of the cyst on the T2W image (*b*) also reflects the presence of blood degradation products. The cyst is sharply demarcated after gadolinium administration (*c*). The foci of blood remain high in signal intensity on postgadolinium images. T1W fat-suppressed SGE (*d*), T2W single-shot echo-train spin-echo (*e*), immediate postgadolinium T1W SGE (*f*), and 90 s gadolinium-enhanced T1W fat-suppressed SGE (*g*) images in a second patient. The pseudocyst is low signal on T1 (arrow, *d*), high signal on T2 (*e*), and does not enhance on early (*f*) or late (*g*) postgadolinium images.

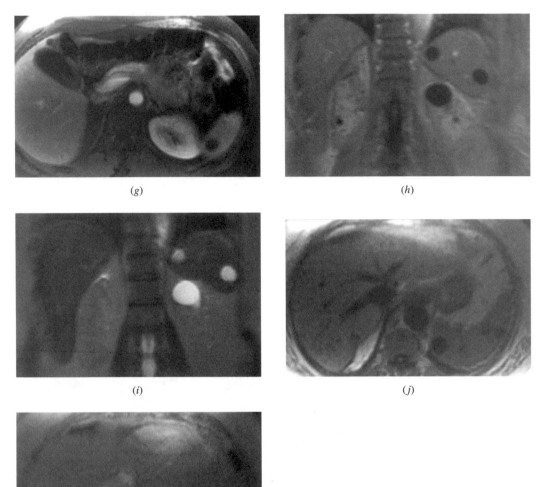

(g)

(h)

(i)

(j)

(k)

FIGURE 5.5 *(Continued)* Coronal T1W single-shot magnetization-prepared gradient-echo (*h*), coronal T2W echo-train spin-echo (*i*), T1W single-shot magnetization-prepared gradient-echo (*j*), and 45 s postgadolinium single-shot magnetization-prepared gradient echo (*k*) images in a third patient with multiple splenic cysts. Renal cysts are also present.

lesser lesion contrast and conspicuity than observed with liver hemangiomas

∘ Hemangiomas may appear isointense to spleen on single-shot echo-train T2W images, due to the lesser contrast-to-noise of this sequence

• Hemangiomas are minimally hypointense to isointense with background spleen on T1W SGE images due to the relatively low-signal intensity of adjacent normal spleen on these images

• Three patterns of contrast enhancement (similar to liver hemangiomas)

∘ Immediate homogeneous enhancement with persistent enhancement on delayed images

▪ Most common with smaller lesions (<1 cm)

○ Peripheral enhancement with progression to uniform enhancement on delayed images (fig. 5.6)

○ Peripheral enhancement with centripetal progression, but persistent lack of enhancement of the central region

▪ A large central scar can appear hypointense on T2W images due to lower fluid content (fig. 5.7)

• Pattern of contrast enhancement different than liver hemangiomas

○ Typically do not demonstrate well-defined nodules on early postgadolinium images

▪ Likely due to differences in blood supply in spleen versus liver

Hamartoma
Background

• Hamartomas are rare and composed of structurally disorganized mature splenic red pulp elements

• Usually single, spherical, and predominantly solid

• Often occur in the midportion of the spleen, arising from the anterior or posterior concave (medial) surface

Imaging

• Mildly low to isointense on T1W images

• Moderately high in signal intensity on T2W images

• Variations

○ Can show heterogeneous signal due, in part, to the presence of cystic spaces of varying size

○ If the composition of fibrous tissue is substantial, hamartomas may have regions of low signal intensity on T2W images

• Gadolinium-enhanced SGE early arterial-venous phase images show intense diffuse heterogeneous enhancement (fig. 5.8)

○ Enhancement becomes homogeneous on more delayed images with signal intensity slightly greater than in background spleen

Mimickers

• Lesion size and enhancement pattern may mimic malignancy

• The early diffuse heterogeneous enhancement permits distinction from hemangioma

• Lesions may also resemble normal splenic parenchyma (fig. 5.8), particularly on delayed equilibrium phase images

Lymphangioma
Background

• Lymphangiomas are composed of collections of small and cystically dilated lymphatic channels

Imaging

• Cystic component shown on T2W images as circumscribed high signal foci

• Splenic lymphangiomatosis is rare and usually appears as a subcapsular multiloculated hyperintense mass on T2W images

○ septa progressively enhance on late-phase post-gadolinium images

Malignant Masses

Lymphoma
Background

• Hodgkin's and non-Hodgkin's lymphomas frequently involve the spleen:

○ 50% rule

▪ Approximately 50% of patients have splenomegaly

▪ Approximately 50% of these patients have splenic lymphoma

▪ Approximately 50% of splenic lymphoma cases show diffuse splenic involvement, and 50% focal/multifocal disease

• Usually see concomitant lymphadenopathy

• Chronic lymphocytic leukemia (CLL) frequently involves the spleen

○ One of the few causes of massive splenomegaly

Imaging

• Lymphoma in the spleen frequently parallels the signal intensity of splenic parenchyma on T1W and T2W images

• Immediate (20 s delay) postgadolinium T1W SGE images provide maximum sensitivity

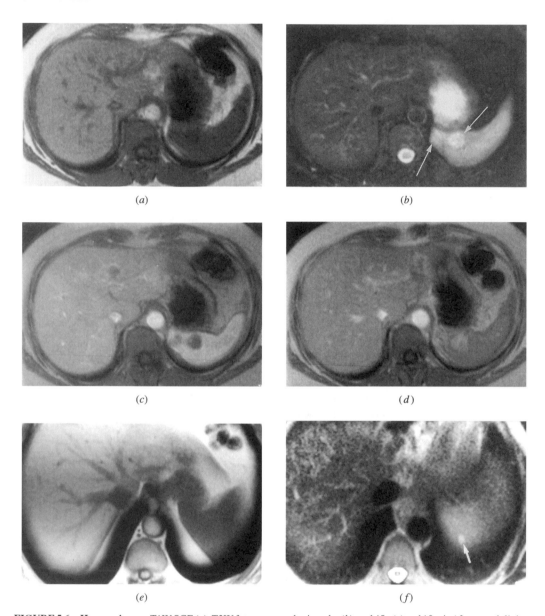

FIGURE 5.6   Hemangiomas. T1W SGE (*a*), T2W fat-suppressed spin-echo (*b*), and 45 s (*c*) and 10 min (*d*) postgadolinium SGE images. Two small (<1.5 cm) hemangiomas are present that are minimally hypointense on T1W images (*a*) and moderately hyperintense on T2W images (arrows, b). Peripheral nodules are present on early postgadolinium images (*c*), and enhancement progresses to uniform high signal intensity by 10 min (*d*). T1W SGE (*e*), T2 fat-suppressed spin-echo (*f*), immediate postgadolinium T1 SGE (*g*), and 90 s postgadolinium T1 fat-suppressed SGE (*h*) images in a second patient. The small hemangioma in the superior aspect of the spleen is isointense on T1, moderately hyperintense on T2 (arrow, *f*), and shows early uniform enhancement (*g*) that persists on the late postgadolinium image (*h*). The hemangioma is better demonstrated on the later postgadolinium image as background splenic enhancement has diminished and is uniform. Early uniform enhancement is common in <1.5 cm hemangiomas.

T1W SGE (*i*), T2W fat-suppressed spin-echo (*j*), immediate postgadolinium T1W SGE (*k*), and 90 s postgadolinium T1W fat-suppressed SGE (*l*) images in a third patient.

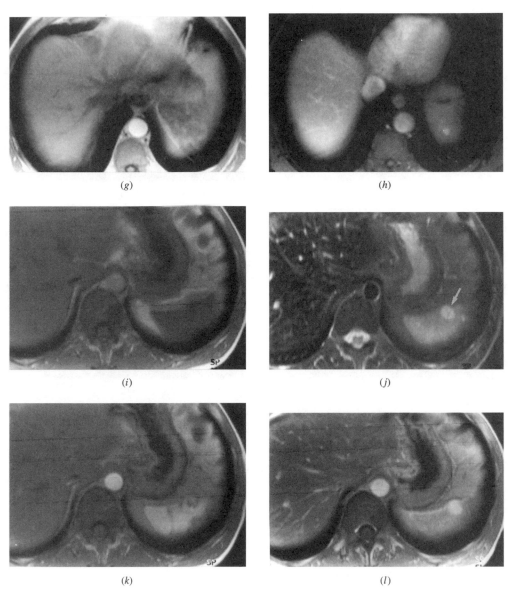

FIGURE 5.6 (*Continued*) The lesion is isointense on T1 (*i*) and moderately hyperintense on the T2W image (arrow, *j*). Note centripetal (*k*, *l*) progressive enhancement of the hemangioma resembling the pattern of a hepatic hemangioma.

- ○ Shown to be superior in sensitivity to contrast-enhanced CT
- Range of appearances on immediate postgadolinium images
  - ○ Diffuse involvement
    - ▪ Large, irregularly enhancing regions of high and low signal intensity (fig. 5.9), in contrast to the uniform bands that characterize normal serpiginous enhancement

- ○ Multifocal involvement
  - ▪ Focal low-signal-intensity mass lesions scattered throughout the spleen
  - ▪ Focal lesions may occur in a background of arciform-enhancing spleen or in a background of uniformly enhancing spleen
  - ▪ Appears as spherical lesions in distinction to the wavy tubular pattern of enhancement of uninvolved spleen

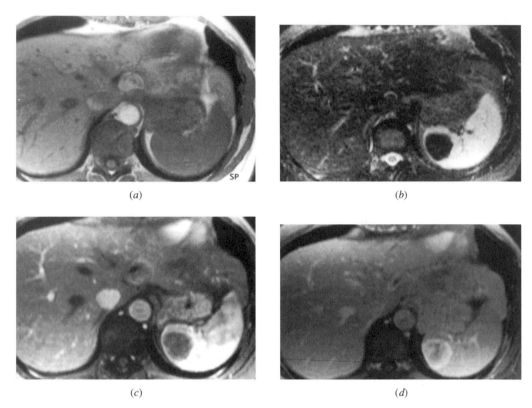

(a)   (b)

(c)   (d)

FIGURE 5.7   Sclerosing hemangioma. T1W SGE (a), T2W fat-suppressed spin-echo (b), immediate postgadolinium T1W SGE (c), and 90 s postgadolinium T1W fat-suppressed SGE (d) images. A 3 cm hemangioma is isointense to the spleen on T1W (a) and markedly hypointense on the T2W image (b). Peripheral nodules of enhancement are present on the early postgadolinium image (c), with moderate progressive enhancement on the delayed postgadolinium (d) images. The combination of hypointensity on T2 with only moderate progression of nodular enhancement on postcontrast T1W images is consistent with a sclerosing hemangioma. (Courtesy of Bert te Strake M.D., Manukau Radiology Institute Ltd. Auckland, New Zealand.)

- Lymphoma nodules may be low in signal intensity compared to background spleen on T2W images (fig. 5.10)
  - A feature distinguishing lymphomas from metastases
- Less frequent appearances
  - Splenomegaly is most often present, but lymphoma may involve normal-sized spleens (fig. 5.11)
  - Lymphoma may also appear as a large mass involving spleen and contiguous organs such as stomach, adrenal, or kidney
    - Characteristically lymphoma can be very infiltrative, crossing tissue barriers, but with minimal destruction of tissues or

vessels, and vessels may remain patent even with large-volume disease
  - Bulky lymphadenopathy is not always present
  - A rare appearance is that of a solitary splenic mass with internal diffuse heterogeneous enhancement on immediate postgadolinium SGE images (fig. 5.12), mimicking a hamartoma
- Alternative contrast agents
  - Superparamagnetic particles also improve the accuracy of diagnosing splenic lymphoma
  - Malignant cells do not take up superparamagnetic particles and do not change in signal intensity

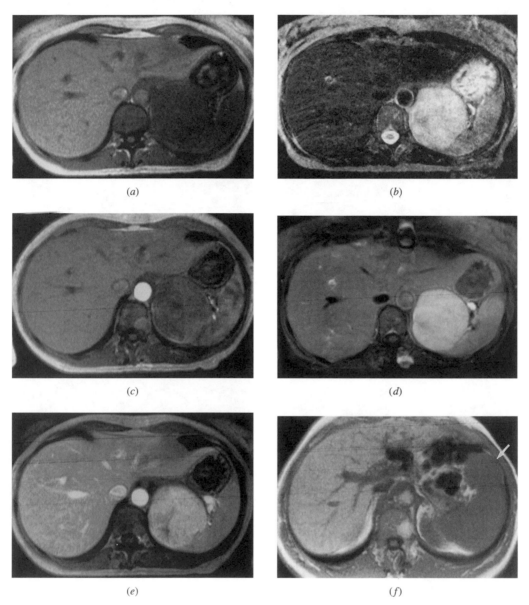

(a) (b) (c) (d) (e) (f)

FIGURE 5.8   Hamartoma. T1W SGE (a), T2W fat-suppressed single-shot echo-train spin-echo (b), immediate post-gadolinium T1W SGE (c), 5 min postgadolinium T1W fat-suppressed spin-echo (d), and 10 min postgadolinium SGE (e) images. A 7 cm mass lesion arises from the posteromedial aspect of the midportion of the spleen that is low in signal intensity on the T1W image (a), moderately high in signal intensity on the T2W image (b), and demonstrates diffuse heterogeneous enhancement on the immediate postgadolinium SGE image (c). On more delayed images (d, e), enhancement becomes more homogeneous and is greater than that of background spleen. T1W SGE (f), T2W fat-suppressed spin-echo (g), and immediate (h), 90 s (i), and 10 min (j) postgadolinium images in a second patient. A 4 cm hamartoma arises from the anterior aspect of the midportion of the spleen (arrow, f). The signal intensity of the hamartoma is very similar to that of background spleen on all imaging sequences. A cleavage plane from spleen is noted on the T2W image (g). On the immediate postgadolinium image (h) the tumor has intense, uniform enhancement, which is different from the arciform enhancement of the normal splenic parenchyma.

T1W SGE (k), T2W fat-suppressed echo-train spin-echo (l), immediate postgadolinium T1W SGE (m), and 90 s gadolinium-enhanced T1W fat-suppressed SGE (n) images in a third patient.

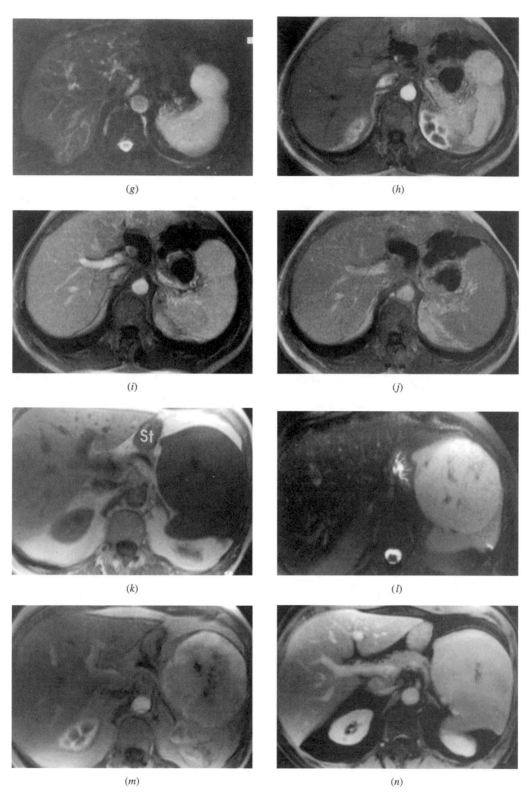

FIGURE 5.8 (*Continued*) A large hamartoma in the anterior aspect of the spleen displaces the stomach (St, *m*) medially. The mass is near isointense to the spleen on all sequences. It shows intense heterogeneous enhancement on the immediate postgadolinium image, similar to the intensity of spleen but with a differing pattern.

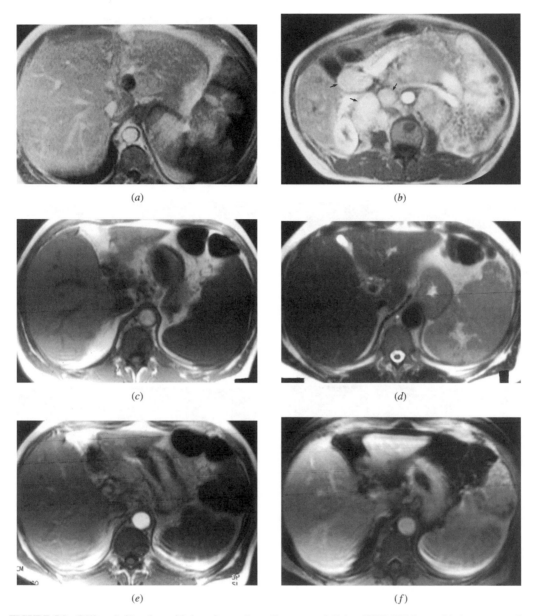

FIGURE 5.9 Diffuse infiltration with lymphoma. Immediate postgadolinium T1W SGE image (*a*) demonstrates irregular regions of high and low signal intensity in the spleen in this patient with non-Hodgkin's lymphoma. Irregular enhancement is observed in the setting of diffuse infiltration. Immediate postgadolinium SGE image (*b*) in a second patient with non-Hodgkin's lymphoma demonstrates irregular enhancement of the spleen consistent with diffuse infiltration. Enhancing lymph nodes (arrows, *b*) are also noted.

T1W SGE (*c*), T2W echo-train spin-echo (*d*), immediate postgadolinium T1W SGE (*e*), and 90 s postgadolinium T1W fat-suppressed SGE (*f*) images in a third patient with B-cell lymphoma infiltrating the spleen. The spleen is homogeneous is signal intensity on T1 (*c*) and is heterogeneous on the T2W image (*d*). Diffuse heterogenous enhancement with large irregular foci of decreased enhancement is appreciated on the immediate postgadolinium image (*e*) that persists on the late image (*f*).

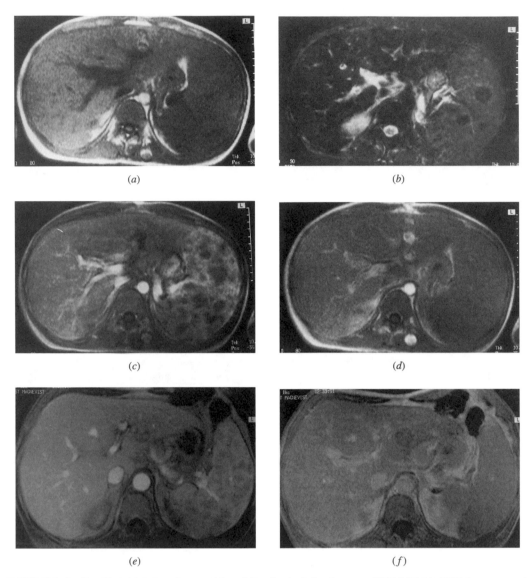

(a)   *(b)*

(c)   *(d)*

(e)   *(f)*

FIGURE 5.10 **Non-Hodgkin's lymphoma with multifocal splenic involvement.** T1W SGE (*a*), T2W fat-suppressed spin-echo (*b*), and immediate (*c*) and 2 min (*d*) postgadolinium SGE images. Splenomegaly is present. Lesions are not apparent on the precontrast SGE image. Several low-signal-intensity focal mass lesions are identified on T2W images, an appearance that is not uncommon for lymphoma but rare for other malignant tumors. Multiple focal masses are most clearly demonstrated on immediate postgadolinium images (*c*). Lymphomatous foci become isointense with background spleen by 2 min after contrast (*d*).

Immediate (*e*) and 90 s (*f*) postgadolinium SGE images in a second patient. Multiple low-signal-intensity masses are identified on the immediate postgadolinium image (*e*). Lesions become isointense with background spleen by 90 s.

○ Adjacent normal spleen takes up iron particles in the reticuloendothelial system (RES)
cells, which causes decreased signal intensity of normal spleen due to T2* effects
■ Best seen on T2*-sensitive imaging such

as single-shot echo-train or longer echo
time SGE imaging
• Chemotherapy-treated lymphoma with response to therapy
○ Can appear as fibrotic nodules

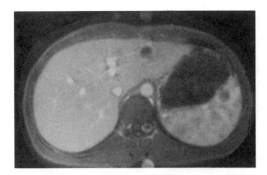

FIGURE 5.11   Hodgkin's lymphoma. Immediate post-gadolinium image demonstrates multiple low-signal-intensity masses within a normal-sized spleen. Rounded lesions are present in a background of arciform-enhancing spleen.

- Low signal intensity on T1W and T2W images
- Minimal to negligible enhancement on early and late postgadolinium images (fig. 5.13)

- CLL
  - Tumor deposits are more infiltrative and less well defined than other lymphomas
  - Deposits are well shown after gadolinium administration and appear as irregular hypointense masses on early postcontrast images (fig. 5.14)
  - Malignancies related to leukemia, such as angioimmunoblastic lymphadenopathy with dysproteinemia, have a similar appearance, with irregular regions of low signal intensity within the spleen on immediate postgadolinium images (Fig. 5.15). Lymphadenopathy is frequently present.

Mimickers
- Metastases
  - Are rarely low in signal intensity on T2W images, as seen with lymphoma, and usually isointense to hyperintense

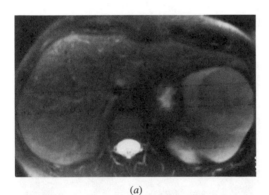

(a)

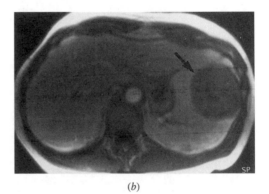

(b)

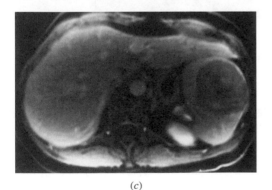

(c)

FIGURE 5.12   Splenic lymphoma presenting as a solitary mass. T2W far-suppressed echo-train spin-echo (a), immediate postgadolinium T1W SGE (b), and 90 s postgadolinium fat-suppressed SGE (c) images. A 6 cm solitary mass arises from the spleen that is mildly heterogeneous and hyperintense on the T2W image (a). The mass enhances moderately in a diffuse heterogeneous fashion on the immediate postgadolinium image (arrow, b) with slightly increased signal intensity by 90 s after contrast (c). The appearance resembles a hamartoma, with diffuse heterogeneous enhancement. Substantially less enhancement is present with this lymphomatous mass than is typically seen with a hamartoma. The patient presented with systemic symptoms, which is a picture in keeping with lymphoma and not hamartoma. The patient did not have retroperitoneal adenopathy, which is another uncommon feature of splenic lymphoma.

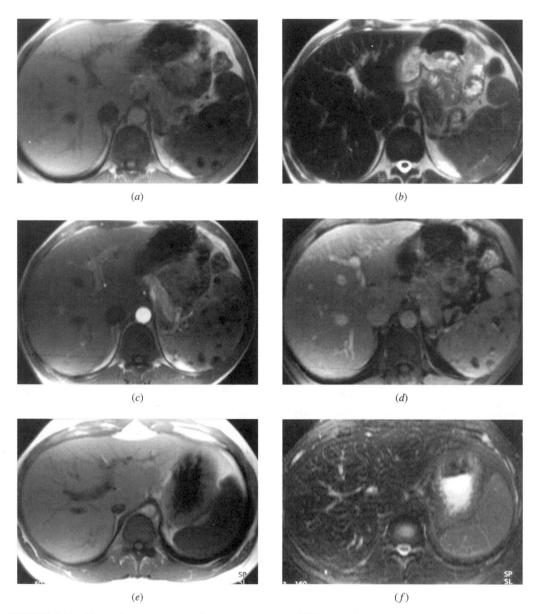

(a) (b)

(c) (d)

(e) (f)

FIGURE 5.13 Chemotherapy-treated splenic lymphoma. T1W SGE (a), T2W single-shot echo-train spin-echo (b), immediate postgadolinium T1W SGE (c), and 90 s postgadolinium T1W fat-suppressed SGE (d) images. Foci of treated lymphoma are hypointense on T1 (a), and hypo to isointense on T2 (b) and demonstrate negligible enhancement on early (c) and late (d) postgadolinium images. The low signal on T2 reflects a diminished fluid content, and fibrous changes result in the diminished enhancement. T1W SGE (e), breath-hold STIR (f), immediate postgadolinium SGE (g), and 90 s postgadolinium SGE (h) in a second patient with Hodgkin's lymphoma receiving chemotherapy.

- Hamartomas
  - Rare solitary lymphoma may show heterogeneous arterial phase enhancement, similar to splenic hamartomas

  - The presence of lymphadenopathy and/or symptoms and signs of systemic disease suggests the diagnosis of lymphoma

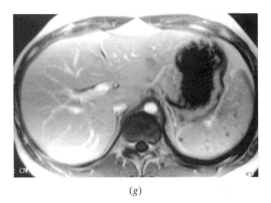
(g)

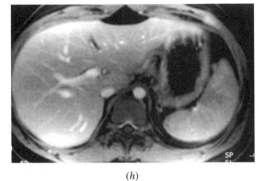
(h)

FIGURE 5.13   (*Continued*) There are multiple small hypointense lesions on T1W (*e*) and T2W (*f*) images, which shows peripheral or diffuse enhancement after contrast administration (*g, h*), reflecting the different stages of the fibrotic process. These lesions remained stable in appearance in follow-up MRI exams (not shown).

Angiosarcoma

Background

- Although rare, this is the most common primary nonlymphoid malignant tumor of the spleen
- Tumors may be single or multiple and demonstrate an aggressive growth pattern
- Hemorrhage is a frequent finding

Imaging

- Commonly demonstrating a variety of signal intensities on T1W images within the mass, due to the varying ages of blood products
- Highly vascular and enhances intensely with gadolinium

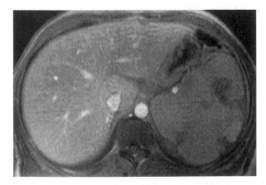

FIGURE 5.14   Chronic lymphocytic leukemia. The spleen is noted to be massively enlarged and contains irregularly marginated focal low-signal-intensity masses on the 45 s postgadolinium T1W SGE image.

Metastases

Background

- Hematogeneous metastases to spleen are rare
- Breast and lung carcinomas and melanoma are the most common primary tumors
- Tumor deposits form as nodules or aggregates of tumor and can disrupt the normal splenic architecture

Imaging

- Splenic metastases are often occult on conventional T1W images
  ○ Melanoma retains melanin production in less than 20% of cases, and may demonstrate high signal on T1W images due to T1 shortening properties of melanin
    ▪ Usually seen as mixed high and low signal on T1W and T2W images
- T2W images usually show masses as slightly hyperintense to spleen
- Maximum sensitivity is on immediate (20 s delay) postgadolinium SGE images (fig. 5.16)
  ○ Metastases are lower in signal intensity than normal splenic tissue
  ○ Images must be acquired within the first 30 s after gadolinium administration because metastases rapidly equilibrate with splenic parenchyma
- Posttreatment metastases

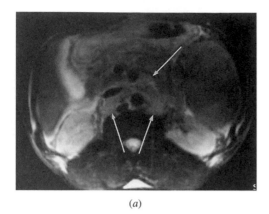

(a)

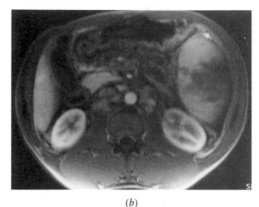

(b)

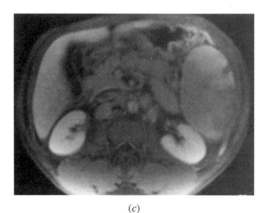

(c)

FIGURE 5.15   Angioimmunoblastic lymphadenopathy with dysproteinemia. T2W fat-suppressed spin-echo (a), immediate postgadolinium T1W SGE (b), and 90 s postgadolinium fat-suppressed SGE (c) images. The spleen is noted to be markedly enlarged. Lymphadenopathy is moderately high in signal intensity of T2W images and is rendered conspicuous because of the suppression of fat signal intensity (arrows, a). Mild enhancement of lymph nodes is noted on immediate postgadolinium SGE (b). Lymph nodes enhance more intensely in the interstitial phase and are more clearly defined by the suppression of fat signal intensity (c). Splenic involvement is demonstrated by irregular, poorly marginated, large regions of diminished enhancement on the immediate postgadolinium image (b). Enhancement of the spleen is more uniform by 90 s after contrast (c), and signal intensity is mildly heterogeneous on the T2W image (a).

- ○ Response to chemotherapy is generally associated with decreased enhancement and diminished signal intensity on T2W images
- Alternative contrast agents
  - ○ Superparamagnetic iron oxide particles render metastases higher in signal intensity than normal spleen

Mimickers
- Lymphoma
  - ○ Lymphoma may be lower in signal on T2W images than spleen, a feature atypical for metastases
- Infarct
  - ○ Demonstrates lack of enhancement on early and late postgadolinium images
  - ○ If centrally located within the spleen, this entity may appear mass-like

- ○ Acute infarcts, particularly in the setting of cirrhosis and portal hypertension, may show unusual peri-infarct splenic enhancement
- ○ Infarct does not enhance centrally, and abnormal peri-infarct enhancement diminishes on later post contrast images

Direct Tumor Invasion
Background
- Direct tumor invasion is most commonly observed with pancreatic cancers including ductal adenocarcinoma, islet cell tumor, and macrocystic cystadenocarcinoma (fig. 5.17)
  - ○ Other primary origins include gastric, colonic, renal, and adrenal sites
- Lymphoma has a particular propensity to involve the spleen in continuity with other organs

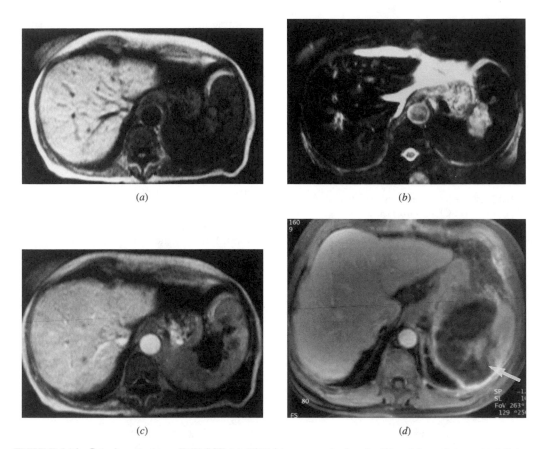

(a)   *(b)*

(c)   *(d)*

FIGURE 5.16   **Splenic metastases.** T1W SGE (*a*), T2W fat-suppressed spin-echo (*b*), and immediate postgadolinium T1W SGE (*c*) images in a woman with endometrial cancer. Metastases are noted throughout the spleen that are mixed hypointense and isointense on the T1W image (*a*), mixed isointense and hyperintense on the T2W image (*b*), and low in signal intensity on the immediate postgadolinium image (*c*). Note that metastases are best shown on the immediate postgadolinium image. The largest metastasis is distinctly demonstrated on the T2W image (*b*). The smaller lesions are poorly shown, despite the presence of iron deposition. Ascites is also present and is low in signal intensity or pre- and postcontrast T1W images and high in signal intensity on the T2W image.

Transverse 90 s postgadolinium fat-suppressed SGE image (*d*) in a second patient demonstrates an expansile destructive lesion (arrow, *d*) in the posterior aspect of the spleen associated with a large subcapsular fluid collection.

Imaging
- Discussed under respective organ systems and tumor types

Miscellaneous

Splenomegaly
Background
- Associated diseases include
  - Venous congestion
    - Portal hypertension
      - Primary (idiopathic—uncommon)
      - Secondary (cirrhosis)
      - Splenic vein thrombosis
  - Neoplastic
    - Leukemia, lymphoma, metastases
  - Infections
- Causes for massive splenomegaly include
  - Portal hypertension, viral (cytomegalovirus, Epstein-Barr virus), leukemia (CLL)

Imaging
- Portal hypertension due to cirrhosis is the most common cause in North America

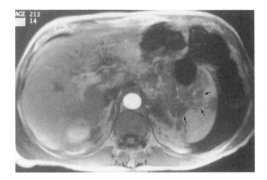

FIGURE 5.17 Direct tumor invasion. Immediate postgadolinium T1W SGE image demonstrates invasion of the splenic hilum by a large infiltrative pancreatic ductal adenocarcinoma (arrows).

○ Immediate postgadolinium images show normal serpiginous splenic enhancement or uniform high-signal-intensity enhancement that exclude malignancy (fig. 5.18)

Infection
- Viral infection may result in splenomegaly
- The three most common viruses to involve the spleen are Epstein-Barr (EBV), varicella, and cytomegalovirus (CMV)
- Histoplasmosis, tuberculosis, and echinococcosis are nonviral infectious agents that involve the spleen in patients with normal or abnormal immune status (fig. 5.19)

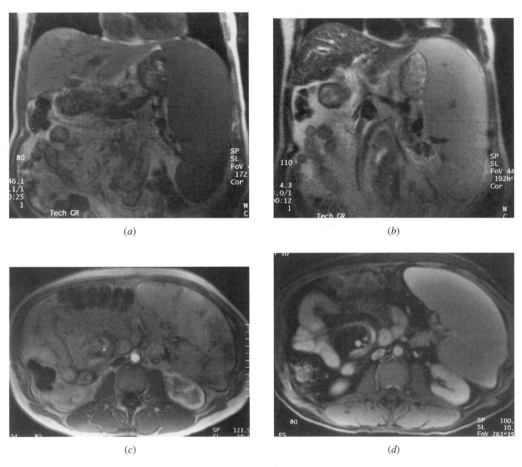

(a)

(b)

(c)

(d)

FIGURE 5.18 Splenomegaly secondary to portal hypertension. Coronal T1W SGE (*a*), coronal T2W echo-train spin-echo (*b*), immediate postgadolinium T1W SGE (*c*), and 90 s postgadolinium fat-suppressed SGE (*d*) images. Massive splenomegaly is demonstrated on all MR images. No focal lesions are present on precontrast T1W (*a*) or T2W (*b*) images. The presence of arciform enhancement on the immediate postgadolinium SGE image (*c*) excludes the presence of malignant disease. At 90 s, the spleen becomes homogeneous in signal (*d*).

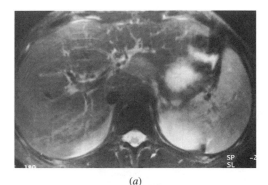

(a)

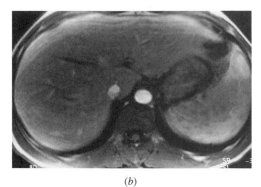

(b)

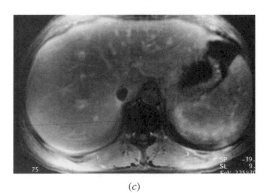

(c)

FIGURE 5.19 Hepatosplenorenal histoplasmosis. T2W fat-suppressed echo-train spin-echo (a), immediate postgadolinium T1W SGE (b), and 90 s postgadolinium fat-suppressed SGE (c) images in a patient with human immunodeficiency virus (HIV) infection. Multiple lesions <1 cm are demonstrated in the liver, spleen, and kidneys. Lesions are poorly visualized on T2W images and appear as small minimally hyperintense lesions (a). On immediate postgadolinium image, lesions appear low in signal intensity (b). By 90 s after gadolinium, lesions enhance more than background tissue (arrows, c)

- In the immunocompromised patient, the most common hepatosplenic infection is fungal infection with *Candida albicans* and cryptococcus
  - Patients with acute myelogenous leukemia are at high risk
  - Multiorgan involvement is common
  - Gastrointestinal tract is almost invariably involved
  - Acute lesions are generally more apparent in the spleen than in the liver
  - Subacute-treated and chronic-healed lesions are more conspicuous in the liver (see chap. 2)

Imaging
- In the acute phase, hepatosplenic candidiasis results in small (<1 cm) well-defined abscesses in the spleen and liver
  - Conspicuous on T2W fat-suppressed images as high-signal-intensity rounded foci (fig. 5.20)

  - Lesions may also be visible on postgadolinium images, but they are usually not visualized on precontrast SGE images
  - MRI is superior to contrast-enhanced CT imaging for the detection of fungal microabscesses

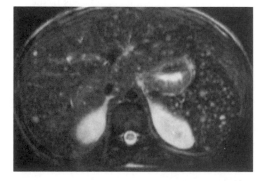

FIGURE 5.20 Hepatosplenic candidiasis. T2W fat-suppressed echo-train spin-echo image demonstrates multiple, well-defined, high-signal-intensity candidiasis abscesses <1 cm in the liver and spleen.

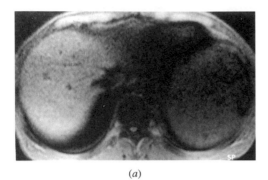

(a)

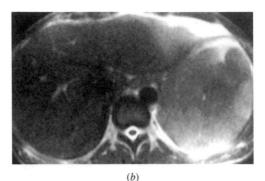

(b)

FIGURE 5.21 Cryptococcal abscess. T1W magnetization-prepared gradient-echo (*a*), T2 fat-suppressed single-shot echo-tain spin-echo (*b*), and coronal 3 min postgadolinium T1W magnetization-prepared gradient-echo (*c*) images in an immunocompromised patient with AIDS and generalized cryptococcal infection. The abscess appears mildly hypointense on T1 (*a*) and mildly hyperintense on T2 (*b*), with subtle signal difference compared to spleen. Lack of enhancement and peripheral ring enhancement (arrow, *c*) are present on the postgadolinium image (*c*), which are features of bacterial and some fungal abscesses.

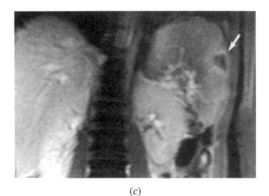

(c)

- Bacterial and fungal abscesses are otherwise rare in the spleen
  - Abscesses appear slightly hypo- to isointense on T1W images and heterogeneous and mildly to moderately hyperintense on T2W images
  - These lesions show intense mural enhancement on early gadolinium-enhanced images often accompanied by increased enhancement of surrounding periabscess tissue
    - Mural enhancement persists on later postgadolinium images (fig. 5.21)

Sarcoidosis
Background
- Histologically characterized by noncaseating granulomatous disease

Imaging
- Lesions of sarcoidosis are small (<1 cm) and hypovascular
- Characteristically low in signal intensity on T1W and T2W images

- Minimal and slowly progressive enhancement on postgadolinium images (fig. 5.22)
- Low signal intensity on T2W images
  - Distinguishes these lesions from acute infective disease

Gamna-Gandy Bodies
Background
- Foci of iron deposition commonly occur in patients with cirrhosis and portal hypertension due to microhemorrhages in the splenic parenchyma
- Rarely associated with blood transfusions

Imaging
- Typical appearance is multiple <1 cm lesions scattered throughout the spleen
- Lesions demonstrate signal void on all pulse sequences (fig. 5.23)
- Susceptibility artifact is demonstrated on gradient-echo images as blooming artifact

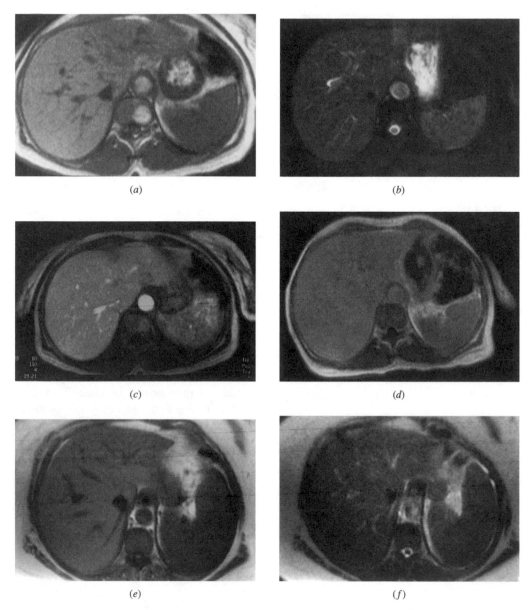

FIGURE 5.22   Sarcoidosis. T1W SGE (*a*), T2W far-suppressed spin-echo (*b*), and immediate (*c*) and 10 min (*d*) post-gadolinium T1W SGE images. Multiple sarcoidosis granulomas, <1 cm, are present in the spleen. Lesions are mildly hypointense to isointense on T1W images (*a*), moderately hypointense on T2W images (*b*), and hypointense on immediate postgadolinium images (*c*), gradually enhancing to near isointensity on delayed postgadolinium images (*d*). Hypointensity on T2W images distinguish these lesions from those of infectious etiologies. (Reproduced with permission from Warshauer DM, Semelka RC, Ascher SM, Nodular sarcoidosis of the liver and spleen: appearance on MR images. *J Magn Reson Imaging* 4:553–557, 1994.)

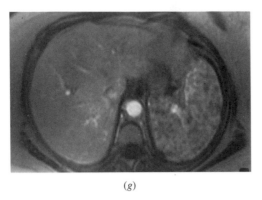

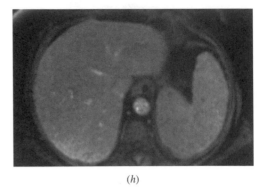

(g)   (h)

FIGURE 5.22 (*Continued*) T1W SGE (*e*), T2W single-shot echo-train spin echo (*f*), immediate postgadolinium T1 single-shot magnetization-prepared gradient-echo (*g*), and 90 s postgadolinium T1W fat-suppressed spin-echo (*h*) images in a second patient. The imaging features are comparable to the above described patient.

○ Lesions appear larger on longer in-phase (TE 4.4 ms at 1.5 T) compared to out-of-phase (TE 2.2 ms) images

  ▪ Calcified granulomas can be signal void on all sequences, but do not change in apparent size comparing in-phase and out-of-phase images

Trauma

Background

• The spleen is the most commonly ruptured abdominal organ in the setting of trauma, which can manifest as

  ○ Subcapsular hematoma
  ○ Contusion
  ○ Laceration with hemorrhage
  ○ Focal infarct or devascularization

• Indications for MR imaging include intolerance to iodinated CT contrast (allergy or renal insufficiency)

Imaging

• Subcapsular or intraparenchymal hematoma secondary to contusion or laceration demonstrates a time course of changes in signal intensity due to the paramagnetic properties of the degradation products of hemoglobin (fig. 5.24)

• Infarcts or devascularization is shown on immediate postgadolinium GRE images as areas of signal void compared to the high signal intensity of vascularized tissue

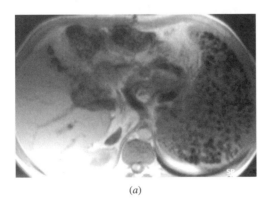

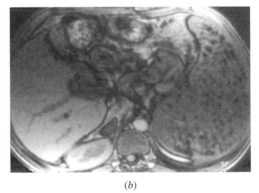

(a)   (b)

FIGURE 5.23   Gamna-Gandy bodies of the spleen. T1W SGE (*a*), T1W out-of-phase SGE (*b*), T2W fat-suppressed single-shot echo-train spin-echo (*c*), immediate postgadolinium T1W SGE (*d*), and 90 s postgadolinium T1W fat-suppressed SGE (*e*) images. Gamna-Gandy bodies are typically multiple and <1 cm in diameter. Gamna-Gandy bodies are near signal void on all imaging sequences, reflecting the magnetic susceptibility effects of iron.

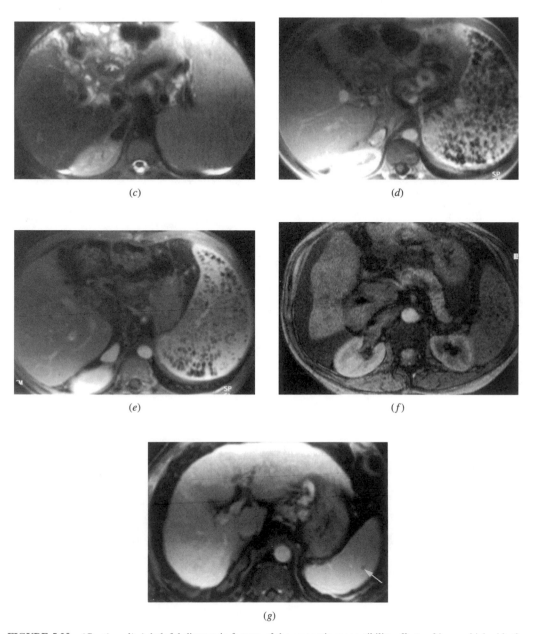

(c) *(d)*

(e) *(f)*

(g)

FIGURE 5.23 *(Continued)* A helpful diagnostic feature of the magnetic susceptibility effects of iron, which aids the distinction from low-fluid-content granulomas, is that the foci of susceptibility artifact appear smaller on the out-of-phase (*b*) compared to the in-phase (*c*) images.

T1-SGE image (*f*) in a second patient with cirrhosis demonstrates multiple <5 mm Gamna-Gandy bodies.

Ninety-second postgadolinium fat-suppressed SGE image (*g*) in a third patient shows a solitary Gamna-Gandy body (arrow, *g*). Note large varices along the lesser curve of the stomach, accentuated with the use of fat suppression.

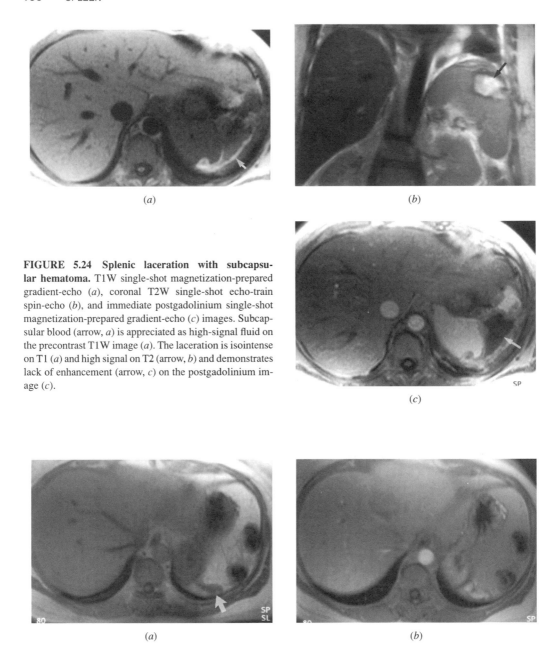

(a)

(b)

FIGURE 5.24 Splenic laceration with subcapsular hematoma. T1W single-shot magnetization-prepared gradient-echo (*a*), coronal T2W single-shot echo-train spin-echo (*b*), and immediate postgadolinium single-shot magnetization-prepared gradient-echo (*c*) images. Subcapsular blood (arrow, *a*) is appreciated as high-signal fluid on the precontrast T1W image (*a*). The laceration is isointense on T1 (*a*) and high signal on T2 (arrow, *b*) and demonstrates lack of enhancement (arrow, *c*) on the postgadolinium image (*c*).

(c)

(a)

(b)

FIGURE 5.25   Splenosis. T1W SGE (*a*), immediate postgadolinium T1W SGE (*b*), and 90 s postgadolinium T1W fat-suppressed SGE (*c*) images. A small elongated mass is present in the left upper abdominal quadrant in a patient with prior splenectomy. The mass is slightly hypointense to the liver on the T1W image (arrow, *a*), with intense enhancement on the immediate postgadolinium image (*b*) and persistent enhancement on the delayed postgadolinium image (*c*). T1W SGE (*d*), coronal T2W echo-train spin-echo (*e*), breath-hold STIR (*f*), immediate postgadolinium T1W SGE (*g*), and 90 s postgadolinium T1W fat-suppressed SGE (*h*) images in a second patient with prior splenectomy. Two splenules are present in the left upper abdomen (arrows, *d*). The masses have an appearance similar to normal spleen, with mild hypointensity on T1 (*d*), moderate hyperintensity on T2 (*e*), and early heterogeneous enhancement (*g*), which becomes more homogeneous on delayed images (*h*).

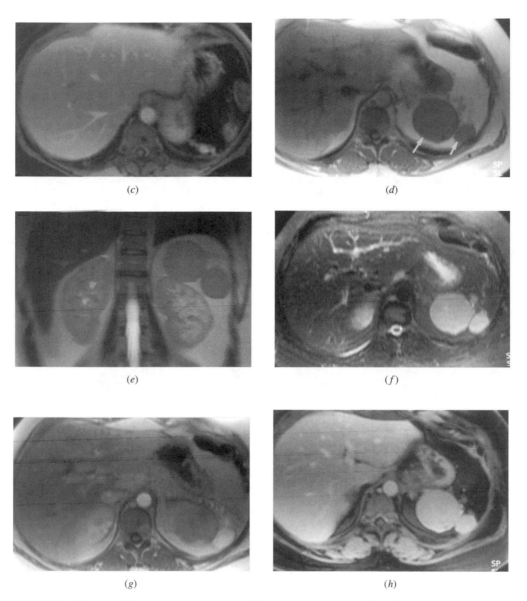

(c) *(d)*

(e) *(f)*

(g) *(h)*

FIGURE 5.25 *(Continued)* Note that the enhancement of the larger mass is less than that of the smaller mass, presumably reflecting a smaller feeding arterial supply.

Splenosis

Background

• Ectopic splenic tissue resulting from splenic injury

Imaging

• Typically solid, well-circumscribed nodules in the abdominal cavity, with signal intensity similar to the normal spleen (fig. 5.25)

Infarcts

Background

• Common occurrence in the setting of obstruction of the splenic artery or one of its branches and in splenomegaly
  ◦ Most common cause is cardiac embol:.

Imaging

• Typically appearing as peripheral wedge-shaped, round, or linear defects that are most

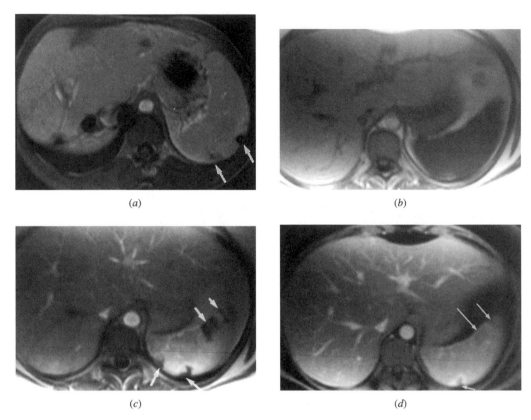

(a)　　　　　　　　　　　　(b)

(c)　　　　　　　　　　　　(d)

FIGURE 5.26　Splenic infarct. One-minute postgadolinium T1W SGE image (a). Peripheral wedge-shaped defects are noted in the spleen (arrows, a) secondary to infarcts.

T1W SGE (b), immediate postgadolinium T1W SGE (c), and 90 s postgadolinium T1W fat-suppressed SGE (d) images in a second patient. An ill-defined posterior subcapsular hyperintensity is present on the T1W image (b). Infarct regions are best seen on postgadolinium images (c, d), and appear as well-defined wedge-shaped defects (arrows, c and d). Peripheral linear enhancement of the capsule may also be appreciated. Note that some of the regions that have no enhancement on the immediate postgadolinium images show delayed enhancement. These are consistent with areas of ischemia.

clearly defined on 1–5 min postgadolinium images as low-signal-intensity wedge-shaped regions (fig. 5.26)

- May occur centrally
- Massive splenic infarcts may appear as diffuse low signal intensity on T1W images and inhomogeneous high signal on T2W images
  ○ Lack of enhancement on early and late postgadolinium images of wedge-shaped regions is the most diagnostic feature

Sickle Cell Disease
Background

- The manifestations of sickle cell anemia vary

and depend on whether the patient is homozygous or heterozygous

Imaging

- Spleen becomes nearly signal void on all sequences due to the sequela of iron deposition from blood transfusions coupled with microscopic perivascular and parenchymal calcifications
- Spleen may become progressively diminished in volume due to repeated infarcts
- These are features usually seen only in homozygous disease

CHAPTER 6

KIDNEYS

BACKGROUND

A useful imaging protocol includes a combination of breath-hold T2W single-shot echo-train coronal and axial images, with at least one plane performed with fat suppression, T1W gradient-echo precontrast axial and coronal, and axial fat-suppressed images, and T1W gadolinium-enhanced arterial capillary and delayed phase images. T1W images using newer 3D GRE combined with gadolinium enhancement has improved spatial resolution for resolving masses and vascular anatomy. T2-like imaging using breath-hold balanced-echo True-FISP imaging may provide additional information for urographic evaluation of the collecting system, with urine having high signal on such images. Additionally, acquisition of pre and postcontrast 3D gradient-echo images performed with identical field of view, resolution, and slice parameters allows for use of the precontrast images as a subtraction mask. The resultant image shows only areas of increased signal due to gadolinium enhancement, which is useful for determining vascularity and tumor within a high signal protein or blood containing renal cyst.

Normal Kidney

- Advantages of MRI include direct multiphase and multiplaner imaging, allowing axial and coronal plane acquisition, and permitting optimal visualization of renal pelvis and poles
- On T1W imaging normal corticomedullary differentiation (CMD) is seen with cortex slightly brighter than skeletal muscle, and medulla relatively dark (fig. 6.1a–h). Inherent CMD is best shown on noncontrast T1W fat-suppressed images.
- On T2W imaging CMD is reversed in contrast to T1W imaging, with brighter signal medulla and lower signal cortex (fig. 6.2a)
- Gadolinium enhancement in the arterial-capillary phase (20 s delay) shows preferential enhancement of the cortex
- The renal medulla begins to enhance at 1–1.5 min postinjection. Excretion of contrast into the renal pelvis commences at 2.5 min

Normal Variants

- Prominent columns of Bertin (fig. 6.3)
- Persistent fetal lobulation (fig. 6.4)

Primer on MR Imaging of the Abdomen and Pelvis, edited by Diego R. Martin, Michele A. Brown, and Richard C. Semelka ISBN 0-471-37340-0 Copyright © 2005 Wiley-Liss, Inc.

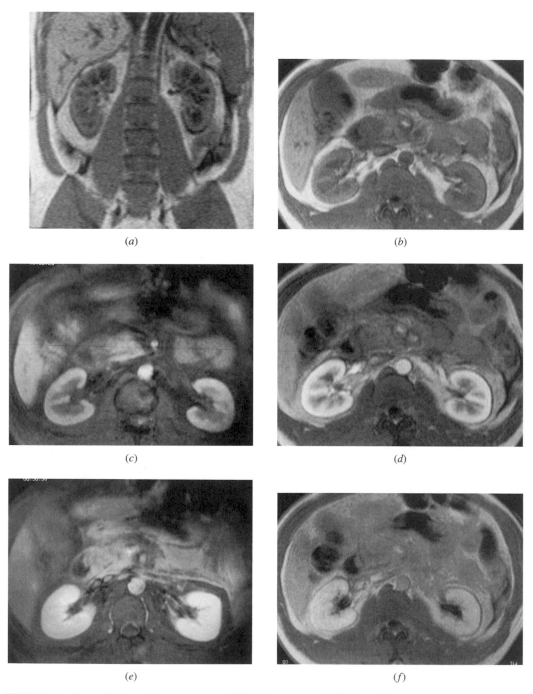

FIGURE 6.1   Normal kidneys. Precontrast coronal SGE (*a*), precontrast SGE (*b*), T1W fat-suppressed spin-echo (*c*), immediate postgadolinium SGE (*d*), gadolinium-enhanced T1W fat-suppressed spin-echo (*e*), 8 min postgadolinium transverse (*f*), and 8.5 min coronal (*g*) gadolinium-enhanced SGE images. Corticomedullary differentiation is shown on precontrast T1W images (*a–c*), and on immediate postgadolinium SGE (*d*) images. Corticomedullary differentiation is most clearly defined on the precontrast T1W fat-suppressed image (*c*) and the immediate postgadolinium SGE image (*d*).

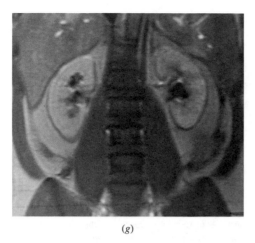

(g)

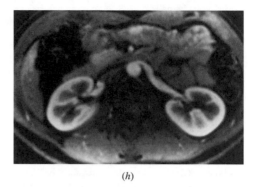

(h)

FIGURE 6.1 (*Continued*) Immediate postgadolinium fat-suppressed SGE image (*h*) in a second patient demonstrates intense cortical enhancement and good demonstration of high-signal-intensity gadolinium-containing left renal vein. Sharp definition of the outer renal cortex is shown because of the suppression of fat.

- Malposition
  - Malrotation (fig. 6.5)
  - Ectopic
    - Ptotic (pelvic) kidney (fig. 6.6)
    - Crossed fused ectopia (fig. 6.7)
- Horseshoe (fig. 6.8)
- Duplication of collecting system (fig. 6.9)
- Hyperplastic kidney (fig. 6.10)

Renal Cysts

- Background
  - MR is the best modality for assessment of cystic lesions

- Renal cysts represent the most common focal lesion in adults
  - As cyst complexity increases, the risk of neoplasm increases
  - Neoplasm features include
    - Irregular and thick septations (>3 mm)
    - Irregular and thick wall or capsule
    - Solid vascular soft tissue components
    - Although CT is the most accurate modality for assessment of calcifications related to cysts, detection of calcium is not necessarily diagnostically important
- Simple Cysts (fig. 6.11)
  - No perceptible wall or septations, and simple free fluid signal internally

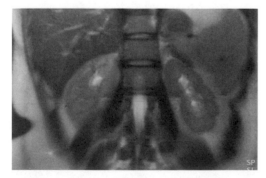

FIGURE 6.2 Fetal lobulation. Coronal single-shot echo-train spin-echo (SS-ETSE) (*a*), and transverse immediate postgadolinium SGE (*b*) images. The coronal SS-ETSE image (*a*) demonstrates an undulating contour of the entire left kidney. The immediate postgadolinium SGE image demonstrates uniform cortical thickness, excluding the presence of a mass.

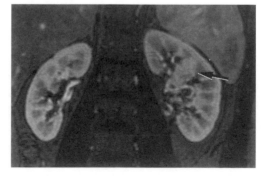

FIGURE 6.3 Prominent column of Bertin. Coronal postgadolinium gradient-echo image. Bertin column (arrow) follows a continuous contour and remains isointense with the renal cortex.

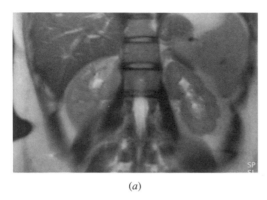

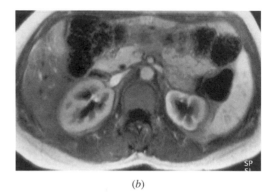

(*a*)   (*b*)

FIGURE 6.4   Fetal lobulation. Coronal single-shot echo-train spin-echo (SS-ETSE) (*a*), and transverse immediate post-gadolinium SGE (*b*) images. The coronal SS-ETSE image (*a*) demonstrates an undulating contour of the entire left kidney. The immediate postgadolinium SGE image demonstrates uniform cortical thickness, excluding the presence of a mass.

- Complex Cysts
  - Septated
    - Low complexity—nonsurgical (fig. 6.12)
    - Moderately high complexity (fig. 6.13)
      - On surgical pathology, this case showed hemorrhage, wall thickening, and calcification, but no malignancy
      - Based on imaging findings, appropriate clinical course requires surgical removal or serial imaging follow-up
      - Calcification can interfere with ultrasound and CT assessment of underlying soft tissue enhancement, but is not problematic on MR
  - Hemorrhagic (figs. 6.14 and 6.15)
    - The majority of hemorrhagic cysts are benign

- Rarely, cystic neoplasm or papillary cystic renal cell carcinoma can present as a hemorrhagic cyst. Therefore, hemorrhagic cysts should be followed by repeat imaging to show stability or resolution. This is especially true for patients with chronic renal failure.
- Cysts with high protein content are generally in distinguishable from hemorrhagic cysts

- Congenital
  - Polycystic Kidney Disease
    - Autosomal dominant (fig. 6.16)
      - Bilateral renal involvement
      - Kidneys massively enlarged with renal architecture distorted by cysts throughout parenchyma

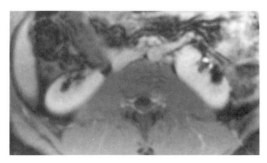

FIGURE 6.5   Malrotation. Postgadolinium T1W fat-suppressed SGE image. The most common form of malrotation is anterior orientation of the pelvis.

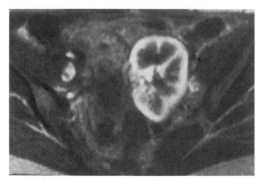

FIGURE 6.6   Pelvic kidney. Immediate postgadolinium SGE image.

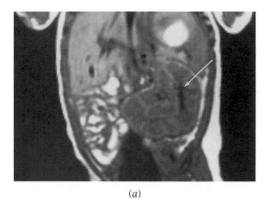 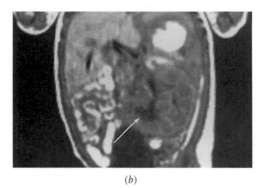

(a)   (b)

FIGURE 6.7   Crossed-fused ectopy. Coronal T1W spin-echo images (*a, b*) demonstrate fusion of a small inferomedial kidney to the normal-sized and -positioned left kidney. Clear depiction is rendered by the definition of CMD. The collecting system of the normally positioned left kidney is normal in size (arrow, *a*), whereas the crossed-fused right kidney has a mildly dilated collecting system (arrow, *b*).

- Hemmorhage into some cysts is invariably present
- Often have coexistent liver cysts, with pancreatic cysts uncommon
- Uncertain increased risk of malignancy over background incidence in general population. Detection of renal neoplasms is more difficult because of the difficulty of distinguishing enhancing tumor from heterogeneous signal hemorrhagic cysts
- Autosomal recessive (fig. 6.17)

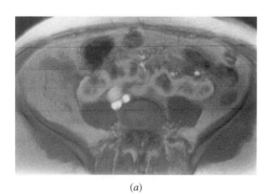 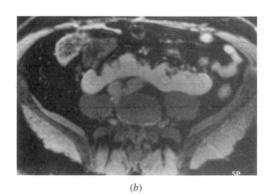

(a)   (b)

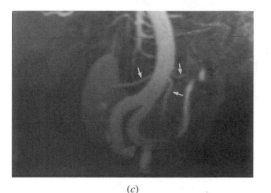

(c)

FIGURE 6.8   Horseshoe kidney. Immediate postgadolinium SGE (*a*) and gadolinium-enhanced T1W fat-suppressed SGE (*b*) images. The presence of corticomedullary differentiation (CMD) on the immediate postcontrast image (*a*) demonstrates that the retroperitoneal mass is a horseshoe kidney and that the isthmus contains functional renal parenchyma. Uniform enhancement of the renal parenchyma is present on later images (*b*). Coronal gadolinium-enhanced 3D FISP demonstrates the horseshoe shape of this anomaly, and the renal arteries are well displayed (arrows, *c*).

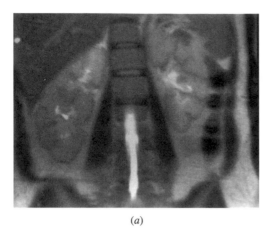

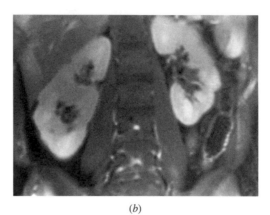

(a)   (b)

FIGURE 6.9   Duplex collecting system. Coronal SS-ETSE (a) and postgadolinium T1W fat-suppressed SGE (b) images demonstrate a patient with a duplicated collecting system in the right kidney. Note the thick column of Bertin separating the two pelves.

- Represents a disease spectrum
- Renal cysts present at birth
- Malformation of the collecting tubules and liver bile ducts leading to cystic dillesionson in kidneys, with cysts <1 cm
- Liver may variably show signs of small cysts, or irregulary dilated ducts, or fibrosis. Pathology always shows hepatic fibrosis.
- Most patients die by 1 year of age, but milder forms occur, with patients living longer, but usually less than 10 years

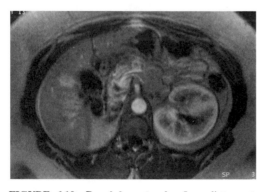

FIGURE 6.10   Renal hypertrophy. Immediate postgadolinium SGE image demonstrates generalized enlargement of the left kidney with uniform thickness of renal cortex. This adult patient had undergone a right nephrectomy.

○ Multicystic Dysplastic Kidney (MCDK) (fig. 6.18)
  - Developmental abnormality with failure of induction of the metanephric kidney by the growing ureteric bud
  - Kidney develops multiple non-connecting cysts. Renal size may be large, abnormality is apparent in the fetus or infant
  - Kidney is non-functional, and eventually atrophies and may disappear
  - Condition is lethal when MCDK occurs in both kidneys
  - Fetal hydronephrosis is distinguished from MCDK by showing fluid filled dilated collecting system spaces that connect
  - Multi-planar single shot echo-train T2W imaging is the most important sequence to evaluate these cysts
○ Tuberous Sclerosis (fig. 6.19)
  - One of the neurocutaneous phakomatoses syndromes
  - Autosomal dominant inheritance, but up to 50% are spontaneous
  - Characterized by developmental delay, epilepsy, and cutaneous lesions
  - Kidneys frequently develop cysts and angiomyolipomas (AML), occuring in 70%–95% of affected individuals, usually

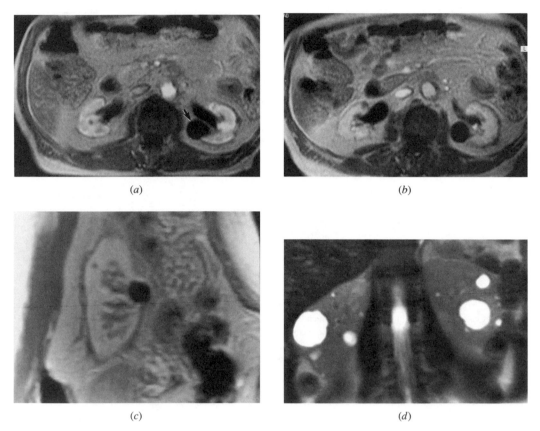

(a)   *(b)*

(c)   *(d)*

FIGURE 6.11   Renal cyst. Immediate (*a*) and 5 min (*b*) postgadolinium SGE images. A cyst is present arising from the posterior aspect of the left kidney. The cyst demonstrates signal void, sharply marginated, and has no definable wall on the immediate postgadolinium image (arrow, *a*). No change in the appearance of the cyst occurs on the delayed postcontrast image (*b*).

Sagittal 5 min postgadolinium SGE image (*c*) of the left kidney in a second patient demonstrates a sharp superior and inferior margin of the renal cyst confirming that it is a simple cyst.

SS-ETSE image (*d*) in a third patient shows multiple bilateral simple renal cysts.

appearing as multiple and bilateral renal lesions
- AML usually exhibit growth, and may undergo hemorrhage
- Uncertain increased risk of renal cell carcinoma (RCC)
  ○ von Hippel–Lindau Disease (fig. 6.20)
    - Another neurocutaneous phakomatoses syndrome
    - Autosomal-dominant inheritance
    - Kidneys frequently develop cysts and often develop adenomas and carcinomas, which may arise in proximity to cysts

- Although renal carcinomas may be multiple with continued new occurrences, these cancers are usually low-grade tumors and may be controlled by nephron-sparing partial nephrectomies
- Breath-hold fat-suppressed T1W SGE postgadolinium imaging is most sensitive for the detection of small tumors
- Patients may also develop hepatic and pancreatic cysts, and rarely pancreatic islet cell tumors
- Patients are well followed by repeat MR scans, avoiding repeat ionizing radiation exposure and iodinated contrast loads

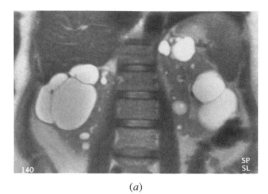

(a)

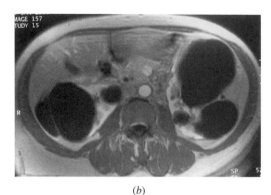

(b)

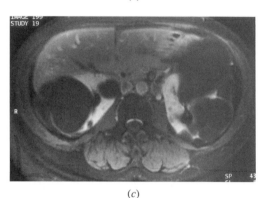

(c)

FIGURE 6.12 Septated renal cysts. Coronal SS-ETSE (*a*), immediate postgadolinium SGE (*b*), and 90 s postgadolinium fat-suppressed SGE (*c*) images. Multiple closely grouped cysts are presented in both kidneys, which create an appearance of multicystic masses (*a*). Renal parenchyma enhances normally (*b*), and the cysts do not change in size and shape on serial postgadolinium images (*b, c*) with no internal enhancement demonstrated.

associated with CT imaging. Ultrasound has insufficient sensitivity and specificity, partly due to the extensive nature of renal lesions.

○ Medullary Cystic Disease (fig. 6.21)
  ▪ Associated with impaired renal function with salt-wasting nephropathy
  ▪ Most often present in adolescent patients
  ▪ Renal parenchyma in the medullary distribution becomes progressively replaced with 1–2 cm cysts
  ▪ Renal cortex atrophies, maintaining a smooth contour
○ Medullary Sponge Kidney (MSK) (fig. 6.22)
  ▪ Characterized by the development of cystic or ectatic distal collecting tubules
  ▪ May form calculi in the ectatic ducts, which may be discharged into the urinary collecting system, with the potential for developing urinary tract obstruction

  ▪ May develop renal tubular acidosis related to impaired function of the distal tubules
  ▪ Pattern of disease is variable, including unilateral, bilateral, diffuse, or segmental
  ▪ May only be demonstrated on postgadolinium interstitial phase T1W images, seen as an exuberant papillary blush (fig. 6.22)
○ Multilocular Cystic Nephroma (fig. 6.23)
  ▪ Rare benign disease, typically unilateral and solitary
  ▪ Often is observed in a bimodal distribution, both in infants from 2 months to 4 years of age, and in young adults over 20 years of age, although earlier reports suggested occurrence was most common in females over 40 years of age
  ▪ Characteristic findings include a large multiseptated cyst with septations up to 4 mm in thickness, with bulging of the lesion into the renal pelvis

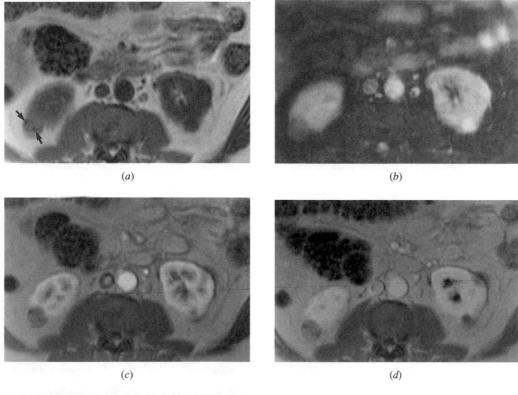

(a) (b)

(c) (d)

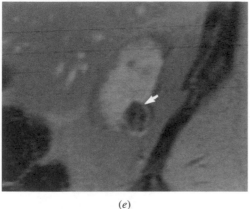

(e)

FIGURE 6.13 Cyst complicated by the presence of calcification, blood, and thickened wall. Precontrast SGE (*a*), T2W fat-suppressed spin-echo (*b*), immediate (*c*) and 8 min transverse (*d*), and 8.5 min sagittal (*e*) postgadolinium SGE images. A lesion arises from the posterior aspect of the right kidney, which is mixed in signal intensity and contains signal void calcifications (arrows, *a*) on the precontrast SGE image. The lesion is mildly low in signal intensity on the T2W image (*b*), which mimics the appearance of a solid tumor. The complicated cyst remains moderate in signal intensity on postcontrast images, but it is sharply defined from adjacent cortex and does not change in size or shape between early (*c*) and late (*d, e*) postcontrast images. The superior margin of the cyst is well defined on the sagittal image (arrow, *e*).

- Cysts can show high signal internally on pregadolinium T1W images due to protein or blood products
- Acquired Cystic Disease of Dialysis (fig. 6.24)
  - Related to long-term end-stage renal disease combined with long-term hemodialysis
  - Kidneys commonly develop multiple cortical cysts 1–2 cm in diameter
  - Kidneys remain small (end stage), and cysts are typically exophytic
  - Commonly a sizable proportion of the cysts will have high signal intensity on T1W images related to protein or hemorrhage
  - Increased risk of RCC
    - RCC is shown on breath-hold T1W SGE images as vascularized tissue showing gadolinium enhancement

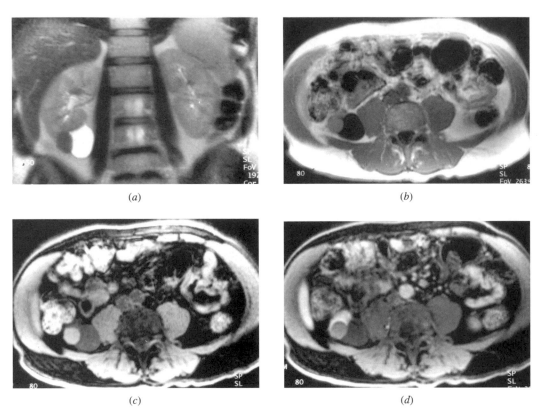

(a)   (b)

(c)   (d)

FIGURE 6.14 **Simple and hemorrhagic cysts.** Coronal SS-ETSE (*a*), axial precontrast T1W SGE (*b*), precontrast T1W fat-suppressed SGE (*c*), and 90 s gadolinium-enhanced T1W fat-suppressed SGE (*d*) images. Exophytic simple and hemorrhagic renal cysts are side-by-side arising from the lower pole of the right kidney. The hemorrhagic cyst shows increased T1 signal (*b, c*) and decreased T2 signal (*a*), signal behavior opposite that of the simple cyst.

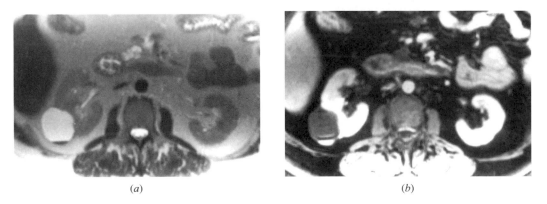

(a)   (b)

FIGURE 6.15 **Hemorrhagic cyst.** SS-ETSE (*a*) and postgadolinium T1W fat-suppressed SGE (*b*) images. A cyst in the right kidney demonstrates layering material that is low signal on T2 (*a*) and increased signal on T1 (*b*), consistent with hemorrhage.

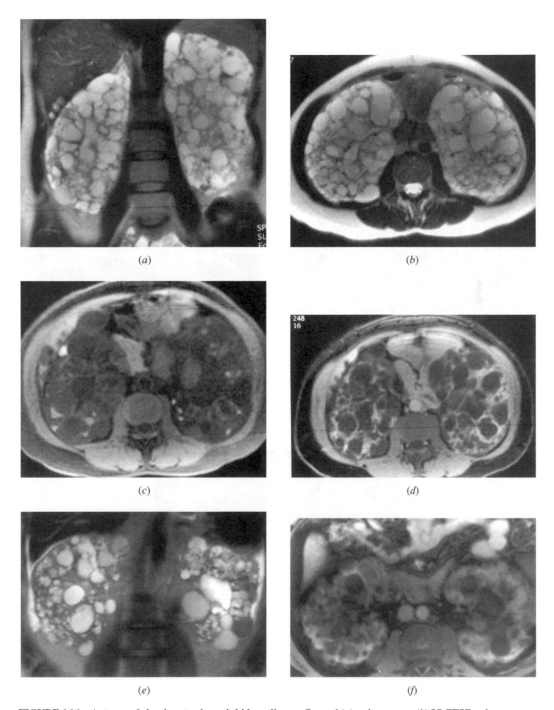

FIGURE 6.16   Autosomal-dominant polycystic kidney disease. Coronal (*a*) and transverse (*b*) SS-ETSE and precontrast (*c*), and postgadolinium (*d*) T1W fat-suppressed SGE images. The kidneys are greatly enlarged with numerous cysts. The majority of the cysts demonstrate increased T2 signal and decreased T1 signal consistent with simple cysts, but a sizable fraction have varying signal consistent with blood products of differing age. Postgadolinium images demonstrate no dominant enhancing areas worrisome for neoplasm.

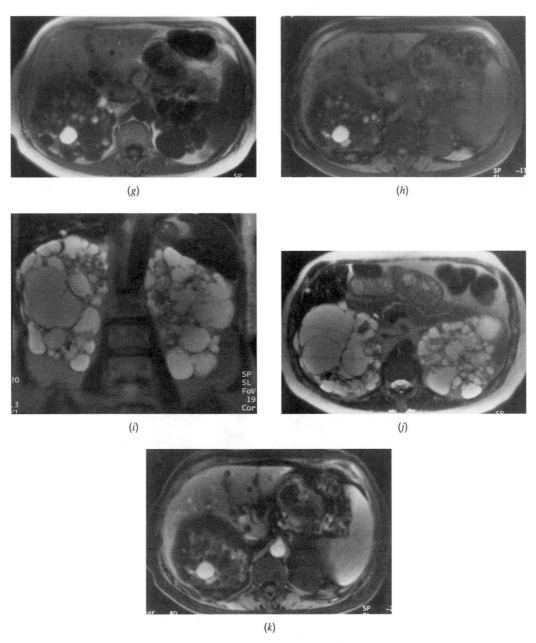

(g) *(h)*

(i) *(j)*

(k)

FIGURE 6.16 *(Continued)* Coronal SS-ETSE (*e*) and axial postcontrast fat-suppressed SGE (*f*) images in a second patient show the same findings described above. Evaluation for neoplasm in cystic kidneys such as these is difficult because of the varying signal of cysts. SGE (g), fat-suppressed SGE (h), coronal SS-ETSE (*i*), transverse SS-ETSE (*j*), and 90 s postgadolinium fat-suppressed SGE (*k*) images in a third patient. The kidneys are massively enlarged and contain multiple cysts of varying sizes scattered throughout the renal parenchyma, distorting renal architecture. Several cysts are high in signal intensity on T1W images (*g*), and the high signal intensity is accentuated on the fat-suppressed T1W image (*h*). The hemorrhagic cysts vary in signal intensity on T2W images (*h, i*), consistent with blood products of varying age. Minimal enhancing parenchyma is apparent after gadolinium (*k*).

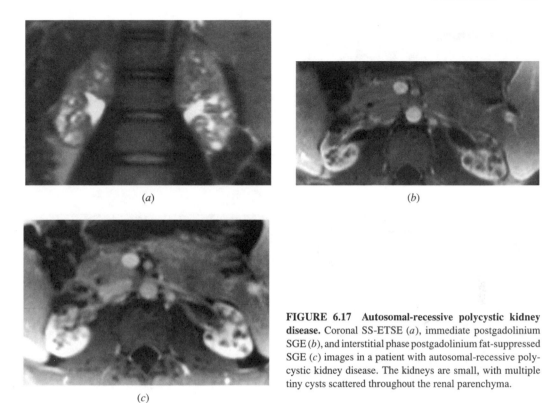

(a)

(b)

(c)

FIGURE 6.17 Autosomal-recessive polycystic kidney disease. Coronal SS-ETSE (*a*), immediate postgadolinium SGE (*b*), and interstitial phase postgadolinium fat-suppressed SGE (*c*) images in a patient with autosomal-recessive polycystic kidney disease. The kidneys are small, with multiple tiny cysts scattered throughout the renal parenchyma.

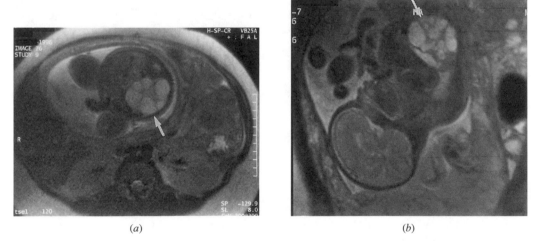

(a)

(b)

FIGURE 6.18 Multicystic dysplastic kidney in fetus. Transverse (*a*) and sagittal (*b*) SS-ETSE images of a fetus demonstrate a multicystic mass in the left renal fossa (arrow, *a*, *b*) with no evidence of organization into a renal collecting system.

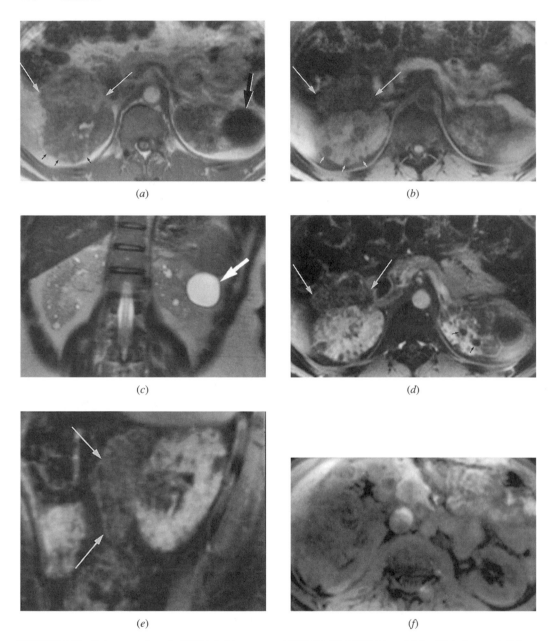

FIGURE 6.19   Tuberous sclerosis. SGE (*a*), fat-suppressed SGE (*b*), SS-ETSE (*c*), and interstitial phase gadolinium-enhanced transverse (*d*) and sagittal (*e*) fat-suppressed SGE images. Numerous varying-size angiomyolipomas are present throughout both kidneys (small arrows, *a*) including a large exophytic angiomyolipoma with multiple high-signal-intensity punctuate foci of fat (long arrows, *a*). Multiple cysts are also present (large arrow, *a*). On the precontrast fat-suppressed image, the numerous small angiomyolipomas (small arrows, *b*) and the large angiomyolipoma (long arrows, *b*) decrease in signal intensity. The numerous angiomyolipomas and cysts (arrow, *c*) are high in signal intensity on the SS-ETSE image (*c*). After gadolinium administration the kidneys are shown to be extensively replaced by angiomyolipomas and cysts (small arrows, *d*). The large exophytic angiomyolipoma (long arrows, *d*, *e*) is well shown on transverse (*d*) and sagittal (*e*) postgadolinium fat-suppressed SGE images.

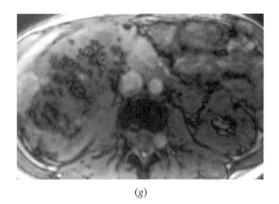

(g)

FIGURE 6.19 (*Continued*) SGE (*f*) and out-of-phase (*g*) images in a second patient demonstrate a large heterogeneous mass within the right kidney and multiple small lesions in the left kidney. Note the dramatic phase-cancellation artifact in both kidneys on the out-of-phase sequence, confirming the presence of fat in numerous angiomyolipomas scattered throughout both kidneys.

- Cysts do not enhance
  - In cases of high signal cysts on T1W images, sensitivity for enhancement may be improved by using 3D GRE T1W pre- and postgadolinium imaging, subtracting the pregadolinium image as a mask. This resulting subtraction image will show signal only where there is enhancement above the background signal of the cyst, thereby revealing vascularized tumor.

Solid Masses

Benign

Angiomyolipoma (AML)
- Background
  - Benign tumors composed of variable amounts of three elements:

  - thick-walled blood vessels
  - smooth muscle
  - mature adipocytes
    - The fat component predominates and is the basis for characterization in 80–90% of lesions
  - Larger tumors have increased risk of undergoing hemorrhage
- Imaging
  - Diagnosis based on detecting fat seen as a mass with
    - Loss of signal on fat-suppressed T1W GRE breath-hold images (fig. 6.25)
    - Signal-void phase cancellation around the periphery of the lesion that abuts renal parenchyma. This signal-void phase cancellation may occupy the entire lesion if it is very small.

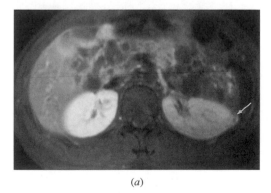

(a)

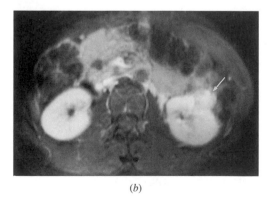

(b)

FIGURE 6.20   von Hippel-Lindau disease. Gadolinium-enhanced T1W fat-suppressed spin-echo images (*a, b*). Two small renal cancers are present in the mid- (arrow, *a*) and lower (arrow, *b*) pole of the left kidney. Multiple pancreatic cysts are also appreciated (*a*).

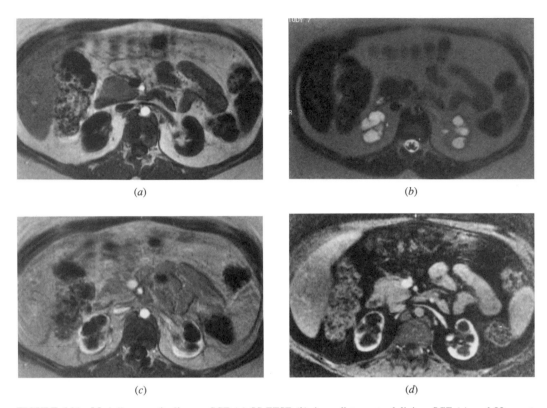

(a)   (b)

(c)   (d)

FIGURE 6.21   Medullary cystic disease. SGE (a) SS-ETSE (b), immediate postgadolinium SGE (c), and 90 s post-gadolinium T1W fat-suppressed SGE (d) images. Multiple cysts measuring <2 cm in diameter occupy the majority of the renal medulla. These simulate the appearance of corticomedullary differentiation on precontrast images (a) in this patient with chronic renal failure. The cysts are homogeneously high in signal intensity on the T2W image (b). After gadolinium administration, cysts in the renal medulla do not enhance and appear nearly signal void (c, d).

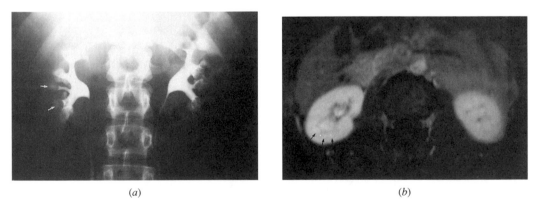

(a)   (b)

FIGURE 6.22   Medullary sponge kidney. Five-minute intravenous urogram (a) and interstitial phase gadolinium-enhanced T1W fat-suppressed spin-echo (b) images. Tubular ectasia is apparent on the intravenous urogram (arrows, a). On the interstitial phase gadolinium-enhanced image (b), prominent papillary enhancement is present (arrows, b).

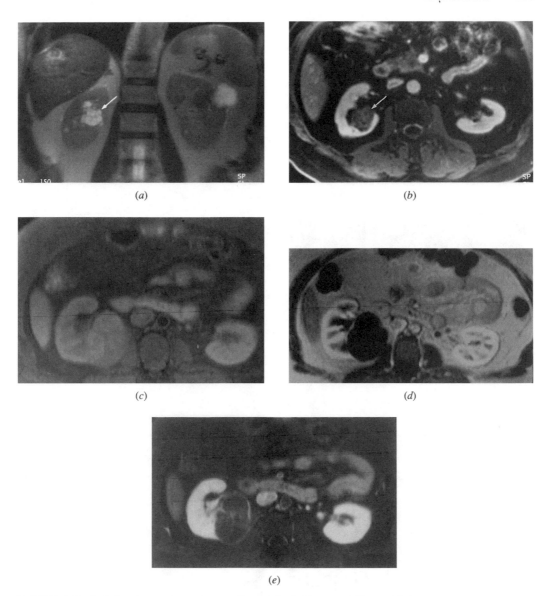

(a)

(b)

(c)

(d)

(e)

FIGURE 6.23 Multilocular cystic nephroma. Coronal SS-ETSE (*a*) and 90 s gadolinium-enhanced fat-suppressed SGE (*b*) images. A well-defined cystic mass arises from the posterior aspect of the right kidney. Internal septations are present, which are low in signal intensity on the T2W image (arrow, *a*) and enhance on the postcontrast T1W image (arrow, *b*). The lesion is noted to bulge into the renal pelvis. These imaging features are typical for multilocular cystic nephroma. This location is also common, arising in the posterior cortex of the kidney at the midrenal level.

T1W fat-suppressed spin-echo (*c*), immediate postgadolinium SGE (*d*), and gadolinium-enhanced T1W fat-suppressed spin-echo images (*e*) in a second patient with multilocular cystic nephroma demonstrate a similar-appearing cystic mass that bulges into the renal pelvis and contains enhancing internal septations. Note that the cyst contents are intermediate in signal intensity on the precontrast T1W image (*c*).

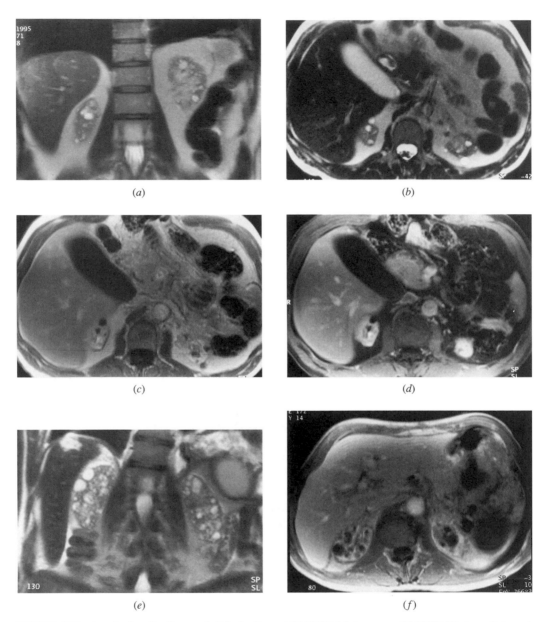

(a)   (b)

(c)   (d)

(e)   (f)

FIGURE 6.24 Acquired cystic disease of dialysis. Coronal SS-ETSE (a), transverse SS-ETSE (b), immediate post-gadolinium SGE (c), and gadolinium-enhanced T1W fat-suppressed SGE (d) images. Multiple cysts <2 cm in diameter are present in both kidneys located predominantly in a superficial cortical location. The capillary phase of enhancement (c) demonstrates minimal parenchymal enhancement and no corticomedullary differentiation. On the gadolinium-enhanced T1W fat-suppressed spin-echo image (d), multiple renal cysts are well shown in background of moderately enhanced atrophic parenchymal tissue. Coronal SS-ETSE (e) and interstitial phase gadolinium-enhanced fat-suppressed SGE (f) images in a second patient on chronic hemodialysis with Alport syndrome. Multiple small cysts are scattered throughout the kidneys.

○ Hemorrhagic products may be seen in acute/subacute cases as variable signal on T1W and T2W images

- Evidence of fat and presence of other characteristic angiomyolipomas in the same or contralateral kidney support the diagnosis
- No evidence of fat in a solitary lesion that contains blood products may obscure the diagnosis
- AML with predominance of vascular/muscle components and absence of fat appears as an enhancing mass lesion
  - Overlap appearance with RCC

○ Mimickers

- RCC with fatty elements
  - Fat in AML is typically diffuse
  - Enhancing AMLs tend to appear uniformly enhancing, contrasting the typically heterogeneous enhancement pattern of RCC
  - Rarely RCC may contain fat, but this generally appears as focal deposits within the mass
    ○ A heterogeneous T1W/T2W signal intensity, irregularly enhancing mass with focal fat shown on fat-suppressed T1W GRE images should be considered suspicious for RCC

Adenoma

- Background
  - ○ Renal adenomas are benign tumors of renal cell origin and typically are small solid neoplasms
  - ○ The relationship of adenomas to renal cell carcinomas is uncertain
  - ○ Adenomas are indistinguishable from papillary renal cell cancers on imaging studies
  - ○ Tumor growth raises the concern of malignancy
  - ○ Suggested imaging follow-up protocol for an indeterminate mass is 3 months, 6 months, 1 year, and yearly thereafter
  - ○ In elderly patients, close observation appears to be prudent to minimize morbidity
  - ○ Oncocytoma is a subtype
    - Benign epithelial tumors
    - Usually solid with central stellate scar

- Imaging
  - ○ Typically small round masses (<4 cm)
  - ○ Slightly hypointense on T1W images
  - ○ Slightly hyperintense on T2W images
  - ○ Enhance diffusely and intensely on early arterial capillary phase images (20 s)
  - ○ Oncocytoma (fig. 6.26)
    - May show on gadolinium-enhanced T1W GRE imaging with early central arterial capillary and venous enhancement with spoke-wheel configuration
    - RCC generally enhances peripherally
      - Overlap in appearance does not facilitate reliable distinction

Malignant
Renal Cell Carcinoma

- Background
  - ○ Renal malignancy is the fifth leading cause of cancer-related mortality in North America and RCC is responsible for 85%
  - ○ MR has been shown to be slightly more sensitive and specific for primary renal tumors and markedly more sensitive and specific for the demonstration of liver metastases than CT
    - Specific indications for contrast-enhanced MRI over CT include
      - CT contrast allergy
      - Impaired renal function
      - Solitary kidney, as with post-RCC resection follow-up imaging
      - Indeterminate lesion on CT
        ○ Hypovascular lesion
        ○ Lesion obscured by calcifications
      - Prior to nephron-sparing surgery for suspected solitary RCC, as CT and ultrasound miss 50% of additional lesions smaller than 1 cm
      - Patients with chronic renal insufficiency screened for tumor development
  - ○ RCC rarely metastasizes before reaching 5 cm in size
  - ○ Growth rates of primary and metastatic lesions may be very slow, in some cases showing no change over a 1-year period
  - ○ Related conditions
    - Chronic renal insufficiency and dialysis (7% risk of RCC)

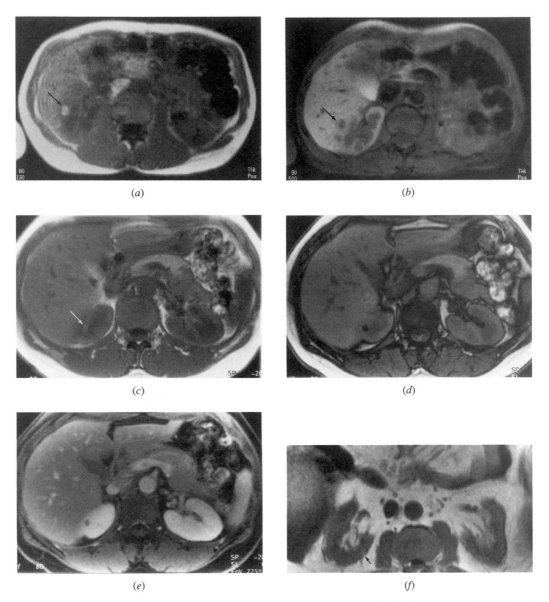

(a)   *(b)*

(c)   *(d)*

(e)   *(f)*

FIGURE 6.25 Small angiomyolipoma. SGE (*a*) and T1W fat-suppressed spin-echo (*b*) images. A small high-signal-intensity lesion arises from the upper pole of the right kidney on the SGE image (arrow, *a*). Fat suppression decreases the signal intensity of this lesion (arrow, *b*), confirming that it represents an angiomyolipoma.

SGE (*c*), out-of-phase SGE (*d*), and interstitial phase gadolinium-enhanced fat-suppressed SGE (*e*) images in a second patient demonstrate a high-signal-intensity tumor on the in-phase image (arrow, *c*) that becomes signal void on the out-of-phase image (*d*) due to phase-cancellation artifact. The lesion is very low in the signal of the postgadolinium fat-suppressed SGE image (*e*).

SGE (*f*), fat-suppressed SGE (*g*) and out-of-phase SGE (*h*) images in a third patient. A 6 mm angiomyolipoma is present in the right kidney that is high in signal intensity on the in-phase image (arrow, *f*), suppresses to low signal intensity on the fat-suppressed image (arrow, *g*), and is signal void on the out-of-phase image (arrow, *h*).

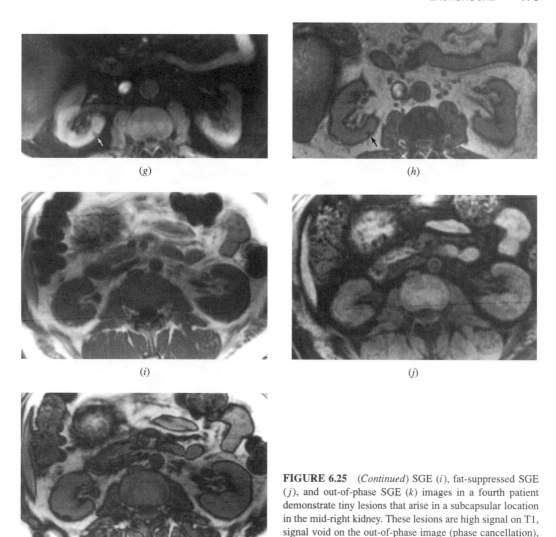

(g)

(h)

(i)

(j)

FIGURE 6.25 (*Continued*) SGE (*i*), fat-suppressed SGE (*j*), and out-of-phase SGE (*k*) images in a fourth patient demonstrate tiny lesions that arise in a subcapsular location in the mid-right kidney. These lesions are high signal on T1, signal void on the out-of-phase image (phase cancellation), and low signal on fat-suppressed images (fat suppression effect).

(k)

- RCC commonly tends to be hypovascular
- Cysts are common in these patients and frequently develop as hemorrhagic or proteinaceous cysts
  - ○ Requires careful analysis by pre- and post-T1W 2D/3D GRE breath-hold gadolinium-enhanced delayed images to determine possible presence of tumor
    - ▪ Using 3D technique, subtraction imaging may further increase sensitivity
      - ▪ If negative for enhancement, hemorrhagic cysts should still be monitored with serial imaging
  - ○ Staging
    - ▪ Robson's staging for RCC
      - • Stage 1: Mass confined within renal capsule (fig. 6.27)
      - • Stage 2: Extension beyond capsule (fig. 6.28)

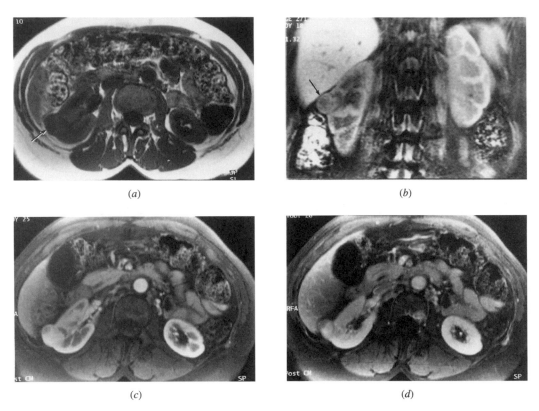

(a)   *(b)*

(c)   *(d)*

FIGURE 6.26   Renal oncocytoma. SGE (*a*), coronal fat-suppressed SGE (*b*), immediate postgadolinium SGE (*c*), and 90 s gadolinium-enhanced fat-suppressed SGE (*d*) images. A well-defined 2 cm mass is present in the right kidney (arrow, *a*, *b*). The majority of the tumor enhances in a moderately intense fashion on the immediate postgadolinium image (*c*) and shows mild peripheral washout by 90 s (*d*). The appearance is indistinguishable from that of a small renal cancer.

- Stage 3
  - ◦ Stage 3a: Extension into renal vein—IVC—right atrium (fig. 6.29)
  - ◦ Stage 3b: Lymph node involvement (fig. 6.30)
  - ◦ Stage 3c: Both vein and lymph node involvement (fig. 6.31)
- Stage 4
  - ◦ Stage 4a: Direct extension through the perirenal fascia into the pararenal space (fig. 6.32)
  - ◦ Stage 4b: Distant metastases (fig. 6.33)
- ◦ Imaging
  - ▪ Slightly hypointense on T1W and irregularly hyperintense on T2W breath-hold images
  - ▪ May appear near isointense to renal cortex on pregadolinium images

- ▪ Gadolinium-enhanced images are essential; most (70%) cancers are hypervascular, showing early intense heterogeneous enhancement. A sizable minority (30%) are hypovascular and exhibit small rounded and linear foci of enhancement throughout the mass. Larger tumors (>5 cm) generally possess hypovascular central areas consistent with necrosis (fig. 6.29).
- ▪ Gadolinium-enhanced T1W images should be obtained, at least in the delayed equilibrium phase, using a breath-hold fat-suppressed 3D GRE sequence
  - • This provides high-resolution imaging of the kidneys, blood vessels, and adjacent abdominal organs, and permits reformatting into additional planes if necessary

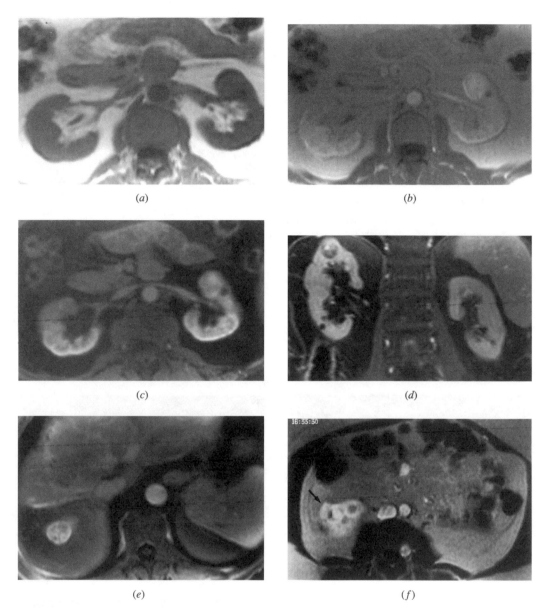

(a)

(b)

(c)

(d)

(e)

(f)

FIGURE 6.27   Renal cell cancer—Stage 1. SGE (a), 45 s postgadolinium SGE (b), 90 s gadolinium-enhanced fat-suppressed SGE (c) images. There is a lesion in the anterior aspect of the mid-pole of the left kidney that is heterogeneous in signal intensity on T1W images and enhances markedly postgadolinium administration, consistent with a renal cell carcinoma. Adjacent to this lesion, a tiny simple cyst is noted.

Coronal (d) and transverse (e) 2–3 min postgadolinium fat-suppressed SGE images in a second patient. A 2 cm renal cell cancer arises from the upper pole of the right kidney that exhibits heterogeneous enhancement on interstitial phase images.

Immediate postgadolinium SGE (f) and 7 min postgadolinium sagittal SGE (g) images in a third patient. A small renal cancer arises from the lower pole of the right kidney. The tumor demonstrates marked enhancement immediately after contrast administration (arrow, f) and diminished enhancement on the delayed postcontrast SGE image (arrow, g).

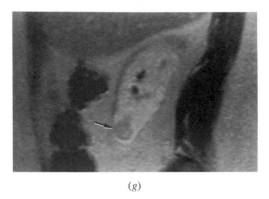

(g)

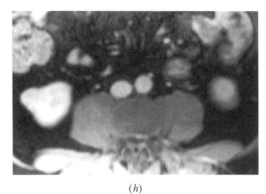

(h)

FIGURE 6.27   (*Continued*) Ninety-second postgadolinium fat-suppressed SGE image (*h*) in a fourth patient. There is a small lesion in the upper pole of the right kidney that shows marked enhancement after administration of gadolinium.

- Precontrast mask image series may be obtained to increase conspicuity of subtle enhancement by subtracting from postcontrast images, which may be useful in the evaluation of high signal cysts
  - Occasionally, small tumors (<2 cm), may show uniform intense, diffuse enhance-

ment on arterial phase images and rapid washout (fig. 6.34)
- Lesions may contain hemorrhage (fig. 6.35)
- Rarely, tumors may appear predominantly cystic (fig. 6.36), and may mimic multilocular cystic nephroma

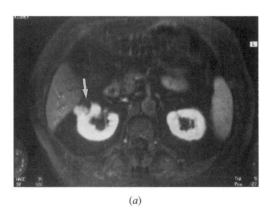

(a)

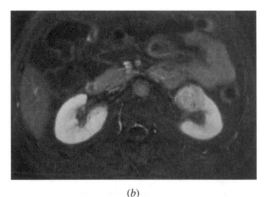

(b)

FIGURE 6.28   Renal cell cancer—Stage 2. Gadolinium-enhanced T1W fat-suppressed spin-echo images in three patients (*a–c*). Stage 2 cancer can vary in size from small (*a*) to large (*c*). Tumors are heterogeneous and lower in signal intensity than adjacent cortex on interstitial phase images. Larger cancers have a propensity to undergo regions of necrosis that appear nearly signal void on postcontrast images (*c*). A simple renal cyst (arrows, *a*) adjacent to the renal cancer is present in the first of these patients.

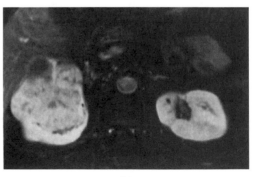

(c)

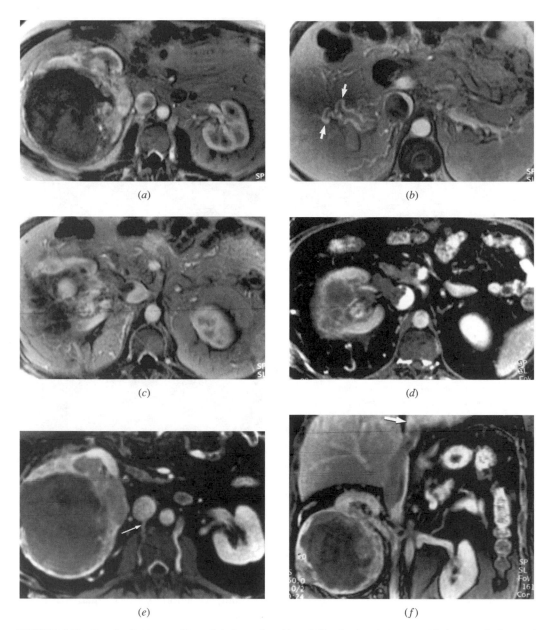

FIGURE 6.29 Renal cell cancer—Stage 3-A. Immediate (*a*) and 45 s (*b, c*) and transverse (*d, e*), coronal (*f, g*), and sagittal (*h*) gadolinium-enhanced T1W fat-suppressed SGE images. A heterogeneous enhancing large renal cancer is present, which originates from the lower two-thirds of the right kidney. An enhancing tumor thrombus is seen within the right renal vein that extends into the inferior vena cava. Direct coronal (*f, g*) and sagittal (*h*) images permit evaluation of the superior extent of thrombus (arrow, *f*).

Extensive vascular parasitization is appreciated (arrow, *b*) around the tumor. Dilated collateral lumbar veins are identified, one of which communicates with the IVC (arrow, *e*) at the level of the lower aspect of the thrombus.

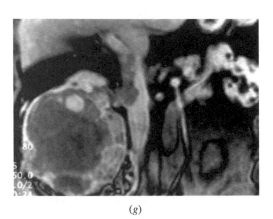

(g)

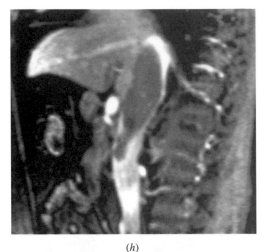

(h)

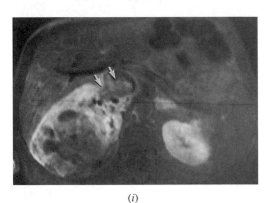

(i)

FIGURE 6.29 (*Continued*) Gadolinium-enhanced T1W fat-suppressed SGE image (*i*) in a second patient. Enhancing tumor thrombus can be appreciated extending along the right renal vein into the IVC (arrows, *i*). Enhancement of tumor thrombus is well shown on fat-suppressed postgadolinium images acquired in the interstitial phase.

- Clear cell RCC is a less aggressive tumor subtype that histologically may develop small amounts of fat, diffuse or focal
  - This may result in a slight drop in signal on out-of-phase images
  - In benign AML, fat is usually higher in quantity, resulting in diffuse marked drop on fat-suppressed images or phase cancellation artifact on out-of-phase imaging

Mimickers
- Column of Bertin (fig. 6.3)
- Fetal lobulations (fig. 6.4)
- Adenoma/oncocytoma (fig. 6.39)
- Extramedullary hematopoeisis
- Cyst with benign nodule (fig. 6.40)
- AML

Transitional Cell Carcinoma
- Background
  - The majority of primary tumors of the urothelium are malignant
  - Transitional cell carcinoma (TCC) is the most common malignancy of the urothelium, accounting for more than 90% of tumors
  - Squamous cell cancer accounts for 8% and adenocarcinoma for less than 1%
  - TCC represents 8% of all renal tumors, usually arises in older patients but rarely occurring in patients younger than 30 years of age
  - TCC of the upper tract is epidemiologically similar to that of the bladder
    - Males are more commonly affected, in a 3-to-1 ratio with females

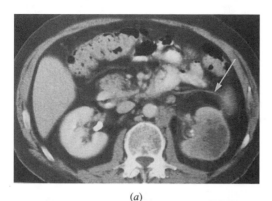

(*a*)

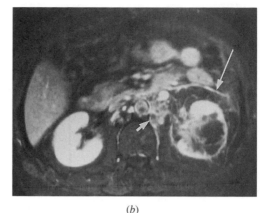

(*b*)

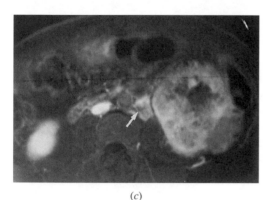

(*c*)

FIGURE 6.30   Renal cell cancer—Stage 3-B. Contrast-enhanced CT (*a*) and interstial phase gadolinium-enhanced T1W fat-suppressed spin-echo (*b*) images. A necrotic 6 cm tumor is present in the left kidney. Enlarged para-aortic nodes are identified on the CT scan. On the postcontrast T1W fat-suppressed image the nodes enhance in a heterogeneous fashion with central low signal intensity (short arrow, *b*), with an appearance similar to that of the primary tumor. Note the thickening of Gerota fascia (long arrows, *a*, *b*) shown on the CT and MR images.

Gadolinium-enhanced TIW fat-suppressed image (*c*) of a Stage 3-B cancer in a second patient demonstrates a heterogeneous necrotic primary renal cancer of the left kidney with central necrosis and para-aorta lymph nodes with a similar heterogeneous appearance (arrow, *c*).

- ▪ Risk factors include analgesics, tobacco, caffeine, chronic infection, and urolithiasis
- ○ 30–50% of cases are multifocal, and 15–25% are bilateral
- ○ Staging
  - ▪ Stage 1: limited to urothelial mucosa and lamina propria
  - ▪ Stage 2: invasion of, but not beyond, pelvic/ureteral muscularis
  - ▪ Stage 3: invasion beyond muscularis into adventitial fat or renal parenchyma
  - ▪ Stage 4: distant metastasis
- • Imaging
  - ○ Usually appear as eccentric filling defects in the renal pelvis (fig. 6.41)
  - ○ May appear as concentric wall thickening
  - ○ Tumors usually spread superficially (fig. 6.42)

- ○ TCC has a propensity to invade renal parenchyma, but invasion may be difficult to detect
- ○ Invasion of or along the IVC may occur
- ○ Although these tumors are hypovascular, they may be moderately high in signal intensity on gadolinium-enhanced interstitial phase fat-suppressed T1W images
- ○ Tumors tend to invade locally with spread to adjacent lymph nodes
- ○ MR urography with gadolinium-enhanced T1W 3D GRE 5–10 min post injection, 2D coronal or axial balanced-echo True-FISP, or single-shot echo-train imaging may show high-signal lumen with a nodular TCC appearing as a filling defect
  - ▪ Associated finding includes hydronephrosis with obstruction above the filling defect

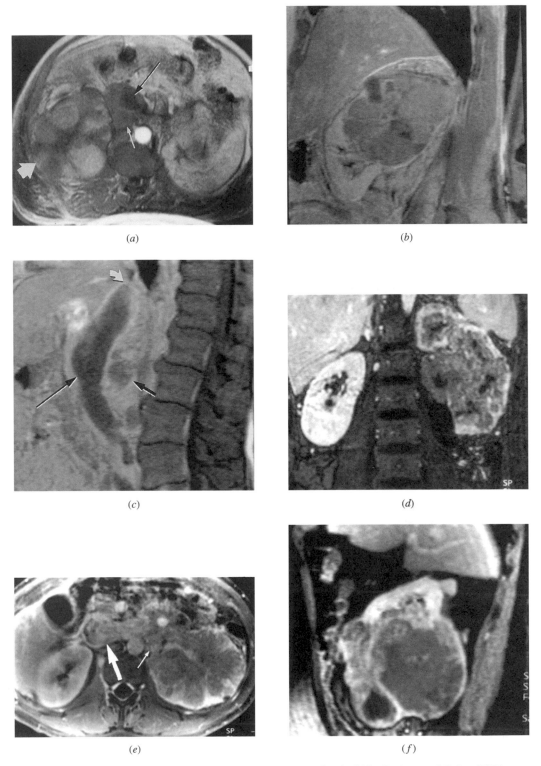

FIGURE 6.31   Renal cell cancer—Stage 3-C. Transverse 45 s (*a*) and sagittal 90 s (*b*, *c*) postgadolinium SGE images. A 7 cm heterogeneously enhancing renal cancer is present in the right kidney (arrow, *a*). Thrombus is present in the IVC (long arrow, *a*, *c*). Retrocaval (short arrows *a*, *c*) and paracaval nodes are identified. The thrombus (long arrow, *c*) is noted to terminate approximately 1 cm below the level of the diaphragm on the sagittal projection (curved arrow, *c*).

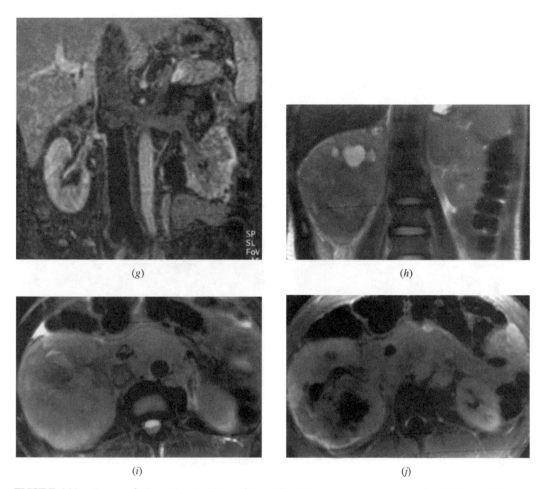

(g)

(h)

(i)

(j)

FIGURE 6.31 *(Continued)* Coronal source image for an MRA (*d*), transverse (*e*) and sagittal (*f*) 2–3 min postgadolinium T1W fat-suppressed SGE and coronal 3D MIP reconstructed MRA (*g*) images in a second patient. A large heterogeneous infiltrative mass is seen involving the lower two-thirds of the left kidney, which invades the left renal vein and extends into the IVC (large arrow, *e*). Regional lymph node metastases are present (small arrow, *e*).

Coronal (*h*) and transverse (*i*) SS-ETSE and 90 s postgadolinium fat-suppressed (*j*) SGE images in a third patient shows a large heterogeneous mass in the right kidney associated with IVC thrombosis and extensive enlarged retroperitoneal lymph nodes.

- Postgadolinium fat-suppressed T1W 2D/3D GRE images show enhancement of the soft tissue nodule and are the most effective MR technique to demonstrate the soft tissue nature of this lesion
  - Evaluation of the entire urothelium with retrograde pyelography is still considered essential to establish the full extent of disease. The role of MR urography is not established at present.

Squamous Cell Carcinoma
- Background
  - Rare malignancy arising from the collecting system urothelium
  - Associated predisposing factors or conditions
    - Calculi in over 50%
    - Leukoplakia or chronic infection
    - Chronic drug exposure to phenacetin
- Imaging
  - Not distinguishable from TCC (fig. 6.43)

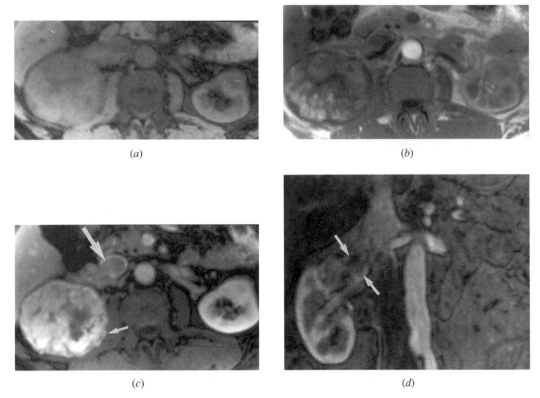

(a)

(b)

(c)

(d)

FIGURE 6.32 Renal cell cancer—Stage 4-A. Precontrast T1W fat-suppressed SGE (*a*), immediate postgadolinium SGE (*b*), 2 min postgadolinium fat-suppressed SGE (*c*), and coronal source image for MRA (*d*) images.

A large cancer arising from the right kidney is present that shows intense heterogeneous enhancement on immediate postgadolinium images (*b*), foci of central necrosis (*c*), tumor thrombus (long arrow, *c*; arrows, *d*), and invasion of the right psoas muscle (short arrow, *c*).

Wilms' Tumor
- Background
  - Wilms' tumor is the most common primary renal tumor in childhood, presenting between 2 and 5 years of age
  - Bilaterality or multicentricity occurs in 10% of cases
  - Areas of hemorrhage, cyst formation, and necrosis are sometimes encountered
  - Microscopically, the classic triphasic composition of cell types is usually identified: blastemal, epithelial, and stromal
  - Wilms' tumors calcify in only 5% of cases (neuroblastomas calcify in 50% of cases)
  - Unilateral Wilms' tumor is associated with a 41% incidence of nephrogenic rests, whereas multifocal Wilms's has a 99% incidence of nephrogenic rests

  - The risk of Wilms' tumor is increased in association with at least three recognizable groups of congenital syndromes
    - WAGR syndrome is characterized by aniridia, genital anomalies, and mental retardation, with a high risk of developing Wilms' tumor
    - Denys-Drash syndrome, consisting of gonadal dysgenesis (male pseudohermaphroditism) and nephropathy leading to renal failure
    - Beckwith-Wiedemann syndrome, characterized by enlargement of body organs, hemihypertrophy, renal medullary cysts, and abnormal cells in the adrenal cortex
    - Staging
      - Stage 1: Tumor confined to the kidney that has been completely excised

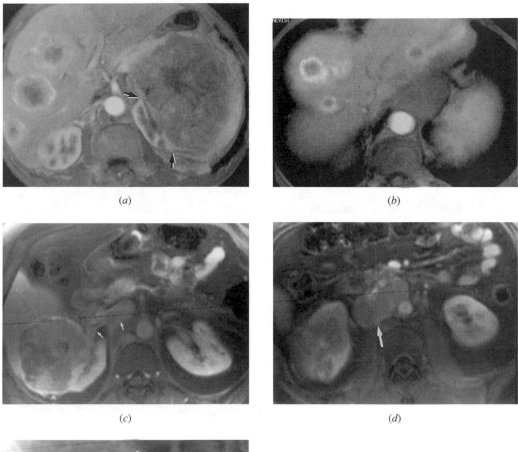

(a)

(b)

(c)

(d)

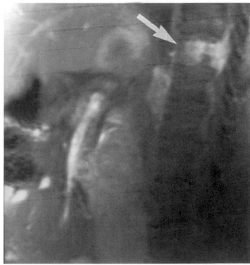

(e)

FIGURE 6.33   Renal cell cancer—Stage 4-B. Immediate postgadolinium SGE images (*a, b*) demonstrate a 12 cm renal cancer arising from the left kidney (arrows, *a*). Multiple hypervascular ring-enhancing liver metastases are noted. Renal cancer metastases to the liver are frequently hypervascular.

Transverse (*c, d*) and sagital (*e*) 2–3 min postgadolinium T1W fat-suppressed SGE images in a second patient. There is a large heterogeneous mass in the lateral aspect of the right kidney that invades the renal vein and extends into the IVC (arrows, *c*). Extensive retroperitoneal adenopathy is also present (arrow, *d*).

Abnormal increased enhancement of the T11 vertebral body is present (arrow, *e*), consistent with metastatic foci. Gadolinium-enhanced fat-suppressed images are effective at demonstrating bone metastasis, revealing them as high-signal focal masses in a dark background of suppressed fatty marrow.

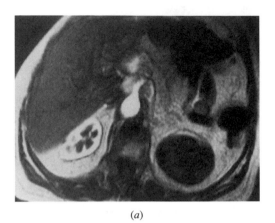

(a)

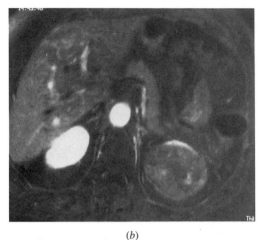

(b)

FIGURE 6.34   Hypovascular Stage 2 renal cell cancer.
Immediate postgadolinium SGE (a) and gadolinium-enhanced T1W fat-suppressed spin-echo (b) images. The tumor shows diminished enhancement immediately after contrast (a). The interstitial phase fat-suppressed image demonstrates small irregular enhancing structures within the mass (b), which distinguishes this lesion from a complicated cyst.

Interstitial phase gadolinium-enhanced T1W fat-suppressed spin-echo image (c) in a second patient shows small irregular enhancing structures in a hypovascular renal cancer arising from the left kidney. The great majority of hypovascular renal cell cancers are of papillary subtype.

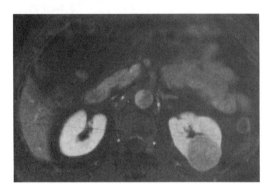

(c)

- Stage 2: Tumor that has extended locally beyond the kidney and has been completely excised
- Stage 3: The presence of residual tumor following surgery that was confined to the abdomen without hematogeneous spread
- Stage 4: Hematogeneous metastases
- Stage 5: Bilateral renal involvement
▪ Metastases occur to the lungs, liver, and lymph nodes
▪ In rare instances, may be highly cystic
▪ Tumors arise from the kidney with an appearance at times indistinguishable from renal cell cancer
▪ Age therefore constitutes a criterion for predicting the histologic diagnosis, since the most common renal malignancy in the pediatric patient is Wilms' tumor

▪ A transition occurs in the midteens after which renal cell cancer is the most common renal tumor
▪ A feature suggestive of Wilms' tumor is large tumor size with extension across the midline
▪ Central necrosis and tumor thrombus are less common in Wilms' tumor compared to renal cell cancer
▪ Wilms' tumor commonly contains central hemorrhage
○ Imaging
  ▪ Wilms' tumors are slightly hypointense on T1W images and slightly hyperintense on T2W images
  ▪ Large cancers are frequently heterogeneous with regions of high signal intensity on T1W images due to the presence of hemorrhage (fig. 6.44)

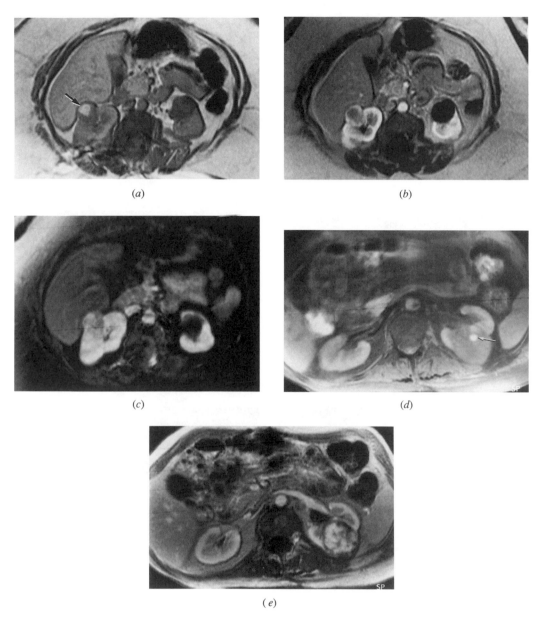

FIGURE 6.35   Stage 2 renal cell cancer with central hemorrhage. Precontrast SGE (*a*), immediate postgadolinium SGE (*b*), and gadolinium-enhanced T1W fat-suppressed spin-echo (*c*) images. Hemorrhage is present in a 2.5 cm stage 2 renal cancer arising from the right kidney, which appears as a high-signal-intensity substance on the precontrast T1W image (arrow, *a*). The tumor shows intense rim enhancement on the immediate postgadolinium image (*b*). Heterogeneous enhancement of the tumor is apparent on the interstitial phase fat-suppressed image (*c*).

Precontrast fat-suppressed SGE (*d*) and immediate postgadolinium SGE (*e*) images in a second patient demonstrate a 5 cm tumor arising in the left kidney. Foci of central high signal intensity on the precontrast image (arrow, *d*) are consistent with hemorrhage. The tumor exhibits an unusual central radiating enhancement pattern on the immediate postgadolinium SGE image (*e*). This pattern of enhancement may be more typical of oncocytoma but was present in this renal cell cancer.

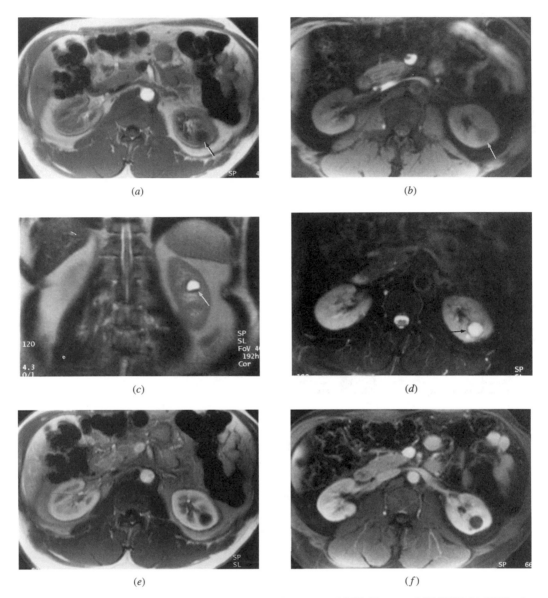

FIGURE 6.36 Purely cystic renal cell cancer. SGE (*a*), fat-suppressed SGE (*b*), coronal SS-ETSE (*c*), T2W echo-train spin-echo (*d*), immediate postgadolinium SGE (*e*), and interstitial phase gadolinium-enhanced fat-suppressed SGE (*f*) images. A well-defined cystic lesion with mural calcification was demonstrated on CT images (not shown). The lesion is well circumscribed and low in signal intensity on T1W images (arrow, *a*, *b*) and high in signal intensity on T2W images and does not enhance after gadolinium administration (*e*, *f*). A low-signal-intensity mural rim on the T2W images (arrow, *c*, *d*) corresponds to calcification as shown on the CT image. At surgery the lesion was considered to represent a cyst, but at histologic examination a thin sheet of tumor cells was present in part of the cyst wall.

- Tumors enhance heterogeneously on postgadolinium images, but tend to be less intensely enhanced and less heterogeneous than renal cell cancer on early postcontrast images

- Nephrogenic rests are typically smaller than 2 cm and enhance minimally on postgadolinium images
- As with renal cancer, tumor thrombus in Wilms' tumor is well shown using

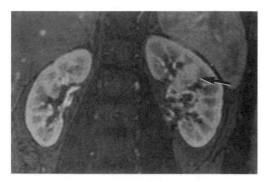

FIGURE 6.37 Prominent column of Bertin. Coronal postgadolinium gradient-echo image. Bertin column (arrow) follows a continuous contour and remains isointense with the renal cortex.

gadolinium-enhanced MR images and can be better defined than on CT images

Lymphoma
• Background
  ○ Non-Hodgkin's lymphoma more common than Hodgkin's in kidney
    ▪ Most commonly B-cell type
  ○ Three basic patterns of involvement occur
    ▪ Direct invasion from adjacent disease, most commonly large retroperitoneal masses (fig. 6.45)
    ▪ Focal masses that may be solitary or multiple (figs. 6.46 and 6.47)
    ▪ Diffuse infiltration (fig. 6.46)

  ○ Renal parenchyma lacks lymphoid tissue, so primary renal lymphoma usually arises from lymphatic tissue in the renal sinus
  ○ Direct extension usually infiltrates through renal capsule
• Imaging
  ○ Generally slightly hypointense relative to renal cortex on T1W images and heterogeneous and slightly hypointense to isointense on T2W images
  ○ Gadolinium enhancement of most lymphomas is mildly heterogeneous and minimal on early postcontrast images and remains minimal on late postcontrast images
  ○ Tumors retain vascularity throughout their stroma even when large (>5 cm), a distinguishing feature from RCC, which typically develops central necrosis
  ○ Cortex-based masses tend to enhance more intensely than other forms of renal involvement, which may reflect the greater blood supply of the cortex
  ○ Solitary focal renal cortical involvement of lymphoma may resemble renal carcinoma
  ○ Distinguishing features between lymphoma and RCC
    ▪ As most forms of lymphoma involve the medulla, these tumors can be distinguished from renal carcinoma, as the latter originate in the renal cortex

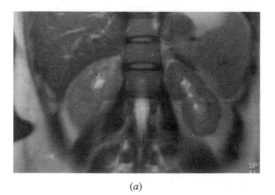

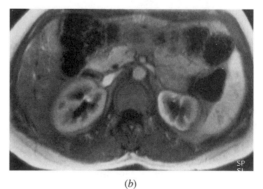

(a)   (b)

FIGURE 6.38 Fetal lobulation. Coronal single-shot echo-train spin-echo (SS-ETSE) (*a*), and transverse immediate postgadolinium SGE (*b*) images. The coronal SS-ETSE image (*a*) demonstrates an undulating contour of the entire left kidney. The immediate postgadolinium SGE image demonstrates uniform cortical thickness, excluding the presence of a mass.

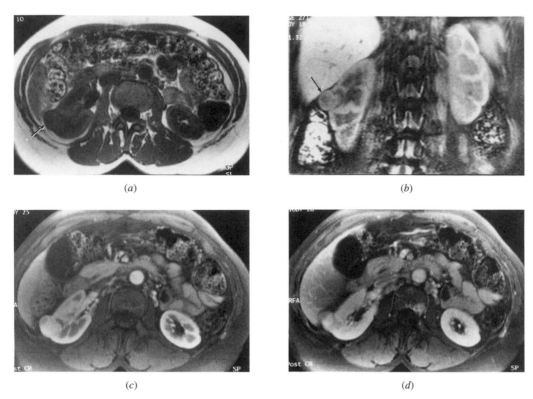

(a)   (b)

(c)   (d)

FIGURE 6.39   Renal oncocytoma. SGE (a), coronal fat-suppressed SGE (b), immediate postgadolinium SGE (c), and 90 s gadolinium-enhanced fat-suppressed SGE (d) images. A well-defined 2 cm mass is present in the right kidney (arrow, a, b). The majority of the tumor enhances in a moderately intense fashion on the immediate postgadolinium image (c) and shows mild peripheral washout by 90 s (d). The appearance is indistinguishable from that of a small renal cancer.

- Larger lymphoma masses are usually centered outside the renal contour
- Even large lymphoma masses do not undergo central necrosis
- Lymphoma shows less marked and less heterogeneous enhancement than RCC
- Vascular extension is not a characteristic of lymphoma
- Lymphoma may encase and squeeze vessels, which may result in diminished renal perfusion—not a feature of RCC
- Direct extension infiltrating the psoas muscle is a feature of lymphoma, whereas RCC may form metastatic hematogenously delivered deposits

Metastases
- The most common primary tumors to metastasize to the kidneys are lung (19.8–23.3%

of cases) and breast (12.3% of cases). Many other tumors may metastasize to the kidneys, but only rarely.
- Imaging
  ○ Can present as solitary, multiple uni/bilateral masses with features otherwise similar to RCC (fig. 6.48)
  ○ Often cortical in location

Infection

Acute Pyelonephritis
- Background
  ○ Most commonly caused by gram-negative bacilli
  ○ Usually develops as an ascending infection from the bladder
- Imaging
  ○ Typical features are striated nephrogram on gadolinium multiphase T1W GRE images

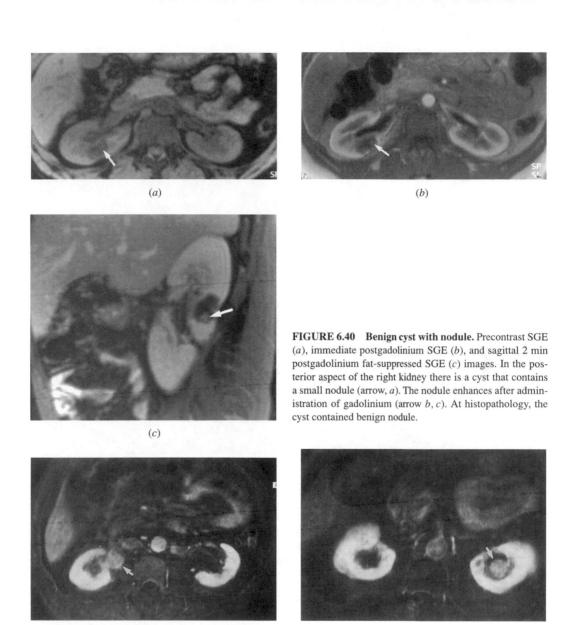

(a)

(b)

(c)

FIGURE 6.40 Benign cyst with nodule. Precontrast SGE (*a*), immediate postgadolinium SGE (*b*), and sagittal 2 min postgadolinium fat-suppressed SGE (*c*) images. In the posterior aspect of the right kidney there is a cyst that contains a small nodule (arrow, *a*). The nodule enhances after administration of gadolinium (arrow *b*, *c*). At histopathology, the cyst contained benign nodule.

(a)

(b)

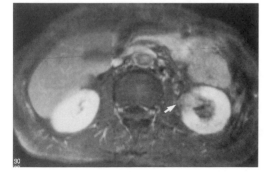

(c)

FIGURE 6.41 Transitional cell cancer—stage 2, focal mass type. Gadolinium-enhanced T1W fat-suppressed spin-echo images in three patients with transitional cell cancer. Tumors are focal rounded masses (arrow, *a–c*) that show heterogeneous mottled enhancement less than neighboring renal cortex. Note that masses have well-defined margins that correspond to lack of infiltration into surrounding fat.

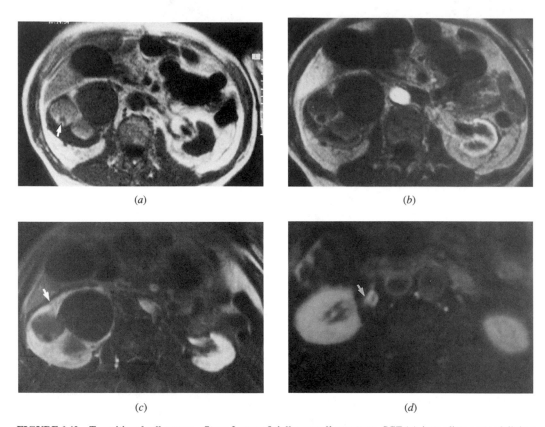

(a) (b)

(c) (d)

FIGURE 6.42 Transitional cell cancer—Stage 3, superficially spreading pattern. SGE (*a*), immediate postgadolinium SGE (*b*), and gadolinium-enhanced T1W fat-suppressed spin-echo (*c*) images. Severe dilatation of the right renal collecting system is present (*a–c*). Blood is identified as high-signal-intensity substance in dilated calyces on the precontrast image (*a*), and a small low-signal-intensity blood clot is also apparent (arrow, *a*). The renal pelvis is filled with a large signal-void blood clot. Diminished cortical enhancement is present on the immediate postgadolinium image (*b*). Thickening of the proximal aspect of the renal pelvis urothelium is noted with invasion of the renal cortex (arrow, *c*), which is best appreciated on the gadolinium-enhanced T1W fat-suppressed spin-echo images (*c*).

Gadolinium-enhanced T1W fat-suppressed spin-echo image (*d*) in a second patient shows increased thickness and intense enhancement of the proximal ureter. Ill-defined external margin of the tumor (arrow, *d*) on the lateral aspect of the ureter wall is consistent with tumor extension into the periureteral fat.

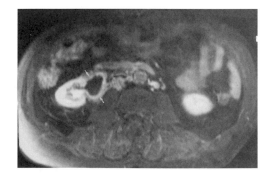

FIGURE 6.43 Squamous cell cancer. Gadolinium-enhanced T1W fat-suppressed spin-echo image demonstrates dilatation of the right renal pelvis with irregularly thickened and intensely enhancing urothelium, which represents squamous cell cancer (arrows). Surrounding peripelvic fat contains ill-defined enhancing tissue consistent with tumor extension.

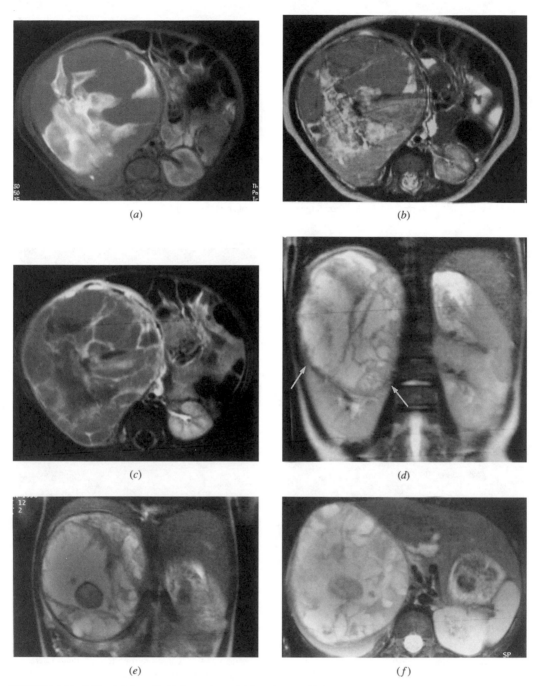

(a)   *(b)*

(c)   *(d)*

(e)   *(f)*

FIGURE 6.44   Wilms' tumor. T1W fat-suppressed spin-echo (*a*), T2W echo-train spin-echo (*b*), and interstitial phase gadolinium-enhanced T1W fat-suppressed spin-echo (*c*) images. A large mass arises from the right kidney and demonstrates central linear regions of high signal intensity on T1W and T2W images, consistent with blood. No substantial central necrosis is identified on the postcontrast images despite the large size of the tumor.

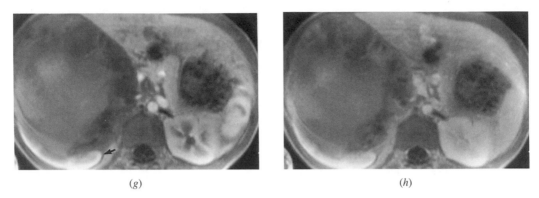

(g)   (h)

FIGURE 6.44 (*Continued*) Coronal SS-ETSE (*d*, *e*), T2W fat-suppressed spin-echo (*f*) and immediate (*g*), and 90 s (*h*) postgadolinium SGE images in a second patient. A large heterogeneous Wilms' tumor arises from the upper pole of the right kidney (arrows, *d*). A rim of posterior normal renal cortex is apparent (arrow, *g*).

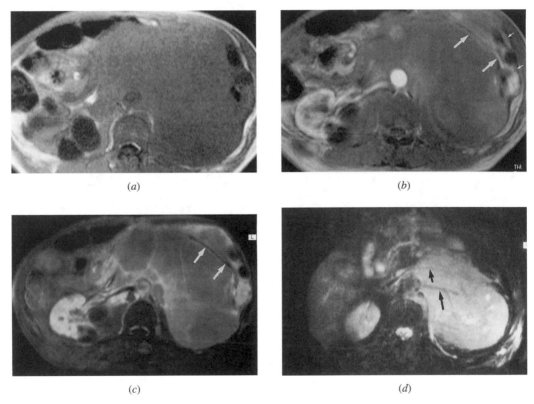

(a)   (b)

(c)   (d)

FIGURE 6.45 Renal lymphoma, large retroperitoneal mass invading kidney. SGE (*a*), immediate postgadolinium SGE (*b*), and gadolinium-enhanced T1W fat-suppressed spin-echo (*c*) images. A large retroperitioneal mass is present that is homogeneous and soft tissue signal intensity on the SGE image (*a*), and enhances minimally on capillary phase (*b*) and interstitial phase (*c*) images. On postcontrast images lymphoma is moderately heterogeneous with no evidence of necrosis. A thin rim of spared renal cortex is evident (small arrows, *b*), and the kidney is displaced anterolaterally. Tumor invades through the renal pelvis into the renal medulla. The renal artery is patent (arrows, *b*, *c*) but encased by lymphoma. Patency is shown by the presence of high-signal-intensity gadolinium in the artery on the immediate postgadolinium SGE image (*b*) and by flow void on the spin-echo image (*c*). In a second patient, a similar appearance of lymphoma is shown on T2W fat-suppressed spin-echo (*d*), immediate (*e*) and 90 s (*f*) postgadolinium SGE, and gadolinium-enhanced T1W fat-suppressed spin-echo (*g*) images. Lymphoma is mildly hyperintense on the T2W image (*d*) and heterogeneous and mildly enhanced on capillary phase (*e*) and interstitial phase (*f*, *g*) gadolinium-enhanced images.

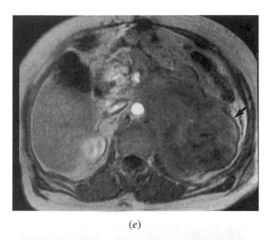

(e)

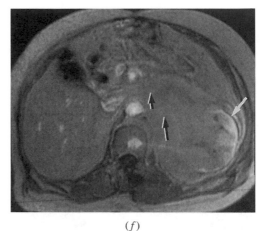

(f)

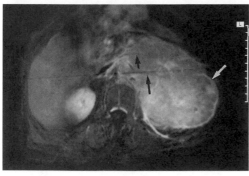

(g)

FIGURE 6.45   (*Continued*) The renal artery (arrow *d*, *f*, *g*) and renal vein (small arrow *d*, *f*, *g*) are encased by tumor but patent. Patency is demonstrated by the presence of high signal intensity on the SGE image (*f*) and signal void on the spin-echo images (*d*, *g*). The involved kidney demonstrates diminished cortical enhancement (arrow, *e*) relative to the normal contralateral right kidney on the capillary phase image (*e*). lymphoma has extensively invaded the medulla, but relative sparing of cortex is observed (white arrow, *f*, *g*).

that radiates from the renal medulla to the cortex, globular renal enlargement, and perinephric fluid best shown on T2W breath-hold imaging (fig. 6.49)
○ Proteinaceous material in the renal tubules may occasionally be visualized as high-signal-intensity substance in the renal medulla on noncontrast fat-suppressed T1W images (see fig. 6.50)

Abscess
• Background
  ○ Typically a complication of pyelonephritis
  ○ Less commonly a result of sepsis and hematogeneous spread, and this form is most frequently associated with
    ▪ Tuberculosis
    ▪ IV drug abuse and bacterial sepsis

○ The diagnosis is not always suspected clinically, as the abscess may result in only minimal or intermittent febrile-septic periods
○ Urine cultures may remain negative or only intermittently positive
• Imaging
  ○ Mass lesion within renal parenchyma showing mixed high/low T2W signal and mixed to low T1W signal
  ○ Postgadolinium T1W images show a nonenhancing central core with marked perinephric enhancement.
  ○ Increased and heterogeneous T2W signal is also associated with inflammation (fig. 6.51). Layering of low-signal material within the abscess is occasionally observed.
• Mimickers
  ○ Renal neoplasms

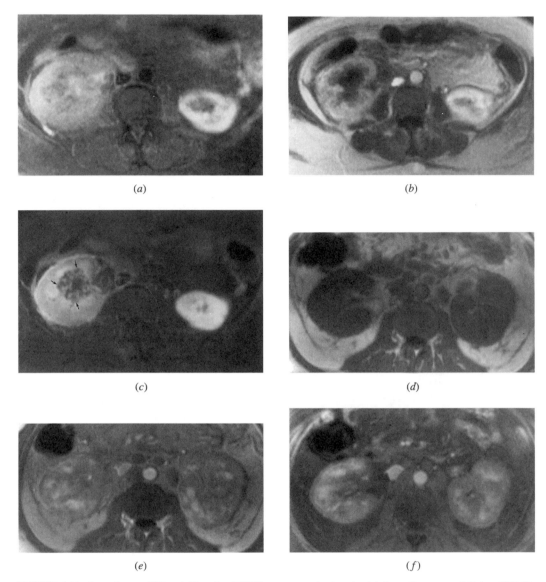

FIGURE 6.46 **Lymphoma, diffuse infiltration.** T1W fat-suppressed spin-echo (*a*), immediate postgadolinium SGE (*b*), and gadolinium-enhanced T1W fat-suppressed spin-echo (*c*) images. The right kidney is enlarged in a generalized fashion (*a–c*). CMD is not well shown on the precontrast T1W image (*a*). On the immediate postgadolinium image (*b*), diminished enhancement of the renal cortex is present. However, the cortex has a normal thickness and uniformity. On the later interstitial phase image increased enhancement is present in the outer medulla, and multiple low-signal-intensity foci (arrows, *c*) are present in the inner medulla, which likely represent focal aggregates of lymphoma. (Reproduced with permission from semelka RC, Kelekis NL, Burdeny DA, Mitchell DG, Brown JJ, Siegelman ES: Renal Lymphoma: Demonstration by MR imaging. *Am J Roentgenol* 166:823–827, 1996.)

Precontrast (*d*), 45 s postcontrast (*e*), and interstitial phase fat-suppressed (*f*) T1W SGE images in a second patient. The kidneys show decreased CMD on noncontrast T1W images. There is also decreased cortical enhancement on the 45 s postcontrast image, with heterogeneous medullary enhancement. The extent of renal enhancement shows negligible changes on the later postcontrast image.

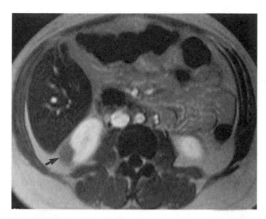

FIGURE 6.47   Granulocytic sarcoma. Transverse 90 s postgadolinium SGE image in a patient with acute myelogenous leukemia. A homogeneous minimally enhanced 2 cm granulocytic sarcoma (arrow) arises from the upper pole of the right kidney. The liver is low in signal intensity secondary to transfusional hemosiderosis.

- Distinction may require correlation with clinical history and follow-up imaging, with the patient on antibiotic therapy, to show interval improvement

Pyonephrosis
- Background
  ○ Represents hydronephrosis combined with infection
  ○ Results from ascending infection of either a preexistent obstructed collecting system or a collecting system that experiences suppurative impaction subsequent to the infection
- Imaging
  ○ Characteristic features seen on T2W images include hydronephrosis, with complex fluid signal in the renal collecting system showing dependent layering of debris

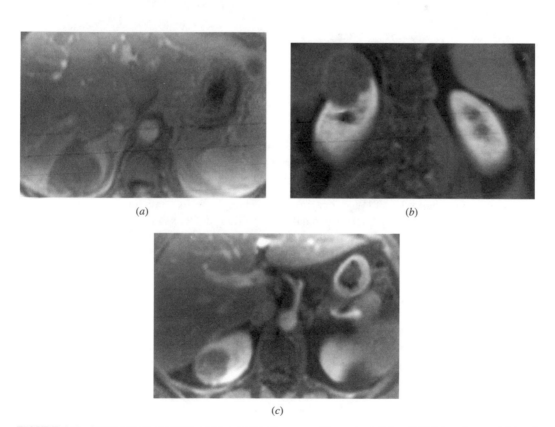

(a)

(b)

(c)

FIGURE 6.48   Renal metastases from ovarian cancer. Transverse 45 s postgadolinium SGE (*a*), and coronal (*b*) and transverse (*c*) 2–3 min postgadolinium T1W fat-suppressed SGE images. A tumor is present in the upper pole of the right kidney that demonstrates mild and heterogeneous enhancement.

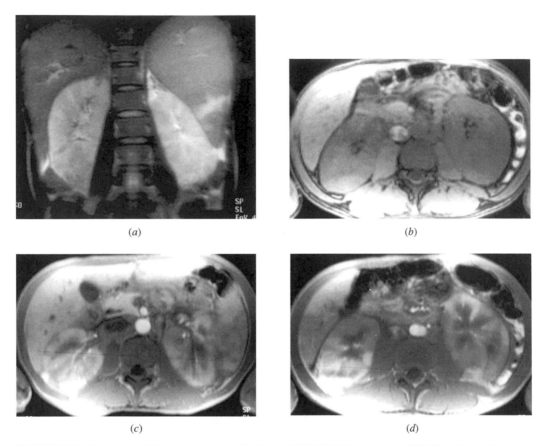

(a)   (b)

(c)   (d)

FIGURE 6.49   Severe acute bilateral pyelonephritis. Coronal SS-ETSE (*a*), precontrast SGE (*b*), and immediate post-gadolinium SGE (*c*, *d*) images. The kidneys are enlarged and demonstrate heterogeneous signal intensity on T1W and T2W images, and heterogeneous enhancement after administration of gadolinium. Note that the heterogeneous enhancement has a striated nephrogram appearance, which is a feature that may be observed in acute pyelonephritis.

○ Gadolinium-enhanced T1W imaging shows enhancement of a thickened renal pelvis urothelium (fig. 6.52)

Candidiasis
• Background
  ○ Usually associated with concomitant liver and spleen involvement
  ○ Risk factors associated with immuno-compromised patients: intensive care unit stay, hematologic malignancy undergoing chemotherapy, diabetes
• Imaging
  ○ Lesions are typically multiple and less than 5 mm
  ○ Highest conspicuity on gadolinium-enhanced T1W GRE images (fig. 6.53)

○ Fungus balls may form and appear as a filling defect within the collecting system, seen as a low-signal focus surrounded by high-signal urine in the renal pelvis on T2W imaging
  ▪ Mimickers include
    • Urolithiasis
    • TCC
      ○ TCC may be diagnosed if filling defect shows enhancement on post-gadolinium T1W images

Xanthogranulomatous Pyelonephritis
• Background
  ○ A result of chronic recurrent pyelonephritis
  ○ Associated with obstruction usually at the level of the major calyces or the pelvis

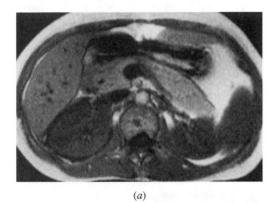

(a)

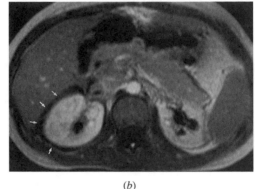

(b)

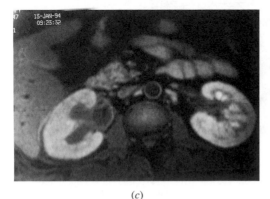

(c)

FIGURE 6.50   Acute pyelonephritis. SGE (*a*) and 2 min postgadolinium SGE (*b*) images. The right kidney is swollen, and perinephric fluid (arrows, *b*) is present. No focal parenchymal abnormalities are identified.

precontrast T1W fat-suppressed spin-echo image (*c*) in a second patient demonstrates striated, cone-shaped regions of high signal intensity in the medulla of the left kidney, consistent with proteinaceous material in acute pyelonephritis. Hydronephrosis of the right kidney is identified.

- ○ At histology, xanthoma cells are identified, which represent foamy macrophages, multinucleated giant cells, and immune cells associated with acute and chronic inflammation
- ○ Proteus infection isolated from the affected kidney in over half of cases
- Imaging
  - ○ Entire kidney or affected renal segments show enlargement and collecting system ectasia, well seen on single-shot echo-train T2W and postgadolinium T1W imaging
  - ○ Low-signal foci in collecting system may be seen on T2W images consistent with calculi
  - ○ Affected renal parenchyma enhances abnormally, showing slow onset, gradually increasing enhancement from arterial through to the late interstitial phase images, and delayed or absence of excretion (fig. 6.54)

- ○ Perinephric inflammatory changes are prominent and may extend into paranephric spaces including involvement of the psoas muscle

Malakoplakia
- Background
  - ○ Malakoplakia (*malakos,* meaning soft; *plakos*, meaning plaques) is a rare chronic granulomatous inflammatory process
  - ○ Associations include
    - ▪ Immunocompromised patients, diabetic patients
    - ▪ Middle-aged females with history of recurrent urinary tract infections
    - ▪ Coliform bacteria identified in over 90%
  - ○ The lower urinary tract is more commonly affected
  - ○ Renal parenchymal involvement is unusual, seen in 16% of cases
  - ○ Pathological assessment

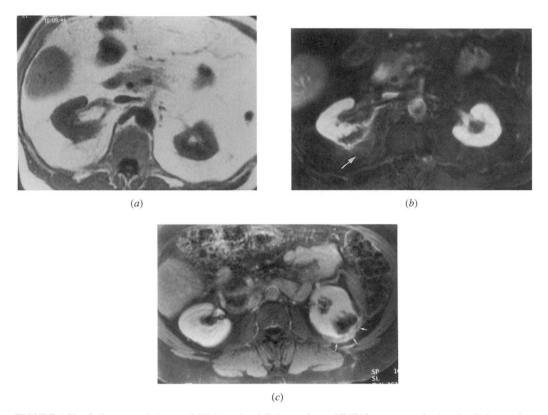

(a)   (b)

(c)

FIGURE 6.51 Solitary renal abscess. SGE (*a*) and gadolinium-enhanced T1W fat-suppressed spin-echo (*b*) images in a patient with a solitary abscess in the posterior aspect of the right kidney. Perirenal stranding is noted on the precontrast image, but the abscess is not well seen. On the gadolinium-enhanced fat-suppressed spin-echo image a signal-void intraparenchymal renal abscess is noted. The inner aspect of the abscess wall is irregular. Prominent perirenal stranding (arrow, *b*) is an important imaging feature of renal abscess.

Three-minute postgadolinium fat-suppressed SGE image (*c*) in a second patient who is a diabetic. A left renal abscess is present that appears as a low-signal-intensity cystic lesion with an irregular wall. Prominent thickening and increased enhancement of adjacent fascia (small arrows, *c*) is present.

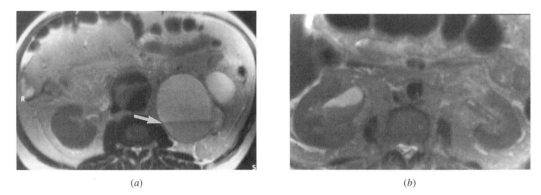

(a)   (b)

FIGURE 6.52 Pyonephrosis. Transverse SS-ETSE image (*a*) demonstrates severe dilatation of the collecting system of the left kidney. Layering of low-signal-intensity debris (arrow, *a*) in the dependent portion of the renal pelvis is a common appearance in infection.

Transverse SS-ETSE image (*b*) in a second patient. There is hydronephrosis of the right kidney with layering of low-signal material consistent with infection within the dilated collecting system. Note also perinephric fluid stranding.

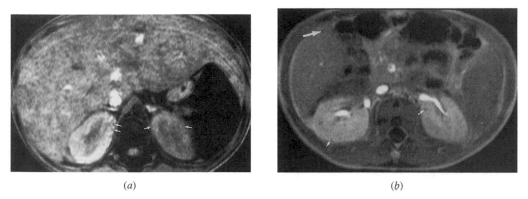

(a)   (b)

FIGURE 6.53   Renal candidiasis. Immediate (a) and 90 s (b) postgadolinium SGE images, in two patients with renal candidiasis. Multiple low-signal-intensity lesions, <5 mm in size, are present in the kidneys of both patients (small arrows, a, b). Extensive hepatic involvement is apparent in the first patient (a), whereas fewer liver lesions are apparent in the second patient (arrow, b).

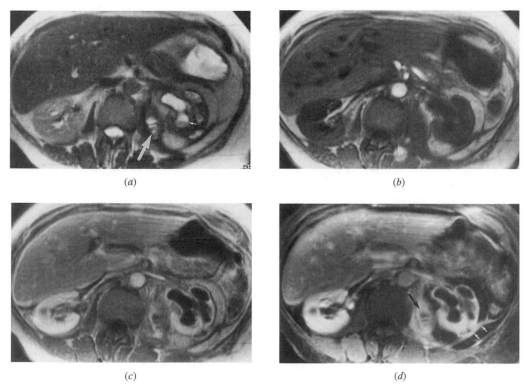

(a)   (b)

(c)   (d)

FIGURE 6.54   Xanthogranulomatous pyelonephritis. SS-ETSE (a), SGE (b) 90 s postgadolinium SGE (c), and 4 min postgadolinium fat-suppressed SGE (d) images. The left renal collecting system is noted to be dilated (a–d). A large extrarenal component of the infection is noted in the psoas muscle (arrow, a, d). Layering of low-signal intensity material (small arrow, a) is noted in calyces on the T2W image (a). No excretion of gadolinium by the involved kidney is apparent on the 4-min postgadolinium image. Inflammatory changes in Gerota fascia and lateral conal fascia (small arrows, d) and psoas abscess are most clearly defined on the gadolinium-enhanced fat-suppressed image (d). The combination of dilatation of the collecting system, lack of contrast excretion, and prominent extrarenal inflammatory changes are features observed for xanthogranulomatous pyelonephritis.

- Urothelium usual site of involvement, with yellow-brown soft plaque and central umbilication
- Less common renal parenchymal lesion shows separate single, multiple, or coalescing nodules, and possible abscess formation
  - Characteristic histology shows Michaelis-Gutmann bodies
- Imaging
  - When presenting as unifocal renal disease, findings appear as an indeterminate mass (fig. 6.55)
  - May require histopathological diagnosis
  - Multifocal malakoplakia may appear as multiple ill-defined regions of lower signal intensity with intervening linear stroma in a mildly enlarged kidney on T2W and T1W SGE images
  - On postgadolinium images, nodules are minimally enhanced, both early and late postcontrast, and intervening linear stroma show progressive enhancement

MR Urography

- A number of approaches may be employed:
  - T2W sequence
    - High-signal urine
    - Urothelium dark
    - Signal of surrounding tissues may be modified:
      - Fat darkened with fat suppression
      - Soft tissues darkened by lengthening TE to above 125 ms
    - Sequence selection includes single-shot echo-train T2W and True-FISP balanced echo
    - Advantages of true-FISP
      - If acquired as 2D, the images are respiratory motion insensitive and may be acquired on even very ill or uncooperative patients
      - Insensitive to artifacts from urine flow
      - Do not require renal excretion of contrast; therefore, effective regardless of degree of impaired renal function

- Multiplanar image acquisition
  - Disadvantages
    - 2D acquisitions are not as well suited to postprocessing
    - 3D acquisition loses the motion insensitivity advantages
  - 3D GRE T1W sequence in combination with delayed image acquisition (10–20 min) gadolinium urinary excretion
    - Urine bright
    - Urothelium enhances, but to a lower signal than concentrated intraluminal excreted gadolinium
    - Surrounding tissues enhance
    - The signal of retroperitoneal fat surrounding the collecting system may be diminished with fat suppression
    - Optional sequences include 3D VIBE
    - Advantages
      - Readily reformated into additional planes
      - Ideally suited for MIP reconstructions and 3D modeling
      - Gadolinium-may be used safely in the setting of impaired renal function
      - Gadolinium-enhanced imaging may show abnormalities of the urothelium, including thickening and tumor nodules associated with TCC
      - This is optimized by acquiring a venous phase image set in which the urothelium is enhanced prior to excretion of contrast into the collecting system (i.e., bright lumen wall seen against dark intraluminal urine)
      - Assessing renal function as manifested by excretion of contrast
    - Disadvantages
      - Motion sensitive
      - Contrast excretion will be delayed if renal function impaired
  - MR urography uses
    - Detection of hydronephrosis and hydroureter and determination of the level of obstruction
    - Characterization of the obstruction
    - May be performed in the setting of impaired renal function or iodinated contrast

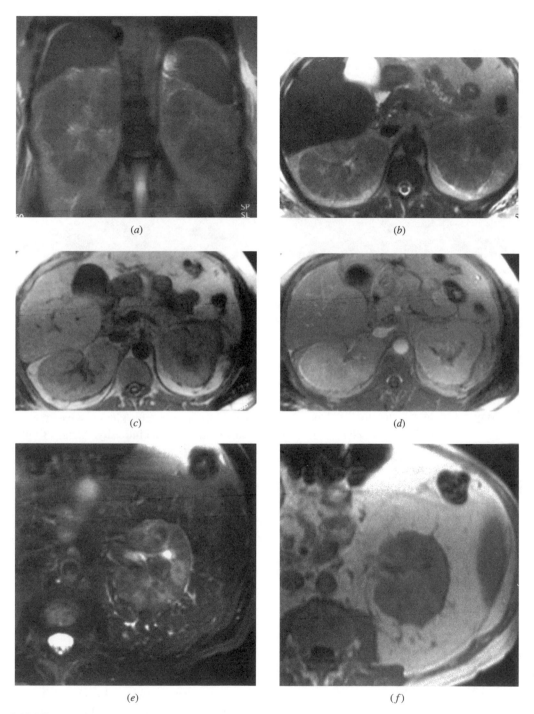

FIGURE 6.55   Malakoplakia. Coronal (*a*) and axial (*b*) SS-ETSE, precontrast SGE (*c*), and 1 min postgadolinium SGE (*d*) images. The kidneys are enlarged with an extensive multinodular appearance. High-signal septations are appreciated on the T2W sequences (*a*, *b*), which enhance after gadolinium administration (*d*).

T2W fat-suppressed echo-train spin-echo (*e*), T1W SGE (*f*), and transverse (*g*) and sagittal (*h*) T1W postgadolinium fat-suppressed SGE images in a second patient.

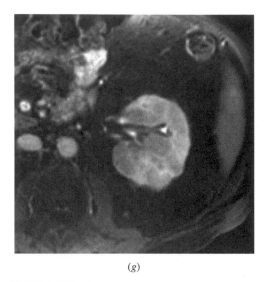

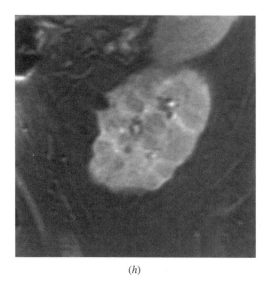

(g) (h)

FIGURE 6.55 (*Continued*) This patient, who had undergone liver transplantation, has a similar appearance of extensive multinodular infiltrate in the kidneys with intervening linear stroma that is high signal on T2 (*e*) and enhances with gadolinium (*g, h*). (Courtsey of Eric Outwater, M.D., University of Arizona.)

allergy, and in young patients to avoid ionizing radiation risks
  ○ Limitations
    ▪ May not demonstrate small calculi, especially if there is no associated ureteral obstruction

Renal Function

- Gadolinium-enhanced dynamic serial imaging of the kidneys demonstrates distinct phases of contrast enhancement based on the location of the bulk of the contrast agent
- The phases of enhancement can be separated into (1) capillary, (2) early tubular, (3) ductal, and (4) excretory
- Evaluation of the concentrating ability of the kidneys may be made by the observation of signal intensity changes in renal tissue based on the presence of gadolinium of varying concentrations (fig. 6.56)
- When dilute, gadolinium renders tissues high in signal intensity, but when highly concentrated, gadolinium renders tissues signal void
- The assessment of these phases of enhancement has been shown to distinguish normal

kidneys and those with dilated nonobstructed collecting systems from acute and chronic obstruction

- Dilated, nonobstructed kidneys have a temporal pattern of signal intensity changes similar to that of normal kidneys because renal transit is not abnormal (fig. 6.57)
- Acutely obstructed kidneys are enlarged and have increased renal transit time
- Chronic obstruction has diminished cortical enhancement and increased transit time (fig. 6.58)
- Functional changes of cortical and medullary enhancement may also be observed in the context of renal ischemia

Diffuse Renal Parenchymal Disease

- Diffuse renal parenchymal diseases are common medical conditions. A variety of disease processes may result in parenchymal disease, and they may be classified into the following broad categories:
  ○ Glomerular disease
  ○ Acute and chronic tubulointerstitial disease
  ○ Diabetic nephropathy and nephrosclerosis

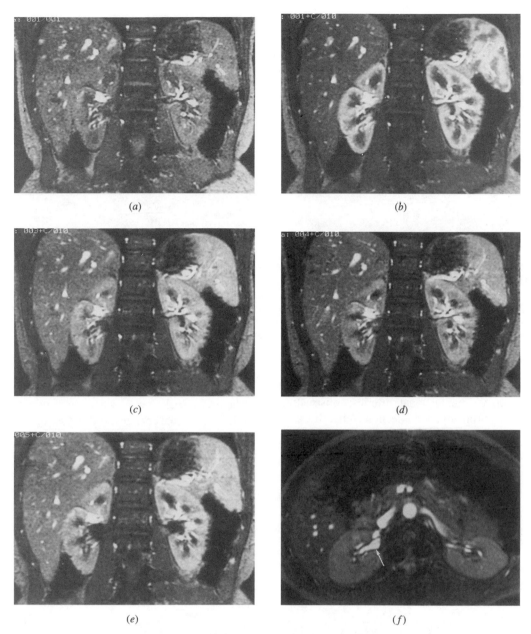

FIGURE 6.56 **Normal renal function.** Precontrast image (*a*). Minimal corticomedullary differentiation is present. Cortical enhancement (capillary) phase image (*b*). Cortex signal intensity is increased by 17%. Corticomedullary differentiation is distinct because of differential blood flow and increased delivery of gadolinium to the renal cortex. Early tubular phase (*c*) image. Signal intensity of medulla is transiently increased, whereas there is little change in cortical signal intensity. Ductal phase image (*d*). Signal intensity of medulla is decreased (6% from vascular phase) because of the concentration of gadolinium in distal convoluted tubules and collecting ducts. There is minimal decrease in cortical signal intensity (2%). Decreased signal intensity is apparent in the inner medulla and therefore mainly represents concentrated gadolinium in collecting ducts. Excretory phase image (*e*). Urine containing concentrated gadolinium appears in renal collecting systems as signal-void fluid. Excretory phase image (*f*) obtained 15 min after injection. No corticomedullary differentiation is present. Urine contains dilute (high signal intensity) gadolinium (arrows, *f*) because of rapid clearance of gadolinium from the body. (Reprinted with permission from Semelka RC, Hricak H, Tomei E, Floth A, Stoller M: Obstructive nephropathy: Evaluation with dynamic Gd-DTPA enhanced MR imaging. *Radiology* 175:797–803, 1990.)

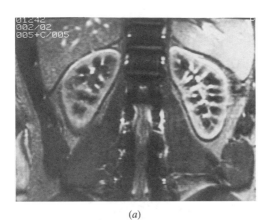

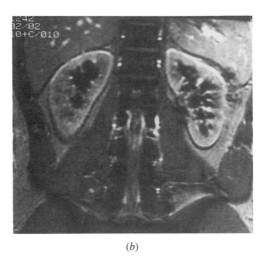

(a)   (b)

FIGURE 6.57 Dilated nonobstructed kidney. Gradient-echo images of subject with a dilated nonobstructed right kidney. Ductal phase image (*a*). Low signal intensity of the medulla appears simultaneously in the dilated nonobstructed right kidney and in the normal left kidney. In the excretory phase image (*b*), excretion of concentrated urine is bilaterally symmetric. Susceptibility-induced image distortion of the renal collecting systems is caused by the high concentration of gadolinium. (Reprinted with permission from Semelka RC, Hricak H, Tomei E, Floth A, Stoller M: Obstructive nephropathy: Evaluation with dynamic Gd-DTPA enhanced MR imaging. *Radiology* 175:797–803, 1990.)

∘ Other forms of microvascular disease; ischemic nephropathy caused by disease of the main renal arteries; obstructive nephropathy; and infectious renal disease

• MRI has played a limited role in the evaluation of diffuse renal parenchymal disease

• There is correlation between renal cortical thickness, signal changes, and diffuse disease

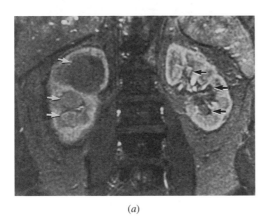

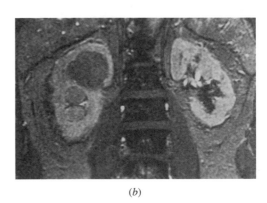

(a)   (b)

FIGURE 6.58 Chronic obstruction. Gradient-echo images of of a subject with a chronically obstructed right kidney and a dilated nonobstructed left kidney. Cortical enhancement (capillary) phase image (*a*). Normal cortical enhancement is appreciated in the left kidney, which demonstrates corticomedullary distinction. Cortical enhancement is lower in the chronically obstructed right kidney with no definition of CMD. Low-signal-intensity gadolinium-free urine is present in both collecting systems (arrows, *a*). On the excretory phase image (*b*), concentrated urine is excreted by the dilated nonobstructed left kidney. There is no apparent excretion by the chronically obstructed right kidney, no development of corticomedullary differentiation, and no significant changes in parenchymal signal intensity from the cortical enhancement phase. (Reprinted with permission from Semelka RC, Hricak H, Tomei E, Floth A, Stoller M: Obstructive nephropathy: Evaluation with dynamic Gd-DTPA enhanced MR imaging, *Radiology* 175:797–803, 1990.)

○ The mean cortex thickness for normal kidney and kidneys with glomerular disease was 8.4 and 7.8 mm, respectively, which were significantly thicker ($p < .01$) than renal cortex in patients with microvascular disease (5.2 mm), tubulointerstitial disease secondary to antineoplastic chemotherapy (5.6 mm), ischemic nephropathy (5.5 mm), and obstructive nephropathy (4.3 mm). Irregularity of the renal cortex was common in microvascular disease (60.9%), infectious renal disease (62.5%), obstructive nephropathy (55.6%), and nonchemotherapy tubulointerstitial disease (53.8%), compared to chemotherapy-induced tubulointerstitial disease (5.9%), glomerular disease (3.8%), and normal kidneys (0%).

○ Diffuse high signal intensity of the entire medulla on delayed postcontrast images was observed in 20.7% of patients with diffuse renal disease and in none of the patients with normal kidneys

○ Combining this information with other imaging findings, such as dilatation of the renal collecting system in obstructive nephropathy or atherosclerotic disease of the aorta in ischemic nephropathy and microvascular disease, allows prediction of the probable underlying type of diffuse renal parenchymal disease

• Glomerular Disease

○ The clinical manifestations are varied and range from asymptomatic urinary abnormalities to acute nephritis, nephrotic syndrome, and chronic renal failure

○ In patients with nephrotic syndrome, the majority have membranous nephropathy, and MRI findings are generally minimal (fig. 6.59)

○ Diffuse increased enhancement resulting in high signal intensity of the medulla may be observed on delayed postgadolinium images

○ In chronic disease, cortical thinning is smooth and regular in contour and medullary atrophy may be substantial (fig. 6.60)

○ Nephrotic syndrome may also be associated with renal vein thrombosis, as can be shown well on SGE images acquired 45–120 seconds after gadolinium (fig. 6.61)

• Tubulointerstitial Disease

○ A variety of underlying etiologies may result in tubulointerstitial disease of which drug-related causes are among the most common

○ Tubulointerstitial disease secondary to analgesic drug overuse results in irregular cortical thinning (fig. 6.62)

○ Tubulointerstitial disease from antineoplastic chemotherapy results in more uniform cortical thinning (fig. 6.63)

  ▪ This presumably reflects the fact that the cortical insult is more constant due to the regular rate of chemotherapy drug administration

• Acute Tubular Necrosis

○ Results from metabolic or toxic etiologies in the majority of cases. Within 1 week of onset of this condition, CMD may be preserved despite substantial elevation of sCr (fig. 6.64).

  ▪ This likely reflects the fact that loss of CMD takes approximately 2 weeks to develop from onset of injury

• Tubular Blockage

○ A number of etiological agents may result in tubular blockage

○ Classical example of diffuse tubular blockage is by Bence Jones proteinuria in multiple myeloma

○ Other causes

  ▪ Rhabdomyolysis leading to myoglobinuria (fig. 6.65)

• Iron Deposition

○ Associated with hemolysis with hemoglobin accumulation in renal glomeruli

○ Sickle cell disease is the most common entity to result in this condition

○ The usual appearance is low signal intensity of the renal cortex due to the T2* shortening effects of iron, best appreciated on gradient-echo or T2W images (fig. 6.66)

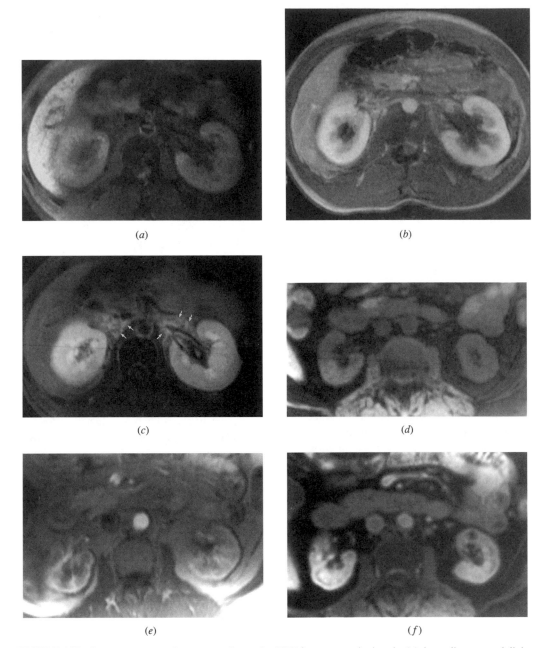

(a)   *(b)*

(c)   *(d)*

(e)   *(f)*

FIGURE 6.59 Recent-onset membranous nephropathy. T1W fat-suppressed spin-echo (*a*), immediate postgadolinium SGE (*b*), and gadolinium-enhanced T1W fat-suppressed spin-echo (*c*) images. CMD is diminished on the precontrast image (*a*). Renal cortex is uniform and of normal thickness on the immediate postgadolinium image (*b*). Diffuse increased enhancement of the medulla is noted on the interstitial phase image (*c*). Enhancing plate-like retroperitoneal tissue is present that extends into the left renal hilum (arrows, *c*). This represents acute benign retroperitoneal fibrosis.

T1W fat-suppressed SGE (*d*), immediate postgadolinium SGE (*e*), and 90 s postgadolinium T1W fat-suppressed SGE (*f*) images in a second patient with chronic renal failure. Decreased corticomedullary differentiation is present on the precontrast fat-suppressed image (*d*), and increased medullary enhancement is appreciated on the interstitial phase image (*f*). Note also a small simple cyst in the left kidney.

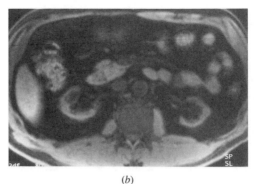

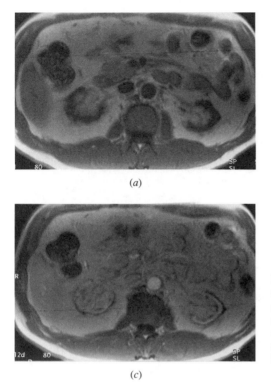

(a)

(b)

(c)

FIGURE 6.60   Chronic membranous glomerulonephritis. SGE (*a*), fat-suppressed SGE (*b*), and immediate postgadolinium SGE (*c*) images. No CMD is appreciated on precontrast images (*a*, *b*). The immediate postgadolinium image (*c*) demonstrates uniform cortical thinning and disproportionate atrophy of the renal medulla. Fat in the renal sinus has increased in volume to supplant the atrophic medulla.

○ On immediate postgadolinium images the T1 shortening effects of gadolinium usually exceed the T2 shortening effects of the iron in the renal cortex, resulting in high-signal-intensity enhanced renal cortex

○ On interstitial phase images, passage of contrast into the tubules and enhancement of the medulla result in signal reversal, with the cortex becoming lower in signal intensity than the medulla. Less commonly,

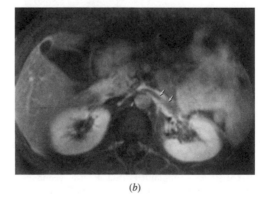

(a)

(b)

FIGURE 6.61   Renal vein thrombosis with nephrotic syndrome. Ninety-second gadolinium-enhanced SGE (*a*) and gadolinium-enhanced T1W fat-suppressed spin-echo (*b*) images. Low-signal bland thrombus is identified in the left renal vein (arrows *a*, *b*). Flow in the vein surrounding the thrombus is identified as high signal intensity on these images. Greater conspicuity of gadolinium in the patent periphery of the vein is apparent on the fat-suppressed image because of suppression of the competing signal intensity of fat (*b*).

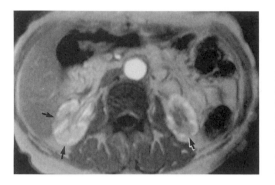

FIGURE 6.62 Tubulointerstitial disease secondary to analgesic abuse. Immediate postgadolinium SGE image demonstrates irregular cortical thinning ranging in thickness from 1 to 4 mm. Regions of extreme cortical thinning are apparent (arrows). (Reproduced with permission from Kettritz U, Semelka RC, Brown ED, Sharp TJ, Lawing WL, Colindres RE: MR findings in diffuse renal parenchymal disease. *J Magn Reson Imaging.* 6:36–144, 1996.)

dilute-concentration iron in the glomeruli may result in a high-signal-intensity renal cortex on precontrast T1W images (fig. 6.67).

○ The spleen in sickle cell disease is also affected with iron deposition, and splenic infarcts are observed

○ Paroxysmal nocturnal hemoglobinuria results in iron deposition in the renal cortex

- Iron deposition in the liver and spleen are variable and related to blood transfusions or portal hypertension
- Parenchymal Changes from Obstruction
  ○ Acute and chronic obstructions are well shown on MR images
  ○ In acute obstruction
    - Kidney size is enlarged, and contrast persists in the renal parenchyma for a

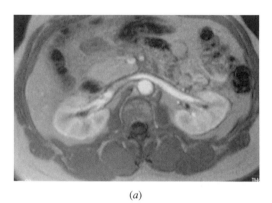

(a)

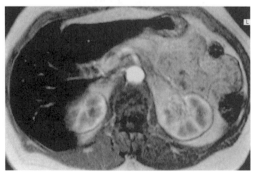

(b)

FIGURE 6.63 Tubulointerstitial disease secondary to chemotherapy. Immediate postgadolinium images in three patients (*a–c*) who have a remote history of antineoplastic chemotherapy. Regualr cortical thinning is present in all patients. Note the low signal intensity of the liver in the third patient (*c*) due to transfusional siderosis.

(c)

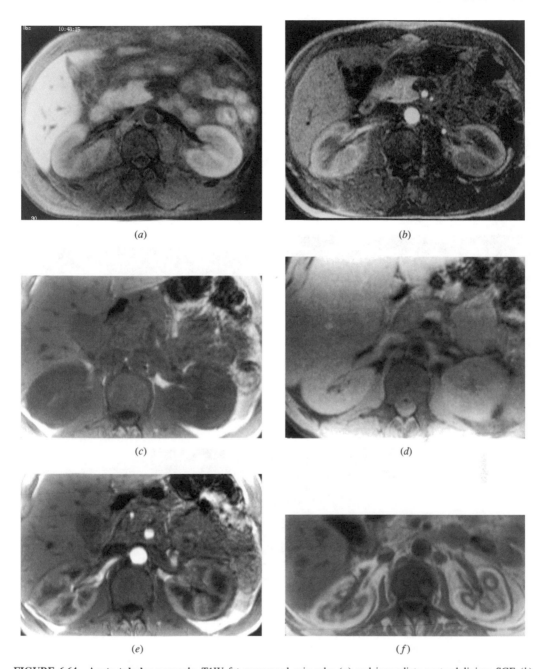

(a)

(b)

(c)

(d)

(e)

(f)

FIGURE 6.64   Acute tubular necrosis. T1W fat-suppressed spin-echo (a) and immediate postgadolinium SGE (b) images. Corticomedullary differentiation is demonstrated on both precontrast (a) and immediate postcontrast (b) images in a patient with acute tubular necrosis and serum creatinine of 6.3 mg/dl. Acute tubular necrosis developed within 1 week before to MRI examination, and the acute nature of the injury presumably accounts for the presence of CMD on the precontrast image.

Precontrast T1W SGE (c), T1W fat-suppressed SGE (d), and immediate postgadolinium SGE (e) images in a second patient, with acute tubular necrosis of 1-week duration, demonstrates globular-shaped kidneys with decreased CMD on precontrast images.

Precontrast T1W SGE image (f) in a third patient shows high signal intensity in the medullar of kidneys on noncontrast T1W images, suggesting infiltration with blood or protein.

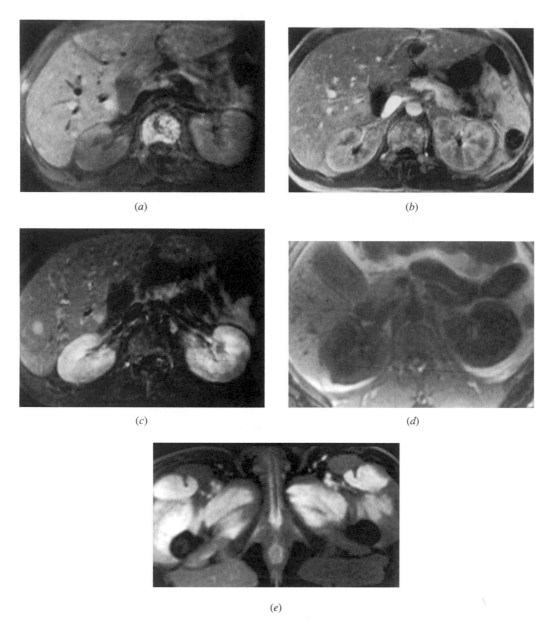

(a)

(b)

(c)

(d)

(e)

FIGURE 6.65   Tubular blockage. secondary to Bence Jones proteinuria. Precontrast T1W fat-suppressed spin-echo (*a*), immediate postgadolinium SGE (*b*), and gadolinium-enhanced T1W fat-suppressed spin-echo (*c*) images. This patient with multiple myeloma has high-signal-intensity lesions in the bone marrow and liver and absent corticomedullary differentiation on precontrast T1W fat-suppressed spin-echo images (*a*). On immediate postgadolinium images (*b*), corticomedullary differentiation is present, but cortical enhancement is not intense. On interstitial-phase T1W fat-suppressed spin-echo images (*c*), diffuse high signal intensity is present in the renal medulla, suggesting the presence of tubular leakage of gadolinium.

Secondary to rhabdomyolysis. Precontrast T1W SGE (*d*) and precontrast T1W fat-suppressed SGE (*e*) images. The kidneys are enlarged with diminished corticomedullary differentiation on the precontrast image. Extensive high signal is present in the muscles of the upper thighs (*e*), which on this noncontrast image reflects diffuse hemorrhagic changes.

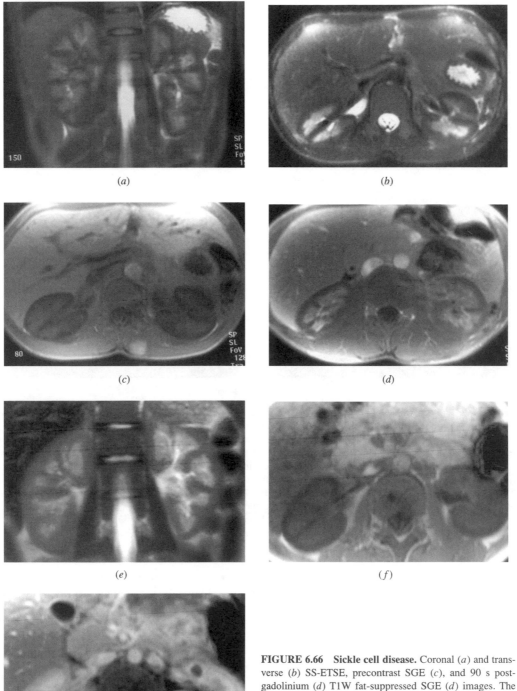

FIGURE 6.66   Sickle cell disease. Coronal (*a*) and transverse (*b*) SS-ETSE, precontrast SGE (*c*), and 90 s postgadolinium (*d*) T1W fat-suppressed SGE (*d*) images. The kidneys are globular shaped, and the renal cortices are low signal on T1W and T2W images, consistent with iron deposition. Coronal SS-ETSE (*e*), precontrast T1W SGE (*f*), and postgadolinium T1W fat-suppressed spin-echo (*g*) images in a second patient reveal similar findings.

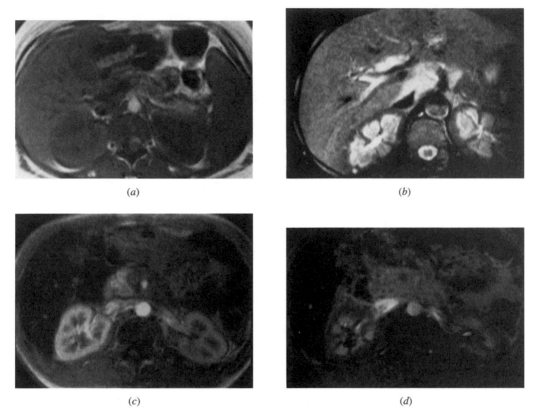

(a)

(b)

(c)

(d)

FIGURE 6.67 Sickle cell disease. SGE (a) image demonstrates preservation of CMD in a patient with sickle cell disease because of the presence of dilute iron in the renal cortex that results in a T1-shortening paramagnetic effect.

T2W fat-suppressed spin-echo image (b) in a second patient demonstrates low signal intensity of renal cortex secondary to accumulation of free hemoglobin. High-signal-intensity celiac and porta hepatic nodes are also present.

Immediate (c) and 2 min (d) postgadolinium SGE images in a third patient. On the immediate postgadolinium image (c), the renal cortex is high in signal intensity, which reflects that the T1-shortening effect of gadolinium exceeds the T2-shortening effects of iron. At 2 min after injection (d), the T2 shortening of iron in the cortex exceeds the T1 shortening of gadolinium, causing diminished signal intensity of the cortex. The relative washout of gadolinium from the cortex coupled with the transit of gadolinium into the medulla results in this signal reversal of cortex and medulla. Signal intensity changes in renal parenchyma on postgadolinium images in patients with sickle cell disease reflect the changing balance on T2-shortening effects of iron and T1-shortening effects of gadolinium.

prolonged period of time, resulting in a prolonged nephrogram phase (fig. 6.68)
- CMD is diminished on immediate post-gadolinium images
○ In chronic obstruction
  - The kidney, which is initially enlarged, with the passage of time gradually decreases in size and develops diminished renal perfusion (fig. 6.69)
  - Renal cortical thinning occurs, and in pure renal obstruction it is usually uniform

- The collecting system generally remains dilated when the kidney atrophies, which permits distinction of chronic obstruction from chronic ischemia
• Reflux Nephropathy and Chronic Pyelonephritis
  ○ Reflux nephropathy represents renal parenchymal changes secondary to urine reflux into the renal collecting system
  ○ Changes of reflux nephropathy are more common in the upper or lower polar regions of the kidneys, due to the presence

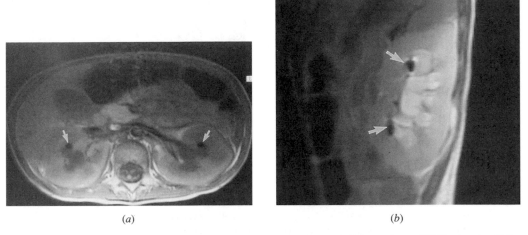

(a)   (b)

FIGURE 6.68   Acute obstruction. T1W spin-echo (*a*) and sagittal-plane gadolinium-enhanced T1W spin-echo (*b*) images. The kidneys are enlarged in a globular fashion. CMD is preserved, reflecting the acuteness of the obstruction (*a*). Gadolinium excreted into the collecting system is dilute and high in signal intensity (*b*). Signal-void foci located in the nondependent portions of the renal collecting system demonstrate blooming artifact (arrows *a*, *b*) that represents air introduced by Foley catheterization.

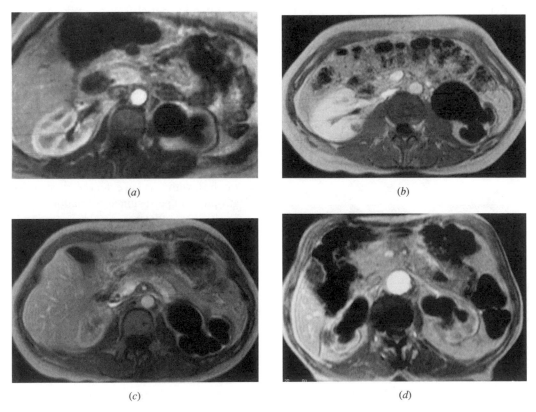

(a)   (b)

(c)   (d)

FIGURE 6.69   Chronic renal obstruction. Immediate postgadolinium SGE images in five patients with chronic renal obstruction (*a–e*). In all cases of unilateral obstruction (*a–c*) the degree of cortical enhancement is less than that of the contralateral normal kidney. Substantial pelvicalyceal dilatation is present in all cases. CMD is diminished, and the cortex is thinned and relatively smooth.

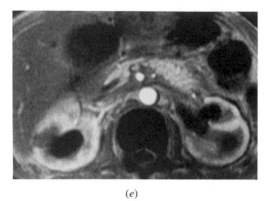
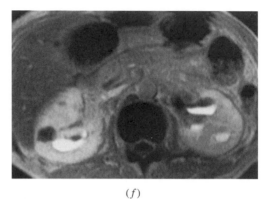

(e)   *(f)*

FIGURE 6.69   (*Continued*) These factors reflect the duration and severity of obstruction. Excreted urine is dilute in the setting of chronic obstruction because kidneys lose concentrating ability. Excretion of dilute gadolinium is shown on a 4 min postgadolinium SGE image (*f*) obtained in the same patient illustrated in (*e*).

of compound papillae or fused tips of the medullary pyramids

- Owing to the fusion of multiple papillae, the papillary tip is flattened or concave
- Renal scarring is a frequent sequela of reflux nephropathy and occurs superficial to dilated calyces (fig. 6.70)
- The renal cortex is thin and usually very irregular
- The hallmark of chronic pyelonephritis is a coarse, discrete corticomedullary scar overlying a dilated blunted or deformed calyx
  - Scarring from ischemic infarcts of arterial origin is distinguished in location and more commonly occurs between calyces

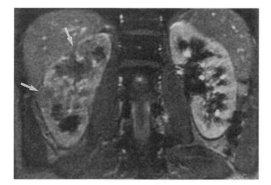

FIGURE 6.70   Reflux nephropathy. Coronal 2.5 min postgadolinium gradient-echo image. Reflux nephropathy of the right kidney is shown by irregular thinning of the renal cortex overlying renal calyces. Damage in this patient is most severe in the upper and midrenal regions (arrows).

- Renal Arterial Disease
  - MRA is the main imaging technique for anatomic vascular imaging (see chap. 9)
  - Disease of the renal arterial system may be thrombotic/arterial wall or embolic in nature
  - Thrombosis/arterial wall disease may be further subdivided into large-vessel, medium-vessel, and small-vessel disease
  - Ischemic nephropathy results from atherosclerotic disease of the main renal artery
  - Multilevel renal artery disease results in kidneys with regions of atrophy (secondary to vascular disease) and region of hypertrophy (secondary to compensatory hypertrophy), with varying extent of global renal atrophy and perfusion abnormalities
  - Small-vessel disease results in multiple small defects in the renal cortex best seen on immediate postgadolinium images; some of the defects may enhance over time, reflecting ischemic changes
  - Acute cortical necrosis
    - Seen in diffuse vascular disease such as systemic lupus erythematosis (SLE)
    - Negligible enhancement of the entire cortex is appreciated on capillary phase images
  - Anatomical changes of renal artery disease are shown on MRA (fig. 6.71), as are the number of arteries and the presence of stenosis (fig. 6.72)

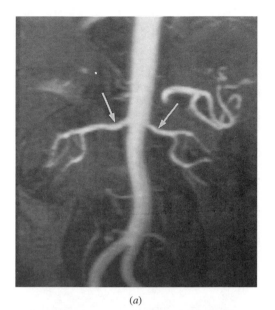

(a)

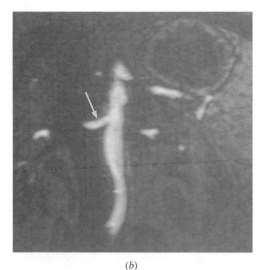

(b)

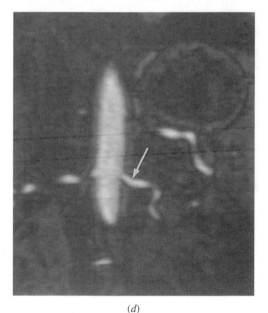

(d)

FIGURE 6.71 MR angiogram with coronal 3D GRE.
Coronal maximum-intensity projection (MIP) reconstructed
image (a) and individual 2-mm-thin 3D GE source images
of right (b) and left (c) renal artery origin. The MIP reconstructed image displays a normal aorta and renal arteries (arrow, a). Areas of stenosis, however, can be masked in reconstructed images. The individual source images of the right
(arrow, b) and left (arrow, c) renal artery are normal.

○ Aortic dissection may also result in changes
  of diminished renal arterial blood flow to
  the kidney fed by the false lumen. This may
  occur either by occlusion/thrombosis of the
  renal artery by the intimal flap or false chan-
  nel, or by decreased arterial flow through
  the renal artery fed by the false lumen. Capillary phase gadolinium-enhanced imaging
  is effective at demonstrating differences in

enhancement between the kidneys, where
one is fed by the true lumen and the other
(usually the left) is fed by the false lumen
(fig. 6.73).
○ Renal artery pseudoaneurysms occur and
  may undergo rupture or may be brought
  to clinical attention because of pressure effects on other structures

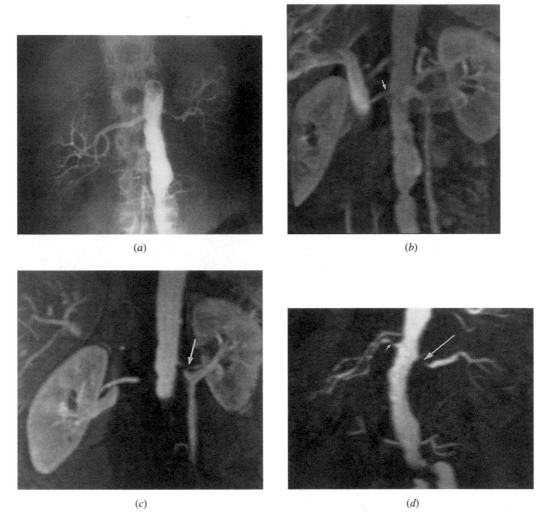

(a) (b)

(c) (d)

FIGURE 6.72 Renal artery stenosis. Angiogram (a) and tailored 3D MIP projections, using an interactively selected volume of interest of a gadolinium-enhanced 3D GE sequence (b, c). Mild stenosis of the right and severe stenosis of the left renal arteries are shown on the angiogram. MIP tailored for the right renal artery demonstrates minimal stenosis (arrow, b). MIP tailored for the left renal artery demonstrates severe stenosis (arrow, c).

Coronal 3D MIP gadolinium-enhanced 3D GE (d) in a second patient demonstrates two right renal arteries with moderate stenosis of the lower artery (short arrow, d) and moderately severe stenosis of a solitary left renal artery (long arrow, d). Breath-hold gadolinium-enhanced MR angiography is efficient at depicting the main as well as accessory renal arteries, which is important for preoperative planning (e.g., surgical repair of atherosclerotic aneurysms of the abdominal aorta).

MIP reconstructed MRA projection (e) and coronal 3D thin-section source (f) images. On the MIP reconstructed image a short segment of right renal artery is not visualized. On the basis of this image it is not clear whether this represents stenosis or occlusion.

○ Renal artery injury sustained by trauma or surgery may result in changes of ischemic nephropathy (fig. 6.74)
   ▪ Associated perirenal hemorrhage is usually present

○ Fibromuscular dysplasia is a disease that affects the main renal arteries
   ▪ Care should be exercised not to misinterpret stepladder image reconstruction artifact for fibromuscular dysplasia

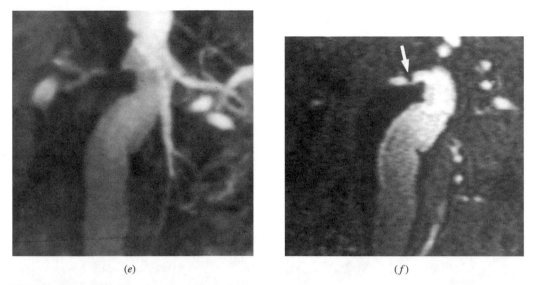

FIGURE 6.72 (*Continued*) The source image (*f*) demonstrates that there is a short segment of high-grade stenosis (arrow, *f*).

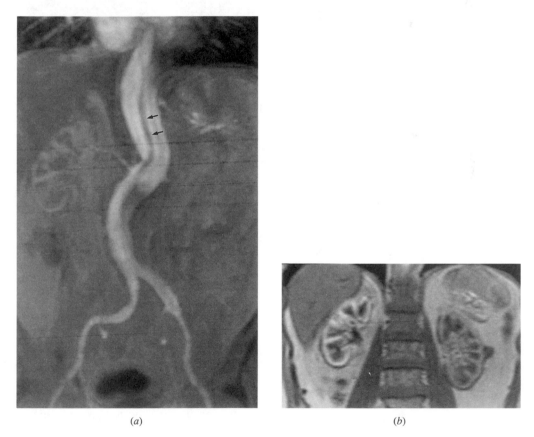

(a) (b)

FIGURE 6.73 Aortic dissection with differential renal perfusion. Coronal MIP reconstructed projection of coronal immediate postgadolinium 2D SGE images (*a*) and coronal 2D immediate postgadolinium source SGE image (*b*). Aortic dissection (small arrows, *a*) is shown on the MIP reconstructed gadolinium-enhanced SGE image (*a*). On an individual coronal source SGE image (*b*), lesser enhancement of the left renal cortex is present, reflecting diminished perfusion of the kidney due to its blood supply arising from the false lumen, which has slower flow.

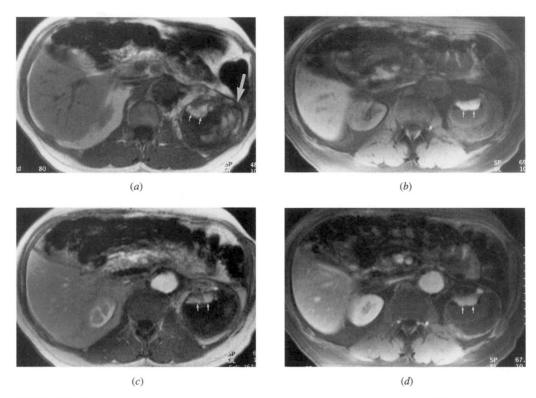

(a)   *(b)*

(c)   *(d)*

FIGURE 6.74   Renal artery injury secondary to abdominal aortic aneurysm surgical repair. SGE (*a*), fat-suppressed SGE (*b*), immediate postgadolinium SGE (*c*), and 90 s postgadolinium fat-suppressed SGE (*d*) images. Abdominal aortic surgery was performed 1 year earlier, in which the left renal artery was injured. The left kidney is atrophic and high in signal intensity on T1W images (small arrows, *a, b*), reflecting intraparenchymal hemorrhage. Associated subcapsular fluid collection and high-signal-intensity perirenal fluid (large arrow, *a*) are present. The kidney remains unchanged in signal intensity on postcontrast images (small arrows, *c, d*).

- Current MRA techniques may not be able to reliably demonstrate subtle changes of fibromuscular dysplasia to supplant angiographic approaches
  - Aortic atheroemboli are the most frequent cause of renal emboli
    - Renal infarction from embolic events tends to occur between calyces and demonstrates well-defined wedge-shaped defects in the renal outline
    - A thin enhancing peripheral rim is present due to enhancement of small vessels in the renal capsule (fig. 6.75)
- Renal Vein Thrombosis
  - Renal vein thrombosis may occur as bland or tumor thrombus
  - Acute thrombosis
    - Kidney enlarges due to tissue swelling secondary to obstructed venous outflow

- A progressive and persistent nephrogram is also observed (fig. 6.76)
  - Chronic thrombosis
    - The kidney is often normal in size

Renal Transplant

- Pretransplant Donor
  - MRI evaluation for vascular and ureteric anatomy
  - Indications
    - Avoids radiation and iodinated contrast exposure
- Posttransplant Recipient
  - Immediate and short-term complications
    - Surgical
      - Renal artery or vein thrombosis
      - Urine leak
      - Ureter implant obstruction and hydronephrosis

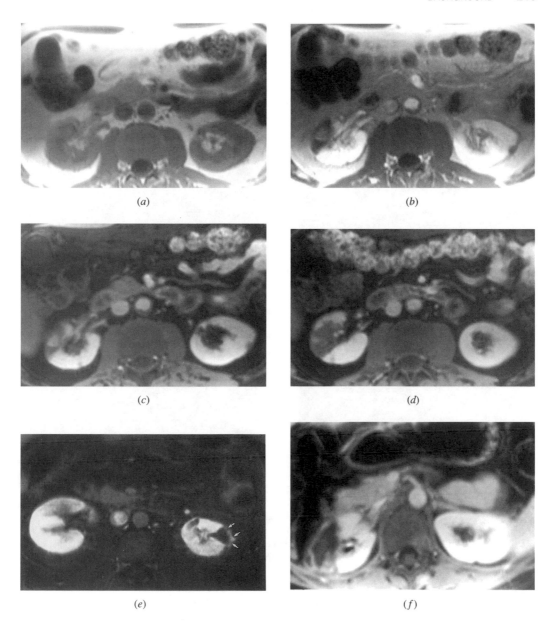

(a)   (b)

(c)   (d)

(e)   (f)

FIGURE 6.75   Renal cortical infarcts. Precontrast T1W SGE (*a*), 45 s postgadolinium SGE (*b*), and 90 s (*c, d*) post-gadolinium fat-suppressed SGE images. There are multiple, peripheral, wedge-shaped areas of decreased enhancement within the kidneys. A focus of central enhancement is noted within a wedge-shaped defect (*b, c*) in the right kidney. The wedge-shaped defects are consistent with areas of infarct, with central sparing in one of the infarcts.

Interstitial phase gadolinium-enhanced T1W fat-suppressed spin-echo image (*e*) in a second patient demonstrates a nearly signal-void wedge-shaped defect in the inferior pole of the left kidney. Linear enhancement peripheral to the wedge-shaped defect (arrows) is due to enhancement of capsular based vessels. This is a classic feature of renal emboli. (Reproduced with permission from Semelka RC, Shoenut JP, Greenberg HM. The Kidney. In: Semelka RC, Shoenut JP (eds.) *MRI of the Abdomen with CT Correlation.* New York: Raven Press, 1993, pp. 91–118.)

Transverse 90 s postgadolinium T1W fat-suppressed spin-echo image (*f*) in a third patient. There is a wedge-shaped defect in the mid aspect of the right kidney consistent with a renal infarction. Note thin capsular enhancement along the outer margin of the defect.

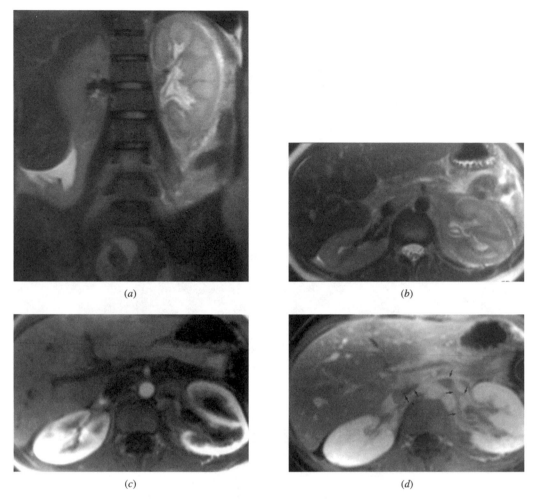

(a) *(b)*

(c) *(d)*

FIGURE 6.76 Acute renal vein thrombosis. Coronal (*a*) and transverse (*b*) SS-ETSE, immediate postgadolinium SGE (*c*), and 90 s postgadolinium T1W fat-suppressed SGE (*d*) images. This pregnant patient presented with severe left flank pain. The left kidney is enlarged, and fluid surrounds the collecting system, consistent with edema. Intraluminal clot is appreciated within the left renal vein extending into the IVC (arrows, *d*).

- Lymphocele
  - Vasculature assessed by using a combination of 3D MRA and gadolinium-enhanced 3D GRE soft-tissue imaging
  - Abnormal fluid collections and hydronephrosis assessed by T2W breath-hold imaging using single-shot echo-train with fat suppression and/or balanced echo (True-FISP, FIESTA, or BFFE) sequences
- Nonsurgical
  - Acute rejection
  - Acute tubular necrosis
- Infection
  - Findings on dynamic gadolinium-enhanced multiphase 3D GRE imaging can show impaired renal corticomedullary perfusion, uptake, and excretion
  - Intermediate and Long-Term Complications
    - Loss of CMD
      - On precontrast T1W fat-suppressed images and immediate gadolinium-enhanced images, CMD has been shown to be associated with normal renal function

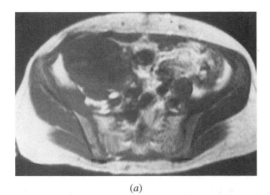

(a)

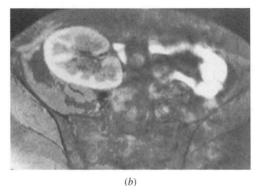

(b)

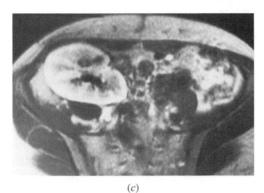

(c)

FIGURE 6.77   Normal transplant kidney. SGE (a), T1W fat-suppressed spin-echo (b), and immediate postgadolinium SGE (c) images of a functioning renal transplant. Normal corticomedullary differentiation is apparent on the SGE image (a), which is clearly defined on the T1W fat-suppressed image (b). Corticomedullary differentiation on the immediate postgadolinium image (c) is consistent with a normal pattern of renal blood flow. (Reprinted with permission from Semelka RC, Shoenut JP, Greenberg HM. The kidney. In: Semelka RC, Shoenut JP, (eds.), *MRI of the Abdomen with CT Correlation.* New York: Raven Press, 1993, pp. 91–118.)

- The presence of CMD demonstrates a strong inverse relationship with serum creatinine
- CMD is diminished and lost in the setting of subacute and long-term impaired renal function (figs. 6.77 and 6.78)
- Diminished CMD is nonspecific, resulting from any cause of impaired renal function including

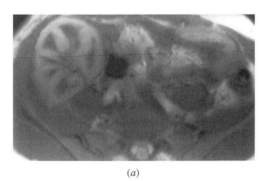

(a)

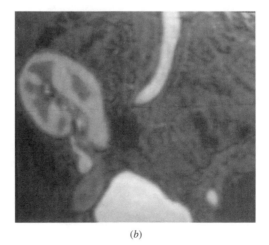

(b)

FIGURE 6.78   Normal transplant kidney. Transverse immediate postgadolinium SGE (a) and coronal 3D MRA source (b) image. The kidney transplant in the right lower quadrant demonstrates normal capillary phase enhancement. No complications were identified.

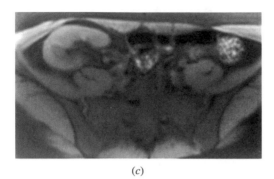
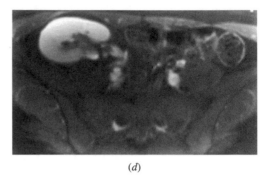

(c)   (d)

FIGURE 6.78 (*Continued*) Precontrast (*c*) and postgadolinium (*d*) T1W fat-suppressed SGE images in a second patient. CMD is present on the noncontrast image. No complications are evident.

- ◦ Subacute or chronic rejection
- ◦ Cyclosporin toxicity
- ◦ Operative complications affecting renal perfusion
- ▪ Impaired perfusion as a measure of reduced glomerular filtration
  - • May be assessed by the observation of impaired corticomedullary perfusion, medullary enhancement, and excretion as shown on arterial, venous, and delayed 3-phase 3D GRE gadolinium-enhanced images, respectively

- • More detailed time course of perfusion and excretion can be obtained by using rapid (e.g., 1 image per second) slice imaging through the kidney during gadolinium injection to obtain better time-resolved kinetics
  - ◦ Early work shows that this method can estimate the single-kidney glomerular filtration rate (GFR) in relation to renal volume, and may be helpful in assessing the viability of a transplanted kidney

CHAPTER 7

ADRENAL GLANDS

BACKGROUND

As with other soft tissues of the abdomen and pelvis, a comprehensive examination of the adrenal glands relies on both T1W and T2W imaging. State-of-the-art imaging should be performed using rapid-acquisition sequences in a breath-hold period. T1W imaging is best performed using GRE breath-hold sequences, which can be acquired with fat suppression to make the adrenal glands more conspicuous. In addition, a single breath-hold dual-echo combination of in-phase and out-of-phase GRE sequence is used for routine examination of the adrenals and represents the most important data acquisitions for evaluating the adrenals. A single breath-hold data acquisition generating both in-phase and out-of-phase echoes is a recent implementation of this method. This technique allows determination of the intracellular lipid content of an adrenal mass, which is important for identifying benign adenomas that normally accumulate lipid.

Gadolinium-enhanced GRE imaging with fat suppression can improve specificity of adrenal mass differentiation and is critical for tumor staging, facilitating assessment of retroperitoneal adenopathy, and for evaluation of adjacent soft tissues including the kidneys, liver, and retroperitoneal blood vessels. Although the in-phase/out-of-phase dual-echo, arterial, and venous phase postgadolinium imaging can be acquired with 2-dimensional (2D) technique, we routinely acquire at least the equilibrium phase imaging using 3D GRE imaging to provide superior spatial resolution and facilitate reconstruction in alternate imaging planes. A key point is that perfusion of an adrenal mass determined by multiphase gadolinium-enhanced T1W imaging can provide important additional information useful for characterization.

The coronal or sagittal plane is useful in the presence of an adrenal mass, to better visualize the relationships with the superior pole of the kidney and the inferior liver edge in cases of right adrenal involvement. T2W imaging should be performed using single-shot echo-train imaging. This technique is motion insensitive, but is best performed during a breath-hold to minimize spatial misregistration between slices. The utility of T2W imaging is

Primer on MR Imaging of the Abdomen and Pelvis, edited by Diego R. Martin, Michele A. Brown, and Richard C. Semelka ISBN 0-471-37340-0 Copyright © 2005 Wiley-Liss, Inc.

TABLE 7.1 Pattern Recognition Adrenal Lesion

	T1 In-Phase	T1 Out-of-Phase	T2	Early Gd	Late Gd	Other Features
Adenoma	↓ - ↑	↓	Ø-↑	Homogeneous intense	Fade	80% drop in signal on out-of-phase 70% have a homogeneous intense capillary blush
Metastases	↓ - ↑	Ø	Ø - ↑	Heterogeneous, variable	Heterogeneous, variable	Heterogeneity increases with increase in lesion size
Pheochromocytoma	↓ - Ø	Ø	↑ - ↑↑	Variable, usually minimal	Variable	Heterogeneous and hyperintense on T2-WI Minimal enhancement with gadolinium
Adrenal cortical carcinoma	↓ - ↑	↓(portions)	↑	↑ Heterogeneous	Fade	Hemorrhagic and necrotic areas Portions of the tumor may drop on out-of-phase images
Lymphoma	Ø	Ø	Ø	Minimal	Minimal	Mild heterogeneity on all sequences

↓↓ Moderately to markedly DECREASED signal intensity
↓ Mildly decreased signal intensity
Ø Isointense
↑ Mildly increased signal intensity
↑↑ Moderately to markedly increased signal intensity

supplemental. Generally, normal adrenal gland and both benign and malignant masses have signal intensity less than fat and between that of liver and spleen. Pheochromocytoma may show very high T2W signal intensity, but this can show overlap with masses of other origins. Pheochromocytoma are also most commonly heterogeneous with moderately high signal intensity on T2W images.

MASS LESIONS

Cortical Masses

Benign
Hyperplasia
Background
- Usually due to secondary response to stimulation, primary hyperplasia is rare

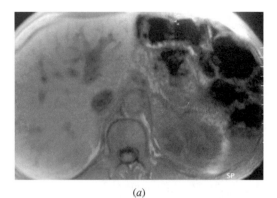

(a)

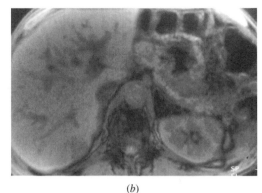

(b)

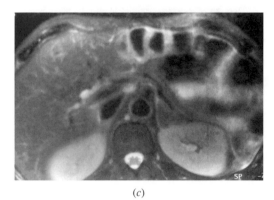

(c)

FIGURE 7.1   Adrenal hyperplasia. T1W SGE (*a*), T1W out-of-phase SGE (*b*), and T2W fat-suppressed single-shot echo-train spin-echo (SS-ETSE) (*c*) images. The left adrenal is diffusely enlarged, and the adrenaliform shape is maintained. It is isointense to the liver on T1 (*a*), drops significantly in signal intensity on out-of-phase SGE (*b*), and is slightly hypointense on T2 fat-suppressed image (*c*). The presence of water and fat in the same voxel results in the findings on out-of-phase images.

- Related conditions include Cushing's syndrome due to adrenocorticotrophic hormone (ACTH)-producing tumor, including Cushing's disease resulting from an ACTH-producing pituitary adenoma
- Also occurs in the setting of hyperthyroidism, acromegaly, diabetes, chronic stress, depression, and other malignancies

Imaging
- Characterized by bilaterally enlarged glands that appear diffusely thickened while retaining an otherwise normal adrenal inverted Y shape (fig. 7.1)
- Unilateral enlargement can occur
- Although enlarged, the glands retain normal signal on T1W, T2W, and postgadolinium-enhanced images, and demonstrate drop in signal intensity on out-of-phase T1W GRE imaging

Mimickers
- Benign adrenal adenoma, which more consistently appears as a defined nodule

Adenoma
Background
- The most common adrenal mass
- Adenomas are usually small neoplasms (<5 cm), with the great majority <2 cm
- Characteristically solitary and well encapsulated
- Clinical evaluation
  ○ Nonhyperfunctioning adenomas are more frequent than functioning adenomas
    ▪ May occur in 2–8% of the general population
    ▪ Increased incidence has been reported in patients who are elderly, obese, hypertensive, or with primary malignancies of bladder, kidney, or endometrium

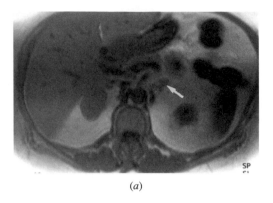

(a)

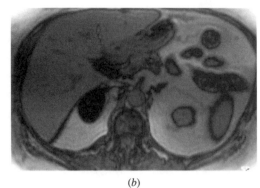

(b)

FIGURE 7.2 Adrenal adenoma—mild capillary blush. T1W SGE (a), T1W out-of-phase SGE (b), and immediate postgadolinium SGE (c) images. Right adrenal adenoma demonstrates signal drop on out-of-phase image and mild capillary blush on immediate postgadolinium image. Note normal left adrenal (arrow, a).

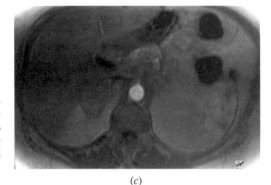

(c)

○ Hyperfunctioning adenomas are usually >2 cm in diameter and commonly are cortisol secreting
  ▪ Responsible for approximately 20% of Cushing's syndrome cases
  ▪ Aldosterone-producing tumors are rare and responsible for most cases of Conn's syndrome
    • Patients present with hypertension, hypokalemia, and low plasma renin

Imaging
• The most accurate method for demonstrating that a mass is an adenoma is to show loss of signal intensity on T1W GRE out-of-phase images (figs. 7.2 to 7.9) which reflects high lipid content
  ○ Similar sensitivity and specificity as for CT, but without ionizing radiation
  ○ Loss of signal intensity should parallel loss of signal in marrow of the adjacent vertebral body

○ Caution should be exercised in using liver as the comparative organ to determine signal intensity loss because the liver may also contain fat
○ The spleen may also be misleading, because in the presence of iron deposition, iron will cause a T2* effect manifesting in a drop in spleen signal on the longer TE in-phase images
○ Renal cortex is less affected by fat or iron deposition and may be a more reliable tissue to use as a visual comparison for signal intensity loss
○ An echo time–adjusted signal intensity drop greater than 20% is diagnostic for adenomas (fig. 7.5), while a 10–20% signal intensity drop is suggestive of adenomas (figs. 7.10 and 7.11)
• Approximately 15% of benign adenomas do not accumulate intracytoplasmic lipid and may retain signal on out-of-phase images (figs. 7.10, 7.12, and 7.13)

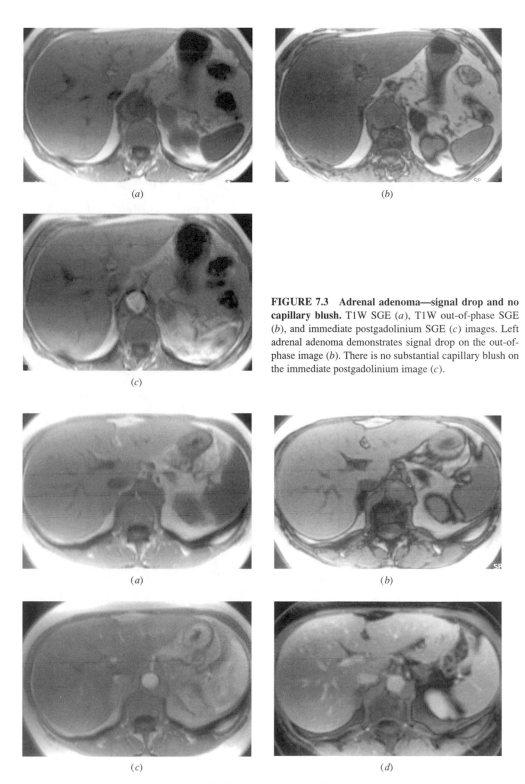

FIGURE 7.3   Adrenal adenoma—signal drop and no capillary blush. T1W SGE (*a*), T1W out-of-phase SGE (*b*), and immediate postgadolinium SGE (*c*) images. Left adrenal adenoma demonstrates signal drop on the out-of-phase image (*b*). There is no substantial capillary blush on the immediate postgadolinium image (*c*).

FIGURE 7.4   Bilateral adrenal adenoma. T1W SGE (*a*), T1W out-of-phase SGE (*b*), immediate postgadolinium SGE (*c*), and 90 s postgadolinium fat-suppressed SGE (*d*) images in a patient with bilateral adrenal adenomas. Note that in this patient both adrenals show signal intensity drop on out-of-phase images, but there is no substantial capillary blush after gadolinium administration (*c*). Late enhancement is mildly heterogeneous (*d*).

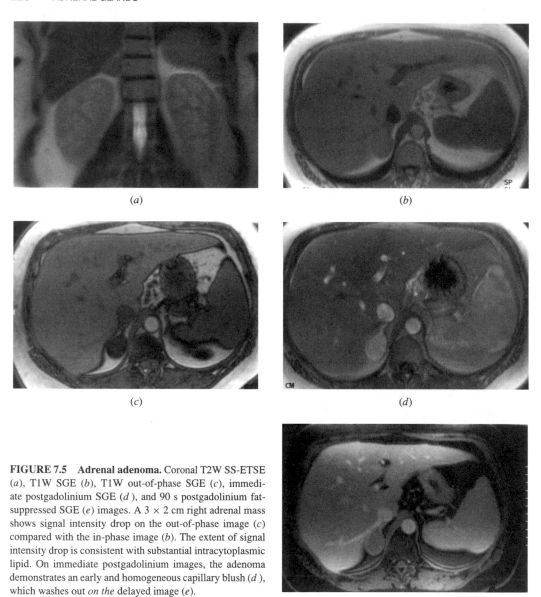

(a)

(b)

(c)

(d)

(e)

FIGURE 7.5   Adrenal adenoma. Coronal T2W SS-ETSE (*a*), T1W SGE (*b*), T1W out-of-phase SGE (*c*), immediate postgadolinium SGE (*d*), and 90 s postgadolinium fat-suppressed SGE (*e*) images. A 3 × 2 cm right adrenal mass shows signal intensity drop on the out-of-phase image (*c*) compared with the in-phase image (*b*). The extent of signal intensity drop is consistent with substantial intracytoplasmic lipid. On immediate postgadolinium images, the adenoma demonstrates an early and homogeneous capillary blush (*d*), which washes out *on the* delayed image (*e*).

- Contrast-enhanced images acquired with 20 s delay often show uniform transient enhancement of the entire lesion on immediate postgadolinium capillary phase images, reported in 70% of cases
  - Uniform enhancement is rare for primary or secondary carcinomas
- Contrast enhancement on immediate postgadolinium images is variable in 30% from minimal (figs. 7.2, 7.3, 7.4, and 7.8) to moderately intense (figs. 7.5 to 7.8), but washout is usually observed by 2–3 min (figs. 7.5 and 7.6)
- Small linear or rounded foci of low or high signal intensity may be present on various MR sequences, representing small areas of cystic change, hemorrhage, or variations of vascularity (fig. 7.14)

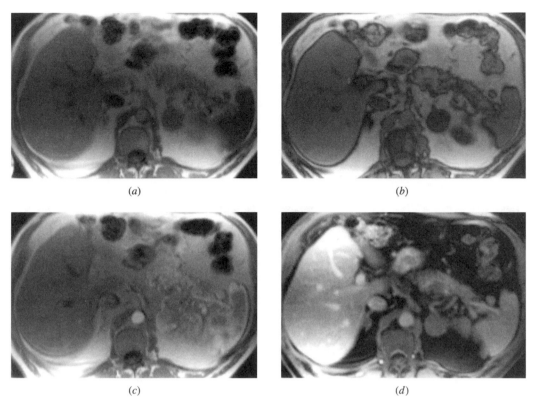

(a) (b)

(c) (d)

FIGURE 7.6   Bilateral adrenal adenoma. T1W SGE (a), T1W out-of-phase SGE (b), immediate postgadolinium SGE (c), and 90 s postgadolinium fat-suppressed SGE (d) images. Bilateral adrenal adenomas, larger on the left side. Both lesions have signal intensity drop on the out-of-phase image (b). There is an intense capillary blush on immediate postgadolinium image (c) and a rapid washout on delayed image (d).

- Malignant disease typically shows heterogeneous enhancement and heterogeneous and variable washout
  - Perfusion characteristics may help further increase sensitivity and specificity, particularly in the 15% of benign cases that do not show lipid accumulation
- Large adenomas may undergo degenerative changes and contain foci of hemorrhage that appear as punctate high-signal-intensity foci on T1W and/or T2W images (fig. 7.14)
- Adenomas are usually homogeneously iso- or hypointense in relation to the normal adrenal gland on T2W images (fig. 7.2), whereas adrenal metastases tend to be mildly hyperintense and heterogeneous

Mimickers
- Benign hyperplasia
- Myelolipoma, with higher abundance of myeloid cells leading to less dense fatty composition and possible signal dropout on out-of-phase images, thus mimicking a benign adenoma
- Nonfatty adenomas may be indistinguishable from a metastasis

Myelolipoma
Background
- Rare benign tumors composed of differentiated adipocytes and hematopoietic cells
- Typically small, unilateral, and high fat content, giving them a pathognomonic appearance on MR images

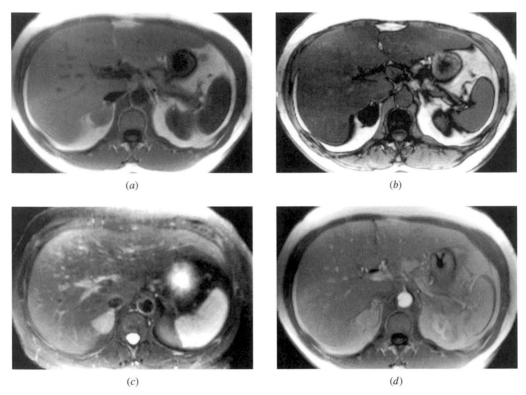

(a)   *(b)*

(c)   *(d)*

FIGURE 7.7   Adrenal adenoma. T1W SGE (*a*), T1W out-of-phase SGE (*b*), T2W single-shot echo-train spin-echo (SS-ETSE) (*c*), and 45 s postgadolinium SGE (*d*) images. Right adrenal adenoma has substantial signal drop from the in-phase (*a*) to the out-of-phase image (*b*) and moderately high signal intensity on fat-suppressed T2 image (*c*). Note the intense homogeneous capillary blush after gadolinium administration (*d*).

Imaging
- High fat content results in the following char-
  acteristics (fig. 7.15):
  ○ Loss of signal on fat-suppressed T1W
    GRE
  ○ High signal on T1W GRE without fat sup-
    pression, similar to retroperitoneal fat
  ○ No drop in signal on out-of-phase GRE
    (TE = 2.2 ms at 1.5 T)
    ▪ Only tissues with a mixture of fat and
      water will drop in signal, as voxels com-
      prised of pure water or pure fat will not
      change in signal
- Larger tumors benefit from coronal/sagittal
  imaging to delineate the lesion from kidney
  and liver
- Occasionally tumor may have proportionately greater abundance of myeloid tissue,
  less fat, and may demonstrate signal drop on
  out-of-phase SGE images

Mimickers
- Lipoma
- Adenoma

Adrenal Cyst
Background
- Uncommon, heterogeneous group of lesions
- Histologically differentiated into 4 types
  ○ Endothelial
    ▪ Along with hemorrhagic pseudocysts, are
      the most common
    ▪ Histologically multilocular, filled with
      clear, milky fluid, with a thin fibrous wall
      lined by a continuous layer of endothelial
      cells

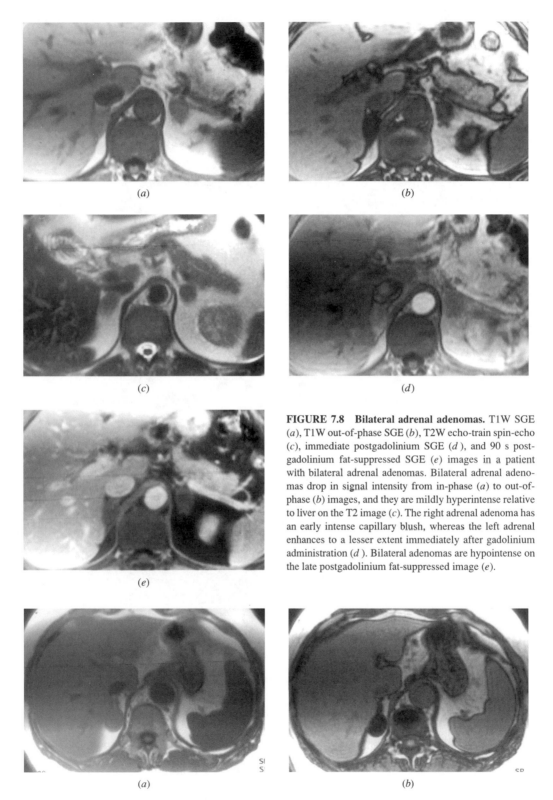

(a)

(b)

(c)

(d)

(e)

FIGURE 7.8 Bilateral adrenal adenomas. T1W SGE (a), T1W out-of-phase SGE (b), T2W echo-train spin-echo (c), immediate postgadolinium SGE (d), and 90 s postgadolinium fat-suppressed SGE (e) images in a patient with bilateral adrenal adenomas. Bilateral adrenal adenomas drop in signal intensity from in-phase (a) to out-of-phase (b) images, and they are mildly hyperintense relative to liver on the T2 image (c). The right adrenal adenoma has an early intense capillary blush, whereas the left adrenal enhances to a lesser extent immediately after gadolinium administration (d). Bilateral adenomas are hypointense on the late postgadolinium fat-suppressed image (e).

(a)

(b)

FIGURE 7.9 Adrenal adenoma with signal drop on out-of-phase image. T1W SGE (a) and T1W out-of-phase SGE (b) images. Substantial signal intensity drop is present on the right adrenal adenoma comparing in-phase (a) to out-of-phase (b) SGE images, consistent with high lipid content.

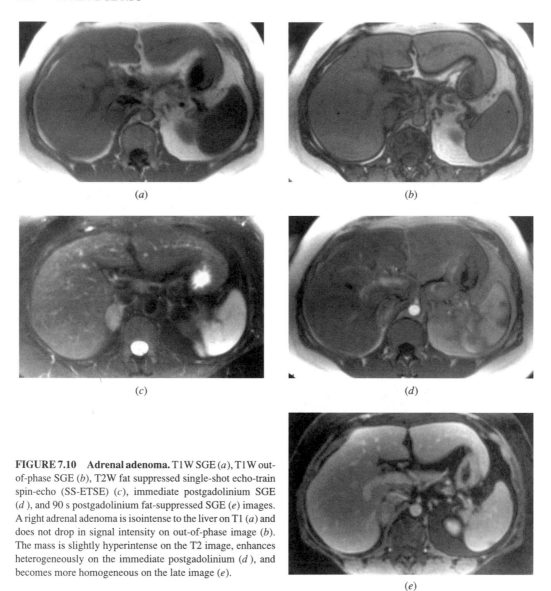

FIGURE 7.10   Adrenal adenoma. T1W SGE (*a*), T1W out-of-phase SGE (*b*), T2W fat suppressed single-shot echo-train spin-echo (SS-ETSE) (*c*), immediate postgadolinium SGE (*d*), and 90 s postgadolinium fat-suppressed SGE (*e*) images. A right adrenal adenoma is isointense to the liver on T1 (*a*) and does not drop in signal intensity on out-of-phase image (*b*). The mass is slightly hyperintense on the T2 image, enhances heterogeneously on the immediate postgadolinium (*d*), and becomes more homogeneous on the late image (*e*).

○ Hemorrhagic (pseudocyst)
  ▪ Hemorrhagic pseudocysts are usually unilocular cystic masses encased in a fibrous capsule and contain amorphous material, blood, and fibrin
  ▪ Microscopic examination reveals numerous irregular, thin-walled vascular channels
○ Epithelial
○ Parasitic

Imaging
• The majority of adrenal cysts and pseudocysts appear low signal on T1W and high signal on T2W images
• Sharply marginated
• No internal gadolinium enhancement
• Pseudocysts resulting from adrenal hemorrhage can show variable signal intensity on T1W and T2W images (fig. 7.16)

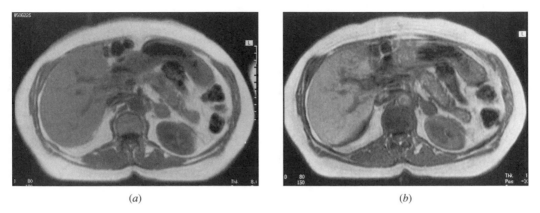

(a)   *(b)*

FIGURE 7.11   Adrenal adenoma—mild signal drop. T1W SGE (*a*) and T1W out-of-phase SGE (*b*) images. Mild signal intensity loss (approximately 15%) is noted from in-phase (*a*) to out-of-phase (*b*) images, which is in the low range for signal intensity drop to diagnose an adrenal mass as an adenoma. The extent of signal intensity drop is consistent with minimal intracytoplasmic lipid.

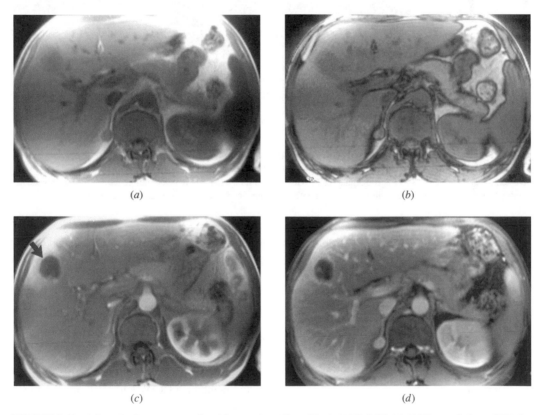

(a)   *(b)*

(c)   *(d)*

FIGURE 7.12   Adrenal adenoma—no signal loss and capillary blush. T1W SGE (*a*), T1W out-of-phase SGE (*b*), immediate postgadolinium SGE (*c*), and 90 s postgadolinium fat-suppressed SGE (*d*) images in a patient with a non-functioning adenoma. The adrenal adenoma is slightly hypointense to the liver on T1 (*a*) and has no signal drop on the out-of-phase image (*b*). After gadolinium administration there is a capillary blush of the adrenal adenoma (*c*) and minimal washout of contrast material on the late image (*d*). A 3.5 cm abscess with a thin capsule is present in the liver (arrow, *c*). Note the intense perilesional enhancement on the immediate postgadolinium image.

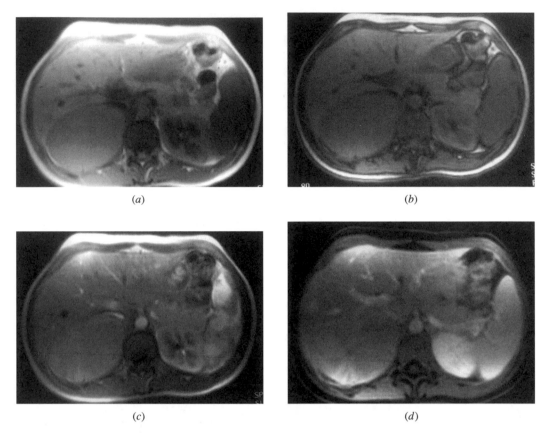

(a) *(b)*

(c) *(d)*

FIGURE 7.13   Large functioning adrenal adenoma. T1W SGE (*a*), T1W out-of-phase SGE (*b*), immediate postgadolinium SGE (*c*), and 90 s postgadolinium fat-suppressed SGE (*d*) images. A right adrenal mass appears hypointense to the liver on T1 SGE (*a*) and does not drop signal on T1 out-of-phase image (*b*). There is a heterogeneous capillary blush after contrast administration (*c*), which diminishes moderately and remains slightly hypointense on late images (*d*).

- Pseudocysts that contain substantial concentration of extracellular methemoglobin from subacute hemorrhage may remain slightly hyperintense on gadolinium-enhanced images
  - Multiphase gadolinium-enhanced images show no change in signal intensity
  - Pseudocysts may be large in size, and coronal/sagittal plane imaging may be useful to demonstrate the location of the mass

Hemangioma
Background
- Uncommon benign vascular tumor composed of mesenchymal cells
- The lesions tend to be large (>10 cm) and have undergone central necrosis and hemorrhage

Imaging
- Postgadolinium T1W GRE images show characteristic intensely enhancing peripheral nodules (fig. 7.17)
  - Do not show central filling in, as is typical of hepatic hemangiomas
    - Likely due to central necrosis secondary to hemorrhage, which is common in adrenal hemangiomas
- Tumors are high in signal intensity centrally on unenhanced T1W and T2W images due to necrosis and hemorrhage

Mimickers
- Adrenal cortical carcinomas or metastases due to the presence of central necrosis and hemorrhage

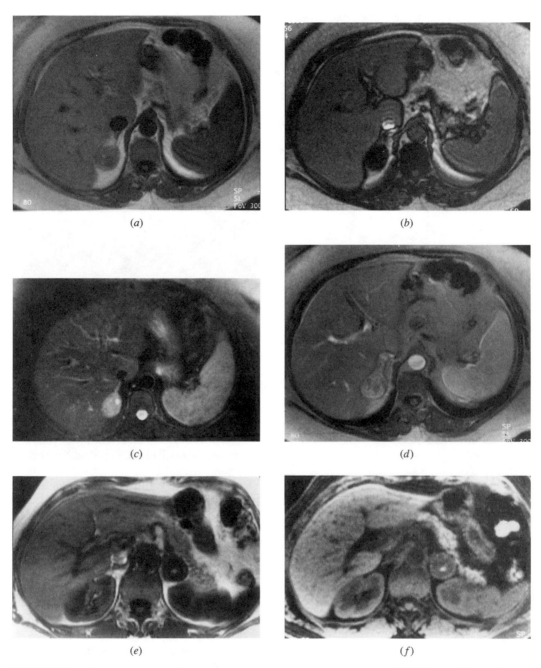

FIGURE 7.14 **Adrenal adenoma with signal intensity drop and minor hemorrhage.** T1W SGE (*a*), T1W out-of-phase SGE (*b*), T2W fat-suppressed spin-echo (*c*), and immediate postgadolinium SGE (*d*) images. Substantial signal intensity drop is present on the right adrenal adenoma comparing in-phase (*a*) to out-of-phase (*b*) SGE images. Small high-signal-intensity foci are present on T1W (*a*) and T2W (*c*) images, which is consistent with hemorrhage. The adenoma enhances intensely on the immediate postgadolinium SGE image (*d*) and contains foci of diminished enhancement that correspond to punctate regions of hemorrhage. T1W SGE (*e*), T1W fat-suppressed SGE (*f*), T2W fat-suppressed single-shot echo-train spin-echo (SS-ETSE) (*g*), immediate postgadolinium SGE (*h*), and 2 min postgadolinium fat-suppressed SGE (*i*) images in a second patient. A 3 cm left adrenal adenoma is present that contains foci of high signal intensity on the T1W image (*e*), which do not suppress with fat suppression (*f*).

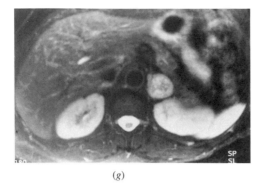

(g)

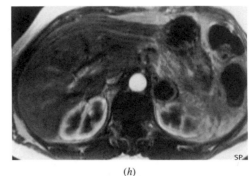

(h)

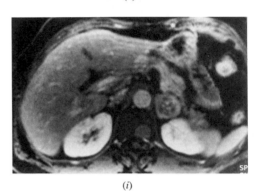

(i)

FIGURE 7.14 (*Continued*) The mass is heterogeneous on the T2W image (*g*) and contains multiple high-signal-intensity foci. A prominent rim of enhancement is present on the immediate postgadolinium image with minimal internal enhancement (*h*). On the interstitial phase gadolinium-enhanced fat-suppressed image (*i*), central punctate high-signal-intensity foci are apparent.

○ Peripheral nodular enhancement distinct from central progressive irregular enhancement of malignant tumor
• Hemorrhagic pseudocysts
  ○ Do not show enhancement

Malignant
Metastases
Background
• Metastases are the most frequent adrenal malignancy (much more frequent than primary adrenal cortical carcinomas, but not more frequent than benign adenomas)
  ○ Most common primary tumors include lung, breast, kidney, pancreas, melanoma, thyroid
• Frequently bilateral
• Metastases do not accumulate lipid, as is observed in adenomas

Imaging
• Absence of lipid results in no signal decrease on T1W out-of-phase images (figs. 7.18 and 7.19)

• Metastases usually show gadolinium enhancement that differs from benign adenomas
  ○ Variable intensity of arterial phase enhancement, although usually mild and most commonly irregular
  ○ Venous and equilibrium delayed phases show variable washout or progressive enhancement but not rapid washout
    ▪ Pattern characterized by coarse irregular lines and patches
    ▪ Best visualized on T1W GRE fat-suppressed equilibrium phase postgadolinium images (fig. 7.18)
• Direct extension of primary tumors may occasionally be seen (fig. 7.18)
  ○ Most frequently observed in pancreatic or renal cancer
• Necrosis and hemorrhage may be seen in larger metastatic masses
  ○ Better shown on MR than CT images (figs. 7.20 and 7.21)
• T2W signal intensity is variable and does not usually add diagnostic specificity

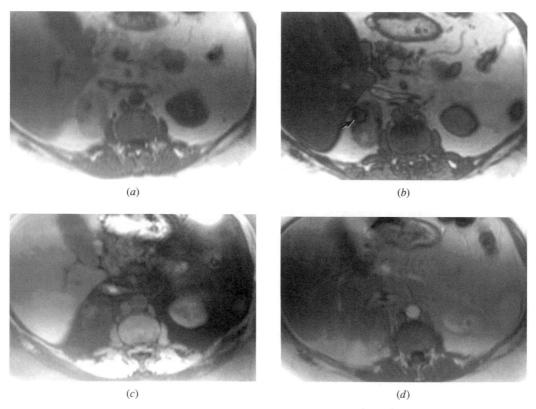

(a)   (b)

(c)   (d)

FIGURE 7.15   Adrenal myelolipoma. T1W SGE (*a*), T1W out-of-phase (*b*), T1W fat-suppressed SGE (*c*), immediate postgadolinium SGE (*d*), and 90 s postgadolinium SGE (*e*) images. The right adrenal myelolipoma is hyperintense on the in-phase (*a*) image and drops in signal on the out-of-phase image (*b*), except for an eccentric focal area that does not drop in signal and possesses a phase-cancellation artifact (arrow, *b*). Myelolipomas may contain focal accumulation of hematopoietic cells within mature adipose tissue, which this focal region represents. The mass is hypointense on T1 fat-suppressed image (*c*), with no suppression of the same focal region. Negligible enhancement on immediate (*d*) and late (*e*) images is appreciated. The predominantly fatty portion of the tumor is low signal on the fat-suppressed image.

○ However, metastases can show proportionately larger central necrosis for a given tumor size compared to adenomas
   ▪ Seen as irregular high- and low-signal central foci

Mimickers
• Benign adenoma with low lipid content
   ○ An adrenal mass that is well marginated but has no signal drop on out-of-phase images is indeterminant for benign adenoma
      ▪ Occurs in 15% of adenomas
      ▪ Similar specificity to a nonenhanced CT study, which would also fail to show low density within the mass

○ Additional information from dynamic gadolinium-enhanced images can increase specificity to over 90–95% and should be included as part of the routine MRI protocol
○ In the setting of known malignancy (breast, lung), around 5% of cases will require follow-up
   ▪ Repeat imaging in 1–3 months to assess for change in size
   ▪ PET scan
   ▪ With the use of in-phase and out-of-phase and gadolinium-enhanced MRI with or without PET, percutaneous biopsies are currently rarely required
   ▪ CT does not have added value

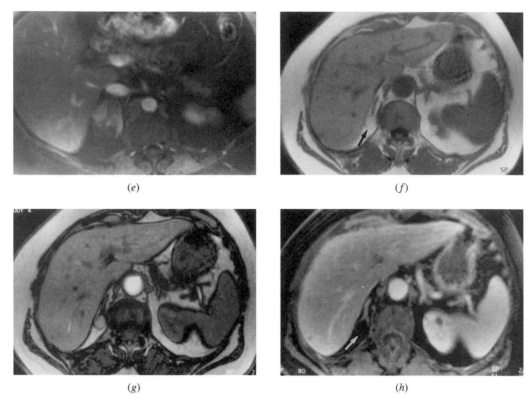

(e)

(f)

(g)

(h)

FIGURE 7.15 (*Continued*) T1W SGE (*f*), T1W out-of-phase SGE (*g*), and 90 s postgadolinium fat-suppressed SGE (*h*) images in a second patient. A 1.8 cm myelolipoma (arrow, *f*) is present of the right adrenal. The tumor is high in signal intensity on the in-phase SGE image because it is composed almost entirely of fat. No drop in signal is present on the out-of-phase image (*g*), reflecting the near complete absence of water protons in the mass. On the fat-suppressed image the mass is near signal void (arrow, *h*), confirming that it is essentially all fat in composition.

Adrenal Cortical Carcinoma
Background
- Very uncommon aggressive tumor
- May contain intracytoplasmic lipid or fatty regions, but heterogeneous in distribution
- The tumor is more common in women, and the age range at presentation is 20–70 years
- Approximately 50% of the tumors present with elevated glucocorticoids with clinical manifestations including hypercortisolism and virilization
- Typically not truly hypersecreting, but rather these are large tumors with some degree of retained capacity to produce hormones that have lost the function of autoregulation

- Adrenal cortical carcinomas typically are considerably larger at presentation (>8 cm) than adenomas
- Areas of necrosis and hemorrhage are frequent

Imaging
- Tumors are frequently necrotic (fig. 7.22) and hemorrhagic
  - These tumors appear heterogeneous and hyperintense on T1W and T2W images, reflecting central necrosis and hemorrhage
  - Necrosis is well shown on gadolinium-enhanced images as signal-void regions
  - Hemorrhage is well shown on precontrast T1W conventional or fat-suppressed images as high-signal-intensity regions (fig. 7.23)

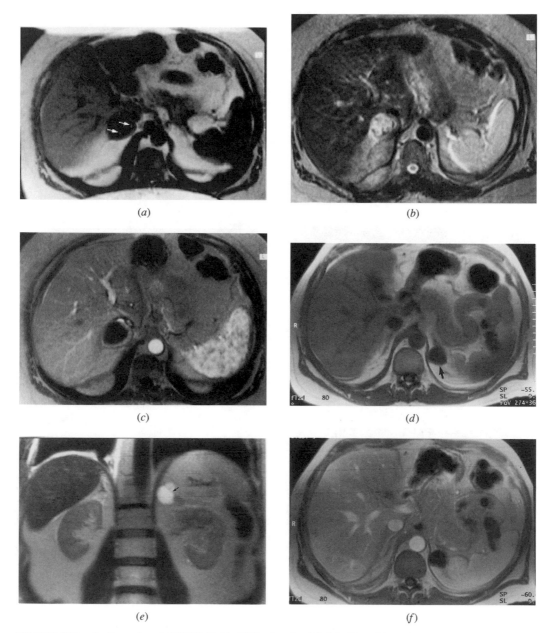

FIGURE 7.16   Cyst/pseudocyst. T1W SGE (*a*), T2W spin-echo (T2-SE) (*b*), and immediate postgadolinium SGE (*c*) images. Small high-signal-intensity foci are noted on the T1 image (arrows, *a*) within the low-signal-intensity pseudocyst, a finding consistent with hemorrhage. The mass is heterogeneous and high in signal intensity on the T2W image (*b*). The heterogeneity reflects the presence of blood products. The lesion is signal void on early (*c*) and late (not shown) postgadolinium images, which are diagnostic features for a cyst.

T1W SGE (*d*), coronal T2W single-shot echo-train spin-echo (SS-ETSE) (*e*), 45 s postgadolinium SGE (*f*), and 90 s postgadolinium fat-suppressed SGE (*g*) images in a second patient. An adrenal pseudocyst is identified arising from the left adrenal (arrow, *d*). The pseudocyst is low in signal intensity on the T1W image (*d*) and high in signal intensity on the T2W image (*e*), and does not enhance on early (*f*) or late (*g*) postgadolinium images.

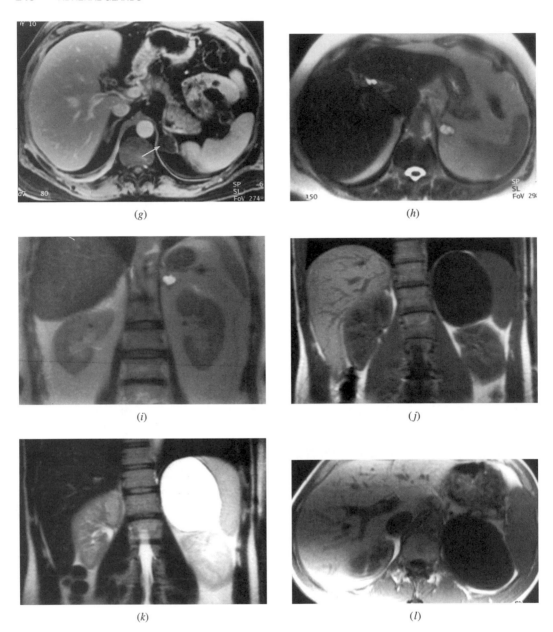

FIGURE 7.16 (*Continued*) Thin septations are present in the pseudocyst (arrow, *e*), which are well shown on the breathing-independent T2W image (*e*) and show faint enhancement on the interstitial phase gadolinium-enhanced fat-suppressed image (arrow, *g*).

T2W single-shot echo-train spin-echo (SS-ETSE) (*h*) and coronal T2W single-shot echo-train spin-echo (SS-ETSE) (*i*) images in a third patient. A pseudocyst in the left adrenal contains septations that are well shown on the snapshot T2W images (*h*, *i*) as hypointense linear structures. Coronal T1W SGE (*j*), coronal T2W single-shot echo-train spin-echo (SS-ETSE) (*k*), T1W SGE (*l*), T1W out-of-phase SGE (*m*), T2W single-shot echo-train spin-echo (SS-ETSE) (*n*), immediate postgadolinium SGE (*o*), 90 s postgadolinium fat-suppressed SGE (*p*), and sagittal postgadolinium SGE (*q*) images in a fourth patient.

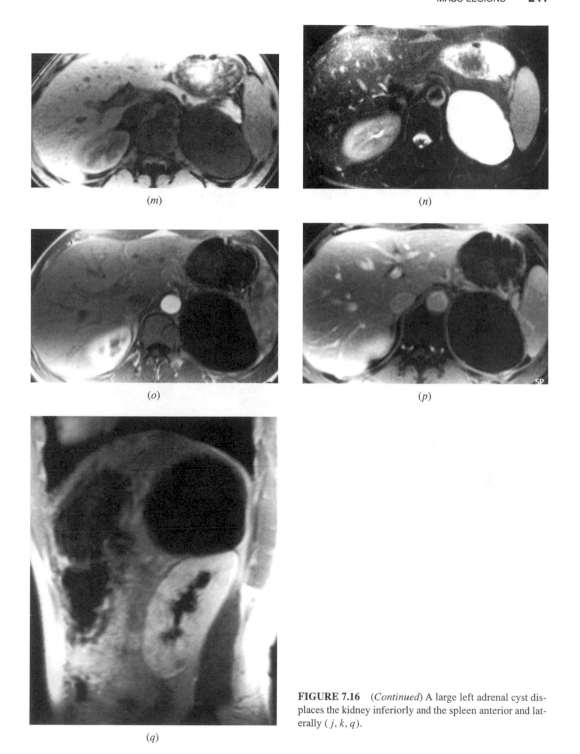

(m)

(n)

(o)

(p)

(q)

FIGURE 7.16 (*Continued*) A large left adrenal cyst displaces the kidney inferiorly and the spleen anterior and laterally (*j, k, q*).

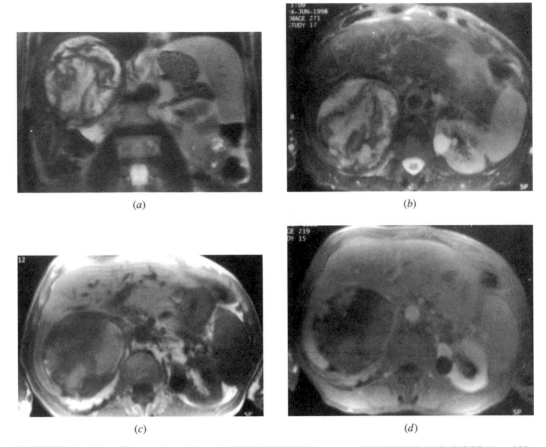

FIGURE 7.17   Adrenal hemangioma. Coronal T2W SS-ETSE (*a*), fat suppressed T2W ETSE (*b*), T1W SGE (*c*), and 90 s postgadolinium fat-suppressed SGE (*d*) images. A large (10 cm) mass is present in the right adrenal, which is heterogeneous and high signal intensity on T2W (*a, b*) and T1W (*c*) images, consistent with hemorrhage and central necrosis. Peripheral enhancing nodules are apparent on the gadolinium-enhanced image (*d*).

- Gadolinium-enhanced GRE images can show peripheral mural-based nodules (fig. 7.24)
- T2W images can exhibit high signal intensity, usually irregular and central, related to necrosis
- Metastases are frequently found at presentation
  - Involvement of regional and para-aortic lymph nodes, lungs, and liver (fig. 7.22) and IVC tumor thrombus (fig. 7.22)
  - Best seen on postgadolinium GRE, particularly fat-suppressed 3D equilibrium phase GRE

Mimickers
- Benign adenomas
  - As carcinomas can be functional, they may contain regions of intracytoplasmic lipid that result in irregular foci of signal intensity loss on out-of-phase images (fig. 7.25)
  - Differentiate from adenoma based on the lack of uniform loss of signal intensity, irregular contrast enhancement, and central necrosis
- Hemangioma
  - Peripheral enhancing nodules can appear similar

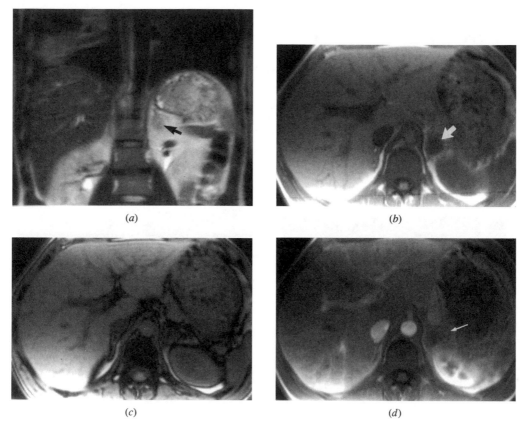

(a)   *(b)*

(c)   *(d)*

FIGURE 7.18   Small left hypovascular adrenal metastasis. Coronal T2W single-shot echo-train spin-echo (SS-ETSE) (*a*), T1W SGE (*b*), T1W out-of-phase SGE (*c*), and immediate postgadolinium SGE (*d*) images. A 1.5 cm metastasis is heterogeneous and moderately high in signal intensity on the T2W image (arrow, *a*). The tumor is hypointense on T1 (*b*) and does not show signal drop on the out-of-phase image (*c*). On immediate postgadolinium image, the tumor demonstrates negligible enhancement with a thin rim (arrow, *d*).

Lymphoma
Background
- Adrenal glands occasionally involved secondarily
- Uni- or bilateral
- Non-Hodgkin's lymphoma is the most frequent cell type
- Retroperitoneal lymphadenopathy is frequently an associated finding

Imaging
- Intermediate signal on T1W images
- Intermediate to minimally hyperintense on T2W images

- Gadolinium enhancement is variable, but is usually minimal on immediate postcontrast images, with increasing enhancement on delayed images (fig. 7.26)
- Retroperitoneal adenopathy and masses in other solid organs; splenomegaly and splenic masses best visualized on gadolinium-enhanced arterial/capillary phase T1W GRE images, including interstitial phase fat-suppressed 3D GRE

Mimickers
- Metastases and primary carcinoma
  ○ Lymphomas tend to show greater uniformity in signal and enhancement for a given

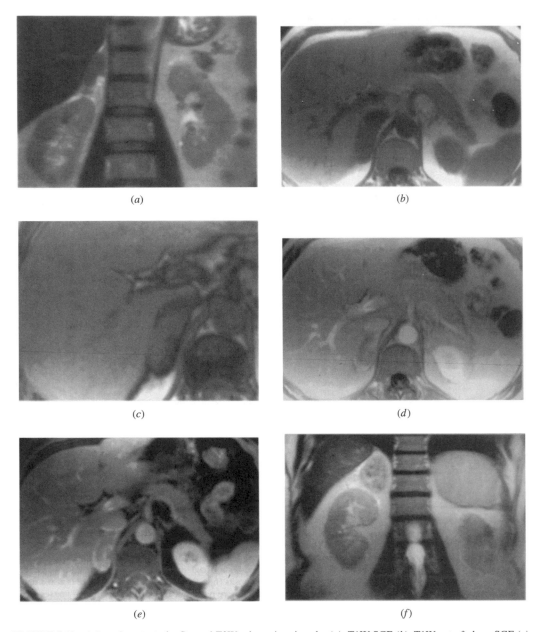

(a)   *(b)*

(c)   *(d)*

(e)   *(f)*

FIGURE 7.19   Adrenal metastasis. Coronal T2W echo-train spin-echo (*a*), T1W SGE (*b*), T1W out-of-phase SGE (*c*), immediate postgadolinium SGE (*d*), and 90 s postgadolinium fat-suppressed SGE (*e*) images in a patient with primary non-small-cell lung cancer. A 5.4 × 2.3 cm oval right adrenal metastasis is slightly hypointense to the liver on the in-phase image (*b*), with no drop in signal on the out-of-phase image. (*c*) After contrast administration, there is peripheral, irregular enhancement of the lesion (*d*, *e*).

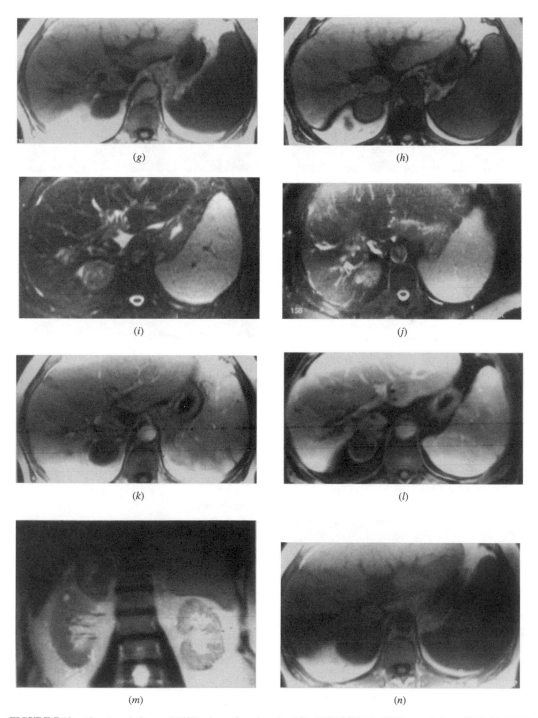

FIGURE 7.19   (*Continued*) Coronal T2W echo-train spin-echo (*f*), T1W SGE (*g*), T1W out-of-phase SGE (*h*), T2W echo-train spin-echo (*i*), STIR (*j*), immediate postgadolinium SGE (*k*), and 90 s postgadolinium fat-suppressed SGE (*l*) images in a second patient, who had primary colon cancer.

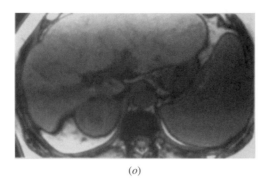

(o)

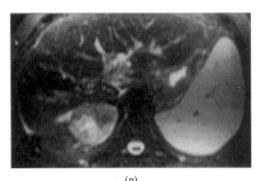

(p)

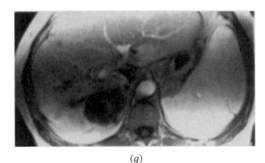

(q)

FIGURE 7.19 (*Continued*) Coronal T2W echo-train spin-echo (*m*), T1W SGE (*n*), T1W out-of-phase SGE (*o*), STIR (*p*), and immediate postgadolinium SGE (*q*) images in the same patient 3 months later. There is no signal loss comparing in-phase (*g*, *n*) and out-of-phase (*h*, *o*) images. On the T2W images, the adrenal lesion appears heterogeneously hypointense with hyperintense foci (*f*, *i*, *j*, *m*, *p*). Interval growth has occurred after 3 months (*m–q*).

size of tumor, with this difference most apparent in larger tumors
- ○ Generally primary adrenal cortical carcinoma and metastases show more irregular enhancement and irregular tissue with larger areas of necrosis

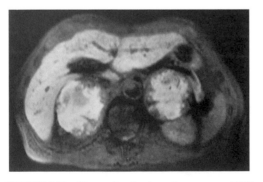

FIGURE 7.20 Hemorrhagic adrenal metastases. T1W fat-suppressed spin-echo image demonstrates high-signal-intensity subacute hemorrhage in bilateral adrenal metastases. Metastasis may undergo hemorrhage, simulating primary adrenal cortical carcinoma.

- ○ Lymphoma is associated with more extensive distribution of retroperitoneal (and other locations) lymphadenopathy

Medullary Masses

Background
- The adrenal medulla is composed of neuroendocrine cells derived from the neural crest
- Represents a part of the paraganglionic system
- Neoplasms arising from the medulla include
  - ○ Pheochromocytoma
  - ○ Neuroblastoma, ganglioglioma, and ganglioneuroblastoma

Pheochromocytoma
Background
- Pheochromocytoma can be defined as a paraganglioma of the adrenal medulla and is a catecholamine-producing tumor

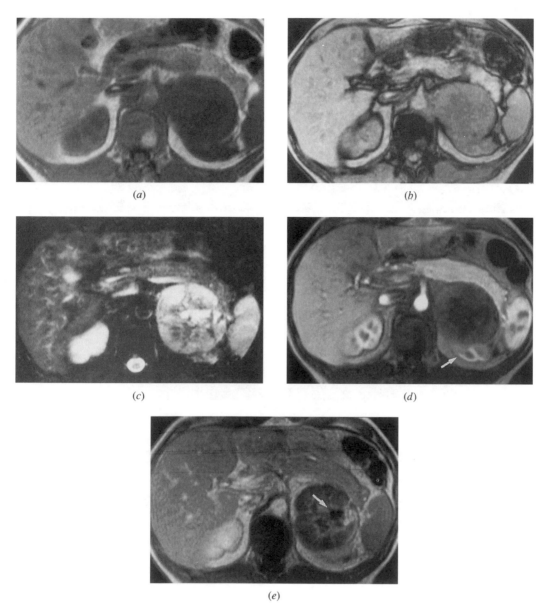

(a)   *(b)*

(c)   *(d)*

(e)

FIGURE 7.21   Large left adrenal metastases. T1W SGE (*a*), T1W out-of-phase SGE (*b*), T2W fat-suppressed spin-echo
(*c*), immediate postgadolinium (*d*), and 3 min postgadolinium SGE (*e*) images. A large (8 cm) left adrenal metastasis is
identified that retains signal intensity from in-phase (*a*) to out-of-phase (*b*) images. The mass is heterogeneous and moderately
high in signal intensity on T2W images, with a central high-signal-intensity region (*c*). On immediate postgadolinium image
(*d*), the mass enhances minimally. On more delayed images, a central low-signal-intensity signal-void region compatible
with necrosis is identified (arrows, *e*) that corresponds to the region of high signal intensity on T2W images. The central
necrosis and heterogeneity demonstrated on T2W and postgadolinium images further confirm the findings on out-of-phase
images corresponding to a malignant mass. Distinction between adrenal metastasis and left kidney is best defined on the
immediate postgadolinium SGE image by the demonstration of corticomedullary differentiation of the kidney (arrow, *d*).

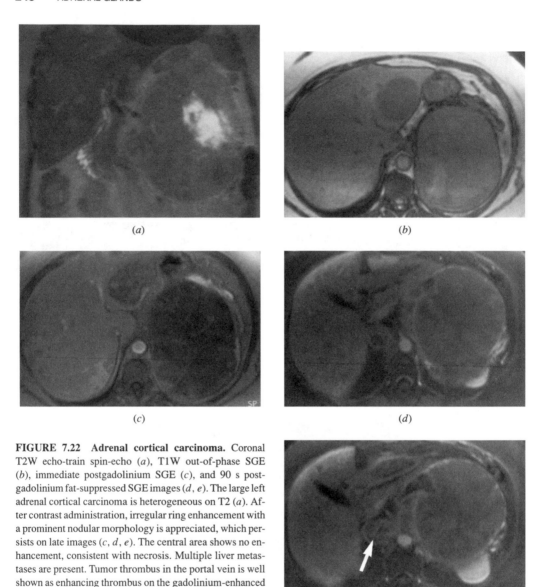

(a)

(b)

(c)

(d)

FIGURE 7.22   Adrenal cortical carcinoma. Coronal T2W echo-train spin-echo (*a*), T1W out-of-phase SGE (*b*), immediate postgadolinium SGE (*c*), and 90 s post-gadolinium fat-suppressed SGE images (*d*, *e*). The large left adrenal cortical carcinoma is heterogeneous on T2 (*a*). After contrast administration, irregular ring enhancement with a prominent nodular morphology is appreciated, which persists on late images (*c*, *d*, *e*). The central area shows no enhancement, consistent with necrosis. Multiple liver metastases are present. Tumor thrombus in the portal vein is well shown as enhancing thrombus on the gadolinium-enhanced fat-suppressed SGE image (arrow, *e*).

(e)

- Tumor cells are arranged in well-defined nests (*Zellballen*) surrounded by fibrovascular stroma
- There is no morphologic marker of malignancy for this tumor other than the presence of metastases
- Arise from the adrenal medulla in 90% of cases

○ Rule of 10%
  ▪ 10% bilateral adrenal
  ▪ 10% malignant
  ▪ 10% extra-adrenal
    • Extra-adrenal pheochromocytomas are malignant in 40% of cases
    • Arise in paraganglia along the course of the sympathetic chain, most frequently

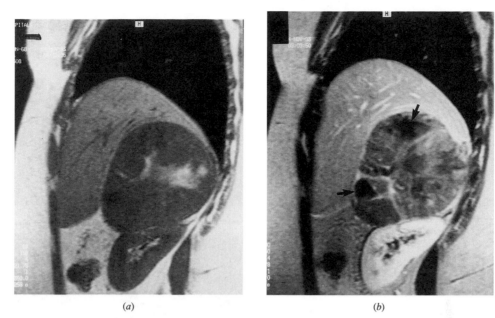

(a)   (b)

FIGURE 7.23   Adrenal cortical carcinoma. Sagittal T1W SGE (*a*) and 90 s postgadolinium SGE (*b*) images in a 25-year-old woman. A 7 cm mass is identified in the right upper abdomen that indents the liver and displaces the right kidney inferiorly. The relationship of the mass to the kidney and liver is clearly defined in profile in the sagittal projection, and the mass is shown to be separate from these organs. High signal intensity is present on precontrast images, a finding consistent with central hemorrhage. The mass enhances heterogeneously after contrast administration and contains signal-void regions of necrosis (arrows, *b*). (Reproduced with permission from Schlund JF, Kenney PJ, Brown ED, Ascher SM, Brown JJ, Semelka RC: Adrenocortical carcinoma: MR imaging appearance with current technique. *J Magn Reson Imaging* 5:171–174, 1995.)

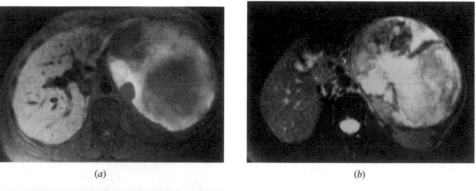

(a)   (b)

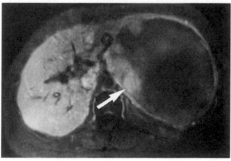

(c)

FIGURE 7.24   Adrenal cortical carcinoma. T1W fat-suppressed spin-echo (*a*), T2W fat-suppressed spin-echo (*b*), and gadolinium-enhanced fat-suppressed spin-echo (*c*) images in a 41-year-old woman. On the precontrast T1W image, central high signal intensity is present in the tumor, which is consistent with blood (*a*). On the T2W image, the tumor is heterogeneous and high in signal intensity because of the presence of central necrosis and blood products of varying age (*b*). Peripheral nodules enhance after contrast administration (arrow, *c*), and the central portion of the tumor remains largely signal void. (Reproduced with permission from Schlund JF, Kenney PJ, Brown ED, Ascher SM, Brown JJ, Semelka RC: Adrenocortical carcinoma: MR imaging appearance with current technique. *J Magn Reson Imaging* 5:171–174, 1995.)

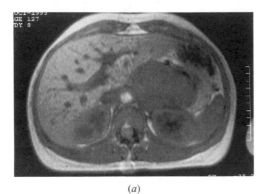

(a)

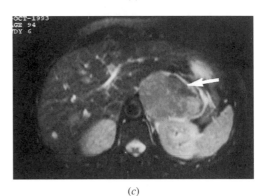

(b)

FIGURE 7.25 Adrenal cortical carcinoma with signal loss on out-of-phase imaging. T1W SGE (a), T1W out-of-phase SGE (b), and T2W fat-suppressed spin-echo (c) images in a 37-year-old woman. On the out-of-phase image, a moderate-sized region of the tumor loses signal (arrow, b) compared to the in-phase image, a finding consistent with fatty tissue. On the fat-suppressed T2W image, (c) the tumor is hyperintense and contains a region of low signal (curved arrow, c), representing fat and corresponding to the region of signal drop on the out-of-phase image (b). (Reproduced with permission from Schlund JF, Kenney PJ, Brown ED, Ascher SM, Brown JJ, Semelka RC: Adrenocortical carcinoma: MR imaging appearance with current technique. *J Magn Reson Imaging* 5:171–174, 1995.)

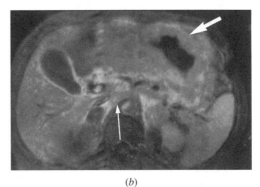

(c)

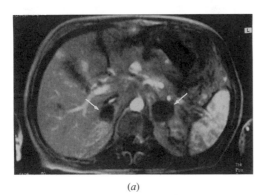

(a)

(b)

FIGURE 7.26 Adrenal lymphoma. Immediate postgadolinium SGE (a) and 4 min fat-suppressed gadolinium-enhanced spin-echo (b) images. Minimal enhancement is present of bilateral lymphomatous involvement of the adrenals on the immediate postgadolinium images (arrows, a). On the more delayed interstitial phase images, mild diffuse heterogeneous enhancement is apparent (b). On the basis of immediate postgadolinium images alone, the adrenal masses could be confused with cysts because of the hypovascularity of the tumors. Diffuse gastric wall involvement (large arrow, b) and retroperitoneal adenopathy (thin arrow, b) are noted.

in a para-aortic or paracaval location including the organ of Zuckerkandl (aortic bifurcation)

- Mediastinal and bladder-wall tumors account for ~2% of tumors
- Typical metastatic sites include lymph nodes, bone, and liver
- Patients present with sustained or paroxysmal hypertension
  - Associated with elevated urinary catecholamines, vanillylmandelic acid (VMA), and metanephron
- Associations
  - Multiple endocrine neoplasia (MEN) type IIA or IIB

- Neurofibromatosis
- von Hippel–Lindau disease
- 75% of patients with MEN-II have bilateral tumors

Imaging
- Pheochromocytomas do not diminish in signal intensity on out-of-phase T1W SGE
- Characteristically hypointense on T1W and hyperintense on T2W images (fig. 7.27)
  - Associated with cystic and hemorrhagic macro/microscopic histological findings
- Pheochromocytomas may appear very bright (e.g., "lightbulbs") on T2W images
  - This finding is of low sensitivity, as the majority are heterogeneous and moderately

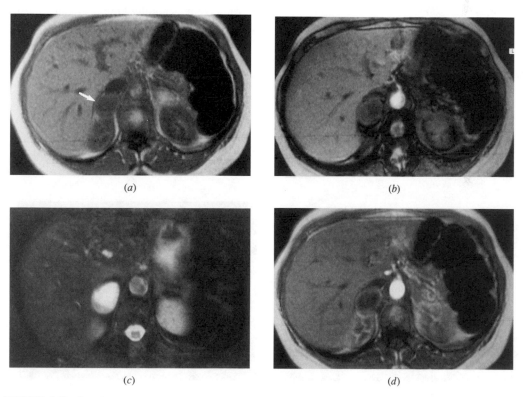

(a) (b)

(c) (d)

FIGURE 7.27 Pheochromocytoma. T1W SGE (*a*), T1W out-of-phase SGE (*b*), T2W fat-suppressed spin-echo (*c*), immediate postgadolinium SGE (*d*), and 2 min postgadolinium SGE (*e*) images. A 2.5 cm pheochromocytoma arises from the right adrenal gland (arrow, *a*), which has a moderate-signal-intensity peripheral rim with a low-signal-intensity center on in-phase (*a*) and out-of-phase (*b*) SGE images. No appreciable drop in signal intensity is present on the out-of-phase image. On the T2W image (*c*), the mass is extremely high in signal intensity, with the peripheral rim appearing slightly low in signal intensity (*c*). On the immediate postgadolinium image, the tumor rim enhances intensely with minimal central enhancement (*d*).

high signal. In rare instances, they may have only moderate signal intensity overlapping with other adrenal tumors.

- A confounding variable is the signal intensity of background fat
  - Lesions become most conspicuous with fat suppression, as shown on T2W fat-uppressed single-shot echo-train (fig. 7.27)
    - Represents an optimal imaging sequence for detecting small tumors and extra-adrenal retroperitoneal tumors
- Cystic pheochromocytomas are as high in signal intensity as cerebrospinal fluid (CSF) on T2W images
- Enhance minimally on immediate post-gadolinium images and demonstrate progressive enhancement on later interstitial phase images (fig. 7.27)
  - Intense early enhancement may be observed

Mimickers
- Cystic pheochromocytomas may be difficult to distinguish from cysts

Neuroblastoma, Ganglioglioma, and Ganglioneuroblastoma
Background

- This group of neoplasms is distinguished by a broad range in differentiation from primitive neuroblastoma at one end of the spectrum to well-differentiated, mature ganglioneuroma at the other end
  - Tumors with intermediary cytological maturation are termed ganglioneuroblastomas
- Neuroblastoma is one of the most common solid tumors of children younger than 5 years of age
  - Most commonly arise from the adrenal medulla or cells in adjacent retroperitoneal tissue
  - In older patients, extra-adrenal sites increase in relative frequency

Imaging: Neuroblastoma
- Tumors are generally high in signal intensity on T2W images and enhance with gadolinium
  - T2W fat-suppressed spin-echo and pre- and postcontrast T1W fat-suppressed spin-echo images in transverse and sagittal planes demonstrate these tumors well (fig. 7.28)
  - Fat-suppressed spin-echo imaging has been recommended rather than fat-suppressed SGE techniques because patients are often too young to cooperate with breath-holding, and spin-echo imaging has a higher

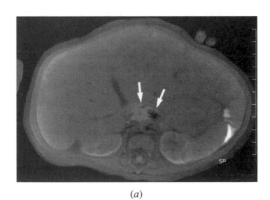

(a)

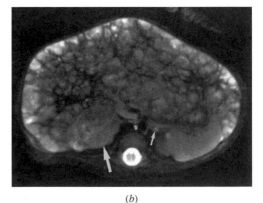

(b)

FIGURE 7.28 Hepatic metastases from neuroblastoma. T1W fat-suppressed spin-echo (a) and T2W fat-suppressed echo-train spin-echo (b) images. The liver is massively enlarged, compressing the pancreas (arrows, a). Multiple liver metastases are present that appear minimally hypointense on T1 and markedly hyperintense on T2. The primary tumor in the right adrenal (large arrow, b) and contralateral involvement of the left adrenal (small arrow, b) have similar signal intensity. Neuroblastoma has a tendency to local infiltration, lymph node metastases, and hematogeneous spread to liver, lungs, and bones.

signal-to-noise ratio, which improves image quality in small patients

- Extension into the neural canal is characteristic
- Encasement of the aorta and IVC is a common feature of advanced disease (fig. 7.28)
- Most common sites of metastatic disease include the skeletal system, liver (fig. 7.29), and lymph nodes
- MRI produces high-intrinsic-contrast resolution that is particularly effective at evaluating both the primary tumor and metastases in pediatric patients who have little body fat

- Multiplanar imaging is helpful for demonstration of extension into the neural canal and invasion of adjacent organs such as liver and kidney (figs. 7.29 and 7.30)
- Neuroblastoma may have an appearance on MRI indistinguishable from adrenal cortical carcinoma in adult patients, with one reported case appearing as a large tumor with central necrosis and hemorrhage, and tumor thrombus in the IVC (fig. 7.29).

Imaging: Ganglioneuromas
- Ganglioneuromas typically occur in older patients, in contrast neuroblastomas

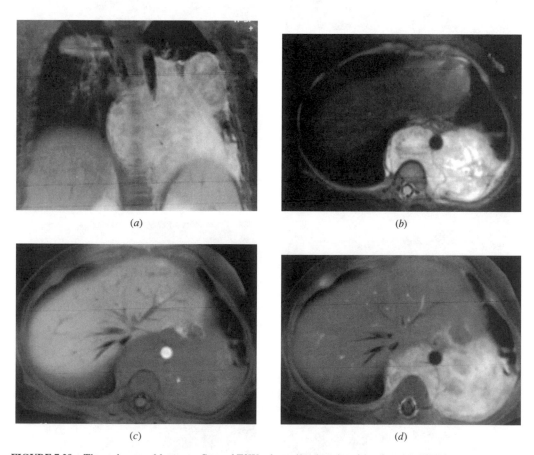

(a)

(b)

(c)

(d)

FIGURE 7.29   Thoracic neuroblastoma. Coronal T2W echo-train spin-echo of the chest (a), T2W fat-suppressed echo-train spin-echo (b), T1W SGE (c), and 90 s fat-suppressed gadolinium-enhanced spin-echo (d) images. A large heterogeneously hyperintense mass arises from the left-side hemithorax (a) and extends into the retrocrural space encasing the descending aorta (b, c, d). After contrast administration, the mass shows diffuse, mildly heterogeneous enhancement on interstitial phase images (d). The posterior mediastinum is the second most common location of neuroblastoma, after adrenal glands.

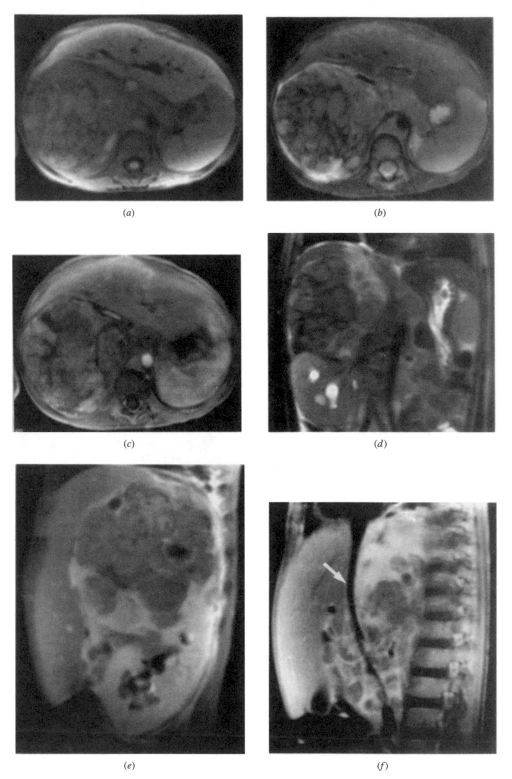

FIGURE 7.30 Large neuroblastoma. T1W SGE (*a*), T2W echo-train spin-echo (*b*), immediate postgadolinium SGE (*c*), coronal T2W echo-train spin-echo (*d*), sagittal 10 min postgadolinium SGE at the level of the left kidney (*e*) and at the level of the IVC (*f*), and immediate postgadolinium SGE at the level of the renal hilum (*g*).

254

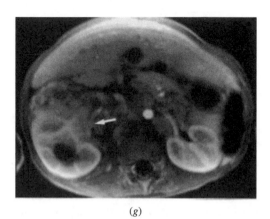

(g)

FIGURE 7.30 (*Continued*) Neuroblastoma arising from the right adrenal displaces the right kidney inferiorly (*d*, *e*) and surrounds the IVC (arrow, *f*) and right renal hilum (arrow, *g*). The tumor has a multinodular appearance with heterogeneous signal intensity on both T1W (*a*) and T2W (*b*) images and peripheral and irregular enhancement on postgadolinium images (*c*, *e*, *f*, *g*).

- Although all tumors may encase vessels, ganglioneuroblastoma and ganglioneuroma tend to be smaller and have better-defined margins (fig. 7.31)
- Tumors are intermediate in signal intensity on T1W images and slightly heterogeneous and high in signal intensity on T2W images
- Enhancement with gadolinium is mildly heterogeneous and moderately intense

Miscellaneous

Inflammatory Disease
Background
- The adrenal glands may be involved in granulomatous disease
  - Most commonly due to histoplasmosis, tuberculosis, and blastomycosis in North America
- Commonly associated with calcification

Imaging
- Signal intensity does not drop on out-of-phase images
- Slight heterogeneity of signal intensity is generally observed on T1W and T2W images
- Minimal heterogeneous enhancement on early postgadolinium images, which progresses over time (fig. 7.32)

Mimickers
- Metastases
- May see signal-void foci associated with calcifications

Adrenal Hemorrhage
Background
- Adrenal hemorrhage occurs secondary to trauma, bleeding diathesis, severe stress including surgery, childbirth, or sepsis

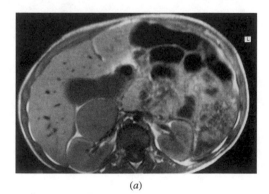

(a)

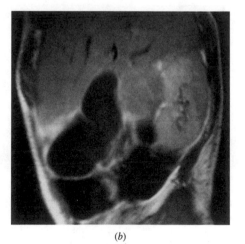

(b)

FIGURE 7.31 Ganglioneuroblastoma. T1W SE (*a*) and sagittal T1W gadolinium-enhanced SE (*b*) images. A well-defined 3 cm extrarenal mass is identified arising anterior to the upper pole of the right kidney. On the sagittal image (*b*), the mass is shown to abut the liver and kidney, with no evidence of invasion.

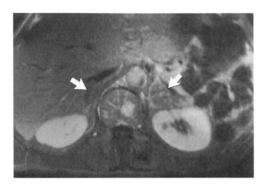

FIGURE 7.32 Tuberculosis involvement of the adrenals. Gadolinium-enhanced T1W fat-suppressed spin-echo image demonstrates bilateral adrenal enlargement with heterogeneous mild enhancement (arrows). (Reproduced with permission from Semelka RC, Shoenut JP: The adrenal glands. In Semelka RC, Shoenut JP (eds.), *MRI of the Abdomen with CT Correlation.* New York: Raven Press, pp. 77–90, 1993.)

Imaging
• Subacute hemorrhage is high in signal intensity on T1W images
  ○ This is more conspicuous on fat-suppressed T1W images (fig. 7.33)
• Decrease in lesion size over time helps to con-

firm that the adrenal enlargement is due to hemorrhage (fig. 7.33)

Mimickers
• Adrenal cortical carcinoma or metastases with central necrosis and hemorrhage
  ○ Carcinoma generally shows distinct stromal enhancement and will not show decrease in size without treatment

Addison's Disease
Background
• Addison's disease results from adrenal insufficiency from a variety of causes

Imaging
• Atrophic glands can be seen with autoimmune disease
• Adrenal hemorrhage may be diagnosed by the demonstration of bilaterally enlarged glands with high signal intensity on T1W images and lack of enhancement
• Enlarged glands without hemorrhage suggests granulomatous disease
• Metastases may uncommonly result in adrenal insufficiency, but generally in the setting of bilateral massive metastases

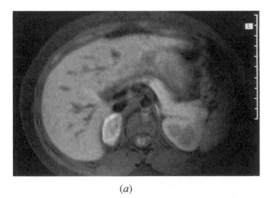
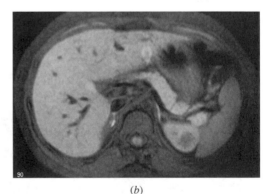

(*a*)   (*b*)

FIGURE 7.33 Adrenal hemorrhage. T1W fat-suppressed spin-echo (*a*) and T1W fat-suppressed spin-echo image obtained 7 weeks later (*b*). The T1W fat-suppressed image acquired 1 week after abdominal trauma (*a*) demonstrates a right adrenal mass with a hyperintense peripheral rim. This appearance is classic for a subacute hematoma. Seven weeks later, the mass has diminished in size and remains high in signal intensity because of persistence of extracellular methemoglobin (*b*).

CHAPTER 8

GASTROINTESTINAL TRACT

BACK GROUND

- Comprehensive bowel examination can be obtained with the combined use of T2W single-shot and breath-hold T1W GRE, without and with fat suppression, and gadolinium-enhanced 2D/3D GRE
- Gadolinium-enhanced imaging should be performed dynamically, but the venous 60–90 s delayed phase images with fat suppression are generally the most valuable
  - Removal of fat signal for detection of enhancing normal and abnormal structures is critical
- Newly available True-FISP sequences obtained in the 2D form may be very helpful in delineation of bowel-wall pathology and overall bowel anatomy, particularly when combined with a water-based intraluminal distending agent
  - Advantages include rapid acquisition, high signal to noise, and motion insensitivity
- Generalized protocol for comprehensive evaluation of the entire abdomen and pelvis may be used for the following bowel indications:
  - Type and severity of inflammatory bowel disease (IBD)
  - Identifying enteric abscesses and fistulae
  - Preoperative staging of malignant neoplasms, including rectal carcinoma
  - Differentiating postoperative and radiation therapy changes from recurrent carcinoma
  - Follow-up evaluation of response of metasta to localized ablative or systemic chemotherapy
- For improved visualization of bowel wall in dedicated examinations, bowel distension should be achieved using either orally or rectally delivered contrast agents to produce either bright or dark lumen
  - Options shown to be most useful for small- and large-bowel imaging are as follows:
    - Fat-suppressed T1W 3D GRE 70 s post-gadolinium plus water by mouth
      - Bowel wall = high signal
      - Lumen = low signal
    - T2W True-FISP 2D without fat suppression plus water by mouth
      - Bowel wall = low signal
      - Lumen = high signal
  - The 3D GRE T1W gadolinium-enhanced fat-suppressed imaging shows several inherent strengths and potential pitfalls
    - Strengths include

Primer on MR Imaging of the Abdomen and Pelvis, edited by Diego R. Martin, Michele A. Brown, and Richard C. Semelka ISBN 0-471-37340-0 Copyright © 2005 Wiley-Liss, Inc.

- Rapid, large field-of-view coverage with high resolution during a single breath-hold
- When using a water-based distending agent, residual gas is also dark and therefore does not interfere with bowel wall visualization
- Can combine with a stool darkening oral agent to make stool signal = distending agent signal, obviating need for bowel cleansing when performing MR colonography
- 3D data set allows reconstruction into other planes and 3D reformatting for fly-through virtual colonoscopy
  - ○ 2D True-FISP without fat suppression provides good quality T2W image of bowel, comparable to single-shot echo-train T2W sequences.
    - ▪ Strengths include
      - Performed without fat suppression results in dark bowel wall sandwiched between intermediate high-signal fat adjacent to bowel serosa and very high lumen signal from water distending agent
      - 2D True-FISP provides motion insensitivity, which is lost if 3D is used
      - True-FISP produces better edge sharpness than single-shot echo-train, higher contrast, and resists flow-void artifacts commonly seen with single-shot echo-train imaging combined with a water distending agent
    - ▪ Drawbacks of this technique include
      - Artifacts related to extreme sensitivity to field inhomogeneity, including air–soft-tissue interfaces at the patient skin surface, and from retained bowel gas
      - Retained bowel gas is dark against dark bowel wall, impairing bowel wall assessment
- Dedicated examination protocol guidelines are suggested as follows:
  - ○ Small Bowel
    - ▪ Indications include
      - IBD, partial obstruction, intussusception, malnutrition, neoplasm search
    - ▪ NPO (nothing by mouth) overnight

- Oral or nasoduodenal administration of distending agent at time of exam (optional—improves distension)
  - 1200 ml water
  - 2.5% mannitol
  - 0.2% Locust Bean Gum
- Image with breath-holding
  - Coronal and axial 2D True-FISP or single-shot echo-train T2W sequence
  - Coronal or axial 3D VIBE (reconstruct in the alternate plane) postgadolinium with 70 s delay
  - Include single-shot echo-train T2W imaging with fat suppression to examine for extra-enteric pathological fluid and to further assess the intraabdominal soft tissues
  - ○ Large Bowel (fig. 8.1)
    - ▪ Indications include
      - Suspected neoplasm, IBD, diverticular disease, postsurgical complications or anatomy, and possibly polyp detection
    - ▪ Standard bowel cleansing preparation starting the day prior to imaging (e.g., oral magnesium citrate and phosphate enemas, or 4 Liters of Go-Lytely orally the evening prior to exam)
    - ▪ At the time of exam, a Foley catheter is placed in the rectum with inflation of the tip balloon, and 2000 ml water is infused under gravity, or to patient tolerance
    - ▪ 3D GRE breath-hold imaging is obtained 70 s after initiation of gadolinium administration at 0.1 mmol/kg at 2 ml/s in the coronal plane with axial reformatting
    - ▪ Optional True-FISP imaging is obtained in 2 or 3 planes both in the supine and prone positions
    - ▪ All imaging is performed using surface phased array coils with a field of view centered in the midabdomen and sufficiently large to capture the entire colon during a single acquisition
    - ▪ Bowel paralysis may be of value for GRE imaging and can be achieved with glucagon or Buscopan administration just prior to contrast injection
    - ▪ Images are viewed on a workstation

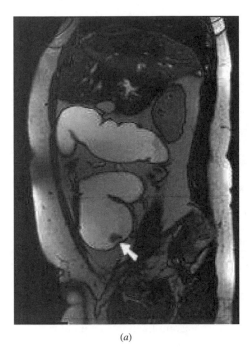

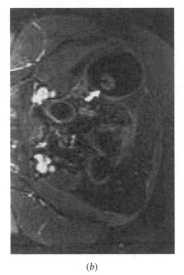

(a)   (b)

FIGURE 8.1   Sagittal True-FISP (*a*) and axial 3D GRE (*b*) gadolinium-enhanced interstitial phase imaging of the cecum in a patient with an inflammatory 6 mm polyp at the tip of the cecum (arrow). These images are from an MR colonography, and the patient received a bowel-cleansing preparation 1 day prior, and 2000 ml water enema at the time of the examination. The polyp is low signal on True-FISP and conspicuous against the high-signal water in the lumen. The polyp enhances on the postgadolinium T1W image and is conspicuous against the low-signal water in the lumen. The combination of these examples of dark and bright lumen techniques can provide increased accuracy.

Esophagus

Overview
- Normal esophageal wall is 3 mm thick
- Lacks a serosal layer, possibly accounting for relative propensity for tumor spread from esophagus to adjacent adventitia and mediastinal structures
- Gadolinium-enhanced fat-suppressed 3D GRE breath-hold imaging has significantly improved visualization of the esophagus and related pathologies

Congenital Abnormalities
Duplication Cysts
- Background
  - Gastrointestinal duplication cysts may occur throughout the alimentary tract
  - Epithelial-lined cysts occur in or adjacent to the wall
- Imaging

  - Typically appear as a small, ovoid, fluid-filled structure in the lower one-third of the esophagus located posteriorly in a periesophageal location or within the esophageal wall
  - Cysts have variable signal intensity on T1W unenhanced fat-suppressed images and may have elevated T1W signal
    - Resulting from protein or mucin
  - Generally high in signal intensity on T2W images
  - Cyst wall enhances after intravenous gadolinium administration, with no internal enhancement

Esophageal Masses

Benign Masses
Leiomyomas
- Background
  - A submucosal tumor of muscularis external smooth-muscle origin

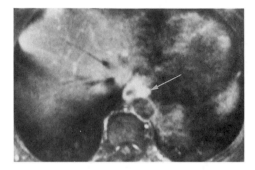

FIGURE 8.2 Esophageal leiomyoma. Gadolinium-enhanced T1W fat-suppressed spin-echo image shows a 2 cm leiomyoma (arrow) arising from the lateral aspect of the distal esophagus. Leiomyomas are the most common benign tumors of the esophagus. (Reprinted with permission from Shoenut JP, Semelka RC, Silverman R, Yaffe CS, Mickflikier AB: The gastrointestinal tract. In Semelka RC, Shoenut JP [eds.], *MRI of the Abdomen with CT Correlation*. New York: Raven Press, pp. 119–143, 1993.)

- ○ The most common benign tumor of the esophagus
- Imaging
  - ○ Demonstrated as small oval masses that are mural based but may be pedunculated
  - ○ Typically isointense with surrounding bowel wall on T1W and T2W images
  - ○ Tumors are hypervascular and enhance greater than adjacent esophageal wall (fig. 8.2)

- Mimickers
  - ○ Benign fibrovascular polyp
    - Most common tumor to cause a polypoid filling defect within the esophageal lumen; diagnosed based on location
  - ○ Squamous cell or adenocarcinoma
    - Leiomyomas generally will be well defined and hypervascular
    - Carcinomas are generally poorly defined and enhance moderately and heterogeneously

Varices
- Background
  - ○ Represents dilated submucosal veins
  - ○ Most commonly associated with portal hypertension, resulting in portosystemic shunts; splenic vein thrombosis also associated with esophageal varices
  - ○ Complications include intraluminal hemorrhage, hematemesis, and hematochezia
- Imaging
  - ○ Best visualized on fat-suppressed 2D or 3D GRE venous or interstitial phase images (fig. 8.3)

Malignant Masses
- Background

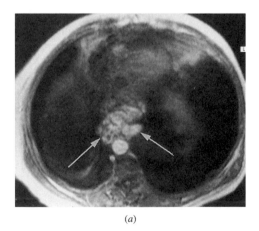

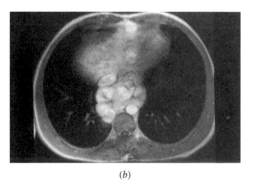

(a)   (b)

FIGURE 8.3 Esophageal varices. Transverse 45 s postgadolinium SGE image (*a*) in a patient with portal hypertension. Enhancing serpiginous tubular structures (arrows) in the lower esophagus represent varices.

Transverse gadolinium-enhanced T1W SGE (*b*) image in a second patient with congenital hepatic fibrosis demonstrates massive esophageal varices.

- Esophagus is lined by epithelial cells from which squamous cell carcinoma can arise, which accounts for approximately 50% of tumors
- Adenocarcinoma accounts for most of the other 50% and is thought to arise from mucosal cells of the stomach or metaplastic mucosa-like cells in the esophagus, as arise in Barrett's esophagus
  - Until 1975, squamous cell carcinoma was proportionally much more common in the United States, and the explanation for the change in relative frequency is unknown
  - Adenocarcinoma ascending from the gastric cardia and crossing the esophageal junction is a cause of secondary achalasia
- Metastases to the esophagus may occur; the most common primaries include lung, breast, and melanoma
- Imaging
  - Optimal visualization is obtained on gadolinium-enhanced fat-suppressed 3D imaging (fig. 8.4)
- Mimickers
  - Metastases
    - May present with identical features

Inflammatory and Infectious Disorders

Reflux Esophagitis
- Background
  - Gastroesophageal reflux is defined as the retrograde flow of gastric and sometimes duodenal contents into the esophagus
  - Associations include hiatal hernia, achalasia, and scleroderma
- Imaging
  - Gadolinium-enhanced T1W fat-suppressed imaging demonstrates distal esophageal wall thickening and enhancement (fig. 8.5)
- Mimickers
  - Radiation esophagitis
    - History shows correlation between radiation portal and affected segment of eshophagus
  - Caustic ingestion
    - History is indicative

- Infectious disease
  - *Candida albicans*, cytomegalovirus (CMV), and herpes simplex virus (HSV) can infect the esophagus, usually associated with immunocompromised conditions related to HIV, bone marrow transplantation, and steroid therapy
- Esophageal carcinoma

Stomach

Overview
- Visualization of the stomach wall benefits from administering an oral distending agent such as water
- Gastric mucosa enhances to a greater extent than mucosa of the remainder of the bowel

Congenital Abnormalities

Overview
- Gastric duplication cysts, congenital heterotopias, and congenital diverticula are relatively rare (fig. 8.6)

Masses

Benign Masses
Polyps
- Background
  - Gastric polyps may be hyperplastic, adenomatous, or hamartomatous
  - They may be isolated findings or associated with a polyposis syndrome
  - Approximately 90% of gastric polyps are hyperplastic and benign
    - Related to gastritis and polyposis syndromes
  - 10% are adenomatous, with approximately 3% having foci of malignant cellular features (risk related to size; approximately 45% are malignant at 2 cm)
    - Associated with chronic gastritis and polyposis syndromes
  - Clinically may present with anemia related to chronic blood loss, iron deficiency, or malabsorption of vitamin B12

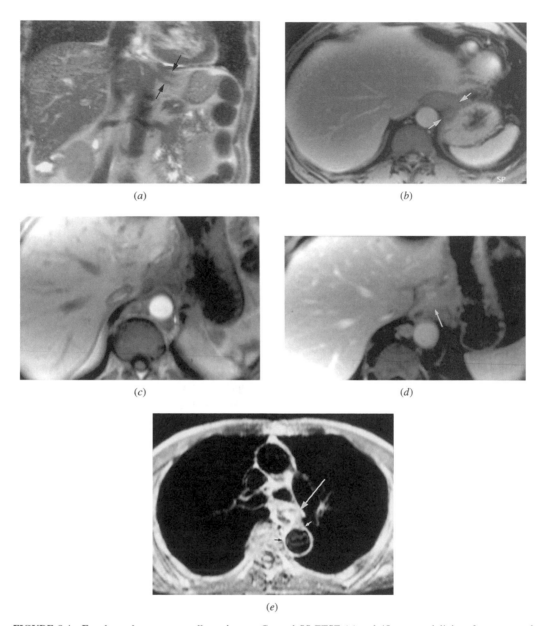

(a) (b)

(c) (d)

(e)

FIGURE 8.4   Esophageal squamous cell carcinoma. Coronal SS-ETSE (*a*) and 45 s postgadolinium fat-suppressed SGE (*b*) images. Increased thickness of the distal esophagus is present on the precontrast image (arrows, *a*). The squamous cell carcinoma of the distal esophagus is clearly defined, and tumor is shown to extend to the gastroesophageal junction (arrows, *b*). Lack of extension into the stomach is well shown by demonstration of normal-enhancing higher-signal gastric mucosa.

Transverse immediate postgadolinium T1W SGE (*c*) and interstitial phase gadolinium-enhanced fat-suppressed SGE (*d*) images in a second patient demonstrate a mass lesion centered in the region of the gastroesophageal junction (arrow, *d*) consistent with distal esophageal squamous cell carcinoma.

Gadolinium-enhanced gated T1W spin-echo image (*e*) in a third patient with squamous cell carcinoma of the midesophagus. A 2 cm cancer (arrow, *e*) is present that shows heterogeneous extension into the aortic wall (small arrows, *e*).

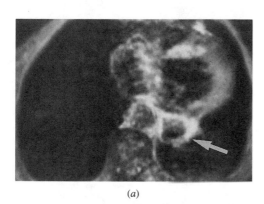

(a)

(b)

FIGURE 8.5   Reflux esophagitis. Gadolinium-enhanced T1W fat-suppressed spin-echo (*a*), gadolinium-enhanced gated transverse (*b*), and sagittal (*c*) T1W spin-echo images in two different patients (*a*) and (*b, c*) with reflux esophagitis. In a patient with achalasia (*a*), balloon dilation for achalasia predisposes to reflux esophagitis. The esophagus appears dilated, and the wall is thickened with increased mural enhancement. The esophagus in a second patient with reflux esophagitis due to hiatal hernia shows increased thickness of the esophageal wall (arrow, *b*) and increased signal intensity of the mucosa. The superior extent of inflamed mucosa (small arrows, *c*) is well shown on the sagittal image (*c*).

(c)

- ○ Hamartomatous gastric polyps may arise in isolation or occur in patients with Peutz-Jeghers syndrome
- Imaging
  - ○ Benign polyps are generally isointense with the gastric wall on unenhanced MR images
  - ○ Adequate distention of the stomach is mandatory in order to distinguish a polyp from a prominent rugal fold
  - ○ Benign polyp enhancement is usually isointense to slightly hyperintense compared to normal gastric mucosa on early postgadolinium images and mildly hyperintense on 2 min postgadolinium images, reflecting retention of contrast in the interstitial space (fig. 8.7)
  - ○ Invasive adenocarcinoma arising in a polyp exhibits more heterogeneous gadolinium enhancement and disruption of the underlying gastric wall

- Mimickers
  - ○ Submuscosal tumors, including leiomyomas, fibromas, hemangiomas, neurogenic tumors, lipomas
    - ▪ Generally can be distinguished by the gastric wall origin
    - ▪ Lipomas show fat signal on all sequences

Bezoar
- Background
  - ○ The word derives from the Arabic *bazahr* or *badzeahr*, meaning antidote, as bezoars were thought to have magical medicinal value
  - ○ Currently refers to accumulated nondigested material in the stomach lumen
    - ▪ Trichobezoar = hair: associated with psychiatric disorder
    - ▪ Phytobezoar = vegetable or plant matter: associated with delayed gastric emptying

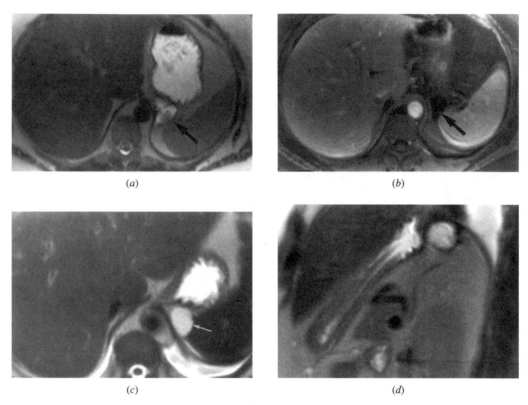

(a)
(b)
(c)
(d)

FIGURE 8.6   Gastric diverticulum. Transverse T2W SS-ETSE (*a*) and 90 s postgadolinium fat-suppressed SGE (*b*) images. A small cystic thin-walled mass (arrow, *a*) is shown, which is high signal intensity and intimately related to the posterior aspect of cardiac portion of the stomach. On the 90 s postgadolinium image (*b*), the diverticulum appears signal void with a thin enhancing wall (arrow, *b*). (Reprinted with permission from Marcos HB, Semelka RC: Stomach diseases: MR evaluation using combined T2W single-shot echo train spin-echo and gadolinium-enhanced spoiled gradient-echo sequences. *J Magn Reson Imaging* 10:950–960, 1999.) Transverse (*c*) and sagittal (*d*) T2W SS-ETSE in a second patient. A small posterior gastric diverticulum (arrow, *c*) is seen in the fundus of the stomach.

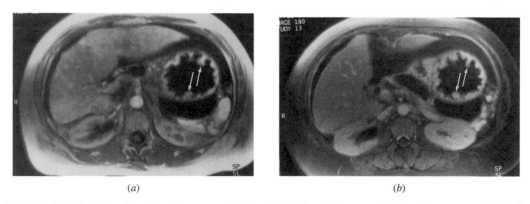

(a)
(b)

FIGURE 8.7   Gastric polyps. Immediate postgadolinium SGE (*a*) and 90 s postgadolinium fat-suppressed SGE (*b*) images in a patient with Gardner syndrome demonstrate multiple enhancing gastric polyps (arrows, *a*, *b*). The polyps possess intense enhancement.

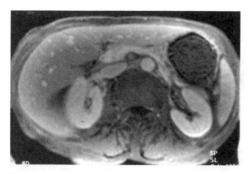

FIGURE 8.8 Gastric bezoar. Transverse interstitial phase gadolinium-enhanced fat-suppressed SGE image. The stomach is distended and filled with debris, which demonstrates a rounded configuration that represents a bezoar.

as seen with diabetes or postvagotomy (fig. 8.8)

Malignant Masses

Adenocarcinoma

- Background
  - The incidence of gastric adenocarcinoma has declined
  - 22,800 Americans are diagnosed with gastric cancer each year
  - Males are affected twice as often as females
  - Associated conditions include atrophic gastritis, pernicious anemia, adenomatous polyps, dietary nitrates
    - Native Japanese have a high incidence of disease, but second-generation immigrants to North America assume a lower incidence similar to background incidence among Americans, likely a result of environmental-dietary etiologic factors
  - Three patterns of growth can be classified
    - Exophytic or polypoid, projecting into the lumen
    - Ulcerated, with a shallow or deeply erosive crater
    - Diffusely infiltrative = linitis plastica
  - Gastric cancer typically metastasizes to regional lymph nodes, liver, peritoneum, and may involve the lungs
  - TNM staging system for gastric carcinoma
    - T—primary tumor
      - Tx: Tumor cannot be assessed
      - T0: No evidence of tumor
      - Tis: Carcinoma in situ
      - T1: Tumor limited to the mucosa or mucosa and submucosa
      - T2: Deep infiltration, involving $<^1/_2$ stomach region
      - T3: Deep infiltration, involving between $^1/_2$ and 1 stomach region
      - T4: Deep infiltration, involving >1 stomach region or directly extending to adjacent structures
    - N—lymph nodes
      - Nx: Regional nodes cannot be assessed
      - N0: No evidence of node involvement
      - N1: Involved nodes within 3 cm of primary mass
      - N2: Involved nodes >3 cm from mass
      - N3: Para-aortic, hepaticoduodenal, or other intra-abdominal nodes involved
    - M—metastases
      - Mx: Metastases cannot be assessed
      - M0: No distant metastases
      - M1: Distant metastases
- Imaging
  - On T1W sequences, gastric adenocarcinoma is isointense to normal stomach and may be apparent as focal wall thickening
  - On T2W images, tumors usually are slightly higher in signal intensity than adjacent normal stomach
  - Collapsed normal gastric wall enhances identically to the remainder of the wall on early and late postgadolinium images, and also exhibits radial organization of enhancing tissue, reflecting collapsed rugal folds (fig. 8.9). Tumors show more heterogeneous enhancement, which may be decreased or increased relative to the gastric wall on early, late, or both sets of images.
  - Linitis plastica carcinoma may enhance only modestly after intravenous contrast (fig. 8.10), although coexistent inflammatory changes may result in greater enhancement

Gastrointestinal Stromal Tumors (GIST)

- Background
  - Smooth-muscle bowel-wall tumors are now referred to collectively as GISTs

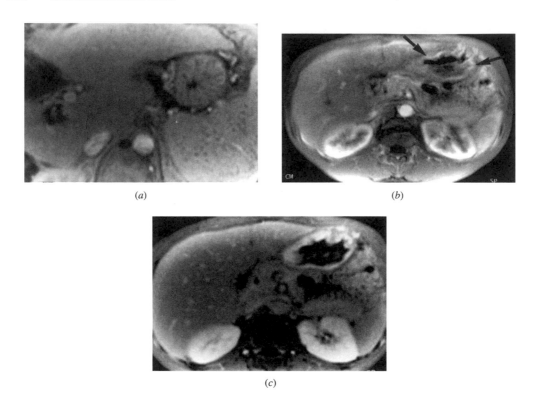

(a)

(b)

(c)

FIGURE 8.9 **Comparison between normal collapsed gastric wall and tumor.** Transverse interstitial phase gadolinium-enhanced fat-suppressed SGE (a) image in a normal patient. Note that the stomach is collapsed and the gastric wall enhancement is homogeneous. Note the symmetric radial fold pattern of the gastric rugae in the collapsed stomach.

Transverse immediate postgadolinium (b) and interstitial phase gadolinium-enhanced fat-suppressed SGE (c) images in a second patient with gastric cancer show diffuse gastric wall thickening and heterogeneous enhancement of the gastric wall. (Reprinted with permission from Marcos HB, Semelka RC: Stomach diseases: MR evaluation using combined T2W single-shot echo train spin-echo and gadolinium-enhanced spoiled gradient-echo sequences. *J Magn Reson Imaging* 10:950–960, 1999.)

- ∘ Stomach is the most common site of occurrence
- ∘ It may be difficult to determine malignant potential from tissue sampling, and benign-appearing tumors may eventually develop malignant behavior
- Imaging
  - ∘ Typically present as a largely exophytic mass arising from the stomach wall
  - ∘ Usually develop central necrosis with hemorrhage
  - ∘ High-grade GISTs are heterogeneous and high in signal on T2W and gadolinium-enhanced fat-suppressed T1W SGE images because of their increased vascularity (fig. 8.11)

- ∘ During the capillary phase of imaging, they show marked enhancement that persists throughout the interstitial phase
- ∘ These tumors may have a thin stalk of attachment to the stomach and may sometimes appear completely separate

Lymphoma
- Background
  - ∘ Primary gastric lymphoma is rare
  - ∘ Approximately 50% of gastrointestinal non Hodgkin's lymphoma (NHL) arise in the stomach, 40% in the small intestine, and 10% in the colon
  - ∘ Infiltration of the gastric wall by tumor cells results in diffuse wall thickening

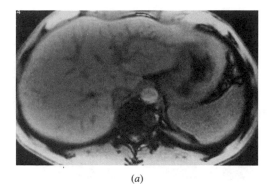

(*a*)

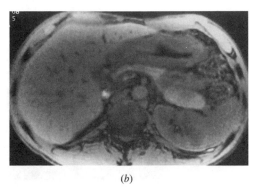

(*b*)

FIGURE 8.10   Gastric adenocarcinoma, linitis plastica.
Fat-suppressed SGE (*a*, *b*) and immediate postgadolinium
SGE (*c*) images. Diffuse relatively homogeneous gastric wall
thickening is present (*a*, *b*). Minimal enhancement is appreciated on the immediate postgadolinium SGE image (*c*).

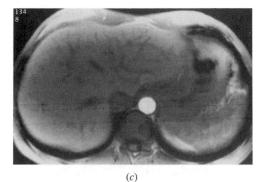

(*c*)

- Imaging
  - Diffuse gastric wall thickening is best seen on single-shot echo-train spin-echo T2W and gadolinium-enhanced fat-suppressed GRE images (fig. 8.12)
    - Stomach often maintains distensibility and capacity
    - Involved regional lymph nodes are best demonstrated on 3D gadolinium-enhanced equilibrium phase fat-suppressed images
  - Hogkins lymphoma may result in a desmoplastic, nondistensible stomach simulating linitis plastica
- Mimickers
  - Linitis plastica resulting from diffuse infiltrating form of gastric carcinoma or metastatic breast carcinoma
    - Preservation of rugal folds and possible thickening is characteristic of lymphoma, while effacement is characteristic of carcinoma due to the associated fibrotic reaction

- Linitis plastica results in rigid narrowing of the stomach

Carcinoid
- Background
  - These are well-differentiated neuroendocrine neoplasms that occur most commonly in the appendix and small bowel
  - Sporadic gastric carcinoid tumors arise throughout the stomach, may be small (<2 cm diameter) submucosal nodules or large tumors that invade deeply and create prominent fibrosis in surrounding tissues
  - Therapy is generally dependent on complete surgical resection
  - In the setting of chronic gastritis and hypergastrinemia, gastrin can stimulate neuroendocrine cells to grow and may promote development of carcinoid
    - These tumors generally occur in the fundus mucosa and tend to regress if the gastrin levels diminish

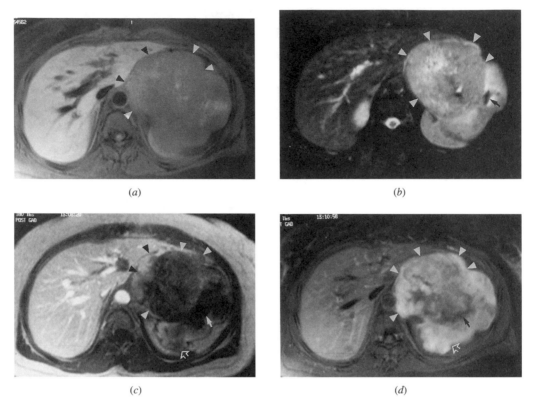

FIGURE 8.11   Gastrointestinal stromal tumor (GIST). T1W fat-suppressed spin-echo (*a*), T2W fat-suppressed spin-echo (*b*), 45 s postgadolinium SGE (*c*), and gadolinium-enhanced fat-suppressed spin-echo (*d*) images. A large exophytic GIST arises from the lesser curvature (arrowheads, *a, b, c, d*) and is contiguous with the spleen. The tumor is heterogeneous and high in signal intensity on the T2W image (*b*) and enhances intensely (*c, d*). Enhancing tumor extends adjacent to the spleen (open arrow, *c, d*). Signal-void areas within the tumor are consistent with necrosis. Air within the gastric lumen is also signal void (solid arrow, *b, c, d*).

- Associated conditions include *Helicobacter pylori* infection, prolonged acid suppression with proton pump inhibitors (such as omeprazole), Zollinger-Ellison syndrome, and MEN type I
- Imaging
  - Carcinoid tumors are near isointense on T1W images, mildly hyperintense and heterogeneous on T2W images, and often show increased enhancement on early and later postgadolinium images (fig. 8.13)

Metastases
- Background
  - Metastases are characteristically submucosal lesions

  - Tumors of neighboring organs, such as esophagus, pancreas, and transverse colon, may involve the stomach by direct extension
  - Carcinomas of lung, breast, melanoma, and lymphoma (fig. 8.14) are the most common primaries that spread hematogeneously
  - Linitis plastica involves diffuse tumor spread and may be observed with breast carcinoma
    - Mimickers
      - Infiltrative form of primary gastric carcinoma, which may have an identical appearance
      - Lymphoma shows preserved rugal folds and retained gastric dispensability

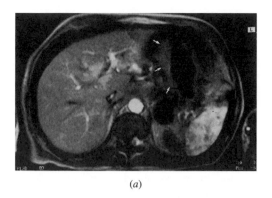

(a)

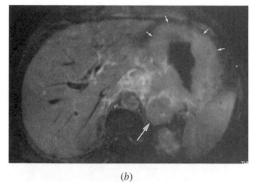

(b)

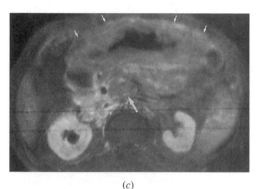

(c)

FIGURE 8.12 Non-Hodgkin's lymphoma of the stomach. Immediate postgadolinium SGE (*a*) and gadolinium-enhanced T1W fat-suppressed spin-echo (*b, c*) images. There is diffuse circumferential lymphomatous infiltration of the stomach wall (short arrows, *a, b, c*). Lymphoma extends to the left adrenal gland (long arrow, *b*). At a lower tomographic section, prominent retroperitoneal lymphadenopathy is present (arrow, *c*), which is commonly observed in the setting of gastric lymphoma.

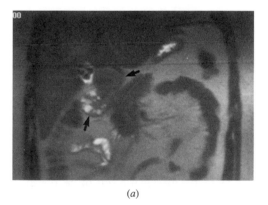

(a)

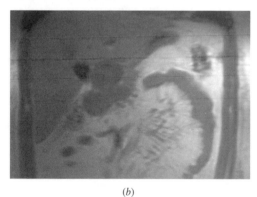

(b)

FIGURE 8.13 Gastric carcinoid. Coronal T2W SS-ETSE (*a*), coronal SGE (*b*), and transverse immediate postgadolinium SGE (*c*) images. This primary carcinoid tumor of the stomach appears as a mass in the wall of the antrum that invades the duodenum and pancreas. The tumor is mixed solid with cystic spaces (arrows, *a*) on T2 and isointense on T1 (*b*) and enhances heterogeneously after contrast administration (arrows, *c*). There are also hepatic metastases that are moderately hyperintense on T2W image and hypointense on precontrast SGE image (*b*) and show homogeneous early enhancement (large arrow, *c*). A simple cyst is also seen in the right kidney.

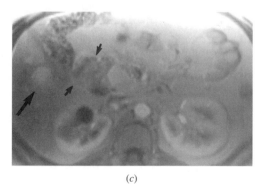

(c)

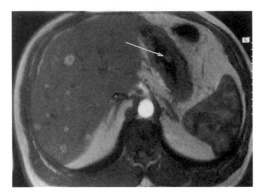

FIGURE 8.14   Melanoma metastasis to the stomach.
Immediate postgadolinium SGE image in a patient with
metastatic melanoma. Malignant melanoma metastasizes
hematogeneously, and in this patient multiple liver metastases and a gastric metastasis (long arrow) are identified.
The metastases are high in signal on this T1W image because of the paramagnetic properties of melanin.

Inflammatory and Infectious Disorders

Gastric Inflammation and Ulceration
- Background
  - *H. pylori* infection has been identified as
    the major etiological factor leading to un-
    derlying gastritis and ulcer promotion
    - Gastritis and ulcers can also be related to
      repeated exposure to alcohol, drugs, bile,
      radiation therapy, and Zollinger-Ellison
      syndrome
  - Benign gastric ulcers usually occur along
    the lesser curvature toward the antrum
  - Approximately 10% of patients have ulcers
    in both the antrum and the duodenum
- Imaging
  - Gastric inflammatory disease in general re-
    sults in increased mural enhancement on
    both early and late gadolinium-enhanced
    images (fig. 8.15)
  - Ulcer craters may be demonstrated on both
    single-shot echo-train spin-echo T2W and
    gadolinium-enhanced fat-suppressed SGE
    images (fig. 8.16)

Small Bowel

Congenital Anomalies
Rotational Abnormalities
- Background

- Intestinal malrotations or nonrotations result from disordered or interrupted embry-
  onic intestinal counterclockwise rotations
  around the axis of the superior mesenteric
  artery
- In rotational abnormalities, the normal rotations and fixations are either incomplete
  or occur out of sequence
- Nonrotation is the most common abnormality and is readily demonstrated by failure
  to demonstrate the duodenum crossing the
  midline below the head of the pancreas,
  the small intestine located in the right abdomen, and the colon situated in the left
  half of the abdomen
- The other types of malrotation occur less
  frequently and include incomplete rotation,
  reversed rotation, and anomalous fixation or
  fusion of the mesenteries
- Imaging
  - Standard imaging protocol, including coro-
    nal T2W single-shot imaging (fig. 8.17), is
    optimal to show bowel anatomy

Diverticulum
- Background
  - Duodenum is the most common site along
    the gastrointestinal tract
    - Congenital diverticula usually contain all
      three layers including the muscularis ex-
      terna
    - Acquired diverticula lack a muscularis
      externa
  - Diverticula of the jejunum and ileum occur
    along the mesenteric side of the bowel
    - This reflects that mesenteric vessels and
      nerves enter potential sites of weakness
      where mucosa may herniate into the
      mesentery
- Imaging
  - T2W single-shot echo-train or True-FISP
    imaging provide excellent visualization of
    bowel, fluid, and gas
  - Diverticula may be demonstrated on MR
    images as air or air fluid–containing
    structures that arise from the bowel
    (fig. 8.18)

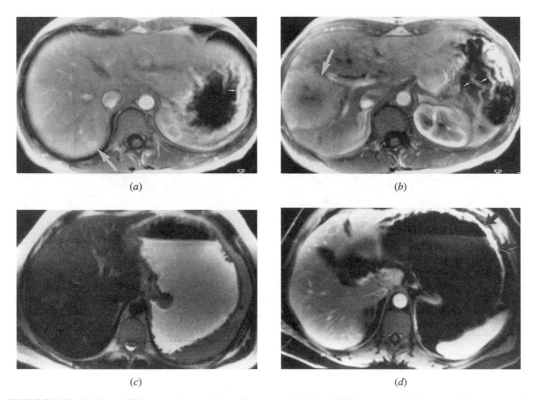

(a)   *(b)*

(c)   *(d)*

FIGURE 8.15   Zollinger-Ellison syndrome. Immediate postgadolinium SGE images (*a, b*). Intense enhancement and increased thickness of gastric rugae are appreciated (small arrows, *a, b*). Hypervascular liver metastases are also present (large arrow, *a, b*).

Transverse T2W SS-ETSE (*c*) and transverse 90 s fat-suppressed postgadolinium SGE (*d*) images in a second patient. There is a marked distension of the stomach and duodenum, and the anterior gastric wall is thickened. On the 90 s postgadolinium fat-suppressed SGE image (*d*), the gastric wall shows intense enhancement (arrows, *b*). (Reprinted with permission from Marcos HB, Semelka RC: Stomach diseases: MR Evaluation using combined T2W single-shot echo train spin-echo and gadolinium-enhanced spoiled gradient-echo sequences. *J Magn Reson Imaging* 10:950–960, 1999.)

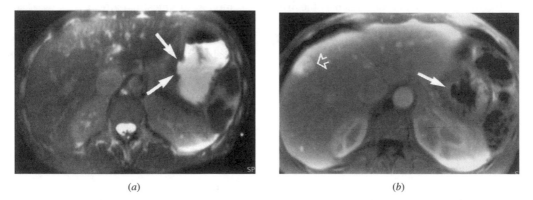

(a)   *(b)*

FIGURE 8.16   Gastric ulcer. Transverse T2W SS-ETSE (*a*) and transverse 1 min postgadolinium SGE (*b*) images. The high signal intensity of gastric contents (orally administered water) deliniates the ulcer crater (arrows, *a*), on the mucosal surface of the lesser curvature. On the 1 min postgadolinium SGE image (*b*), the ulcer shows mildly increased enhancement (arrow, *b*). A 2 cm hemangioma is incidentally noted as an intensely enhancing mass lesion in the liver on the 1 min postgadolinium image (open arrow, *b*). (Reprinted with permission from Marcos HB, Semelka RC: Stomach diseases: MR evaluation using combined T2W single-shot echo train spin-echo and gadolinium-enhanced spoiled gradient-echo sequences. *J Magn Reson Imaging* 10:950–960, 1999.)

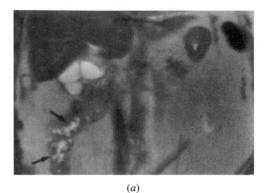
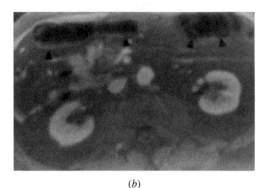

(a)   (b)

FIGURE 8.17   Rotational abnormalities of small bowel. Coronal T2W SS-ETSE (*a*) and transverse 90 s postgadolinium fat-suppressed SGE images. Coronal T2 (*a*) demonstrates that small bowel is predominantly located in the right side of the abdomen (arrows). The 90 s postgadolinium fat-suppressed SGE image demonstrates that the third and fourth portions of the duodenum are located to the right of midline (arrows, *b*). Note that the large bowel is in a normal location (arrowheads). (Reprinted with permission from Marcos HB, Semelka RC, Noone TC, Woosley JT, Lee JKT: MRI of normal and abnormal duodenum using half-Fourier single-shot RARE and gadolinium-enhanced spoiled gradient-echo sequences. *Magn Reson Imaging* 17:869–880, 1999.)

○ Change in size of the diverticulum may be observed between sequences in an MRI examination reflecting contraction and expansion

Meckel's Diverticulum
• Background
  ○ Represents a remnant of the omphalomesenteric duct (vitelline duct)
  ○ Normally this duct is obliterated by the fifth week of gestation
  ○ Occurs in 2% of the general population and within 25 cm of the ileocecal valve along the antimesenteric border
  ○ Most patients remain asymptomatic
  ○ Complications
    ▪ If the diverticulum contains acid-secreting epithelium of gastric mucosa, ulceration and bleeding may result
    ▪ Intussusception and inflammation
• Imaging
  ○ Detection may be difficult
  ○ The presence of gastric mucosa in 10–20% of Meckel's diverticulum cases may result in marked enhancement on immediate (capillary phase) and interstitial phase postgadolinium images (fig. 8.19)

Atresia and Stenosis
• Background
  ○ Intestinal atresia results in complete absence of a portion of bowel or closure by an occluding mucosal diaphragm, while congenital stenosis represents a narrowing of an intestinal segment by fibrosis or stricture
  ○ Both may cause intestinal obstruction
  ○ Duodenal atresia represents the most common gastrointestinal atresia
  ○ Approximately 25% of cases will have associated congenital anomalies including malrotation of the gut and Meckel's diverticulum
• Imaging
  ○ T2W single-shot echo-train spin-echo images (fig. 8.20) and True-FISP images offer excellent depiction of these abnormalities and have the advantage of motion insensitivity, which is important in younger patients

Masses

Benign Masses
Overview
• Small-bowel tumors are relatively rare

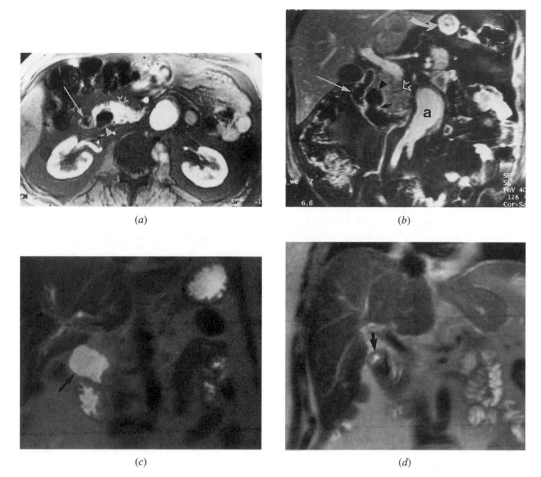

FIGURE 8.18 Duodenal diverticulum. Transverse immediate (*a*), and coronal 90 s (*b*) postgadolinium fat-suppressed SGE images. An air- and fluid-containing diverticulum (arrowhead, *a*, *b*) is interposed between the duodenum (long arrow, *a*, *b*) and the head of the pancreas (open arrow, *a*, *b*). On the coronal image, a neck (short arrow, *b*) connecting the diverticulum to the duodenum is well shown, which confirms that the lesion represents a diverticulum and not a cystic mass in the head of the pancreas. Duodenal diverticula are common and usually incidental findings. The normal gastric wall (curved arrow, *b*) enhances more intensely than normal small bowel. An abdominal aortic aneurysm (a, b) is also present. Coronal T2W SS-ETSE (*c*, *d*) in two other different patients demonstrate fluid-containing duodenal diverticula (arrow, *c*, *d*).

- Adenomas, leiomyomas, and lipomas constitute the three most common primary benign small intestinal tumors
- Tumors increase in frequency from proximal to distal small bowel

Polyps
- Background
  - Hamartomatous, hyperplastic, and inflammatory polyps are benign nonneoplastic lesions; adenomatous polyps are true neoplastic tumors containing dysplastic epithelium and are precursors to carcinoma
  - Polyps are infrequently symptomatic and are usually incidental findings
  - Clinically evident polyps may present with pain, obstruction, or bleeding, and are the most common cause for adult intussusception
  - Adenomatous polyps of the small intestine are rare, with <0.05% of all gastrointestinal adenomas arising in the small intestine

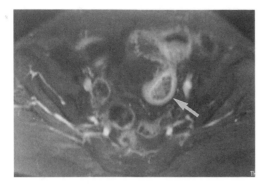

FIGURE 8.19 Meckel diverticulum. Gadolinium-enhanced T1W fat-suppressed spin-echo image in a patient with lower gastrointestinal bleeding. A teardrop-shaped Meckel diverticulum (arrow) extends from a loop of mildly dilated ileum. The inner wall of the diverticulum enhances to a greater extent than adjacent small bowel and colon. This allows detection of the diverticulum, and the degree of enhancement is consistent with the presence of gastric mucosa.

- Multiple adenomas occur in the setting of Gardner's and familial polyposis syndromes
- Small-bowel hamartomas occur commonly in Peutz-Jeghers syndrome and rarely in juvenile polyposis syndromes

- Imaging
  - Small-bowel polyps appear as enhancing masses on gadolinium-enhanced fat-suppressed SGE images (fig. 8.21)

Neurofibromas
- Background
  - Primary neurogenic tumors of the gastrointestinal tract are rare
  - Neurofibromas consist of neoplastic cells arising from the nerve sheath
  - Neurofibromatosis type 1 predisposes individuals to an increase risk of a variety of gastrointestinal lesions, including neurofibromas, schwannomas, smooth-muscle tumors, and neuroendocrine tumors of the duodenum and ampullary region
- Imaging
  - These tumors appear as intraluminal masses that enhance to a comparable extent as bowel wall (fig. 8.22)

Leiomyomas
- Background
  - The frequency of small-bowel leiomyoma is comparable to that of adenoma

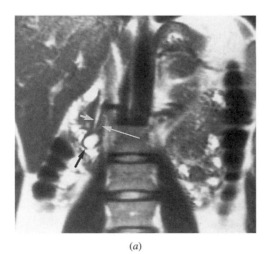

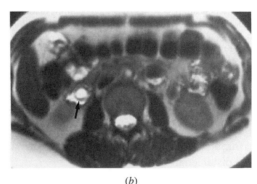

(a)   (b)

FIGURE 8.20   Choledochocele. Coronal (*a*) and transverse (*b*) T2W SS-ETSE images in a patient with recurrent bouts of pancreatitis. A high-signal-intensity choledochocele (black arrow, *a*, *b*) protrudes into the duodenum. The SS-ETSE image clearly defines the cystic nature of the lesion, which excludes an ampullary tumor, and demonstrates the relationship to the common bile duct (small arrow, *a*) and the pancreatic duct (long arrow, *a*). (Courtesy of Susan M Ascher, MD, Dept Radiology, Georgetown University Medical Center.)

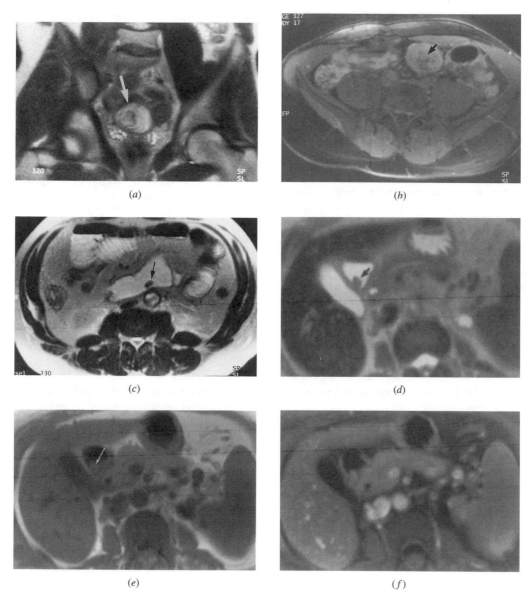

FIGURE 8.21   Small bowel polyps. T2W SS-ETSE (*a*) and gadolinium-enhanced fat-suppressed SGE (*b*) images of a hamartoma in Peutz-Jeghers syndrome. A bowel-within-bowel appearance (arrow, *a*) is identified on the T2W image (*a*) in the proximal jejunum because of intussusception. The intussusception is caused by a hamartomatous polyp that has acted as a lead point. The hamartoma is shown as a 1 cm uniformly enhancing mass (arrow, *b*) on the gadolinium-enhanced fat-suppressed SGE image (*b*). T2W image (*c*) in a second patient demonstrates a 1 cm polyp (arrow, *c*) within a slightly dilated loop of duodenum.

T2W SS-ETSE (*d*), SGE (*e*), and 90 s postgadolinium fat-suppressed SGE (*f*) images in a third patient. T2 image shows a low-signal-intensity mass (arrow, *d*) measuring 1.5 cm located in the descending portion of the duodenum. Note that the high signal intensity of intraluminal fluid within the duodenum clearly deliniates the polyp, which appears moderately low in signal intensity. Comparing precontrast (*e*) and postgadolinium (*f*) images, enhancement of the polyp is demonstrated, showing it to remain comparable in signal to the duodenal wall, reflecting the tissue nature of the polyp. (Reprinted with permission from Marcos HB, Semelka RC, Noone TC, Woosley JT, Lee JKT: MRI of normal and abnormal duodenum using half-Fourier single-shot RARE and gadolinium-enhanced spoiled gradient-echo sequences. *Magn Reson Imaging* 17:869–880, 1999.)

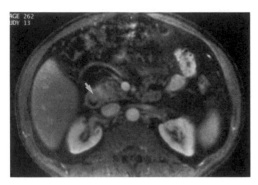

FIGURE 8.22 **Neurofibroma of duodenum.** Transverse 90 s postgadolinium fat-suppressed SGE image in a patient with type 1 neurofibromatosis. A 1 cm intraluminal mass (arrow) arises in the second part of duodenum. This mass enhances to the same extent as the duodenal wall, reflecting the tissue composition of the neurofibroma. The patient expired, and at autopsy multiple cutaneous and gastrointestinal neurofibromas were found. (Reprinted with permission from Semelka RC, Marcos HB: Polyposis syndromes of the gastrointestinal tract. *J Magn Reson Imaging* 11:51–55, 2000.)

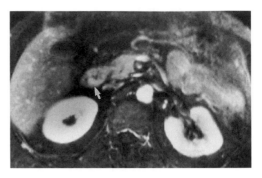

FIGURE 8.23 **Duodenal leiomyoma.** Gadolinium-enhanced T1W fat-suppressed spin-echo image shows a uniformly enhancing mass (arrow) protruding into the duodenum. When intraluminal, leiomyomas are indistinguishable from polyps. (Reprinted with permission from Shoenut JP, Semelka RC, Silverman R, Yaffe CS, Mick-flikier AB: The gastrointestinal tract. In Semelka RC, Shoenut JP [eds.]. *MRI of the Abdomen with CT Correlation.* New York: Raven Press, pp. 119–143, 1993.)

- ○ Leiomyomas are smooth-muscle proliferations that usually originate in the submucosa or muscularis externa and present as solitary lesions
- ○ Depending on their location, they may protrude into the lumen or produce a mass effect on adjacent bowel
- ○ As leiomyomas enlarge, they may undergo central necrosis and bleeding
- • Imaging
  - ○ Uniform enhancement greater than that of adjacent bowel is observed on postgadolinium images (fig. 8.23)
- • Mimickers
  - ○ Polyps may be indistinguishable

Malignant Masses

Adenocarcinomas
- • Background
  - ○ Small-bowel tumors account for only 1% of all gastrointestinal malignancies, and half are adenocarcinomas
  - ○ The most common site for small-bowel adenocarcinoma is the duodenum, usually in close proximity to the ampulla
    - ▪ May present with obstructive jaundice

- • Imaging
  - ○ The combined use of T2W single-shot echo-train spin-echo and gadolinium-enhanced fat-suppressed SGE imaging has resulted in reproducible good image quality for the evaluation of small-bowel neoplasms
  - ○ Duodenal neoplasms are particularly well shown due to the relatively fixed position of the duodenum in the anterior pararenal space
  - ○ The most consistent MR imaging feature that permits tumor detection is that tumors enhance in a heterogeneously moderate fashion on interstitial phase gadolinium-enhanced images (fig. 8.24)

Gastrointestinal Stromal Tumor (GIST)
- • Background
  - ○ Approximately 25% occur in the small bowel, with 50% arising from the stomach
  - ○ Tumors may be large and ulcerating
- • Imaging
  - ○ Gadolinium-enhanced SGE or fat-suppressed SGE images demonstrate heterogeneous and substantial enhancement of the primary tumor (fig. 8.25)

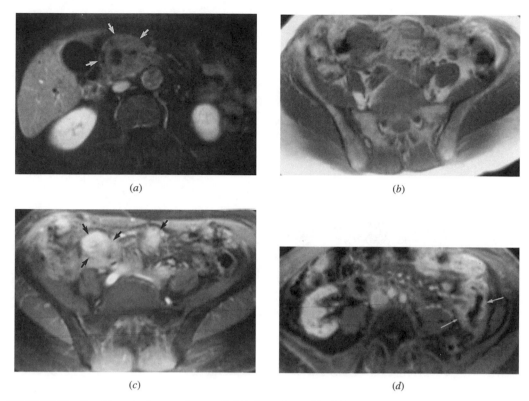

FIGURE 8.24   Small-bowel adenocarcinoma. Gadolinium-enhanced T1W fat-suppressed spin-echo (*a*), SGE (*b*), and postgadolinium T1W fat-suppressed spin-echo (*c*) images in two different patients (*a*) and (*b*, *c*) with small-bowel adenocarcinoma. In the first patient (*a*), the size and extent of a large duodenal tumor (arrows, *a*) are well shown on the gadolinium-enhanced fat-suppressed image. In the second patient (*b*, *c*), the neoplasm is difficult to identify on the precontrast SGE image (*b*) because it is isointense with background bowel. On the gadolinium-enhanced fat-suppressed SGE image (*c*), the distal jejunal tumors are conspicuous (arrows, *c*) because they are higher in signal intensity and heterogeneous compared with background bowel.

Transverse 90 s postgadolinium fat-suppressed SGE image (*d*) in another patient with adenocarcinoma of the jejunum. Irregular thickening and enhancement of a segment of proximal jejunum is apparent (arrows, *d*).

- ○ Arterial phase postgadolinium SGE is particularly effective at detecting liver metastases because these tend to be hypervascular and are often small

Lymphoma
- • Background
  - ○ Arises in the submucosa and represents 1% of all bowel tumors
  - ○ Primary gastrointestinal non-Hodgkin's lymphomas are most commonly of B-cell type and appear to arise from B cells of mucosa-associated lymphoid tissue (MALT) (fig. 8.26)
  - ○ Terminal ileum is the most common site affected

- • Imaging
  - ○ Patterns
    - ▪ Diffusely infiltrating lesions that often produce transmural wall thickening with effacement of overlying mucosal folds
    - ▪ Polypoid lesions that protude into the lumen
    - ▪ Large, exophytic, fungating masses that are prone to ulceration and fistula formation
  - ○ Lymphoma generally appears as moderately enhancing thickened loops of bowel and large tumor masses that invest the bowel. A characteristic feature is that despite large-volume disease, lymphoma usually does not result in obstruction (fig. 8.27).

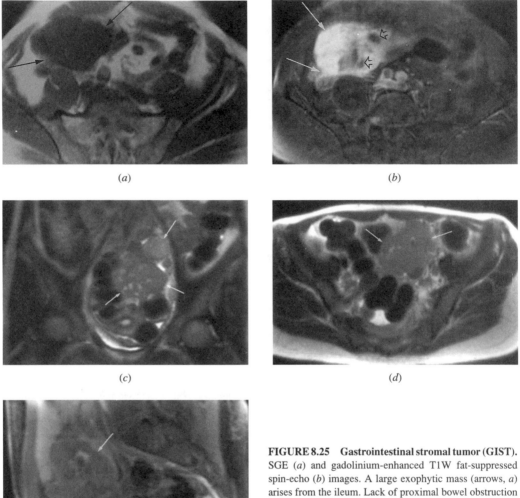

(a) *(b)*

(c) *(d)*

(e)

FIGURE 8.25 Gastrointestinal stromal tumor (GIST).
SGE (*a*) and gadolinium-enhanced T1W fat-suppressed
spin-echo (*b*) images. A large exophytic mass (arrows, *a*)
arises from the ileum. Lack of proximal bowel obstruction
is consistent with its eccentric origin. The tumor's large size
coupled with intense enhancement (arrows, *b*) and regions
of necrosis (open arrows, *b*) are typical features of GIST.
Coronal (*c*) and transverse (*d*) T2W SS-ETSE and sagittal
interstitial phase gadolinium-enhanced fat-suppressed SGE
(*e*) images in a second patient with small-bowel GIST also
show large heterogeneous lobulated masses (arrows, *c–e*)
in the pelvis.

◦ The presence of splenic lesions and mesenteric and retroperitoneal lymphadenopathy
support the diagnosis

Carcinoid
- Background
  ◦ The most common primary neoplasm of the
  small bowel

◦ Tumors are well-differentiated neuroendocrine neoplasms that occur primarily in
the distal ileum, in which location they are
almost always malignant
◦ Presentations include bleeding, bowel obstruction or intussusception
◦ Particular to ileal carcinoids are regional
mesenteric metastases and vascular sclerosis

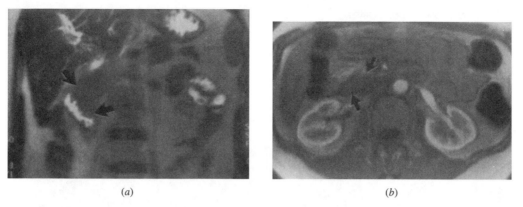

(a)   (b)

FIGURE 8.26   Duodenal MALToma. Coronal T2W SS-ETSE (*a*) and immediate postgadolinium fat-suppressed SGE (*b*) images. T2W image demonstrates irregular thickening of the superior aspect of the duodenal wall caused by a paraduodenal mass (arrows, *a*). Postgadolinium image shows a mass that is interposed between the third portion of the duodenum and the head of the pancreas. This mass shows mild heterogeneous enhancement compared to duodenal wall and pancreas, which permits a good distinction between mass and pancreas. Low-grade lyphoma (MALToma type) was proven by endoscopic biopsy. (Reprinted with permission from Marcos HB, Semelka RC, Noone TC, Woosley JT, Lee JKT: MRI of normal and abnormal duodenum using half-Fourier single-shot RARE and gadolinium-enhanced spoiled gradient-echo sequences. *Magn Reson Imaging* 17:869–880, 1999.)

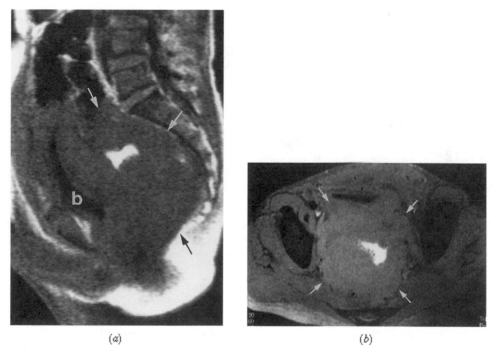

(*a*)   (*b*)

FIGURE 8.27   Small intestine lymphoma. Sagittal SGE (*a*), T1W fat-suppressed spin-echo (*b*), sagittal 45 s postgadolinium SGE (*c*), and gadolinium-enhanced T1W fat-suppressed spin-echo (*d*) images in a patient with diffuse lymphomatous infiltration of the distal jejunum and ileum. A large pelvic mass (arrows, *a*, *b*) is seen on precontrast images. After intravenous gadolinium, minimal enhancement of the mass is present on early postgadolinium images (*c*), and heterogeneous, slightly greater enhancement is present on the interstitial phase image (*d*). Minimal enhancement on early postgadolinium images with slight increase and minimal heterogeneous enhancement on more delayed images are common imaging findings for lymphoma in general. The relationship of the mass to adjacent structures can be assessed by imaging in multiple planes. The rectum (arrows, *c*, *d*) is displaced and compressed by the tumor. Despite extensive disease, there is no proximal small-bowel obstruction, a characteristic finding with small intestine lymphoma. High signal intensity within the pelvic mass is consistent with hemorrhage. Bladder, b.

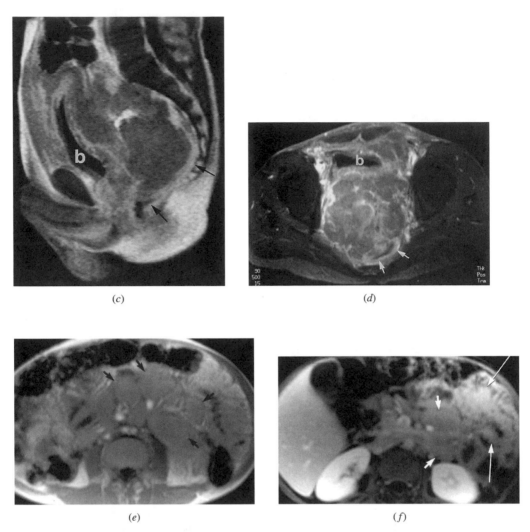

(c)

(d)

(e)

(f)

FIGURE 8.27 (*Continued*) Transverse gadolinium-enhanced SGE (*e*) and interstitial phase gadolinium-enhanced fat-suppressed SGE (*f*) images in a second patient with non-Hodgkin's lymphoma. Bulky mesenteric lymphadenopathy (small arrows, *e, f*) is observed as well as thickening of small-bowel loops (long arrows, *f*).

- ○ Liver metastases are responsible for the carcinoid syndrome, which is characterized by vasomotor instability, intestinal hypomotility, and bronchoconstriction
- • Imaging
  - ○ The primary tumor may be quite small, with the accompanying lymphadenopathy and desmoplastic reaction in the root of the mesentery presenting as the only visible manifestation of disease
  - ○ Larger primary tumors may cause asymmetric bowel-wall thickening and en-

hance in a moderate heterogeneous fashion following intravenous gadolinium (fig. 8.28)
- ○ The characteristic desmoplastic changes in the mesentery and retroperitoneum that occur in response to the secretion of serotonin and tryptophan are low in signal on both T1W and T2W images and show negligible enhancement after contrast
- ○ Liver metastases are often hypervascular and high in signal intensity on T2W images,

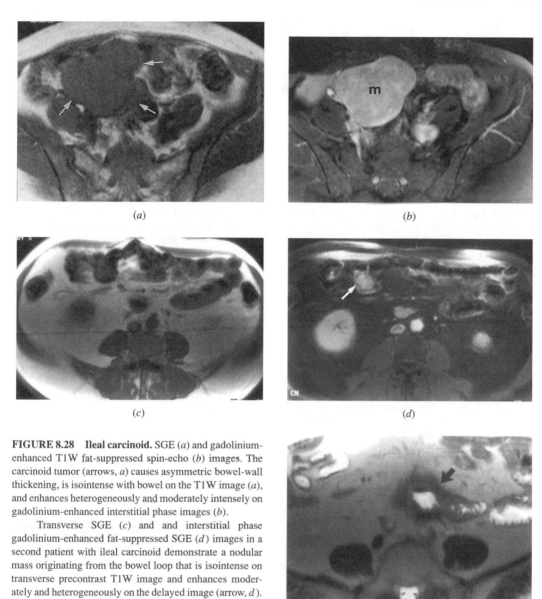

FIGURE 8.28 Ileal carcinoid. SGE (*a*) and gadolinium-enhanced T1W fat-suppressed spin-echo (*b*) images. The carcinoid tumor (arrows, *a*) causes asymmetric bowel-wall thickening, is isointense with bowel on the T1W image (*a*), and enhances heterogeneously and moderately intensely on gadolinium-enhanced interstitial phase images (*b*).

Transverse SGE (*c*) and and interstitial phase gadolinium-enhanced fat-suppressed SGE (*d*) images in a second patient with ileal carcinoid demonstrate a nodular mass originating from the bowel loop that is isointense on transverse precontrast T1W image and enhances moderately and heterogeneously on the delayed image (arrow, *d*).

Transverse T2W SS-ETSE (*e*) in a third patient shows irregular circumferential thickening small bowel consistent with carcinoid tumor.

possessing intense ring or uniform enhancement on immediate postgadolinium SGE images
  ○ Occasionally carcinoid liver metastases are hypovascular and appear nearly isointense with liver on T2W images and demonstrate faint ring enhancement on immediate postgadolinium SGE images

Metastases
• Background
  ○ Tumors arising in the mesentery, pancreas, stomach, or colon may involve the small intestine through contiguous extension (fig. 8.29)
  ○ Metastases to the small intestine from melanoma and carcinomas of the lung,

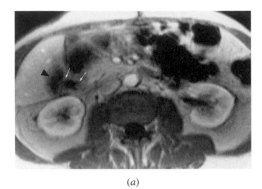
(a)

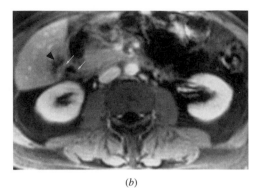
(b)

FIGURE 8.29 Colon cancer liver metastasis with invasion of the duodenum. Immediate postgadolinium SGE (*a*) and 90 s postgadolinium fat-suppressed SGE (*b*) images in a patient with colon cancer metastasis to liver and duodenum. A peripheral hepatic metastasis (arrowhead, *a*, *b*) transgresses the liver capsule to directly invade the adjacent duodenum (arrows, *a*, *b*).

testes, adrenal glands, ovary, stomach, large intestine, uterus, cervix, liver, and kidney have been reported
○ Ovarian tumors are the most common cause of disseminated serosal implants
• Imaging
○ On gadolinium-enhanced fat-suppressed T1W GRE images, metastases are moderately high in signal intensity in contrast to the low signal intensity of intra-abdominal fat
○ Peritoneal spread of tumor can cause irregularly thickened peritoneal or serosal tissue (fig. 8.30) and characteristically involves the concave mesenteric small bowel

○ Hematogenous metastatic spread of carcinomas from distant cancers such as breast and lung occur, and lesions often involve the antimesenteric border of the small bowel and may appear as intramural masses (fig. 8.31)

Inflammation, Infection, and Diffuse Disorders

Inflammatory Bowel Disease (IBD)
• Background
○ Crohn's disease is the most common inflammatory condition to affect the small bowel

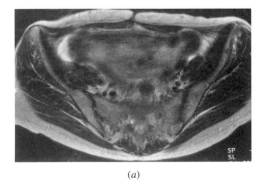
(a)

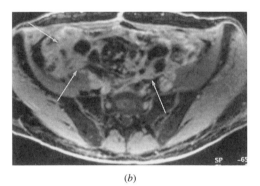
(b)

FIGURE 8.30 Ovarian carcinoma metastases to the peritoneal and serosal surfaces. Transverse 512-resolution T2W echo-train spin-echo (*a*) and 90 s postgadolinium fat-suppressed SGE (*b*) images highlight the improvement in disease detection afforded by breath-hold gadolinium-enhanced fat-suppressed SGE. On the high-resolution T2W image, bowel motion degrades image quality; no metastatic disease can be identified. On the gadolinium-enhanced fat-suppressed SGE image (*b*), the acquisition during suspended respiration avoids breathing artifact and minimizes bowel motion. Enhancement of irregularly thickened tissue along the peritoneum and serosal surface of bowel (arrows, *b*) is consistent with widespread metastatic disease.

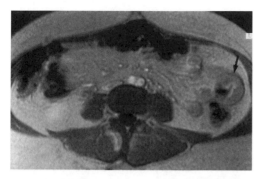

FIGURE 8.31   Hematogeneous metastases. Transverse 45 s postgadolinium SGE image demonstrates an eccentric mural tumor in the midjejunum (arrow). This tumor was a hematogeneous metastasis from uterine leiomyosarcoma.

- ○ The incidence is greatest in the second and third decades of life, with bimodal distribution and with a smaller subset of patients presenting in later adult years
- ○ Associations include genetic predisposition, with risk factors including family history of IBD and Ashkenazi Jewish ancestry
- ○ Etiologic factors appear to include autoimmune effector mechanisms
- ○ Symptoms include watery diarrhea, crampy abdominal pain, weight loss, and fever
- ○ Regional involvement
  - ▪ 70% have involvement of the terminal ileum (TI)
    - • 30% isolated to TI
    - • 40% involving TI and cecum
  - ▪ 15–20% have isolated colon disease
  - ▪ 5% have disease affecting duodenum or jejunum
  - ▪ Crohn's disease is characterized pathologically by
    - • Transmural involvement by chronic inflammation, fibrosis, and noncaseating granulomas
    - • Skip lesions: intervening segments of healthy bowel
    - • Creeping fat: inflammation and fibrosis predominantly involving adjacent mesenteric fat
- • Imaging
  - ○ Gadolinium-enhanced fat-suppressed T1W and single-shot T2W images with and without fat suppression are important for de-

tecting and characterizing Crohn's disease (fig. 8.32)
- ○ Possible findings on T1W images:
  - ▪ Bowel-wall thickening with increased enhancement on delayed postgadolinium fat-suppressed images
  - ▪ Stranding extending into the mesenteric border fat and increased size and number of vessels
  - ▪ Accordion-like retraction and thickening of folds, asymmetrically involving the mesenteric side of the small bowel and creating a tethered appearance
  - ▪ Reactive enlarged draining mesenteric nodes
  - ▪ Fistula formation
  - ▪ Abscess
- ○ Possible findings on T2W images
  - ▪ Bowel-wall thickening with increased signal in and adjacent to the abnormal bowel
  - ▪ Fluid accumulation in adjacent intraperitoneal and mesenteric spaces
- ○ The combination of gadolinium-enhanced fat-suppressed T1W and T2W images can be used to determine disease activity and severity
  - ▪ Severe acute disease demonstrates moderately intense enhancement on capillary phase images in addition to interstitial phase fat-suppressed images
  - ▪ Moderate to mild forms of acute disease show lesser capillary phase enhancement, but prominent interstitial phase enhancement
  - ▪ Quiescent disease shows capillary phase enhancement comparable to normal bowel and minimally increased interstitial phase enhancement in conjunction with bowel-wall thickening and development of fibrosis
  - ▪ Acute-on-chronic disease tends to appear as increased enhancement on early and late images (reflecting severity as described above), which may primarily affect the inner aspect of a thickened bowel wall.
  - ▪ Complementary information may be provided by fat-suppressed single-shot T2W

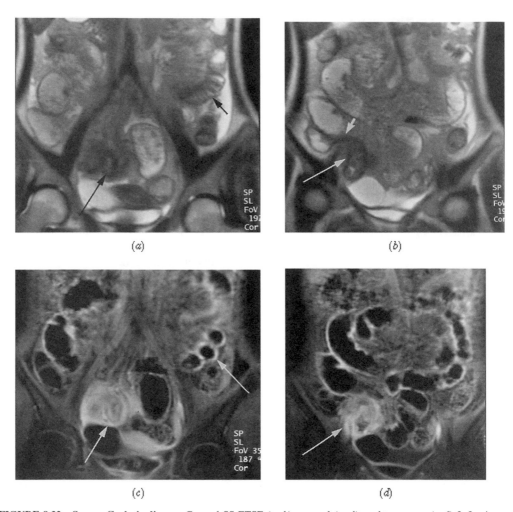

(a)

(b)

(c)

(d)

FIGURE 8.32 Severe Crohn's disease. Coronal SS-ETSE (*a*, *b*), coronal (*c*, *d*), and transverse (*e*, *f*) 2–3 min post-gadolinium fat-suppressed SGE images in a patient with severe disease.

images where severe and acute disease exhibits high signal and quiescent disease is more isointense with unaffected bowel

Ulcerative Colitis
- Background
  - Ulcerative colitis primarily affects the large bowel and primarily affects the mucosa
  - Involvement of the ileocecal valve may lead to a patulous valve and reflux ileitis
- Imaging
  - Inflammation of the TI appears as inflammatory changes on gadolinium-enhanced

fat-suppressed T1W images, usually isolated to the distal most portion of this bowel segment
  - The large bowel will demonstrate pancolic disease changes (see section colon, ulcerative colitis)

Gluten-Sensitive Enteropathy (Celiac Disease, Celiac Sprue)
- Background
  - This is an immunologically mediated inflammatory disease of the small bowel arising in response to dietary glutens, producing a malabsorption syndrome

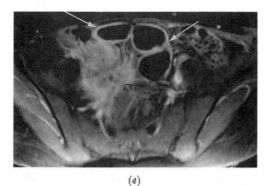
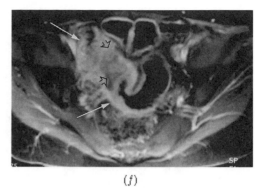

(e)   (f)

FIGURE 8.32 (*Continued*) Coronal T2W images from midabdominal plane (*a*) and 2 cm more anterior (*b*) demonstrate thickened loops of distal small bowel (long arrows, *a*, *b*). The terminal ileum is well shown at its entry into the cecum (small arrow, *b*). Coronal gadolinium-enhanced fat-suppressed SGE images acquired from similar tomographic sections, respectively, demonstrate substantial enhancement of the thickened loops of bowel and surrounding tissues. An enhancing fistulous tract (arrow, *d*) is apparent close to the ileocecal valve. Transverse gadolinium-enhanced images demonstrate intense enhancement of multiple loops of bowel, including loops with wall thickness of 4 mm (arrows, *e*). On the more inferior tomographic section, narrowing of distal ileum is apparent (long arrows, *f*), which accounts for the mild dilation of more proximal loops (arrows, *e*). Inflammatory mesenteric changes are evident (hollow arrows, *e*, *f*). Normal-appearing proximal jejunum (small arrow, *a*) is appreciated on the T2W image.

- ○ GSE likely results from a specific immunologic hyperactivity to a constituent of dietary gluten
- ○ The diagnosis can be made through jejunal biopsy and is based on the presence of mucosal atrophy, with blunting or complete loss of villi, in conjunction with mucosal inflammation
- Imaging
  - ○ T2W single-shot echo-train spin-echo images may demonstrate an abnormal mucosal fold pattern of the small bowel, associated with an increase of intraluminal fluid (fig. 8.33)

Scleroderma
- Background
  - ○ Scleroderma, or progressive systemic sclerosis, is a connective tissue disease that commonly involves the GI tract
  - ○ Patchy destruction of the muscularis propria in the small intestine occurs, mainly involving the duodenum and jejunum. There is also degeneration of both circular and longitudinal muscle layers and replacement by collagen tissue.

- Imaging
  - ○ Dilation is the most common finding on imaging studies (fig. 8.34)
  - ○ Additional characteristic features include
    - ▪ Sacculation with formation of pseudodiverticula
    - ▪ Retention of normal or increased number of bowel folds per unit length
  - ○ Pearl
    - ▪ Small-bowel dilation associated with increased number of folds is a hallmark of scleroderma. (e.g., fig. 8.34*a*)

Pouchitis
- Background
  - ○ A continent ileostomy pouch is often fashioned for patients after total colectomy
  - ○ The creation of an ileal pouch changes the main function of this part of the small intestine from absorption to fecal storage
    - ▪ Stasis and bacterial overgrowth may occur, leading to pouchitis
    - ▪ Most commonly seen in Crohn's patients
- Imaging
  - ○ MRI features include an enhancing and thickened pouch wall and inflammatory

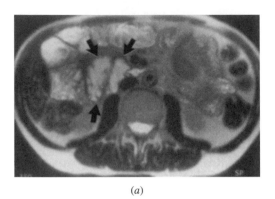

(a)

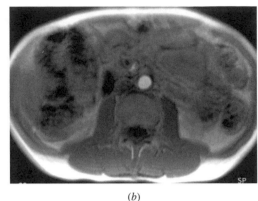

(b)

FIGURE 8.33   Gluten-sensitive enteropathy. T2W SS-ETSE (*a*), immediate postgadolinium SGE (*b*), and 90 s postgadolinium fat-suppressed SGE (*c*) images. T2W image demonstrates an abnormally prominent mucosal pattern in the duodenum associated with an increase in intraluminal fluid (short arrows, *a*). The duodenal mucosa enhances normally, which reflects a lack of vascular changes related to the disease process. Upper gastrointestinal endoscopy with biopsy was performed, and histopathologic examination established the diagnosis of gluten-sensitive enteropathy. (Reprinted with permission from Marcos HB, Semelka RC, Noone TC, Woosley JT, Lee JKT: MRI of normal and abnormal duodenum using half-Fourier single-shot RARE and gadolinium-enhanced spoiled gradient-echo sequences. *Magn Reson Imaging* 17:869–880, 1999.)

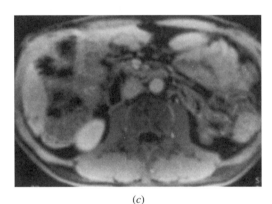

(c)

stranding in the fat adjacent to the pouch (fig. 8.35)

Fistula
- Background
  - Etiologic conditions include infection, inflammation, neoplasia, radiation therapy, and ischemia (embolic, thrombotic, or vasoconstrictive)
    - Important disease considerations include Crohn's disease, diverticulitis, radiation therapy for cervical cancer
- Imaging
  - The appearance of a fistula will depend on its contents and the degree of inflammation (fig. 8.36)
  - Fluid-filled tracts are high in signal intensity on T2W images, whereas gas-filled tracts are signal void

- Fat suppression combined with intravenous gadolinium highlight the enhancing fistulous tract wall amid the surrounding low-signal-intensity suppressed intra-abdominal fat
- Focal discontinuity of the involved organ wall at the site of tract penetration is diagnostic

Radiation Enteritis
- Background
  - The small intestine is the most sensitive segment of the gastrointestinal tract to radiation injury
  - Enteritis can be seen with doses of 45 Gy
  - Most commonly associated with radiation therapy for gynecological malignancy
    - The distal jejunum and ileum are the most common sites affected

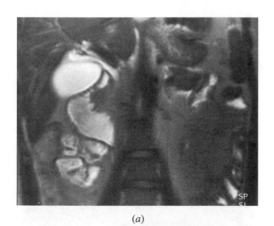

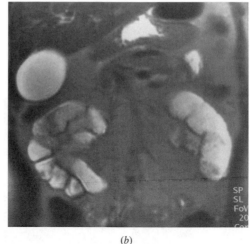

(a)   (b)

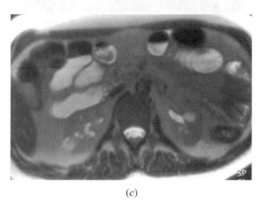

(c)

FIGURE 8.34 Scleroderma. Coronal (*a, b*) and transverse (*c*) T2W SS-ETSE images show dilatation of the duodenum and multiple small-bowel loops without evidence of obstruction.

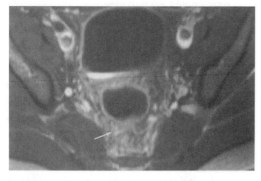

FIGURE 8.35 Pouchitis. Gadolinium-enhanced T1W fat-suppressed spin-echo image demonstrates slight thickening of the pouch with stranding in the surrounding fat (arrow).

- Microscopic inspection shows sloughed villi with mucosal hemorrhage, edema, focal necrosis, and inflammation present within hours to days following therapy
- Early postradiotherapy complications include ulceration, necrosis, bleeding, perforation, and abscess formation
- The development of chronic radiation enteritis is variable, arising months to years after the radiation event
  - This is a progressive disease resulting from underlying vascular damage, leading to bowel atrophy and fibrosis
  - Complications include strictures, fistulae, bowel fixation with angulation, and obstruction
- Imaging
  - Gadolinium-enhanced fat-suppressed SGE imaging is the most effective technique to

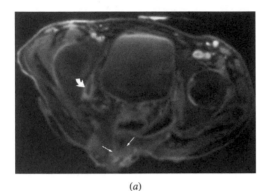

(a)

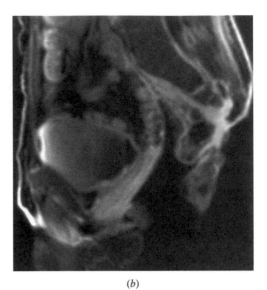

(b)

FIGURE 8.36   Pelvic fistulas in a patient with Crohn's disease. Transverse (*a*) and sagittal (*b*) interstitial phase gadolinium-enhanced fat-suppressed SGE images. There is a large decubitus ulcer associated with destruction of the coccyx and lower part of the sacrum. Extensive pelvic cutaneous fistulas appear as enhancing track walls (arrows, *a*). An abscess of the obturator internus muscle is present (curved arrow, *a*).

demonstrate diffuse early ischemic and inflammatory changes of radiation enteritis and to show late fibrotic changes and strictures
- It is also critical to discriminate radiation changes from recurrent tumor (fig. 8.37). In general, radiation changes show uniform circumferential bowel-wall thickening, whereas recurrent tumor exhibits asymmetrical involvement with prominent solid mass tissue extending beyond the confines of the bowel wall.

Ischemia and Hemorrhage
- Background
  - Ischemia and hemorrhage may occur in tandem or as isolated events
  - Ischemia, regardless of etiology, leads to wall edema secondary to capillary leakage (fig. 8.38)
  - There is a range of findings and sequelae of ischemia, depending on severity:
    - Mild
      - Transient event with complete recovery to morphologically normal bowel

- Severe acute
  - Perforation
  - Hemorrhage
- Severe chronic
  - Fibrosis and stricture formation
- Imaging
  - MRI findings parallel the severity of blood flow compromise on gadolinium-enhanced T1W images
  - Early changes include mural thickening with increased enhancement on late postcontrast images (fig. 8.39)
  - Increased enhancement on immediate postgadolinium images reflects leaky capillaries
  - Necrotic bowel with hemorrhage and portal venous gas can be demonstrated (fig. 8.39)
  - Vascular compromise or thrombosis may be well shown on early (less than 1 min) postgadolinium images (fig. 8.40)
  - MRA can be performed to examine the SMA at the origin and proximal extent (see chap. 9)
  - Bowel-wall hemorrhage from trauma or ischemia can result in high signal intensity

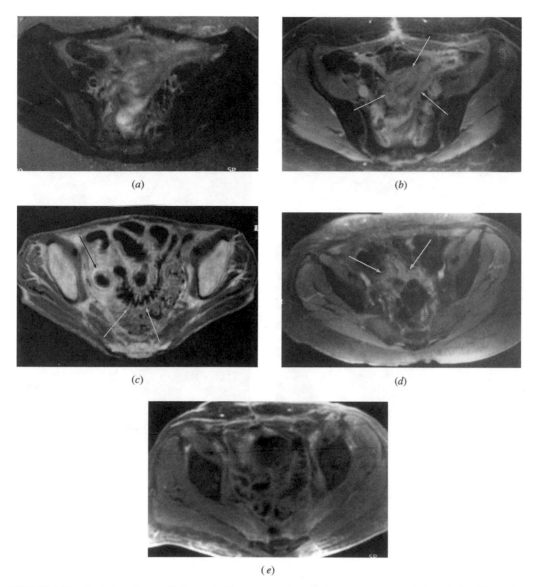

FIGURE 8.37 Small intestine radiation enteritis versus metastatic disease. Transverse 512-resolution T2W echo-train spin-echo (*a*), 90 s postgadolinium fat-suppressed SGE (*b*), and 90 s postgadolinium SGE (*c*) images in two patients (*a, b*) and (*c*) with radiation enteritis, respectively. In the first patient, the T2W echo-train spin-echo image (*a*) is degraded by blurring artifact secondary to peristalsis. Breath-hold technique coupled with gadolinium-enhanced fat-suppressed imaging at the same level highlights postradiation therapy changes of the small bowel: diffuse, symmetric wall thickening with increased enhancement (arrows, *b*). Similar changes are noted in the second patient after radiation therapy (arrows, *c*).

Transverse 90 s postgadolinium fat-suppressed SGE image (*d*) in a third patient, who has recurrent ovarian cancer, demonstrates irregular focal thickening of small bowel. Note the difference between the symmetric and uniform bowel thickening associated with radiation changes (*b, c*) and the more focal and asymmetric changes produced by metastatic disease to the small bowel (arrows, *d*).

Transverse gadolinium-enhanced interstitial phase fat-suppressed SGE (*e*) image in a fourth patient after radiation therapy for colon cancer shows circumferential small-bowel thickening.

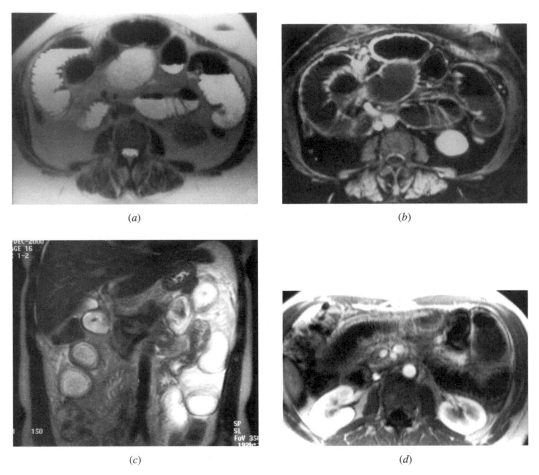

(a)

(b)

(c)

(d)

FIGURE 8.38   Small-bowel ischemia. T2W SS-ETSE (*a*) and interstitial phase gadolinium-enhanced fat-suppressed SGE (*b*) images in a patient with encarcerated hernia. Multiple dilated enhancing loops of small bowel with increased mural enhancement are observed. Air-fluid levels are identified on T2W image (*a*).

on both T1W and T2W images, due to the presence of extracellular methemoglobin. This is most conspicuous on fat-suppressed noncontrast T1W images (fig. 8.41).

Hypoproteinemia
- Background
  - Hypoproteinemia most commonly results from cirrhosis, malabsorption states, and malnourishment
  - This condition can manifest in diffuse bowel edema due to diminished oncotic pressure and fluid shift from the intravascular to the interstitial spaces

- Imaging
  - Generalized bowel-wall thickening is usually most pronounced in the jejunum
  - Dolinium-enhanced fat-suppressed T1W images show wall thickening in conjunction with negligible enhancement (fig. 8.42)

Intussusception
- Background
  - Intussusception is characterized by the telescoping of one intestinal segment into another
    - The invaginating bowel segment is referred to as the intussusceptum

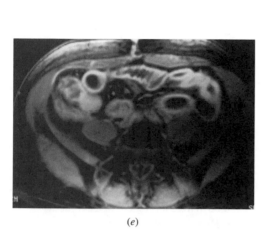

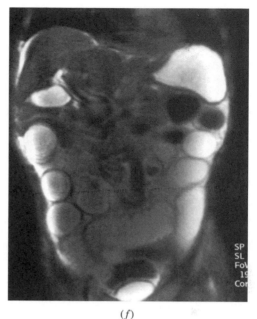

(e)   (f)

FIGURE 8.38   (*Continued*) Coronal T2W SS-ETSE (*c*), immediate postgadolinium T1W SGE (*d*), and interstitial phase gadolinium-enhanced fat-suppressed SGE (*e*) images in a second patient, who underwent radiotherapy for cervix cancer. Small bowel dilatation with increased thickness and enhancement is present. Operative finding were consistent with multiple adhesions and bowel ischemia.

Coronal T2W SS-ETSE (*f*) image in a third patient shows diffuse, markedly dilated small-bowel loops.

- The bowel segment into which the prolapse has occurred is referred to as the intussuscipiens
  ○ Intussusceptions are commonly transient and not associated with symptoms, and do not have underlying pathology in this setting
  ○ Symptomatic intussusceptions in adults present as a result of mechanical obstruction, bowel ischemia, and/or hematochezia

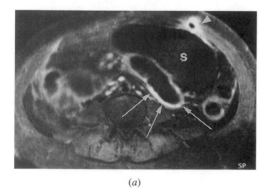

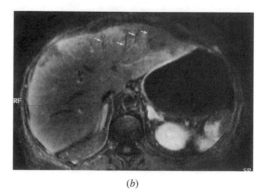

(a)   (b)

FIGURE 8.39   Small-bowel ischemia. Gadolinium-enhanced T1W fat-suppressed spin-echo images (*a*, *b*). The patient had undergone previous small-bowel resection. Increased enhancement of a loop of proximal small bowel (arrows, *a*) is present. The stomach (S, *a*) also contains regions of increased mural enhancement. Increased enhancement results from leaky capillaries in ischemic bowel disease. Portal venous gas (small arrows, *b*) is an ominous finding suggesting bowel necrosis. Susceptibility artifact (arrowhead, *a*) is noted within the anterior abdominal wall.

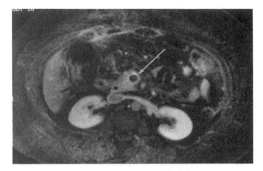

FIGURE 8.40 Superior mesenteric vein (SMV) thrombosis. Transverse 90 s postgadolinium fat-suppressed SGE image demonstrates signal-void thrombus in the SMV with increased enhancement of the SMV wall (arrow), which was caused by infection associated with thrombosis.

- Predisposing factors include masses, motility disorders, and gluten-sensitive enteropathy
- Imaging
  - Intussusception is clearly demonstrated on T2W single-shot echo-train spin-echo images facilitated by the presence of abundant fluid in the dilated bowel proximal to the obstructing intussusception outlining the lower-signal-intensity intussusceptum (fig. 8.43)
    - True-FISP imaging may provide similar-quality imaging of these bowel findings

Graft-versus-Host Disease (GVHD)
- Background
  - This condition results in the setting of transplantation (organ or bone marrow) from an imperfectly immunologically matched donor, where the donor immune cells mount an immune rejection attack on host tissues, due to HLA-type differences between host and donor cells
  - Acute GVHD involves the gastric antrum, small bowel, and colon, and occurs within 7 to 100 days following transplantation
    - Histologically shows loss of normal intestinal mucosal architecture with ulceration, mucosal denudation, and submucosal edema
  - Chronic GVHD may follow the acute form or occur insidiously and is usually associated with esophageal involvement
    - Histologically shows esophageal involvement with sloughed and hyperemic mucosa
- Imaging
  - In acute GVHD, MR images may show diffuse bowel-wall thickening with increased enhancement of the inner wall layers (fig. 8.44)
  - Chronic GVHD may lead to desquamative esophagitis with formation of webs and strictures

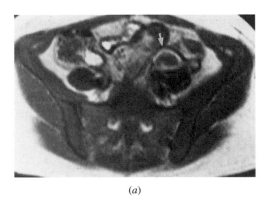

(a)

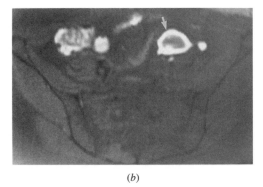

(b)

FIGURE 8.41 Submucosal hemorrhage. SGE (*a*) and T1W fat-suppressed spin-echo (*b*) images in a woman status posthysterectomy who had undergone vigorous intraoperative bowel retraction. Increased signal intensity in the bowel wall on the SGE image (arrow, *a*) becomes more conspicuous after fat suppression (arrow, *b*). (Reprinted with permission from Shoenut JP, Semelka RC, Silverman R, Yaffe CS, Mickflikier AB: The gastrointestinal tract. In Semelka RC, Shoenut JP [eds.]. *MRI of the Abdomen with CT Correlation*. New York: Raven Press, pp. 119–143, 1993.)

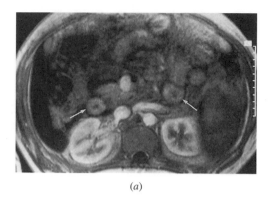

(a)

(b)

(c)

FIGURE 8.42   Small-bowel edema in cirrhosis. Immediate postgadolinium SGE (*a*), 90 s postgadolinium SGE (*b*), and T2W single-shot echo-train spin-echo (*c*) images in three patients with cirrhosis. Ascites and diffuse thickening of multiple loops of small bowel (arrows, *a*) are present. Third spacing of fluid secondary to hypoproteinemia accounts for the bowel-wall thickening. High-signal submucosal edema is well shown on the single-shot T2W image (arrow, *c*).

Large Bowel

- The rectum is a fixed retroperitoneal structure and the pelvis is generally less prone to motion artifacts from respiration, facilitating high-resolution longer-acquisition-time imaging, such as T2W short echo-train multishot imaging with a 512 matrix
  - This technique is particularly useful for the evaluation of rectal carcinoma: in assessing the extent of bowel-wall involvement by tumor, determining the relationship of tumors to adjacent structures, and distinguishing tumor recurrence from fibrosis
  - The layers of the rectal wall can also be visualized on gadolinium-enhanced T1W fat-suppressed images (fig. 8.45)
  - Transition between rectum and anal canal can be determined by the observation that the rectum contains intraluminal air and the anal canal is collapsed

- The use of intraluminal contrast to distend the colon improves detection of mucosal abnormalities (see Overview at the beginning of this chapter)

Congenital Abnormalities
Malrotation
- Nonrotation, the most common rotational abnormality, was discussed earlier for small bowel. In this condition the large bowel occupies the left side of the abdomen.

Duplication
- Background
  - Colonic duplications represent a congenital longitudinal division of the developing gut and may be limited to a single segment of large bowel or can involve the entire colon
  - Symptoms may depend on whether there is communication of the duplication with the remainder of the colon

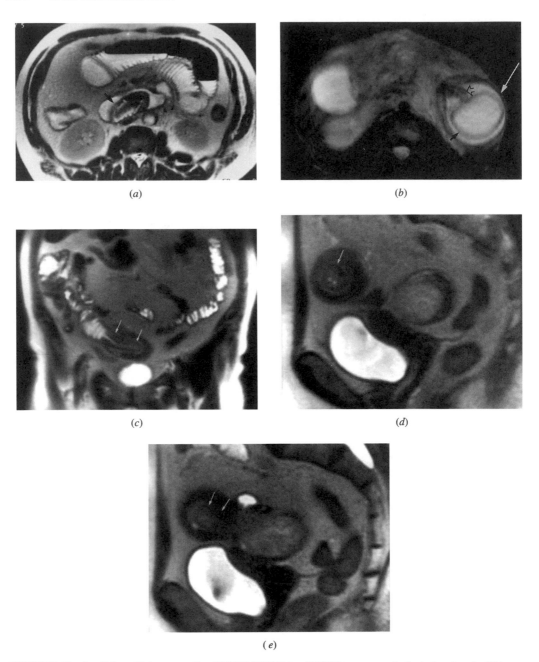

FIGURE 8.43   Small-bowel intussusception. T2W SS-ETSE (*a*) and T2W fat-suppressed echo-train spin-echo (*b*) images in two patients. In the first patient, the T2W image (*a*) provides clear definition of the bowel-within-bowel appearance (arrow, *a*) of intussusception. In the second patient (*b*), respiratory and bowel motion degrades the majority of the peritoneal cavity. However, the dilated, relatively fixed, hypotonic loop of the intussuscipiens (long arrow, *b*) is relatively well shown. The intussusceptum (short arrows, *a*) is clearly shown, and its mesentery (hollow arrow, *b*) is also appreciated. In this second patient adequate visualization of the intussusception occurred in this non-breath-hold study because of the hypotonicity of the involved bowel segments.

Coronal (*c*) and sagittal (*d*, *e*) T2W SS-ETSE images in a third patient. The bowel-within-bowel appearance (arrows, (*c–e*) is clearly demonstrated. (Courtesy of N. Cem Balci, Florence Nightingale Hospital, Istanbul, Turkey.)

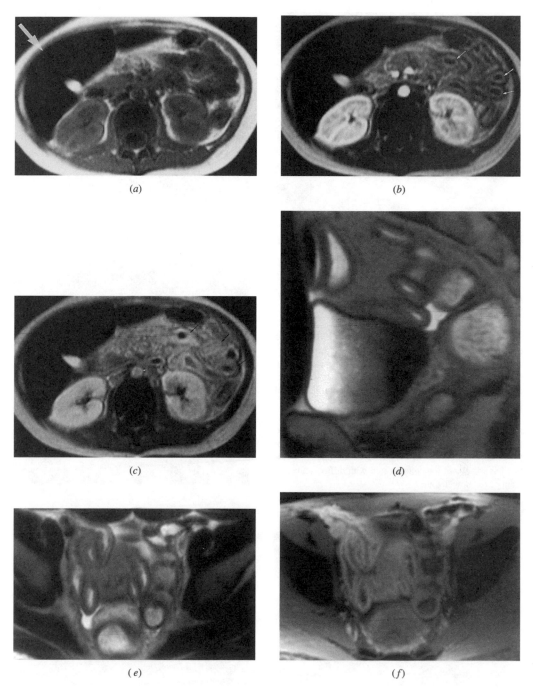

FIGURE 8.44 Graft-versus-host disease. SGE (*a*), immediate (*b*), and 90 s (*c*) postgadolinium SGE images in a patient status post bone marrow transplant. Unenhanced images suggest thickening of multiple loops of small bowel. Immediately after intravenous contrast, intense mucosal enhancement of multiple loops of small bowel (arrows, *b*) is appreciated. On the interstitial phase image (*c*), enhancement has spread to involve the majority of the wall (arrows, *c*). This enhancement pattern reflects hyperemia and capillary leakage, respectively. The decreased signal intensity of the liver (arrow, *a*) is consistent with iron overload secondary to multiple blood transfusions. (Reprinted with permission from Ascher SM, Semelka RC: MRI of the gastrointestinal tract.

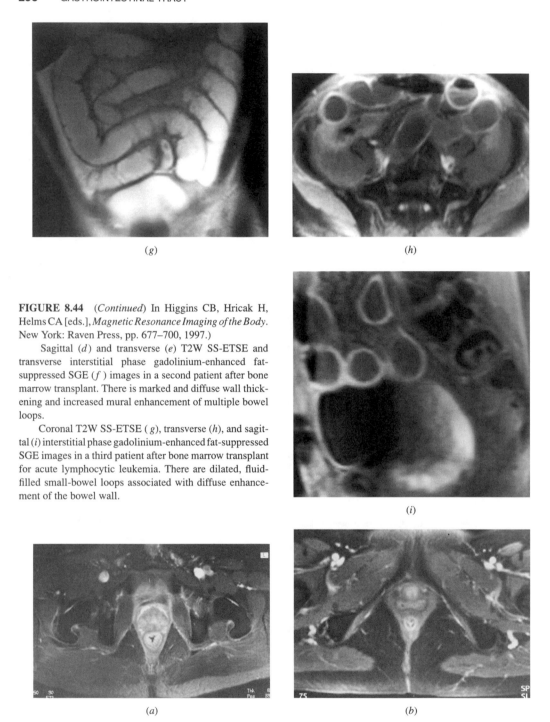

(g)

(h)

FIGURE 8.44 (*Continued*) In Higgins CB, Hricak H, Helms CA [eds.], *Magnetic Resonance Imaging of the Body.* New York: Raven Press, pp. 677–700, 1997.)

Sagittal (*d*) and transverse (*e*) T2W SS-ETSE and transverse interstitial phase gadolinium-enhanced fat-suppressed SGE (*f*) images in a second patient after bone marrow transplant. There is marked and diffuse wall thickening and increased mural enhancement of multiple bowel loops.

Coronal T2W SS-ETSE (*g*), transverse (*h*), and sagittal (*i*) interstitial phase gadolinium-enhanced fat-suppressed SGE images in a third patient after bone marrow transplant for acute lymphocytic leukemia. There are dilated, fluid-filled small-bowel loops associated with diffuse enhancement of the bowel wall.

(i)

(a)

(b)

FIGURE 8.45   Normal rectum and anal canal. Gadolinium-enhanced T1W fat-suppressed spin-echo image (*a*) in a man highlight the different layers of the rectum (from inner layer to outer layer): high-signal-intensity mucosa, low-signal-intensity muscularis mucosa and lamina propria, high-signal-intensity submucosa, and low-signal-intensity muscularis propria. The rectum contains air within the lumen.

Gadolinium-enhanced T1W fat-suppressed spin-echo image (*b*) in a woman demonstrates the same enhancement features of the anal canal. Note that the anal canal is collapsed and does not contain air.

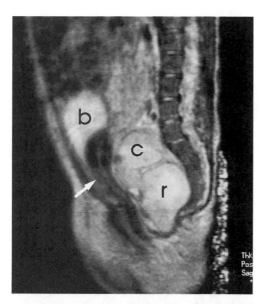

FIGURE 8.46   Colonic duplication. T2W spin-echo image in a patient with colonic duplication. The uterus (arrow) and bladder (b) are anteriorly displaced by two fluid-filled viscous structures that represent the rectum (r) and the duplication cyst (c).

- Patients with right colon duplication are at risk for intussusception
- Imaging
  - Two colonic lumens are identified in parallel (fig. 8.46), which is well shown on single-shot T2W or True-FISP images

Anorectal Anomalies
- Background
  - Most cases of anorectal anomalies occur in association with other congenital malformations
  - MRI has been successful in evaluating these patients, since it directly demonstrates the rectal pouch and sphincter muscles in multiple planes, and facilitates exact determination of the location and developmental status of the sphincter muscles as well as identification of associated anomalies of the kidneys and spine
  - MRI is also valuable for postoperative assessment of the neorectum and sphincteric muscles (figs. 8.47 and 8.48)

Masses

Benign Masses
Adenoma
- Background
  - Adenomas are mucosal origin lesions and are the most common form of colorectal polyp, representing the most common large-bowel neoplasm
    - Most adenocarcinomas arise from adenomatous polyps
  - Three basic types of adenomatous polyps are discerned histopathologically: tubular, tubulovillous, and villous
  - Villous adenomas are characterized by a neoplastic growth composed of fine fingerlets or villi that project from the muscularis mucosae to the outer tip of the adenoma and are associated with a higher rate of malignancy

Polyps and Polyposis Syndromes
- Multiple colonic adenomas are seen in association with familial adenomatous polyposis or Gardner's syndrome, whereas multiple colonic hamartomas may be seen in Peutz-Jeghers syndrome or juvenile polyposis syndromes
  - Familial adenomatous polyposis syndrome
    - Autosomal-dominant disorder
    - Characterized by numerous adenomas affecting primarily the colon and the rectum
    - Risk of malignant transformation to colorectal carcinoma approaches 100%
    - Increased risk of developing peri-ampullary duodenal carcinoma
  - Gardner's syndrome (possibly a variant of familial polyposis)
    - Autosomal-dominant disorder
    - Diffuse adenomatous polyps
    - Approaching 100% risk of colon malignancy
    - Osteomas
    - Soft-tissue abnormalities, including desmoid tumors
  - Peutz-Jeghers syndrome
    - Autosomal-dominant disorder

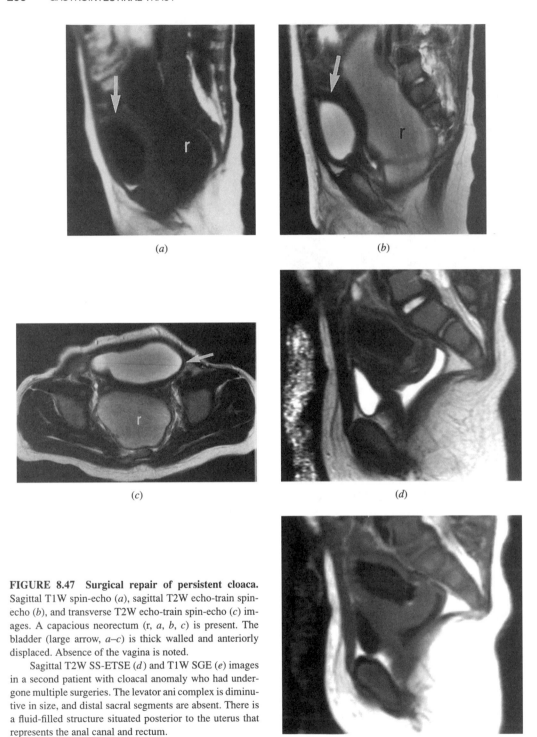

FIGURE 8.47 Surgical repair of persistent cloaca.
Sagittal T1W spin-echo (*a*), sagittal T2W echo-train spin-echo (*b*), and transverse T2W echo-train spin-echo (*c*) images. A capacious neorectum (r, *a, b, c*) is present. The bladder (large arrow, *a–c*) is thick walled and anteriorly displaced. Absence of the vagina is noted.

Sagittal T2W SS-ETSE (*d*) and T1W SGE (*e*) images in a second patient with cloacal anomaly who had undergone multiple surgeries. The levator ani complex is diminutive in size, and distal sacral segments are absent. There is a fluid-filled structure situated posterior to the uterus that represents the anal canal and rectum.

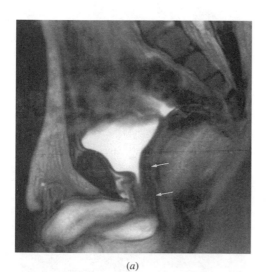

(a)

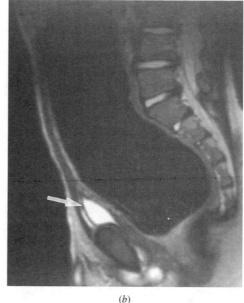

(b)

(c)

FIGURE 8.48   Reconstructed imperforate anus. Sagittal T2W SS-ETSE (a) image in a 1-year-old boy shows that the anal canal (arrows, a) is situated in an anterior location, just posterior to the prostate. The levator ani muscle is intact.

Sagittal T2W echo-train spin-echo images in a second (b) and a third (c) patient demonstrate a markedly dilated air-filled rectum, compressing and displacing the bladder anterosuperiorly (arrow, b).

- Skin and mucosal pigmented macules
- Gastrointestinal hamartomas found in small bowel in 95% of patients, colon and stomach in 25%
- Hamartoma polyps are benign, but patients have other associated multiorgan tumor risks
- Stomach or duodenal adenocarcinoma develops in 3%
- Ovarian cysts or neoplasms in 5%

○ Three distinct syndromes are associated with juvenile polyps
- Juvenile polyposis, gastrointestinal juvenile polyposis, and Cronkhite-Canada syndromes
- Hamartomas are common to all three syndromes
• Imaging
○ Gadolinium-enhanced fat-suppressed SGE and T2W single-shot echo-train images can

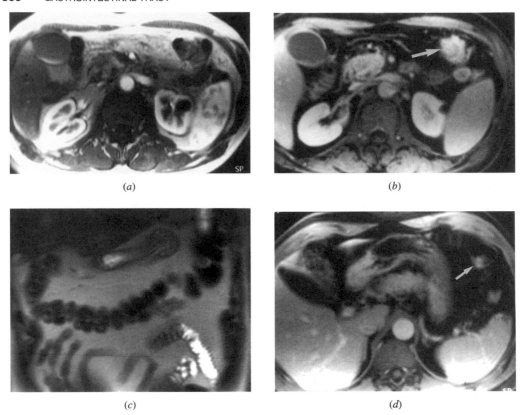

(a) (b)

(c) (d)

FIGURE 8.49 Villous adenoma. Immediate postgadolinium SGE (a) and interstitial phase gadolinium-enhanced fat-suppressed SGE (b) images. A polypoid mass is seen within the distal transverse colon. The mass enhances minimally on immediate postgadolinium images (a) and in a moderately intense fashion with mild heterogeneity on 2 min postgadolinium images (arrow, b).

Coronal T2W SS-ETSE (c) and transverse interstitial phase gadolinium-enhanced fat-suppressed SGE (d) images in a second patient with villous adenoma of transverse colon (arrow, d) demonstrates a similar appearance to the previous patient. Most tumors show moderately intense enhancement with mild heterogeneity on 2 min postgadolinium interstitial phase images, reflecting a larger and more irregular interstitial space than adjacent normal bowel.

demonstrate polyps as small as 5–10 mm (figs. 8.49 and 8.50)
- Multiple techniques of MR colonography are in development (see Overview at beginning of chapter)

Lipoma
- Background
  - Lipomas are the second most common benign neoplasm of the large bowel, and the most common mesenchymol benign tumor
  - Arise from the submucosa
  - Most are asymptomatic
  - Most commonly arise in the cecum, ascending colon, and sigmoid colon
  - Other mesynchymol tumors are rare and include leiomyomas, hemangiomas, and neurofibromas
- Imaging
  - Demonstration of the fat signal within lipomas with T1W and fat-suppressed T1W sequences is pathognomonic
  - High in signal intensity on T1W images and diminished in signal intensity on fat-suppressed T1W images (fig. 8.51)
  - Additional use of out-of-phase SGE may demonstrate fat-water black ring phase

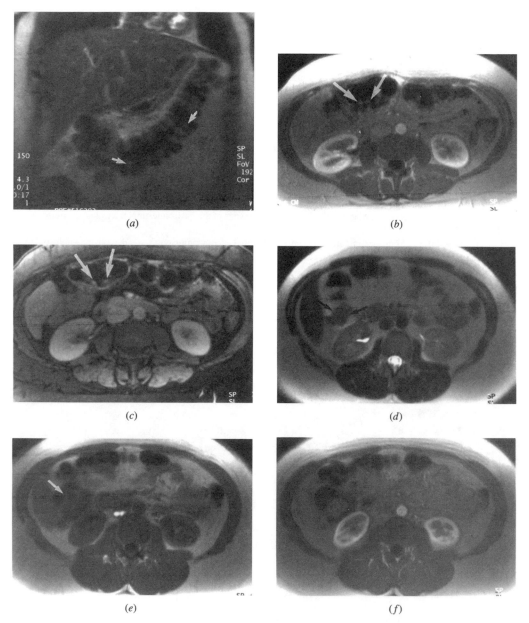

FIGURE 8.50 Familial adenomatous polyposis syndrome. Coronal T2W SS-ETSE (*a*), immediate postgadolinium SGE (*b*), and interstitial phase gadolinium-enhanced fat-suppressed SGE (*c*) images. Numerous polyps are seen measuring <1 cm in diameter in the transverse colon (arrows, *a*). The signal void of the air in the colon provides good contrast from the soft tissue polyps on the T2W image (*a*). The polyps are mildly enhanced (arrows, *b*) on the immediate postgadolinium image (*b*). Polyps demonstrate persistent enhancement on interstitial phase images (arrows, *c*). This patient underwent total colectomy, which demonstrated numerous adenomatous polyps. Transverse T2W SS-ETSE (*d*), SGE (*e*), and immediate postgadolinium SGE (*f*) images in another patient with familial polyposis syndrome. A 2.5 cm polyp is present that arises in the ascending colon. The high signal intensity of the fluid contents of the colon permits good delineation of the low signal intensity of the polyp on the SS-ETSE image (arrows, *d*). The polyp is isointense to the bowel wall on the precontrast T1W image (arrow, *e*). On the early postgadolinium image, the polyp shows mild heterogeneous enhancement comparable to the bowel wall. Note the intense enhancement of the normal renal cortex, which is greater than the enhancement of the bowel wall or the polyp.

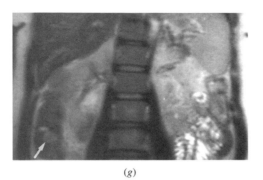

(g)

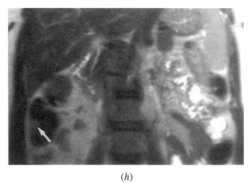

(h)

FIGURE 8.50 (*Continued*) This patient underwent sigmoidoscopy with biopsy followed by total colectomy (Reprinted with permission from Semelka RC, Marcos HB: Polyposis syndromes of the gastrointestinal tract. *J Magn Reson Imaging* 11:51–55, 2000.)

Coronal SS-ETSE (*g, h*) images in a third patient with familial adenomatous polyposis demonstrate polypoid lesions in the cecum (arrow, *g, h*).

cancellation surrounding the polyp (fig. 8.51)

- Lipomas may also act as a lead point for intussusceptions (fig. 8.52)
- Nonneoplastic lesions show an inflamed mucosa or hyperplastic epithelium

- Neoplastic mucoceles are classified as mucinous cystoadenoma or mucinous cystadenocarcinoma
  - Mucinous cystoadenocarcinoma will spread to local lymph nodes and by peritoneal seeding

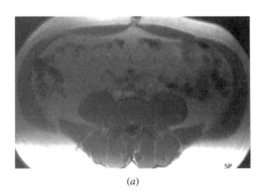

(a)

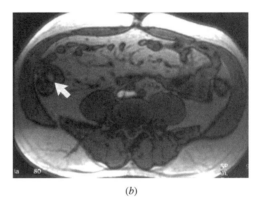

(b)

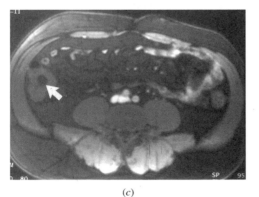

(c)

FIGURE 8.51 Cecal lipoma. Precontrast SGE (*a*), precontrast out-of-phase SGE (*b*), and 90 s postgadolinium fat-suppressed SGE (*c*) images. A 2 cm mass in the cecum is high in signal intensity in the precontrast SGE image (arrow, *a*) and demonstrates a phase-cancellation artifact in the out-of-phase SGE image (arrow, *b*). Markedly diminished signal intensity of the mass is noted on postcontrast fat-suppressed SGE image (arrow, *c*). (Reprinted with permission from Chung JJ, Semelka RC , Martin DR, Marcos HB: Colon diseases: MR evaluation using combined T2W single-shot echo train spin-echo and gadolinium-enhanced spoiled gradient-echo sequences. *J Magn Reson Imaging* 12:297–305, 2000.)

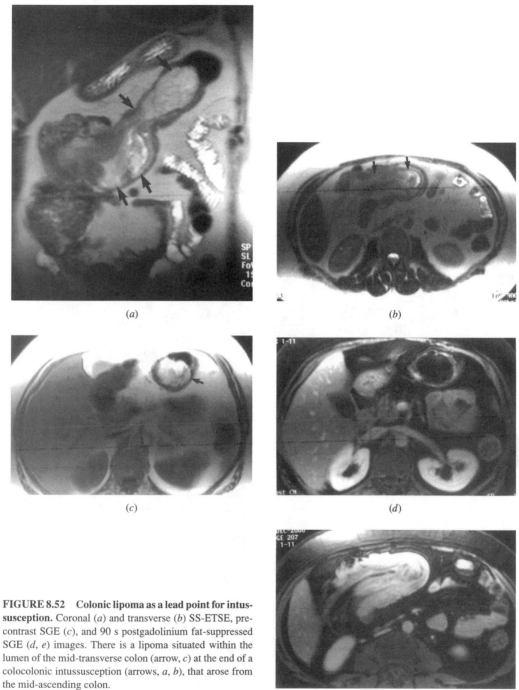

FIGURE 8.52   Colonic lipoma as a lead point for intussusception. Coronal (*a*) and transverse (*b*) SS-ETSE, precontrast SGE (*c*), and 90 s postgadolinium fat-suppressed SGE (*d*, *e*) images. There is a lipoma situated within the lumen of the mid-transverse colon (arrow, *c*) at the end of a colocolonic intussusception (arrows, *a*, *b*), that arose from the mid-ascending colon.

▪ Pseudomyxoma peritonei is a form of peritoneal spread

○ Given the overlap in appearance and the risk of cyst rupture, mucoceles should be prophylactically removed

• Imaging

○ T2W single-shot echo-train spin-echo images show a high-signal-intensity tubular structure in the region of the appendix (fig. 8.53)

○ Mucoceles have higher signal intensity than simple fluid on T1W sequences due to pro-

tein in solution, and the wall will enhance with gadolinium administration, appearing thin if uncomplicated by inflammation or tumor

Malignant Masses

Adenocarcinoma

• Background

○ Adenocarcinoma of the colon is the most common gastrointestinal tract malignancy, the third most common cancer in North

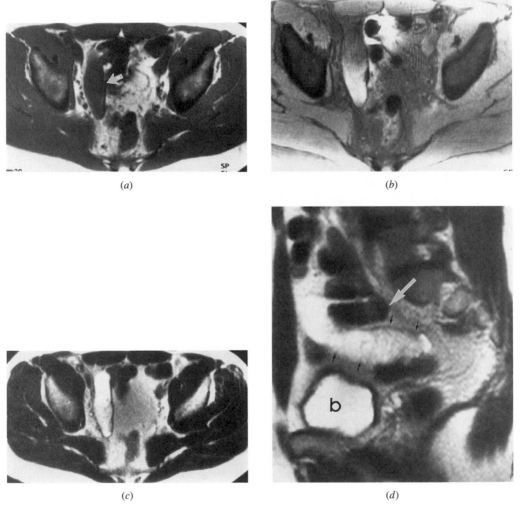

(a)

(b)

(c)

(d)

FIGURE 8.53   Mucocele of the appendix. SGE (*a*), fat-suppressed SGE (*b*), SS-ETSE (*c*), sagittal SS-ETSE (*d*), and immediate postgadolinium fat-suppressed SGE (*e*) images. An oblong-shaped mucocele of the appendix is present (arrow, *a*) that contains high-signal-intensity material in the dependent portion of the cyst on the T1W image (*a*), which is accentuated with the application of fat suppression (*b*). The mucocele is high in signal intensity on the T2W image, with slight heterogeneity in the dependent portion (*c*).

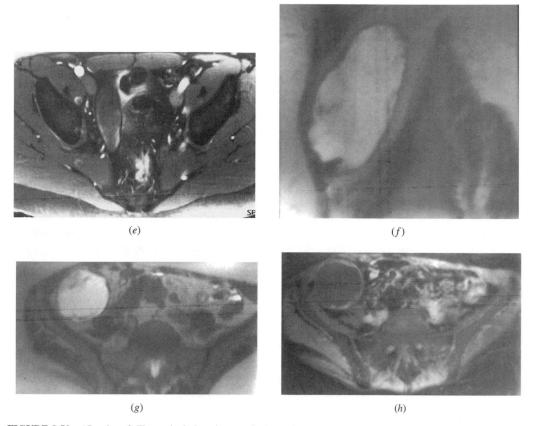

(e)

(f)

(g)

(h)

FIGURE 8.53 (*Continued*) The sagittal plane image (*d*) shows the orientation of the mucocele (small arrows, *d*) to the base of the cecum (arrow, *d*) and the relationship to the bladder (b, *d*). No appreciable enhancement of the mucocele wall is noted on the postgadolinium image (*e*), which excludes the diagnosis of abscess.

Sagittal (*f*) and transverse (*g*) SS-ETSE and interstitial phase gadolinium-enhanced SGE (*h*) images in a second patient show a large cystic mass in the lower right quadrant of the abdomen extending into the pelvic inlet. Note the presence of septations and a thin rim enhancement.

America, and the most common cause of cancer death
- Incidence increases with age
- 138,000 new cases per year
- Overall 5-year survival is 50–60%
◦ High-risk conditions include
- Familial adenomatous polyposis, Gardner's syndrome, ulcerative or Crohn's colitis
◦ Cancers occur most often in the rectosigmoid colon
◦ Tumors may be polypoid, plaque-like, or circumferential, causing narrowing in an apple core configuration
◦ Symptoms reflect tumor location and morphology, with most patients reporting a combination of change in bowel habits, bleeding, pain, and weight loss
◦ Tumor markers include carcinoembryonic antigen (CEA), which is elevated in approximately 20% of cases and may be used to follow tumor therapy
◦ Staging is generally performed with TNM system and is as follows:
- T—primary tumor
  - Tx: Tumor cannot be assessed
  - T0: No evidence of primary tumor
  - Tis: Carcinoma in situ
  - T1: Limited to the mucosa or mucosa and submucosa
  - T2: Extension to muscle or muscle and serosal

- T3: Extension beyond the colon to immediately contiguous structures
- T3a: Without fistula formation
- T3b: With fistula formation
- T4: Deep infiltration occupying more than one region but not more than one region, or extending to neighboring structures
  - N—lymph nodes
    - Nx: Nodes cannot be assessed
    - N0: No evidence of node involvement
    - N1: Regional nodes involved
    - N2, N3: Not used
    - N4: Beyond regional lymph nodes
  - M—metastases
    - Mx: Distant metastases cannot be assessed
    - M0: No distant metastases
    - M1: Distant metastases
- Imaging
  - Malignant lymph nodes may not be enlarged greater than 10 mm at the time of diagnosis
    - More than five lymph nodes that measure <1 cm in a regional distribution related to the tumor correlates well with tumor involvement
  - The combination of T2W single-shot echo-train spin-echo and gadolinium-enhanced fat-suppressed SGE images results in optimal assessment of the colon above the rectum (figs. 8.54 and 8.55)
  - Gadolinium-enhanced fat-suppressed SGE imaging is valuable in demonstrating perirectal tumor extension, regional lymph nodes, and seeding of peritoneum by tumor
  - When performing a combined abdominal-pelvic two-stage examination, the abdominal gadolinium-enhanced imaging should be done first to obtain multiphase arterial and venous imaging of the liver for metastatic staging, followed by the T1W gadolinium-enhanced pelvic imaging, which is now performed in the interstitial phase
    - T2W pelvic imaging can be acquired at the beginning of the study, prior to the abdominal study, to avoid having signal

changes in the bladder due to excreted gadolinium concentrating in the bladder. However, pelvic imaging can be performed in the presence of gadolinium in the bladder if necessary, where the gadolinium in the dependent aspect of the bladder can be used to produce useful contrast to look for posterior bladder wall extension in the setting of a metastatic rectal mass (fig. 8.56).
  - Surface coils should be used, and current MR systems are available, facilitating multistation coil placement to allow coverage of the pelvis and the abdomen without having to move these coils, performing all patient centering from software control
- Employing phased-array surface multicoils with current systems may obviate the need for endorectal coil imaging for anatomic evaluation
- Challenges associated with endorectal probes include
  - Probe alters anatomy by exerting a direct mass effect
  - Probe induces contractions in the sigmoid and rectum, causing artifacts on motion-sensitive pelvic imaging
  - May slide superior to the anal verge and thereby not include the distal rectum in the field of view
  - Additional time requirements for coil placement, and is generally not favored by patients (or staff)
- Potential benefits of the endorectal coil
  - High-resolution visualization of the rectal wall (fig. 8.57)
- Gadolinium-enhanced fat-suppressed T1W 2D/3D GRE interstitial phase imaging is sensitive for direct bone invasion or bone metastases
- Posttherapy inflammatory fibrosis, as observed following radiation of the pelvis, can lead to gadolinium enhancement of the sacrum that persisits up to 1.5 to 2 years
  - Elevated T2W signal usually diminishes to normal earlier than diminution of abnormal enhancement

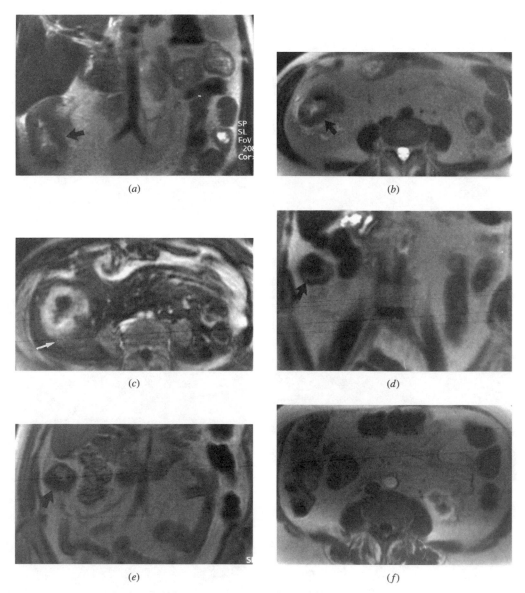

FIGURE 8.54   **Colon adenocarcinoma, ascending colon.** Coronal (*a*) and transverse (*b*) SS-ETSE and 90 s postgadolinium fat-suppressed SGE (*c*) images. Irregularly thickened bowel wall with intermediate signal intensity representing cancer is noted in the ascending colon (arrow, *a, b*). The cancer enhances in a moderate and slightly heterogeneous fashion. Pericolonic fat infiltration is demonstrated in the ascending colon on postcontrast fat-suppressed SGE image as enhancing strands of tissue (arrow, *c*).

Coronal SS-ETSE (*d*), coronal precontrast SGE (*e*), and transverse immediate postcontrast SGE (*f*) images in a second patient also demonstrate an irregular thickening of the ascending colon wall (arrow, *d–f*). There is no evidence of pericolonic fat infiltration with sharp external margins to the tumor.

- Mimickers
  - Differentiation between posttherapy fibrosis and recurrent malignancy is challenging

- In general, radiation changes are more linear and affect structure (bowel/bladder) in a more uniform fashion, whereas recurrent cancer is more nodular and involves

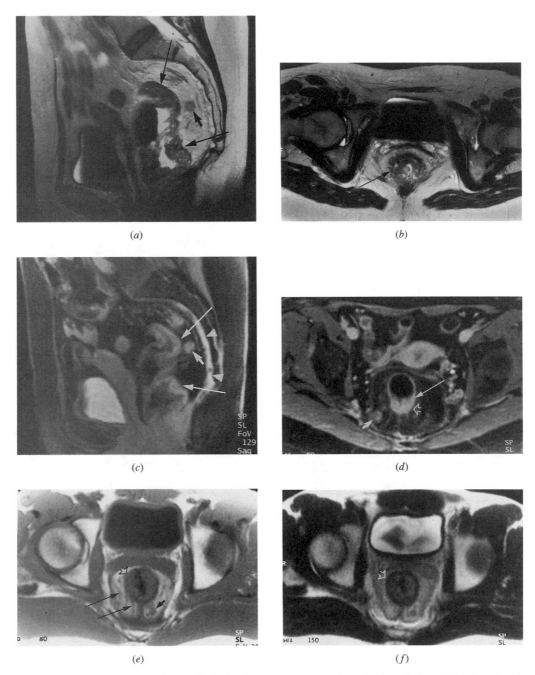

FIGURE 8.55   Rectal adenocarcinoma. Sagittal and transverse postgadolinium high-resolution T2W echo-train spin-echo (*a, b*) and sagittal and transverse postgadolinium fat-suppressed SGE (*c, d*) images in a patient with advanced colon cancer. A large rectal cancer is present (long arrows, *a, c*). The craniocaudal extent of tumor is well shown on sagittal images (*a, c*). The tumor extends inferiorly in the rectum (arrow, *b*) to the anal verge. Lymphovascular extension with involved lymph nodes (small arrows, *a, c, d*) is present. At the superior margin, the tumor is mainly posterior in location (hollow arrow, *d*). The transition from normal colon to tumor (long arrow, *d*) is clearly shown. Presacral spread of tumor is shown as enhancing tissue on the sagittal gadolinium-enhanced fat-suppressed image (arrowheads, *c*).

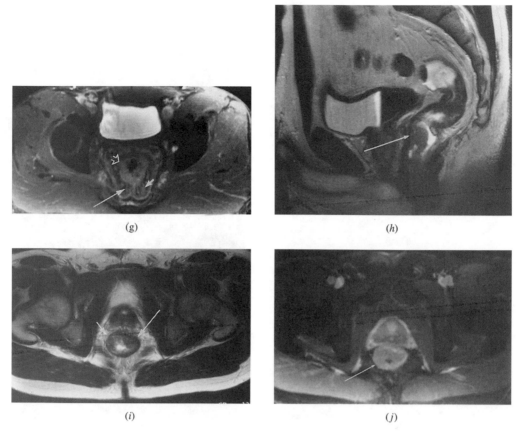

(g)

(h)

(i)

(j)

FIGURE 8.55 (*Continued*) SGE (*e*), SS-ETSE (*f*), and postgadolinium fat-suppressed SGE (*g*) images in a second patient with rectal adenocarcinoma and similar imaging findings. The rectal tumor (hollow arrows, *e, f, g*), lymphovascular extension (long arrows, *e, g*), and perirectal lymph nodes (short arrow, *e, g*) are well shown.

Sagittal and transverse postgadolinium 512-resolution T2W echo-train spin-echo (*h, i*) and interstitial phase gadolinium-enhanced fat-suppressed SGE (*j*) images in a third patient. Asymmetric tumor involvement of the rectal wall is apparent on the 512-resolution T2W images (long arrow, *h, i*). Tumor penetrates the full thickness of the right aspect of the rectum (short arrow, *i*). This is shown by interruption of the muscular wall that appears low signal intensity on the T2W image (long arrow, *i*). On the gadolinium-enhanced fat-suppressed SGE image, lower-signal-intensity tumor (arrow, *j*) penetrates the full thickness of the higher-signal-intensity wall. Postgadolinium T2W imaging is a novel technique for assessing possible bladder invasion. Enhancing tumor is conspicuous against the low signal intensity produced by concentrated gadolinium excreted into the bladder. In this case, the bladder is spared.

structures asymmetrically, although overlap exists
- PET imaging may not be more accurate
  than MR for this evaluation, as fibrosis
  can be active on PET-FDG imaging. In
  the future, MR spectroscopic evaluation
  may show additional value.

Squamous Cell Carcinoma
- Background
  ○ Squamous cell cancer occurs in the anal

canal, and its imaging characteristics re-
semble those of adenocarcinoma.
- Imaging
  ○ Evaluation of local and distant spread is
    well performed by gadolinium-enhanced
    fat-suppressed SGE images (fig. 8.58).

Lymphoma
- Background
  ○ Primary non-Hodgkin's lymphoma ac-
    counts for approximatelly 0.5% of all

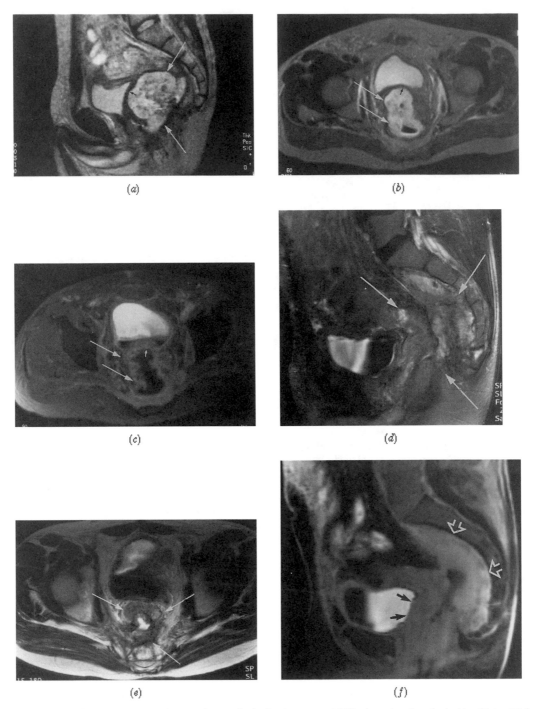

FIGURE 8.56   Recurrent rectal adenocarcinoma. Sagittal and transverse T2W echo-train spin-echo (a, b) and interstitial phase gadolinium-enhanced T1W fat-suppressed spin-echo (c) images. A large heterogeneous mass occupies the rectal fossa, a finding consistent with recurrence. Recurrent tumors are usually moderately high in signal intensity on T2W images (long arrows, a, b) and enhance moderately after intravenous contrast (long arrows, c). Central necrosis is well shown on the gadolinium-enhanced T1W fat-suppressed image. The tumor is contiguous with the bladder wall (short arrow, a–c), but the low signal intensity of the bladder wall on the T2W images shows that the bladder wall is not invaded.

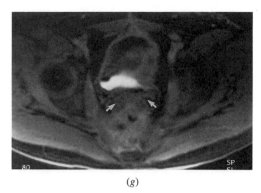

(*g*)

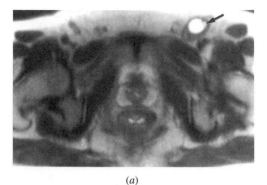

(*a*)

FIGURE 8.56 (*Continued*) Sagittal and transverse post-gadolinium 512-resolution T2W echo-train spin-echo (*d*, *e*) and sagittal and transverse interstitial phase gadolinium-enhanced fat-suppressed SGE (*f*, *g*) images in a second patient with recurrent rectal tumor. The 512-resolution T2W images show a large heterogeneous tumor in the rectal bed (arrows, *d*, *e*). Low-signal-intensity urine reflects concentrated gadolinium dependently. The gadolinium-enhanced fat-suppressed SGE images (*f*, *g*) demonstrate extensive recurrent disease involving the rectal fossa, rectovesical space (arrows *f*, *g*), presacral space (open arrows, *f*), and sciatic foramina.

colorectal malignancies and may be seen in patients with HIV infection or chronic ulcerative colitis
° The cecum is the most common site of

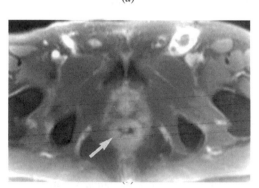

FIGURE 8.58   Squamous cell carcinoma of anal canal. T2W SS-ETSE (*a*) and interstitial phase gadolinium-enhanced SGE (*b*) images. There is a diffuse wall thickening of the anal canal associated with stranding in the perianal fat, which is consistent with cancer (arrow, *b*). Note the necrotic left inguinal lymph node, which contains central high signal on T2 (arrow, *a*) and is centrally low signal with intense peripheral enhancement on postgadolinium fat-suppressed T1W image.

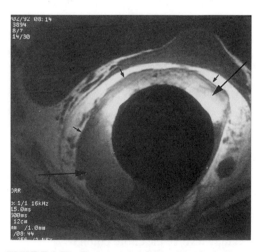

FIGURE 8.57   Endorectal coil imaging of rectal cancer. Gadolinium-enhanced T1W image demonstrates a T2 rectal cancer (long arrows). Preservation of low-signal-intensity muscular wall (short arrows) along the outer margin of the tumor confirms lack of full-thickness involvement. (Courtesy of Rahel A. Kubik Huch.)

involvement followed by the rectosigmoid colon
° Secondary involvement of the colon occurs in the setting of widespread disease
• Imaging
° Diffuse nodularity with wall thickening, and mildly heterogeneous enhancement may be seen after intravenous gadolinium administration (fig. 8.59)
° Coexistent lymphadenopathy and splenic lesions may aid in the diagnosis and is best demonstrated on postgadolinium T1W 2D/3D GRE imaging
° Most frequent presentation includes single or multiple masses

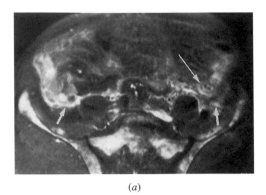

(a)

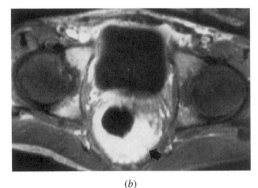

(b)

FIGURE 8.59   Colonic lymphoma. Gadolinium-enhanced T1W fat-suppressed spin-echo images (*a*, *b*) in two patients with lymphoma. In the first patient, with Burkitt's lymphoma (*a*), there is enhancing soft tissue in both paracolic gutters (arrows, *a*), thickening of the descending colon (long arrow, *a*), and ill-defined stranding in the mesentery. Note the diffuse enhancing bone marrow involvement. The second patient (*b*) has HIV infection and a primary rectal lymphoma (arrow, *b*). HIV patients are at risk for developing primary large-bowel lymphoma. (Reprinted with permission from Shoenut JP, Semelka RC, Silverman R, Yaffe CS, Mickflikier AB: The gastrointestinal tract. In Semelka RC, Shoenut JP [eds.], *MRI of the Abdomen with CT Correlation.* New York: Raven Press, pp. 119–143, 1993.)

Carcinoid Tumors
* Background
  * The rectum is a common location for carcinoid tumor (fig. 8.60), and 55% are primary
* Imaging
  * Gadolinium-enhanced T1W GRE imaging is important and is also required for assessment of liver metastases (fig. 8.60)

Melanoma
* Background
  * Primary melanoma is rare and carries a poor prognosis
* Imaging
  * Owing to the paramagnetic effects of melanin, the lesion can have characteristic high signal intensity on T1W images (fig. 8.61)
  * Tumors may demonstrate ring enhancement after gadolinium administration

Metastases
* Background
  * Ovaries, stomach, and pancreas represent the most common primary malignancies, which result in serosal metastases
  * Peritoneal disease spread represents the most common cause of large-bowel metastases

* Lung and breast carcinoma are potential sites of origin for hematogenous metastases
  * In the setting of previously treated colon carcinoma, a new large-bowel mass most likely represents a metachronous primary mass or peritoneal seeding
  * The rectum can be involved by direct extension of tumor from adjacent structures, such as prostate, cervical, or bladder carcinoma
* Imaging
  * Colorectal involvement is well shown on gadolinium-enhanced fat-suppressed T1W images as heterogeneously enhancing tissue (fig. 8.62)

Inflammation and Infection
Ulcerative Colitis (UC)
* Background
  * UC is an inflammatory disease limited to the large bowel
  * The disease originates in the rectum, extends proximally and contiguously, and may involve the entire colon
  * Skip lesions do not occur, representing one discriminating feature between UC and Crohn's disease
  * The incidence of ulcerative colitis is greatest in the second, third, and fourth decades

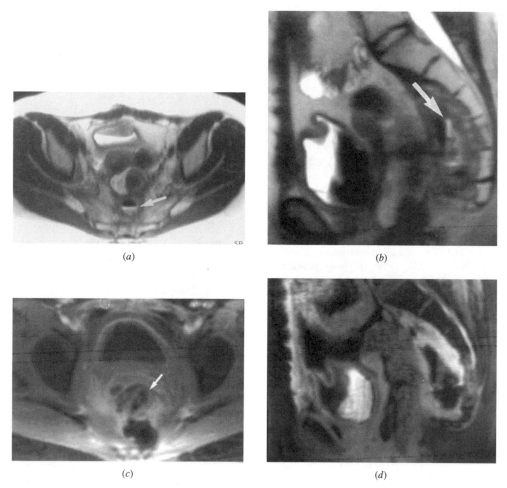

FIGURE 8.60 Rectal carcinoid recurrence associated with abscess. Transverse (*a*) and sagittal (*b*) postgadolinium T2W SS-ETSE and transverse (*c*) and sagittal (*d*) interstitial phase gadolinium-enhanced T1W SGE fat-suppressed images. There is thickening and enhancement of the rectal wall (arrow, *c*) associated with soft-tissue stranding within the pelvis. An air-fluid level is present in the presacral space (arrow, *a, b*), which is consistent with a small abscess.

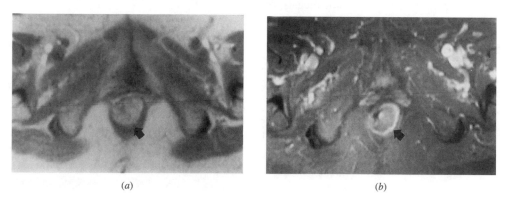

FIGURE 8.61 Anorectal malignant melanoma. SGE (*a*) and gadolinium-enhanced T1W fat-suppressed spin-echo (*b*) images in a patient with melanoma. Melanoma may be bright on T1W sequences (arrow, *a*) because of the paramagnetic properties of melanin. Rim enhancement is apparent after contrast and allows accurate determination of mural extent (arrow, *b*). (Reprinted with permission from Shoenut JP, Semelka RC, Silverman R, Yaffe CS, Mickflikier AB: The gastrointestinal tract. In Semelka RC, Shoenut JP [eds.], *MRI of the Abdomen with CT Correlation*. New York: Raven Press, pp. 119–143, 1993.)

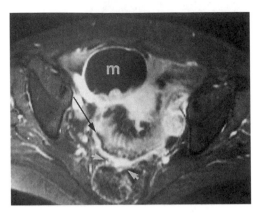

FIGURE 8.62 Ovarian carcinoma metastatic to colon. Gadolinium-enhanced T1W fat-suppressed spin-echo image in a patient with metastatic ovarian carcinoma. A complex cystic mass (m) encases the sigmoid colon (long arrow) and invades the rectum (short arrows). Tumor extension is clearly defined as enhancing tissue in a background of suppressed fat. (Reprinted with permission from Shoenut JP, Semelka RC, Silverman R, Yaffe CS, Mickflikier AB: The gastrointestinal tract. In Semelka RC, Shoenut JP [eds.], *MRI of the Abdomen with CT Correlation*. New York: Raven Press, pp. 119–143, 1993.)

of life, with a Caucasian, Jewish, and female predominance
- Family history is reported in up to 25% of cases
○ Etiology appears multifactorial, but likely represents an autoimmune disease
○ Symptoms include intermittent diarrhea and rectal bleeding
○ Severe cases may develop toxic megacolon

○ Chronic UC is associated with an increased risk of colon cancer, usually approximately 10 years following initial presentation
○ Histologically, disease is restricted to the mucosa, with edematous inflammatory tags of residual mucosa surrounded by sloughed mucosa, resulting in pseudopolyps
○ In longstanding disease, longitudinal shortening with loss of haustral folds may occur most prominently in the descending colon and sigmoid, and leads to an ahaustral straightened "lead pipe" appearance
• Imaging
○ Imaging with combined T2W and fat-suppressed gadolinium-enhanced 2D/3D T1W sequences
○ Diagnostic features include (fig. 8.63)
- Rectal involvement with contiguous retrograde disease
- Serosal/pericolic regions are not involved
- Submucosal sparing, which appears as a dark stripe sandwiched between intensely enhancing inflamed mucosa and the enhancing serosal layer. Crohn's disease, in contrast, shows transmural enhancement.
- Vasa rectae may be prominent, but there is no evidence of mesenteric fibrosis or transmural inflammation, peribowel lymph nodes, fistulas, and abscesses, as seen with Crohn's disease
- Colon may appear foreshortened, tubular, and rigid, creating "lead pipe" appearance

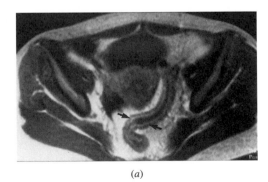

(a)

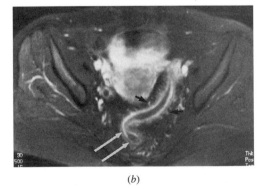

(b)

FIGURE 8.63 Ulcerative colitis. Immediate postgadolinium SGE (*a*) and gadolinium-enhanced T1W fat-suppressed spin-echo (*b*) images in a patient with ulcerative colitis. Increased enhancement on the immediate postgadolinium image (*a*) reflects increased capillary blood flow observed in severe disease. On the interstitial phase image (*b*), there is marked mucosal enhancement with prominent vasa rectae (short arrows, *b*) and submucosal sparing (long arrows, *b*).

most easily appreciated in sigmoid colon. Crohn's disease, in contrast, tends to show preserved colonic redundancy despite inflammatory changes.

○ Toxic megacolon diagnostic criteria require both clinical and imaging features

■ Clinical presentation must include severe illness with abdominal pain, debilitating bloody diarrhea, fever, and leukocytosis

■ MR findings include pancolitis seen as abnormal bowel-wall enhancement involving the entire colon, marked dilation, and thin wall (fig. 8.64). Colon may be thick walled if toxic colon has occurred in the setting of chronic disease. Also, the severity of the disease may mask submucosal sparing by the extensive capillary leakage.

• Mimickers
  ○ Rectal UC and rectal Crohn's may be indistinguishable
    ■ Crohn's often shows disease elsewhere, especially the small bowel, and attention should be paid to the terminal ileum to support a diagnosis of Crohn's disease
    ■ Perianal fistulae in Crohn's disease and not UC
  ○ Infectitious colitis, antibiotic-related colitis

Crohn's Colitis
• Background
  ○ See section on small-bowel Crohn's disease
  ○ Isolated colon involvement is noted in approximately 25% of patients
  ○ MRI is an effective imaging modality for evaluating colonic fistulae, a potential complication typical of Crohn's disease

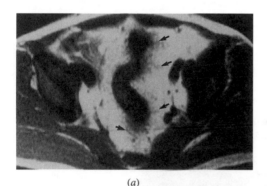

(a)

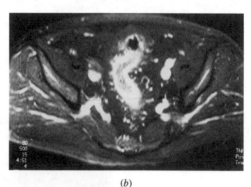

(b)

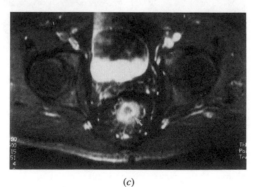

(c)

FIGURE 8.64   Ulcerative colitis, toxic colon. SGE (*a*) and gadolinium-enhanced T1W fat-suppressed spin-echo (*b*, *c*) images. The precontrast image shows irregular low-signal-intensity strands (arrows, *a*) related to a thick-walled sigmoid colon. After contrast there is marked mural enhancement. Enhancement of the pericolonic strands reflects prominent vasa rectae. Submucosal sparing is apparent (arrow, *c*), which is a feature of ulcerative colitis. Note the very intense enhancement of the colon wall, which appears to involve full thickness in the sigmoid colon. This is consistent with patient's presentation of toxic colon.

○ Perirectal fistulae may be a particularly debilitating cause of symptoms, and therapy directed to fistulae is a critical aspect of patient management

○ The relationship of fistulae to the levator ani muscle may require a combination of transverse, coronal, and sagittal plane images

• Imaging
  ○ Diagnostic criteria include
    ▪ Persistence of colonic redundancy and haustrations in pancolonic disease

▪ Transmural enhancement, which at times may show the most intense enhancement in the submucosal layer—a layer that is spared in ulcerative colitis (figs. 8.65 and 8.66)

▪ Crohn's disease frequently develops perianal and perirectal fistulae that may communicate with the perineum

  • This can be well visualized by multiplanar T2W and T1W imaging (fig. 8.67), and high-resolution (e.g., 512 matrix) T2W imaging combined with

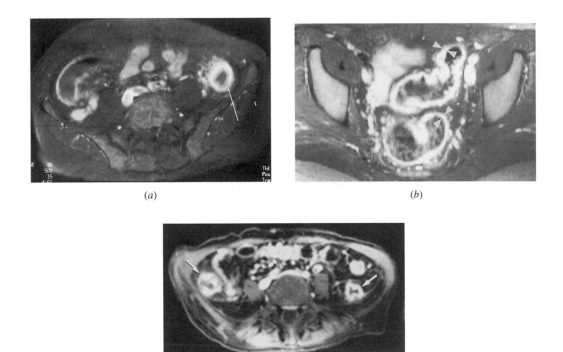

(a)   (b)

(c)

FIGURE 8.65   Crohn's colitis. Gadolinium-enhanced T1W fat-suppressed spin-echo image (*a*) demonstrates transmural enhancement with greater enhancement of the submucosa (arrow, *a*) than the other bowel wall layers, which is diagnostic of Crohn's disease and excludes the diagnosis of ulcerative colitis.

In a second patient with Crohn's colitis, gadolinium-enhanced T1W fat-suppressed spin-echo image (*b*) shows full-thickness enhancement of the sigmoid colon (arrowheads, *b*). The distribution of colon involvement is compatible with ulcerative colitis. However, the colon has remained redundant with persistence of haustrations despite severe disease. These findings combined with transmural enhancement are consistent with Crohn's colitis. Note the enhancing pericolonic inflammation in both patients. (Reprinted with permission from Shoenut JP, Semelka RC, Magro CM, Silverman R, Yaffe CS, Mickflikier AB: Comparison of magnetic resonance imaging and endoscopy in distinguishing the type and severity of inflammatory bowel diseases. *J Clin Gastroenterol* 19:31–35, 1994.)

Interstitial phase gadolinium-enhanced T1W SGE (*c*) image in a third patient with Crohn's colitis shows thickening and enhancement of the ascending and descending colon (arrows, *c*).

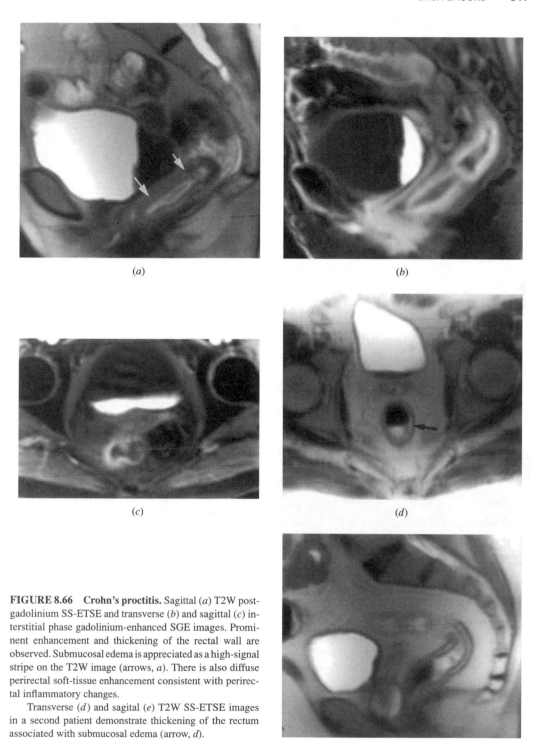

FIGURE 8.66 **Crohn's proctitis.** Sagittal (*a*) T2W post-gadolinium SS-ETSE and transverse (*b*) and sagittal (*c*) interstitial phase gadolinium-enhanced SGE images. Prominent enhancement and thickening of the rectal wall are observed. Submucosal edema is appreciated as a high-signal stripe on the T2W image (arrows, *a*). There is also diffuse perirectal soft-tissue enhancement consistent with perirectal inflammatory changes.

Transverse (*d*) and sagital (*e*) T2W SS-ETSE images in a second patient demonstrate thickening of the rectum associated with submucosal edema (arrow, *d*).

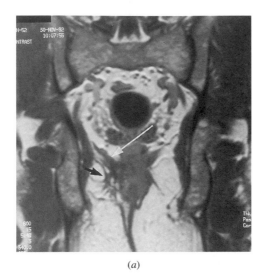

(a)

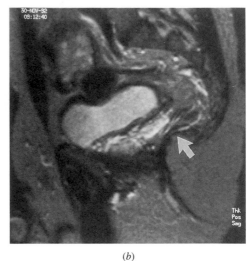

(b)

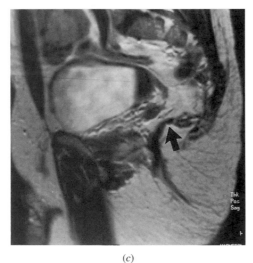

(c)

FIGURE 8.67   Perianal fistula. Coronal T1W spin-echo (*a*), sagittal T2W spin-echo (*b*), and gadolinium-enhanced T1W spin-echo (*c*) images. A complex fistula (arrow, *a*) is present in a right perianal location that extends to the levator ani muscle (long arrow, *a*). The fistula is low in signal on T1W (arrow, *a*), T2W (arrow, *b*), and postgadolinium (arrow, *c*) images, reflecting its chronic fibrotic nature.

fat-suppressed T1W 3D GRE gadolinium-enhanced interstitial phase imaging may provide highly detailed anatomic information
- ○ Mimickers
  - ▪ UC may resemble Crohn's disease in patients receiving rectal anti-inflammatory enemas
    - • The rectum and distal large bowel may appear relatively uninvolved, mimicking a noncontiguous pattern of disease typical of Crohn's disease
    - • Clinical history and correlation with findings is required

Diverticulitis
- • Background
  - ○ Diverticula occur throughout the colon and tend to be most numerous in the sigmoid colon (fig. 8.68)
  - ○ Inflamed diverticula favor the left colon
  - ○ Hemorrhagic diverticula tend to occur in the right colon
- • Imaging
  - ○ MR imaging is sensitive for, detection of diverticulosis (fig. 8.68), diverticulitis (fig. 8.69), and diverticulitis complicated by abscess formation (fig. 8.70)

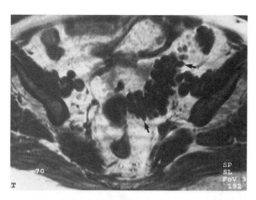

FIGURE 8.68   Diverticulosis. SGE image demonstrates multiple signal-void sacculations arising from the sigmoid colon consistent with diverticulosis. Diverticula are common and often incidental findings. Complications of diverticula include diverticulitis and frank abscess. (Reprinted with permission from Ascher SM, Semelka RC: MRI of the gastrointestinal tract. In: Higgins CB, Hricak H, Helms CA [eds.], *Magnetic Resonance Imaging of the Body*, Raven Press, pp. 677–700, 1997.)

  ○ Diverticulitis is shown by the presense of intense mural enhancement, prominent extramural enhancing tissue, and abscess formation

Appendicitis
• Background
  ○ Although CT imaging and ultrasound have replaced barium enema in the workup of

appendicitis, MRI has several features that make it an attractive alternative
  ▪ High-contrast resolution for inflammatory processes is useful in cases that are equivocal on CT or difficult to visualize on CT due to paucity of retroperitoneal and mesenteric fat
    • This may be of particular value in pediatric-age patients
  ▪ Patients are often young, and MR avoids ionizing radiation associated with CT
  ▪ Technique of choice in pregnant patients
○ Imaging
  ▪ On fat-suppressed T1W gadolinium-enhanced images, the inflamed appendix and surrounding tissues show marked enhancement (fig. 8.71) in combination with elevated signal on fat-suppressed T2W imaging
  ▪ Inflammatory stranding in the surrounding fat is well visualized on unenhanced T1W SGE images obtained without fat suppression
  ▪ If complicated by abscess, the abscess wall will show enhancement with intravenous contrast administration, whereas the cavity remains signal void (fig. 8.72)

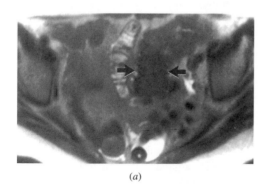
(a)

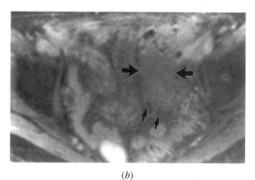
(b)

FIGURE 8.69   Diverticulitis. T2W SS-ETSE (*a*) and 90 s postgadolinium fat-suppressed SGE (*b*) images. Marked concentric wall thickening of an 8 cm segment of sigmoid colon is noted on the T2W SS-ETSE image (arrows, *a*). The thickness of the colon wall measures up to 1 cm. Moderate contrast enhancement and marked wall thickening in the sigmoid colon (large arrows, *b*) are shown with small diverticula (small arrow, *b*) on the postcontrast fat-suppressed SGE image. (Reprinted with permission from Chung JJ, Semelka RC, Martin DR, Marcos HB : Colon diseases: MR evaluation using combined T2W single-shot echo train spin-echo and gadolinium-enhanced spoiled gradient-echo sequences. *J Magn Reson Imaging* 12:297–305, 2000.)

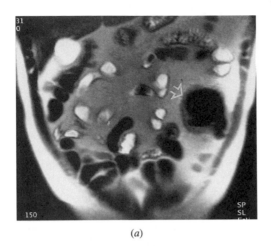

(*a*)

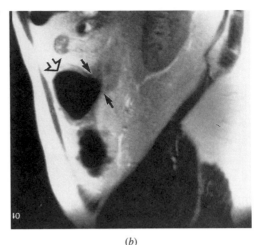

(*b*)

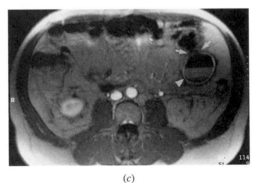

(*c*)

FIGURE 8.70   Diverticular abscess. Coronal (*a*) and sagittal (*b*) SS-ETSE, and immediate postgadolinium SGE (*c*) images. An air- and fluid-containing collection (open arrow, *a*, *b*) originates from the descending colon (solid arrows, *b*, *c*), a finding consistent with a diverticular abscess. On the immediate postgadolinium-image the inner wall of the abscess (arrowhead, *c*) enhances. An air-fluid level is apparent on the transverse image (*c*).

Infectious Colitis
- Background
  - Pseudomembranous colitis is caused by *Clostridium difficile* and is defined as an acute colitis characterized pathologically by the formation of an adherent inflammatory "membrane" (pseudomembrane) overlying areas of mucosal damage
  - This disease occurs as a sequela of broad-spectrum antibiotic use
  - The severity of the disease varies from mild to life-threatening
  - Typhlitis is an inflammatory disorder of the cecum seen in immunocompromised patients, including patients with AIDS, and neutropenic patients
  - Other infectious agents that target the colon include Shigella, Salmonella, *Escherichia coli*, amebiasis, and cholera

  - Patients with AIDS are prone to cytomegalovirus colitis and *Mycobacterium avium*-intracellulare, and frequently develop proctitis
  - Opportunistic infection leads to rectal-wall thickening and stranding in the perirectal space, and perirectal abscesses may develop
- Imaging
  - In most cases of clinically significant infectious inflammation of the colon, gadolinium-enhanced T1W fat-suppressed GRE images demonstrate bowel-wall thickening with increased enhancement and can show abscess formation (figs. 8.73 and 8.74)
  - Unenhanced T1W GRE imaging is effective for showing perirectal stranding, which appears low in signal intensity in a background of high-signal-intensity fat

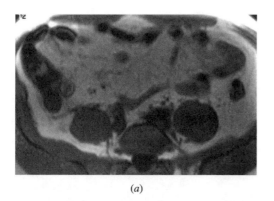

(*a*)

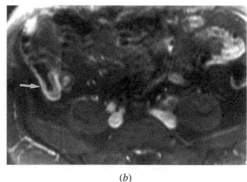

(*b*)

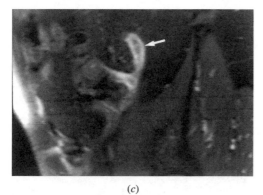

(*c*)

FIGURE 8.71 Acute appendicitis. SGE (*a*), transverse (*b*), and sagittal (*c*) interstitial phase gadolinium-enhanced fat-suppressed SGE images demonstrate a small-caliber tubular structure in the lower right quadrant with intense mural enhancement. The findings are consistent with acute appendicitis. The direct multiplanar imaging permits display of a long segment of the inflamed retrocecal abscess on the sagittal projection (*c*).

Radiation Enteritis

- Background
  - ∘ The gastrointestinal tract is one of the most radiosensitive tissues due to high cell mitotic activity resulting from high rate of mucosal cell turnover

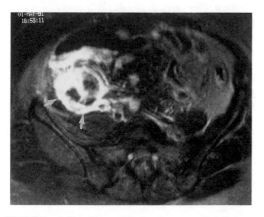

FIGURE 8.72 Appendiceal abscess. Gadolinium-enhanced T1W fat-suppressed spin-echo image demonstrates a low-signal-intensity appendiceal abscess with a prominent enhancing rim (arrow).

- ∘ Radiation injury also manifests induction of vasculitis that can cause ischemia, which may develop into chronic permanent vascular insufficiency
- ∘ Pathologically the bowel wall develops submucosal edema, ulceration, and inflammatory polyps
- ∘ Chronic radiation injury may show the histological features of mucosal, submucosal, and smooth-muscle atrophy and fibrosis, resulting in stricture formation
- ∘ The rectum is the most susceptible segment of large bowel to develop radiation enteritis for reasons that include
  - ▪ The pelvis is the most commonly radiated portal in the abdomen and pelvis, for treatment of prostate, gynecological, and rectosigmoid malignancies
  - ▪ The rectum is fixed in position
- Imaging
  - ∘ High-resolution T2W images demonstrate the findings of submucosal edema in acute radiation enteritis (figs. 8.75 and 8.76)

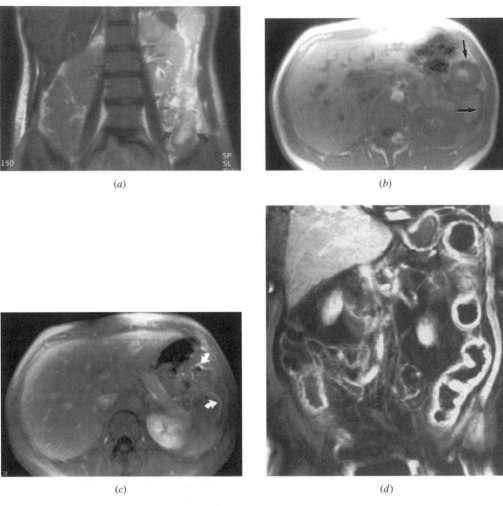

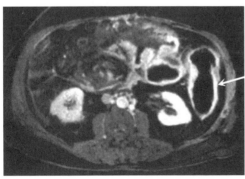

FIGURE 8.73 Pseudomembranous colitis. T2W SS-ETSE (*a*) and precontrast SGE (*b*) and 90 s postgadolinium fat-suppressed SGE (*c*) images. Diffuse bowel wall thickening is noted in the descending colon on the coronal T2W image (arrows, *a*). Circumferential bowel wall thickening is seen in the splenic flexure of the large bowel on precontrast SGE image (arrows, *b*). Moderately increased enhancement and wall thickening of the splenic flexure is noted on the postcontrast fat-suppressed SGE image (arrows, *c*). (Reprinted with permission from Chung JJ, Semelka RC, Martin DR, Marcos HB: Colon diseases: MR evaluation using combined T2W single-shot echo train spin-echo and gadolinium-enhanced spoiled gradient-echo sequences. *J Magn Reson Imaging* 12:297–305, 2000.)

Coronal (*d*) and transverse (*e*) interstitial phase gadolinium-enhanced fat-suppressed SGE images in a second patient demonstrate diffuse thickening of the descending colon (arrow, *e*) with intense mural enhancement. (Courtesy of Russel Low, MD, Sharp Clinic, San Diego, CA.)

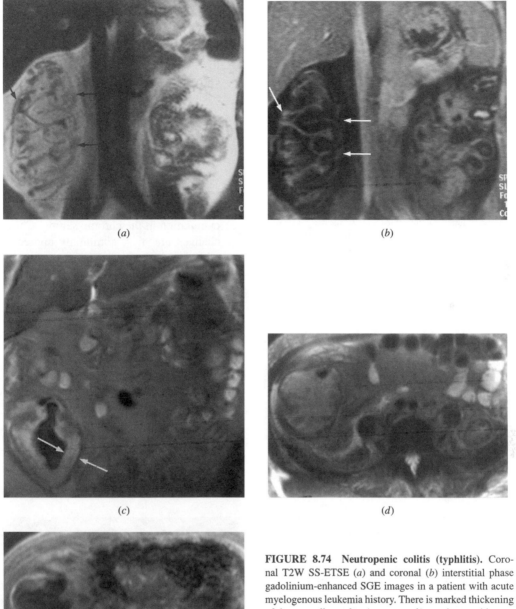

(a)

(b)

(c)

(d)

(e)

FIGURE 8.74 Neutropenic colitis (typhlitis). Coronal T2W SS-ETSE (a) and coronal (b) interstitial phase gadolinium-enhanced SGE images in a patient with acute myelogenous leukemia history. There is marked thickening of the ascending colon (arrows, a, b) consistent with neutropenic colitis. Small-bowel thickening and ascites are also present. Coronal (c) and transverse (d) T2W SS-ETSS and transverse interstitial phase gadolinium-enhanced SGE (e) images in a second patient after chemotherapy. The cecum shows dilatation with marked thickening and enhancement of the wall (arrows, c).

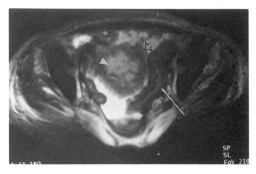

FIGURE 8.75 Radiation enteritis. Transverse 512-resolution T2W echo-train spin-echo image in a patient after radiation therapy. The sigmoid colon is thick walled with marked submucosal edema (arrow). The circumferential and symmetric nature of the bowel wall changes are suggestive of radiation enteritis. Note the thick-walled bladder (open arrow) and its heterogeneous contents (arrowhead), findings consistent with hemorrhagic cystitis, another sequela of radiation therapy. Free pelvic fluid is also present.

○ Fat-suppressed gadolinium-enhanced T1W imaging will show progressive abnormal wall enhancement that can be associated with leaky capillaries in the presence of active inflammation, and due to fibrosis in the chronic irreversible phase of injury
  ▪ There is a wide range of findings in the degree of T2W and T1W signal changes among patients, and these findings are not specific for radiation. Clinical correlation is necessary.
○ Bone marrow changes are appreciated on sagittal images of the pelvis, representing edema in the acute setting and fatty accumulation in the chronic setting. Chronic changes are most commonly appreciated with sharply demarcated abnormal marrow signal within the radiation portal.

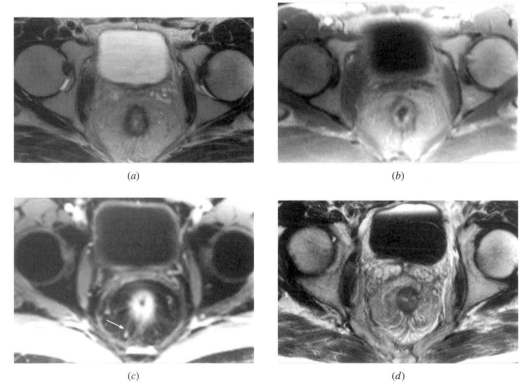

(a)

(b)

(c)

(d)

FIGURE 8.76 Radiation proctitis. Transverse T2W ETSE (*a*), immediate postgadolinium SGE (*b*), and interstitial phase gadolinium-enhanced SGE (*c*) images. The rectal wall is thickened with multiple radiating soft tissue strands (arrow, *c*) in the perirectal fat. There is intense enhancement of the rectum consistent with radiation-induced inflammation. Abundant perirectal fat is also appreciated.

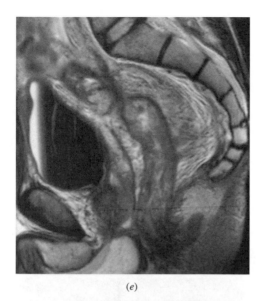

(e)

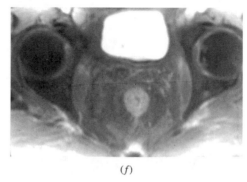

(f)

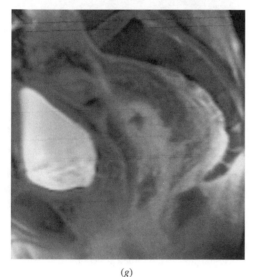

(g)

FIGURE 8.76 (*Continued*) These findings are consistent with postradiation changes. Transverse (*d*) and sagittal (*e*) T2W ETSE and transverse (*f*) and sagittal (*g*) interstitial phase gadolinium-enhanced SGE images in a second patient after radiation therapy show substantial thickening of the rectal wall with extensive linear strands in the enlarged perirectal fat.

- ▪ Well shown as high-signal marrow on T1W images, and marked drop in signal on fat-suppressed T1W images of the sacrum, relative to adjacent nonradiated marrow in the lumbar spine

Rectal Surgery
- • Background
  - ○ Most rectal surgery is performed for either tumor resection or surgical treatment of IBD

- ○ Abdominoperineal resection (APR) is performed for tumors that are distal in the rectum in which a tumor-free distal margin may not be achievable otherwise
- ○ Following APR, anteriorly located pelvic structures reposition more posteriorly, including the bladder, prostate, seminal vesicles, and uterus
- ○ The pelvis may be packed with omental fat at surgery, in order to prevent small bowel from filling the potential space, particularly

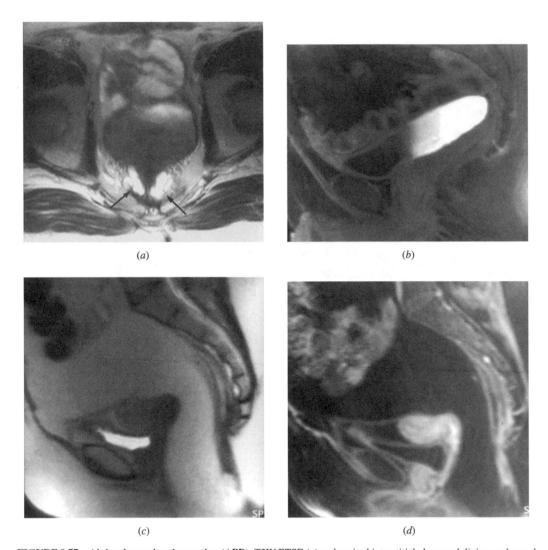

(a)   *(b)*

(c)   *(d)*

FIGURE 8.77   Abdominoperineal resection (APR). T2W ETSE (*a*) and sagittal interstitial phase gadolinium-enhanced fat-suppressed SGE (*b*) images. The bladder and the seminal vesicles (arrows, *a*) are shifted posteriorly in the pelvis.

Sagittal T2W SS-ETSE (*c*) and sagittal interstitial phase gadolinium-enhanced fat-suppressed SGE (*d*) images in a second patient show increase of pelvic fat consistent with omental packing.

when postoperative radiation therapy is planned
- Imaging
  - Rectal imaging can be achieved using the combination of T2W single-shot echo-train and fat-suppressed gadolinium-enhanced T1W interstitial phase imaging. This facilitates depiction of surgical changes (fig. 8.77) and allows assessment for complica-

tions including inflammation, leakage, or abscess formation.
  - If necessary, high-resolution (e.g., 512 matrix) imaging can be performed using T2W shorter echo-train spin-echo imaging plus or minus fat suppression
    - Water enema may also be given through a small Foley catheter, to provide intraluminal contrast that will be bright on T2W and dark on T1W images, as discussed at the beginning of this chapter

CHAPTER 9

RETROPERITONEUM

- MRI Technique
  - Combination of breath-hold and breathing-independent sequences acquired in at least two different planes, including
    - Fat-suppressed T2W
    - Precontrast T1W SGE or 3D GRE
    - Gadolinium-enhanced fat-suppressed T1W GRE
  - MR angiography (MRA) optimized 3D GRE imaging dynamically timed to capture the arterial phase is used for imaging the major retroperitoneal arteries
- MRA Technique
  - Techniques classified as bright blood or black blood
  - In the abdomen and pelvis the most commonly employed techniques use bright blood gadolinium-enhanced imaging with breath-hold 3D GRE
    - Phase contrast is another method for refocusing flowing blood signal and can be used for special applications such as to assess renal vessel or aortic flow (fig. 9.1)
  - Gadolinium is administered at 0.1–0.2 mmol/kg body weight at a rate of 2 ml/s followed by a saline flush of 20–30 cc

- Typically 0.2 mmol/kg (or 40 cc per patient at 1.5 T) or 0.1 mmol/kg (or 20 cc per patient at 3.0 T)
  - A dual-syringe power injector is critical to ensure reproducible results
  - Timing of interval between start of injection and start of sequence acquisition
    - All current systems provide a timing slab function
      - A thick slab is placed over the vessel of interest, for example, a coronal or sagittal slab over the upper abdominal aorta, and images are acquired and displayed in near real time at a rate of 0.5–1 frame per second
    - All current systems provide MRA 3D GRE sequences with reordered k-space filling such that the central k-space will be acquired first
      - Central k-space provides the contrast information for the images
    - Contrast is injected into an arm vein while timing slab images are simultaneously acquired
    - When contrast is visualized in the aorta, the patient is instructed to stop breathing and the 3D MRA GRE sequence is started

Primer on MR Imaging of the Abdomen and Pelvis, edited by Diego R. Martin, Michele A. Brown, and Richard C. Semelka ISBN 0-471-37340-0 Copyright © 2005 Wiley-Liss, Inc.

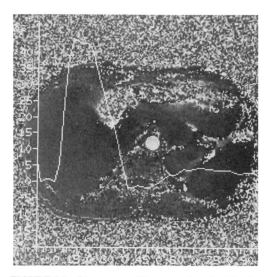

FIGURE 9.1 Phase map of the normal aorta. The abdominal aorta (encircled) appears high in signal intensity on this phase map in the systolic phase of antegrade blood flow. A blood velocity tracing obtained throughout the cardiac cycle is superimposed on the phase image, demonstrating the normal velocity profile of blood in the abdominal aorta. (Reproduced with permission from Semelka RC, Shoenut JP, Kroeker MA: The retroperitoneum and the abdominal wall. In: Semelka RC, Shoenut JP [eds.], *MRI of the Abdomen with CT Correlation.* New York: Raven Press, pp. 13–41, 1993.)

- Current MR systems also provide bolus chase function
  - Two- or three-station examinations with automated capacity to image one station, then move to and image adjacent stations, following the gadolinium bolus down the aorta and into the lower extremities (fig. 9.2)
- Potential pitfall of bolus chase is that the calf veins may be filled by the time the third station images are acquired
  - An alternative technique is to image the calf arteries first, using 30 cc an axial or coronal timing slab placed over the popliteal arteries, and imaging three consecutive MRA acquisitions to obtain arterial and venous phase images
    - The abdominal aorta and upper leg vessels can be imaged with a two-

station examination performed after the calf study using a second dose of gadolinium
- A subtraction mask image set is acquired prior to the second contrast administration to subtract residual gadolinium signal in the veins (venous contamination is generally not a problem in the larger vessels of the abdomen and pelvis, where anatomic delineation is relatively straightforward)
- Tourniquets applied to the upper thighs allow delayed filling of veins, which diminishes venous contamination
- Although the built-in whole-body coil is easier to use, multistation surface coils will significantly improve signal-to-noise (fig. 9.2)
- Although experience with 3 T scanners is still under development, it appears that increased signal from this system can facilitate use of the whole-body coil and decrease volume of contrast injected by up to 50% while preserving image quality
- Image processing
  - 3D MRA images can be processed using maximum intensity projection (MIP) rendering (e.g., fig. 9.3) to acquire any desired projection
  - Selected multiplanar reformation (MPR) of the origin of specific vessels is also of value (e.g., renal arteries)

Aorta

Aortic Aneurysm
- Background
  - Incidence of 21 per 100,000
  - Mostly infrarenal
  - Important diagnostic information for patient management includes
    - Maximum outer wall-to-outer wall diameter
    - Longitudinal length
    - Relationship to renal, common iliac, and femoral arteries

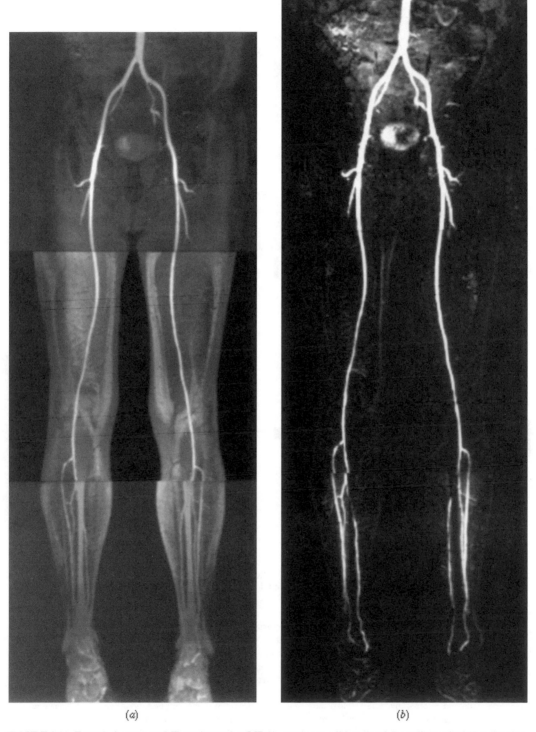

(a)   (b)

FIGURE 9.2   Extended-coverage MR angiography (MRA). Aortic run-off 3-station 3-D gradient-echo MRA showing normal (*a* and *b*), abnormal (*c*, right side), and conventional fluoroscopic digital subtraction angiogram (*c*, left side).

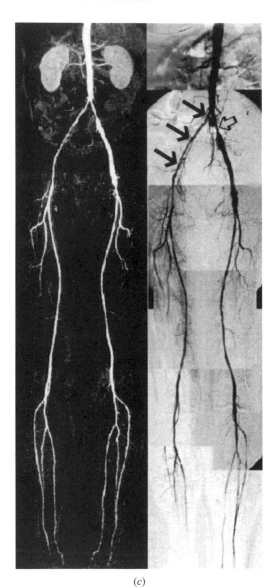

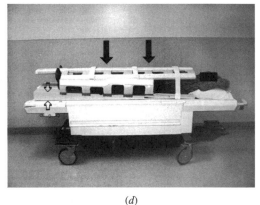

(c)   (d)

FIGURE 9.2   (*Continued*) A normal patient was sacnned using a peripheral vascular 3-station phased-array coil (*d*) having 2 cm overlaps between upper and middle (junction at the midsuperficial femoral artery), and again between middle and bifurcation into the peroneal and posterior tibital arteries). A bolus of 0 lower stations (junction at the distal end of the common peroneal trunk, just above 0.2 mmol/kg gadolinium) was administered intravenously at a rate of 2 cc/s after a 15 s timed injection, based on bolus timing (see text). Each acquisition required 32 s, using 4 mm slice thickness constructions. The data were processed by maximum intensity projection (MIP) software analysis and are shown with no background subtraction and with soft-tissue window and level (*a*), and after background subtraction using a high-contrast window and level (*b*) to eliminate soft tissues. Surgical planning often requires soft-tissue visualization for spatial reference (*a*), although vascular detail may be more easily appreciated after removal of the soft tissue (*b*). Image *c* compares an MRA run-off study performed as in *a* and *b*, but with atherosclerotic irregular narrowing demonstrated over a long segment of right common and external iliac artery, and a short segment of proximal to mid-left common iliac artery. Nearly identical results are demonstrated on a conventional fluoroscopic angiogram using iodinated contrast agent, performed on the same patient, and shown on the right (arrows, right common and external iliac artery, hollow arrow: proximal left common iliac artery).

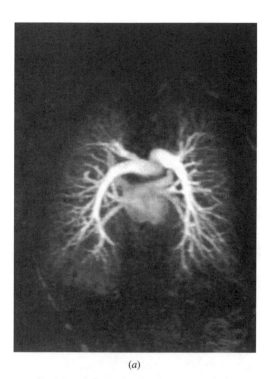

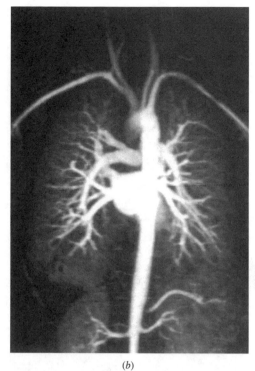

(a)   (b)

FIGURE 9.3 ⏐ **Normal pulmonary MRA.** Coronal 3D gradient-echo (a and b) images. The acquisition of image data over a short time period, after rapid injection of a small volume of gadolinium contrast, allows better temporal resolution, obtaining an image with contrast predominantly within the pulmonary arteries and just starting to fill pulmonary veins and left atrium. The image acquired immediately after the pulmonary angiogram (b) shows contrast within the pulmonary veins, left atrium, aorta, and major aortic arch vessels and starting to fill the renal arteries.

- Surgical repair feasible if infrarenal in location with 1–1.5 cm space between top of aneurysm and most inferior renal artery
  - Variant anatomy important for presurgical assessment
    - For example, anterior or circumaortic left renal vein
  ∘ Complications
    - Spontaneous rupture, with risk significantly increased when diameter is >6 cm
    - Atherosclerotic stenosis of the aorta or major branches
      - Renal arteries resulting in hypertension and renal insufficiency
      - SMA resulting in bowel ischemia, abdominal pain, and malabsorption
    - Aortitis

- Imaging
  ∘ Comprehensive examination includes a combination of T2W and T1W gadolinium-enhanced MRA as well as soft-tissue optimized imaging (fig. 9.4)
  ∘ T2W single-shot echo-train with and without fat suppression to visualize overall aortic anatomy and assess abnormal elevated signal around the aorta or end organs (e.g., bowel loops) that can be associated with inflammation in the setting of aortitis (or bowel ischemia)
    - Flow-void effect makes vascular lumen dark in the presence of normal flow
      - Mural thrombus will have mixed intermediate to high signal (and possibly elevated signal on precontrast T1W GRE)

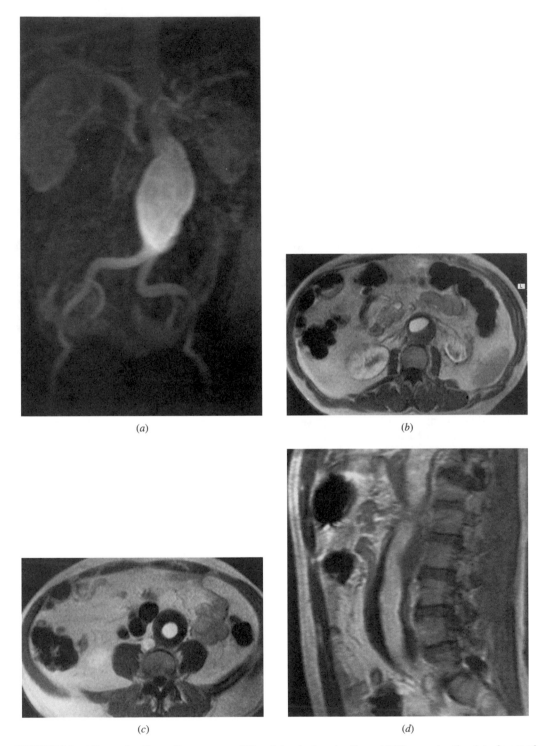

(a)   *(b)*

(c)   *(d)*

FIGURE 9.4   Atherosclerotic aortic aneurysm of the abdominal aorta. Coronal MIP reconstruction (*a*) of a set of gadolinium-enhanced 2 mm thin-section coronal 3D gradient-echo sections in a patient with an infrarenal aortic aneurysm. The MIP images demonstrate a large fusiform infrarenal aortic aneurysm. The aneurysm is shown not to extend into the common iliac arteries.

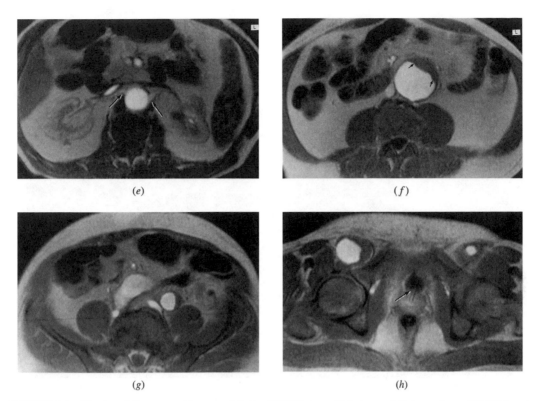

(e)

(f)

(g)

(h)

FIGURE 9.4 (*Continued*) Transverse 45 s postgadolinium SGE (*b*), interstitial phase gadolinium-enhanced SGE (*c*), and sagittal interstitial phase SGE (*d*) images in a second patient. An abdominal aortic aneurysm containing high-signal-intensity gadolinium in the lumen and low-signal-intensity wall thrombus is evident on the 45 s postgadolinium SGE image (*b*). The left kidney is small and demonstrates delayed enhancement of a uniform thin cortex, findings consistent with left renal artery stenosis. Note that the signal intensity of the cortex and medulla of the right kidney has equilibrated at this tubular phase of enhancement. Good delineation of the patent lumen and mural thrombus is provided by gadolinium enhancement on early postgadolinium SGE images (*b, c*), whereas imaging in the sagittal plane demonstrates the longitudinal extent of disease.

Immediate postgadolinium (*e*) and transverse (*f, g, h*) and sagittal (*i*) interstitial phase gadolinium-enhanced SGE images in a third patient. The abdominal aorta ia normal in diameter at the level of the origins (arrows, *e*) of the renal arteries. At lower tomographic levels (*f–h*), enlargement of the aortic lumen with sharp demarcation of the high-signal-intensity patent lumen and low-signal-intensity wall thrombus (small arrows, *f*) is noted. Involvement of the infrarenal aorta (*f*), common iliac arteries (*g*), and common femoral arteries (*h*) is demonstrated. A Foley catheter is also noted in place (arrow, *h*). The sagittal interstitial phase image provides direct visualization of the site of maximal anteroposterior diameter (arrow, *i*) with depiction of low-signal-intensity thrombus (small arrows, *i*) in the anterior aortic wall. The origin of the superior mesenteric artery (thin arrow, *i*) is also demonstrated.

- ○ T1W 3D MRA is performed in the coronal plane for optimal visualization of the renal arteries with MIP reconstruction into multiple views including sagittal
  - ■ If the patient has suspected bowel ischemia, the sagittal plane may be used for plane of image acquisition
  - ■ Acquisition time should be kept under 20 s to ensure that the time is shorter than the patient's ability to breath-hold, and image slab slice reconstruction should be no greater than 3–4 mm thickness
    - • If unavoidable, the MRA can be acquired with quiet breathing, as the aorta does not experience much respiratory movement, but renal artery visualization will be impaired

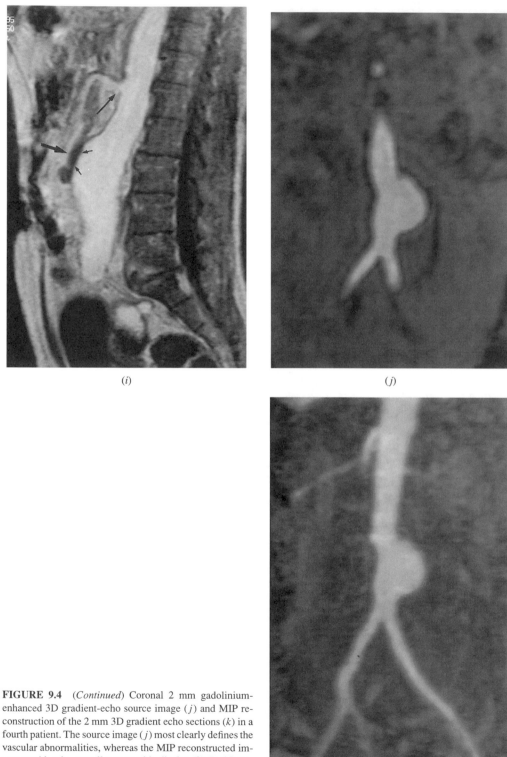

(i)

(j)

FIGURE 9.4 (*Continued*) Coronal 2 mm gadolinium-enhanced 3D gradient-echo source image (*j*) and MIP reconstruction of the 2 mm 3D gradient echo sections (*k*) in a fourth patient. The source image (*j*) most clearly defines the vascular abnormalities, whereas the MIP reconstructed image provides the overall topographic display (*k*). In this patient, a saccular infrarenal aortic aneurysm is clearly shown.

(k)

- 3D MRA should be followed with fat-suppressed 3D GRE representing an interstitial phase data acquisition for optimized visualization of soft tissues including the aorta and surrounding retroperitoneum
  - Also provides excellent venographic examination of the IVC, SMV, portal and splenic veins
  - Aortitis shows enhancement of strand-like tissue encasing the involved aorta and extending into the adjacent para-aortic retroperitoneal fat (fig. 9.5)

○ Additional T2W-like imaging can be obtained using True-FISP
  - This sequence can provide bright blood angiographic overview images due to high signal from fluid in blood, and high resistance to flow void or in-flow saturation effects
  - Acquired as a 2D sequence, this method is a slice-by-slice technique, and like T2W single-shot methods, it is very robust and motion insensitive
  - Can be used for an overview of anatomy and pathology, and for scout images to set up the MRA

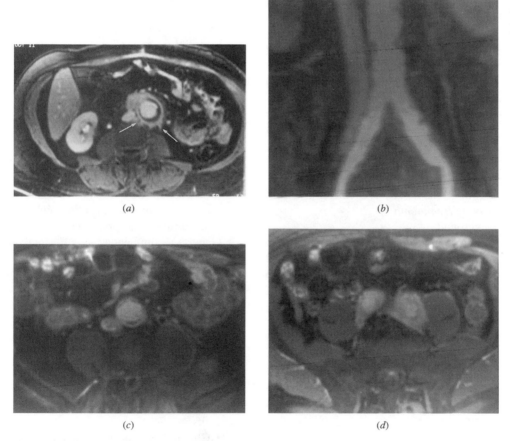

(a) (b)

(c) (d)

FIGURE 9.5 Inflammatory aortitis. Interstitial phase gadolinium-enhanced fat-suppressed SGE image (*a*). An aortic aneurysm is present with diffusely thickened wall and enhancing ill-defined tissue that projects (arrows) into the retroperitoneal fat surrounding the aneurysm. Enhancement of the lumen and nearly signal-void mural thrombus is also shown.

Coronal 3D MIP reconstruction (*b*) and transverse gadolinium-enhanced fat-suppressed SGE (*c, d*) images in a second patient demonstrate dilatation of the infrarenal aorta and common iliac arteries. Note the homogeneous enhancing tissue surrounding these vessels, consistent with perianeurysmal inflammation.

Aortic Dissection
- Background
  - Aortic dissection usually originates in the thoracic aorta
  - Underlying causes include atherosclerosis and hypertension
  - MRI with MRA is accurate and avoids nephrotoxic effects of iodinated contrast used for CT or X-ray angiography
  - Standard angiography may miss a dissection with complete thrombosis of the false or true lumen, as this technique demonstrates only lumen with flow
- Imaging (fig. 9.6)
  - Breath-hold gadolinium-enhanced 3D gradient-echo images provide sharp detail and demonstrate the full extent of dissection, the entry site, the location of the intimal flap, and the relation of the visceral vessels to the true and false lumen (fig. 9.7)
  - The abdominal aortic extension is evaluated better on transverse than on sagittal or coronal plane images. Transverse images may also be obtained using transverse MPR data reconstruction of the source MRA images.

Penetrating Aortic Ulcers and Intramural Dissecting Hematoma
- Background
  - Penetrating aortic ulcers result from ulcerated atherosclerotic plaques that penetrate the internal elastic lamina and may lead to hematoma formation within the media of the aortic wall, false aneurysm, and finally transmural rupture of the aorta
  - Most common locations
    - Descending thoracic and upper abdominal aorta
  - Conventional angiography is often unable to show the intramural dissection and thrombus
- Imaging
  - Intramural hematoma is high in signal intensity on both T1W and T2W images, and can be differentiated from chronic mural thrombus which is low in signal intensity

  - MRA and 3D GRE gadolinium-enhanced T1W soft-tissue imaging optimally shows the lumen, plaque ulceration and wall thickening, and nonenhancing mural thrombus (fig. 9.8)

Aortoiliac Atherosclerotic Disease—Thrombosis
- Background
  - Occlusion of the abdominal aorta and its branches may occur in advanced thrombotic disease or dissection
- Imaging
  - Gadolinium-enhanced MRA or fat-suppressed SGE images may demonstrate gross atherosclerotic changes of the aorta and iliac arteries (fig. 9.9)
  - Gadolinium-enhanced SGE images permit clear distinction between high-signal-intensity patent lumen and low-signal-intensity thrombosed lumen

Postoperative Aortic Graft Evaluation
- Background
  - Imaging is performed to assess for possible complication
    - Occlusion; hemorrhage with pseudoaneurysm; infection; fistulae such as aortoenteric fistula formation
  - General recommendation is for interval of 4 weeks between surgical placement of clips and MR examination to avoid the possibility of dislodgement of a vascular clip by the magnetic field
  - Stents are used increasingly more often to treat infrarenal aortic aneurysms, particularly in nonsurgical candidates
- Imaging
  - MRA may provide information regarding patency and different classifications of leaks
    - Clip and stent artifacts have been significantly reduced with current generation of low ferromagnetic surgical appliances, but magnetic susceptibility artifact still occurs

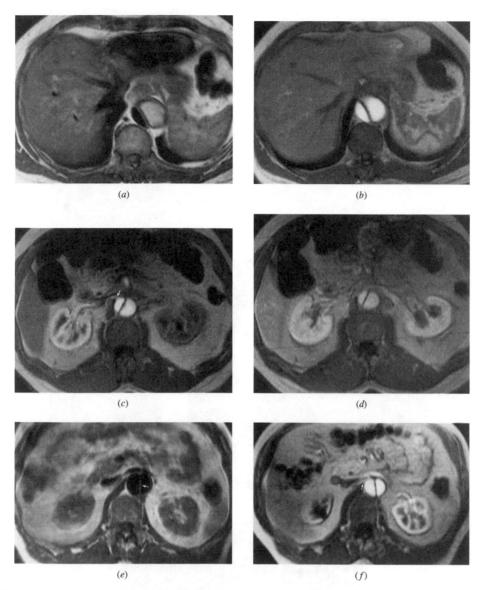

(a)   *(b)*

(c)   *(d)*

(e)   *(f)*

FIGURE 9.6 Aortic dissection with perfusion differential between the kidneys. T1W spin-echo (*a*) and immediate (*b*, *c*) and 90 s (*d*) postgadolinium SGE images. The T1W spin-echo image (*a*) shows enlargement of the abdominal aorta, which contains an intimal flap and has a true and a false lumen. High signal intensity is noted in the false lumen because of slow flow. Note that the true lumen has a biconvex configuration because of the higher blood pressure. The immediate postgadolinium SGE image (*b*) acquired at the same tomographic levels shows enhancement of both lumens with sharp demarcation of the intimal flap. The false lumen enhances substantially less than the true lumen on the immediate postgadolinium SGE image (*c*) at a lower tomographic level because of diminished contrast delivery secondary to slow flow in the false lumen. The right renal artery (arrow, *c*) is demonstrated originating from the true lumen. Intense cortical enhancement of the right kidney and minimal cortical enhancement of the left kidney is evident, reflecting the origin of the left renal artery from the false lumen. Note that on the 90 s postgadolinium SGE image (*d*), lumen and kidneys enhance to the same extent. T1W spin-echo (*e*) and immediate postgadolinium SGE (*f*) images in a second patient with aortic dissection. The T1W spin-echo image shows an aortic aneurysm with an intimal flap (arrow, *e*). Both lumen are signal void on this image, reflecting higher blood velocity in the false lumen than ovserved in the first patient. The right lumen has a biconvex configuration consistent with the true lumen. High flow in both lumen is also reflected as equal enhancement on the immediate postgadolinium SGE image. The origin of the right renal artery (arrow, *f*) from the true lumen is well shown. Immediate postgadolinium SGE images in patients with aortic dissection provide hemodynamic information that is helpful in determining true and false lumens and abdominal organ arterial perfusion.

337

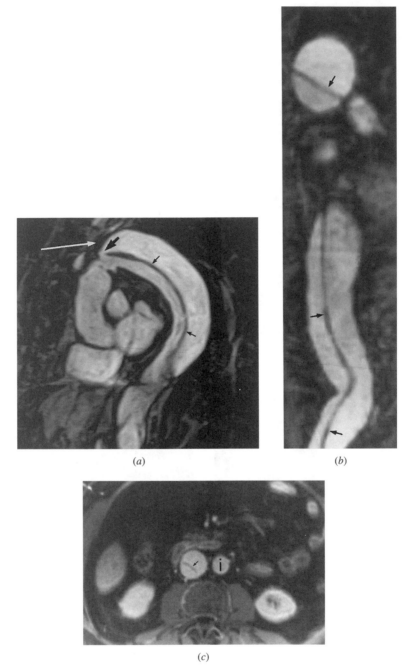

(a)

(b)

(c)

FIGURE 9.7   Aortic dissection. Gadolinium-enhanced 2 mm thin-section 3D gradient-echo image (a) obtained in an oblique sagittal plane through the center of the lumen of the aortic arch, coronal multiplanar reconstruction (b) from the set of gadolinium-enhanced 2 mm thin oblique sagittal 3D gradient-echo sections, and transverse interstitial phase gadolinium-enhanced fat-suppressed SGE images (c) in a patient with type B aortic dissection. The oblique sagittal gadolinium-enhanced 3D gradient-echo image (a) demonstrates an aortic dissection originating in the thoracic aorta. The intimal flap (small arrows, a–c) is readily demonstrated as a low-signal-intensity curvilinear structure. The entry site (arrow, a) is identified immediately distal to the origin of the left subclavian artery (long arrow, a). The multiplanar reconstruction (b) outlines the course of the dissection and demonstrates the intimal flap (small arrows, b) from the thoracic to the abdominal aorta.

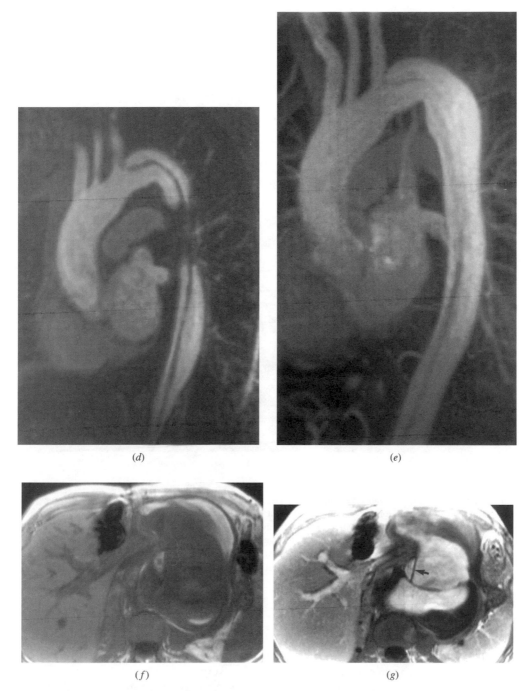

(d)

(e)

(f)

(g)

FIGURE 9.7 (*Continued*) The intimal flap is well seen on the interstitial phase gadolinium-enhanced fat-suppressed SGE image (*c*) at the level of the abdominal aorta. Incidental note is made of a left-sided IVC (i, *c*).

Coronal 2 mm gadolinium-enhanced 3D gradient-echo source image (*d*) and 3D MIP reconstruction of the 2 mm 3D gradient-echo sections (*e*) from a second patient show similar features of an aortic dissection.

Transverse SGE (*f*) and immediate postgadolinium SGE (*g*) images in a third patient. There is a large, complex abdominal aortic saccular aneurysm associated with thrombus and dissection. The intimal flap is clearly shown (arrow, *g*) after contrast administration.

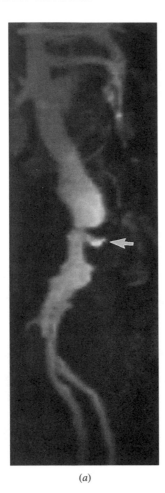

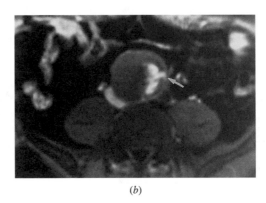

(a)   (b)

FIGURE 9.8   Penetrating aortic ulcer. Lateral MIP projection of a set of gadolinium-enhanced 2 mm coronal 3D gradient-echo sections (*a*) and transverse interstitial phase gadolinium-enhanced fat-suppressed SGE (*b*) images. An atherosclerotic aneurysm of the infrarenal abdominal aorta is present. An ulceration of the atherosclerotic plaque (arrow, *a*, *b*) is demonstrated on the lateral MIP projection. On the interstitial phase gadolinium-enhanced fat-suppressed SGE image (*b*), the diameter of the aortic aneurysm and the presence of mural thrombus are well evaluated. The depth of the ulceration in relation to the outer aortic wall is appreciated. Interstitial phase gadolinium-enhanced fat-suppressed SGE images provide information on the aortic wall and the surrounding tissues that are not available on MR angiographic images.

- Use of shortest TR and TE gradient-echo imaging and the fastest performance gradients reduce the severity of dephasing metal-related susceptibility artifacts
- Metal artifacts may preclude use of MRA, and they require imaging by contrast-enhanced CT provided renal function is not a contraindication
  ○ Infection
    - High signal on T2W images and evidence of stranding pattern of persistent or increasing enhancement on post-gadolinium T1W images around the graft repair should dramatically diminish or be absent beyond 3 months post-surgery
- Abscess formation is easily identified on fat-suppressed gadolinium-enhanced T1W GRE images within the retroperitoneum or peritoneum (see also section on peritoneum infection) (fig. 9.10)

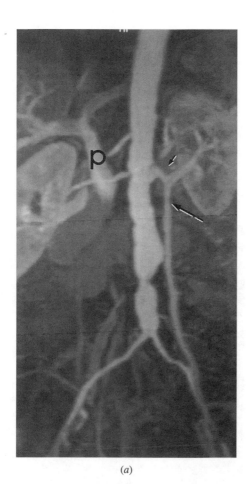

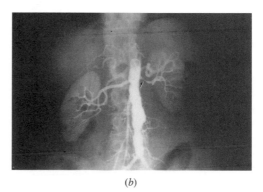

(a)   (b)

FIGURE 9.9   Atherosclerotic disease of the abdominal aorta. Coronal 3D MIP reconstruction of gadolinium-enhanced 2 mm source images (a) and anteroposterior conventional arteriography image (b). Diffuse atherosclerotic disease of the abdominal aorta with irregularity of the contour and focal stenotic and dilated segments is demonstrated on the 3D MIP image (a). Close correlation of the MRI findings with the intra-arterial catheter angiographic image (b) is present. The image acquisition timing in this case was slightly delayed, and the 3D gradient echo images were acquired during the capillary rather than the arterial phase of enhancement, as evidenced by the presence of enhanced portal vein (p, a) and right renal vein. Enhancement of the left renal vein partially masks a stenosis (small arrow, a, b) of the left renal artery. Targeted 3D MIP reconstructions of the left renal artery revealed this stenosis. Note early retrograde filling of the left ovarian vein (arrow, a).

Coronal 3D MIP reconstruction of gadolinium enhanced 2 mm source images (c) in a second patient shows irregular contour of the aorta (small arrows, c) due to diffuse atherosclerotic changes. Note normal renal arteries (long arrow, c) bilaterally. The common hepatic artery (short arrow, c) and splenic artery (hollow arrow, c) are also demonstrated.

Inferior Vena Cava

- Background
  - CT examination of the IVC above the renal arteries can often lead to the appearance of incomplete contrast opacification due to mixing of enhanced renal venous blood and unenhanced infrarenal venous blood

- Contrast-enhanced CT (CECT) imaging of the infrarenal veins is challenging due to the requirement of sufficient image acquisition delay to allow for contrast recirculation and the diminution of contrast density that results from excessive delay

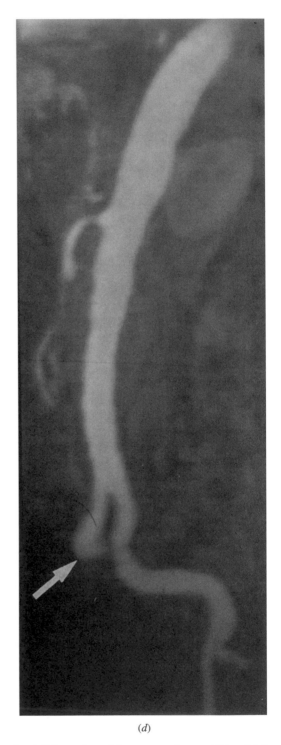

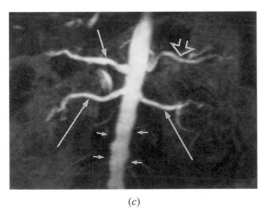

(c)   (d)

FIGURE 9.9   (*Continued*) Coronal 3D MIP reconstruction of gadolinium-enhanced 2 mm source images (*d*) in a third patient demonstrates slight irregularity of the abdominal aorta associated with stenoses of the celiac axis and superior mesenteric artery and occlusion of the right common iliac artery (arrow, *d*).

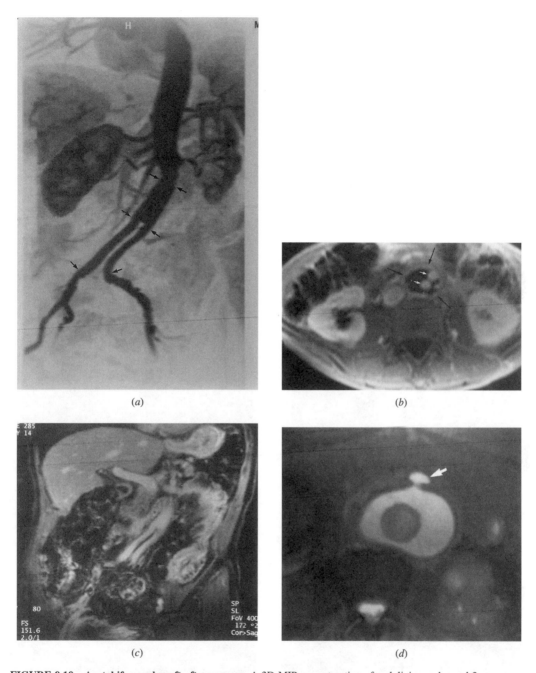

(a)

(b)

(c)

(d)

FIGURE 9.10   Aortobifemoral graft after surgery. A 3D MIP reconstruction of gadolinium-enhanced 2 mm source images (*a*) and transverse (*b*) and coronal (*c*) interstitial phase gadolinium-enhanced fat-suppressed SGE images in a patient with Marfan's syndrome 1 month after surgery. The MIP image (*a*) demonstrates an abdominal aortic aneurysm with a maximal diameter of 4.5 cm at the level of the upper pole of the left kidney. More distally within the abdominal aorta, an aortoiliac graft is identified (small arrows, *a*). Irregularity of the luminal contour is noted distal to the graft because of atherosclerotic disease. The transverse 1 min postgadolinium fat-suppressed SGE image shows the patent lumens of the limbs of the graft (small arrows, *b*) surrounded by low-signal-intensity postoperative fluid contained within the wall (arrow, *b*) of the native aorta. The patency of the graft is also shown on the coronal interstitial phase gadolinium-enhanced fat-suppressed SGE image (*c*).

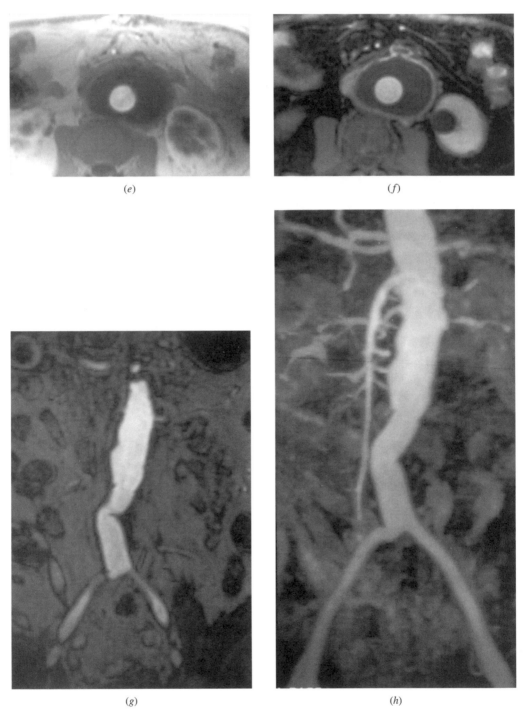

(e)

(f)

(g)

(h)

FIGURE 9.10 (*Continued*) T2W fat-suppressed SS-ETSE (*d*), immediate postgadolinium SGE (*e*), and interstitial phase gadolinium-enhanced fat-suppressed SGE (*f*) images in a second patient, with recent history of aortobifemoral graft surgery, demonstrate the presence of perigraft fluid. A small pocket of fluid is noted along the incision margin of the aneurysm (arrow, *d*). Coronal immediate postgadolinium 2 mm 3D gradient-echo source image (*g*) and MIP reconstruction of the 2 mm 3D source images (*h*) demonstrate a normal appearance for the vascular graft.

○ MRV imaging of the IVC depends on the same principle imaging strategies as MRA, with the main difference being timing

▪ MRV can be performed by delaying the timing until recirculation has occurred and a relative equilibrium phase has been achieved, shown by compa-

rable signal intensity of arteries and veins

▪ High signal from gadolinium renders MRV technically not challenging

○ The most common indications include

▪ Thrombus detection and characterization as bland versus tumor (figs. 9.11, 9.12, and 9.13)

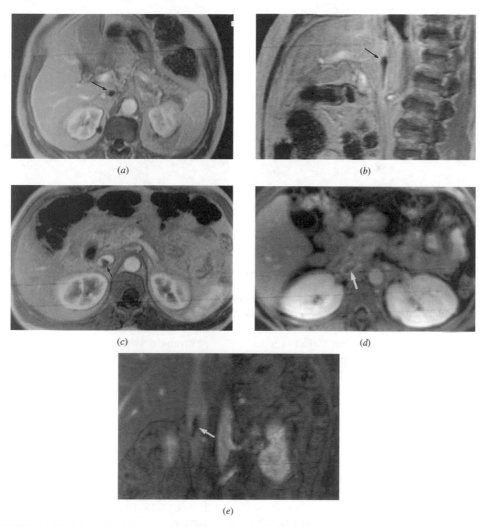

FIGURE 9.11 IVC thrombosis. Transverse 45 s (*a*) and sagittal 90 s (*b*) postgadolinium SGE images. Bland thrombus (arrow, *a*, *b*) appears nearly signal void on gadolinium-enhanced SGE images. The 45 s postgadolinium SGE image (*c*) in a second patient demonstrates low- to intermediate-signal-intensity thrombus (arrow, *c*) attached to the posterior wall of the IVC. The combination of intense enhancement of the IVC on gadolinium-enhanced SGE images with multiplanar imaging renders MRI an excellent, minimally invasive modality for the assessment of venous thrombosis.

Gadolinium-enhanced interstitial phase SGE images (*d*, *e*) in a third patient show a nonocclusive low-signal-intensity structure (arrows, *d*, *e*) within the lumen of the infrahepatic IVC consistent with thrombus. Imaging in two planes is useful to verify patency or thrombosis of vessels.

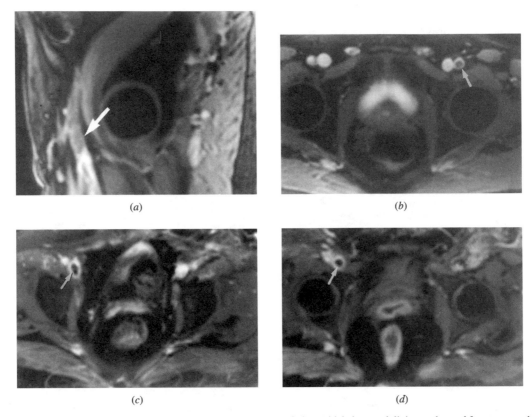

(a)   (b)

(c)   (d)

FIGURE 9.12   Venous thrombosis. Sagittal (*a*) and transverse (*b*) interstitial phase gadolinium-enhanced fat-suppressed SGE images demonstrate nonenhancing very low-signal-intensity tissue (arrows, *a*, *b*) within the lumen of the left external iliac vein consistent with venous thrombus. Transverse interstitial-phase gadolinium-enhanced fat-suppressed SGE images (*c*, *d*) in a second patient show the same finding within the right common femoral vein (arrows, *c*, *d*).

- Superimposed thrombophlebitis versus tumor extension is a challenging diagnosis
  - The clinical picture provides differentiating information
  - Anatomical relationships (fig. 9.14)
- Imaging
  - Same principles as for MRA, but delayed timing is used with a broad timing window of 2–10 min postgadolinium administration
  - Careful to distinguish low signal from inflowing blood from thrombus. Differentiating features:
    - low-signal flowing blood is often central in location, amorphous and varying shape from acquisition to acquisition and mildly low signal

  - thrombus is often well marginated with consistent appearance from acquisition to acquisition, including different planes
  - blood thrombus possesses a very low signal

Retroperitoneal Masses

Benign Masses
- Background
  - Benign retroperitoneal tumors are rare relative to malignancies
  - Differential diagnosis includes
    - Inflammatory
      - Retroperitoneal fibrosis
      - Inflammatory pseudotumor (inflammtory myofibroblastic tumor)
    - Benign lymphadenopathy

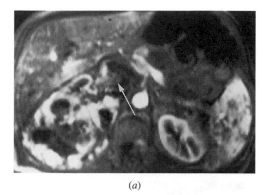

(a)

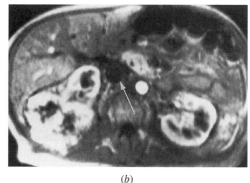

(b)

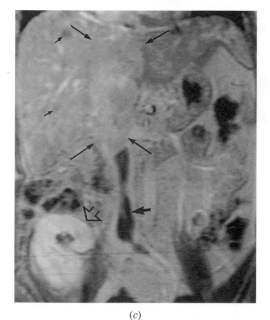

(c)

FIGURE 9.13 Tumor and blood thrombus. Immediate postgadolinium SGE images (*a*, *b*). A large hypervascular renal cell carcinoma is present in the right kidney. Extension into the inferior vena cava is depicted on the higher tomographic level image (*a*), with tumor thrombus (long arrow, *a*) demonstrating heterogeneous enhancement. The SGE image at a lower tomographic level demonstrates blood thrombus (long arrow, *b*) to be nearly signal void. MRI using postgadolinium SGE images can reliably differentiate tumor from bland thrombus.

Interstitial phase gadolinium-enhanced SGE image (*c*) in a second patient shows a renal cell carcinoma with enhancing tumor thrombus (long arrows, *c*) and signal-void blood thrombus (arrow, *c*) extending distally to the left common iliac vein. Multiple hepatic metastases (small arrow, *c*) and a renal transplant (hollow arrow, *c*) are also noted.

- Retroperitoneal hemorrhage
- Extramedullary hematopoiesis
- Benign neoplasms
  - Neural
    - Neurilemoma
    - Plexiform neurofibroma
    - Paraganglioma
  - Hemangioma
  - Lymphangioma
  - Lipoma
- Imaging
  - The combination of T2W single-shot and breath-hold T1W GRE with and without fat suppression and fat-suppressed gadolinium-enhanced T1W interstitial phase images provides a comprehensive evaluation with specific features noted as follows:
  - *Retroperitoneal Fibrosis*
    - Background
      - This is most frequently an idiopathic disease, but may be related to drugs (e.g., methysergide), inflammatory aortic aneurysm, retroperitoneal hemorrhage, infection, surgery, radiation therapy, mediastinal fibrosis, sclerosing cholangitis, Riedel's thyroiditis, and orbital and sinus pseudotumors

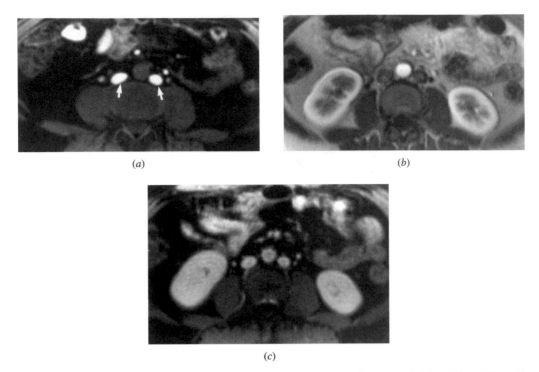

(a)

(b)

(c)

FIGURE 9.14 Duplicated IVC. Noncontrast fat-suppressed SGE (*a*), immediate postgadolinium (*b*), and interstitial phase gadolinium-enhanced SGE (*c*) images in a patient with duplicated IVC. The noncontrast T1W image shows high-signal time-of-flight effects in venous structures on the inferior sections of the data acquisition. The bilateral IVCs (arrows, *a*) are clearly appreciated with the time-of-flight effects. The capillary phase image (*b*) shows lack of enhancement of the IVCs early postcontrast, which then become opacified on the interstitial phase image (*c*). Combining morphologic and directional flow information on the precontrast images with dynamic temporal flow information on serial postgadolinium SGE images permits evaluation of congenital vascular variations and malformations.

- Imaging
  - Acute form has high T2W signal and intense enhancement (fig. 9.15) with infiltrative, wispy, ill-defined margins
  - Chronic form has low T2W signal, minimal enhancement, and is more oval and sharply demarcated in morphology (fig. 9.16)
  - Results in tissue encasement of the aorta and possibly IVC and ureters
  - Envelops the aorta circumferentially, but does not lift the aorta from the spine
  - Lymphoma can completely encase the aorta and will characteristically lift the aorta from the spine
  - *Inflammatory pseudotumor*, currently termed inflammatory myofibrobastic

tumor, is a rare entity with nonspecific imaging features that overlap with malignant disease. It is generally minimally low in signal intensity on T1W images, heterogeneous and moderately high in signal intensity on T2W images, and demonstrates moderately intense diffuse heterogeneous enhancement on immediate postgadolinium GRE images (fig. 9.17).
  - *Benign lymphadenopathy* may occur secondary to inflammatory or infectious disease and nodes are best visualized on fat-suppressed 3D GRE gadolinium-enhanced interstitial phase images
    - Castleman's disease (fig. 9.18), also known as giant lymph node hyperplasia, is an unusual cause for benign lymphadenopathy

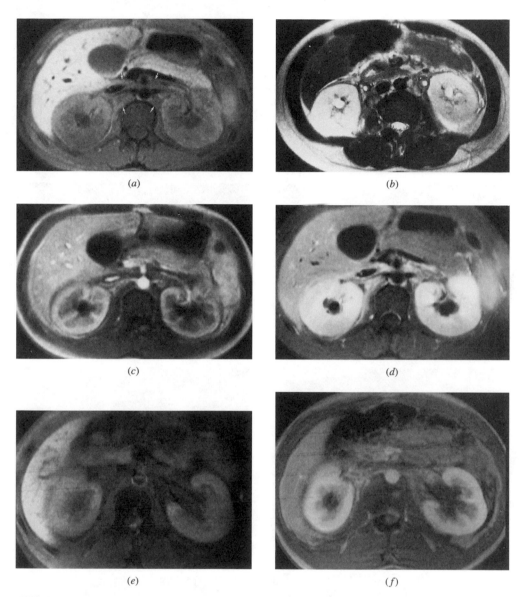

FIGURE 9.15 Acute benign retroperitoneal fibrosis. T1W fat-suppressed spin-echo (*a*), T2W spin-echo (T2-SE) (*b*), immediate postgadolinium SGE (*c*), and delayed postgadolinium T1W fat-suppressed spin-echo (*d*) images. The aorta, IVC, renal arteries, and ureters are encased by soft tissue (arrows, *a*), which is low in signal intensity on T1W (*a*) and heterogeneously high in signal intensity on T2W (*b*) images and has ill-defined margins. There is bilateral hydronephrosis and ureteral dilatation (*b*) caused by ureteral obstruction at a lower level. The fibrous tissue demonstrates heterogeneous enhancement on the immediate postgadolinium SGE image (*c*), which progresses on the more delayed T1W fat-suppressed spin-echo image (*d*).

Precontrast T1W fat-suppressed spin-echo (*e*), immediate postgadolinium SGE (*f*), and gadolinium-enhanced T1W fat-suppressed spin-echo (*g*) images in a second patient with biopsy-proven membranous glomerulonephritis and benign retroperitoneal fibrosis. Ill-defined extensive infiltrative soft tissue is present in the retroperitoneum. The fibrous tissue is low signal on the precontrast T1W image (*e*), demonstrates moderate heterogeneous enhancement on the immediate postgadolinium image (*f*), and is more conspicuous on the gadolinium-enhanced T1W fat-suppressed spin-echo image (*g*) because of the removal of the competing high signal intensity of the fat and progressive enhancement of the fibrous tissue. Corticomedullary differentiation is absent in both kidneys on the precontrast T1W fat-suppressed spin-echo image (*e*) because of elevated serum creatinine level.

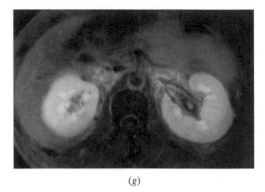

(g)

FIGURE 9.15 (*Continued*) Corticomedullary differentiation, however, is present on the immediate postgadolinium
SGE image (*f*), reflecting some preservation of renal function.
Increased medullary enhancement is shown in both kidneys on
the gadolinium-enhanced T1W fat-suppressed spin-echo image (*g*), reflecting tubulointerstitial damage.

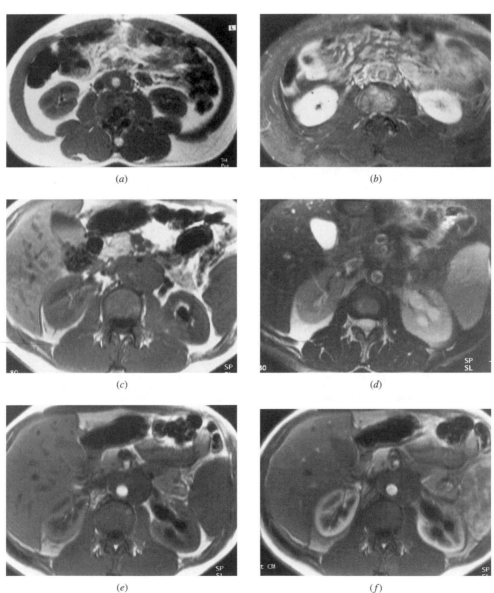

(a)

(b)

(c)

(d)

(e)

(f)

FIGURE 9.16 **Chronic benign retroperitoneal fibrosis.** SGE (*a*) and interstitial phase gadolinium-enhanced
fat-suppressed spin-echo (*b*) images. Low-signal-intensity oval-shaped tissue surrounds the aorta.

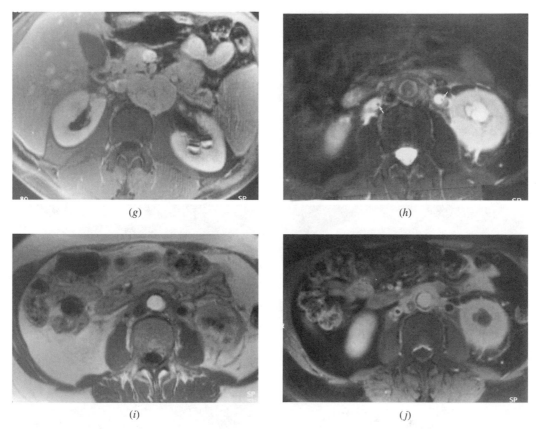

(g)   *(h)*

(i)   *(j)*

FIGURE 9.16 (*Continued*) The fibrous tissue has well-defined margins and shows minimal enhancement on the gadolinium-enhanced T1W fat-suppressed spin-echo image (*b*), findings that are typical of mature fibrous tissue. SGE (*c*), T2W echo-train spin-echo (*d*), arterial-phase (*e*) and capillary phase (*f*) postgadolinium SGE, and 90 s postgadolinium fat-suppressed SGE (*g*) images in a second patient. The fibrotic tissue is oval shaped with well-defined margins and encases the aorta. Note that, despite its size, the tissue does not substantially displace the aorta anteriorly. The fibrotic tissue is low in signal-intensity on the T1W image (*c*) and heterogeneously low with focal areas of high signal intensity on the T2W image (*d*), demonstrates minimal enhancement on the arterial phase (*e*) and capillary phase (*f*) postgadolinium SGE images, and enhances moderately on the more delayed fat-suppressed SGE (*g*) image. Delayed enhancement is characteristic of relatively mature fibrous tissue. Greater enhancement of the fibrotic tissue in the second patient reflects a more active stage in the transition between acute and chronic fibrosis than in the first patient. The pyelocalyceal system of the left kidney is dilated because of concomitant ureteral obstruction.

T2W echo-train spin-echo (*h*), immediate postgadolinium SGE (*i*), and interstitial phase gadolinium-enhanced fat-suppressed SGE (*j*) images in a third patient. Again noted is relatively well-marginated oval tissue encasing the aorta, IVC, and both ureters. The fibrous tissue is heterogeneously low in signal intensity on the T2W image (*h*) and demonstrates minimal enhancement on the immediate postgadolinium SGE image (*i*), progressing to moderate enhancement on the interstitial phase gadolinium-enhanced fat-suppressed SGE image (*j*), indicating mature fibrous tissue. Bilateral ureteral obstruction with hydronephrosis is present, and signal-void ureteral stents (arrows, *h*) are demonstrated in both ureters on the T2W image (*h*). The majority of the fibrous tissue is located anterior to the aorta and IVC, and these vessels are not displaced substantially anteriorly.

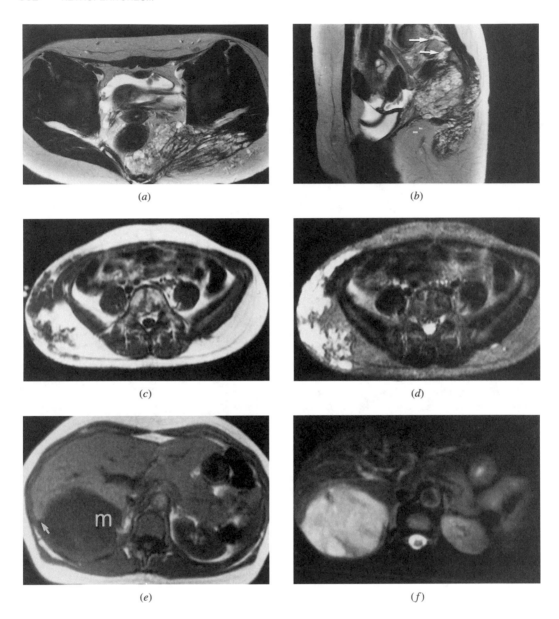

(a)   *(b)*

(c)   *(d)*

(e)   *(f)*

FIGURE 9.17   **Benign retroperitoneal tumors.** Transverse (*a*) and sagittal (*b*) 512-resolution T2W echo-train spin-echo images in a patient with plexiform neurofibroma of the pelvis and neurofibromatosis type 1. The plexiform neurofibroma appears as a large heterogeneous mass that occupies the majority of the left posterior pelvis and infiltrates the left gluteus maximus and pyriformis muscles. Extension into the sacral neural foramina is present (arrows, *b*). T1W spin-echo (*c*) and T2W spin-echo (*d*) images in a second patient demonstrate an extensive plexiform neurofibroma in the right subcutaneous tissues that is low in signal intensity on the T1W image (*c*) and high in signal intensity on the T2W image (*d*). The tumors are high in signal intensity on the T2W images in both patients, which is characteristic for tumors of neural origin.

    SGE (*e*), T2W fat-suppressed echo-train spin-echo (*f*), and immediate postgadolinium SGE (*g*) images in a patient with inflammatory pseudotumor arising from the renal capsule. A large mass (mass = m, *e*) is noted posterior to the liver.

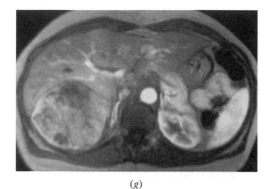

(g)

FIGURE 9.17 (*Continued*) The mass is well marginated, heterogeneous, and low in signal intensity on the T1W image (*e*) and moderately high in signal on the T2W image (*f*) and demonstrates intense diffuse heterogeneous enhancement on the immediate postgadolinium SGE image (*g*). The posterior liver margin at the interface with the mass forms an obtuse angle consistent with an extrahepatic origin of the mass. The right kidney (not shown) was displaced but not invaded by the mass. Inflammatory pseudotumor may have an aggressive appearance that mimics the appearance of a malignant tumor.

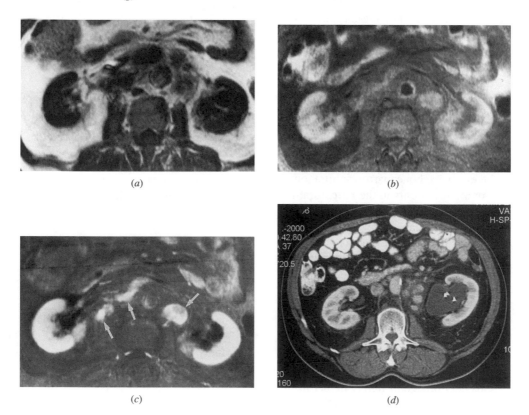

(a)

(b)

(c)

(d)

FIGURE 9.18 **Castleman's disease.** SGE (*a*), T1W fat-suppressed spin-echo (*b*), and gadolinium-enhanced T1W fat-suppressed spin-echo (*c*) images. Enlarged retroperitoneal lymph nodes are present. The lymph nodes are low in signal intensity on the SGE image (*a*) and intermediate to moderate in signal intensity on the T1W fat-suppressed spin-echo image (*b*), with several of them demonstrating substantial enhancement (arrows, *c*) on the gadolinium-enhanced image (*c*). Ill-defined stranding is also present in the retroperitoneum (*a*). (Reproduced with permission from Semelka RC, Shoenut JP, Kroeker MA: The retroperitoneum and the abdominal wall. In Semelka RC, Shoenut JP [eds.], *MRI of the Abdomen with CT Correlation.* New York: Raven Press, pp. 13–41, 1993.)

Iodine-contrast enhanced spiral CT image (*d*) in a second patient demonstrates enlarged lymph nodes and ill-defined retroperitoneal tissue. Associated hydronephrosis is present because of entrapment of the ureters by strandy tissue. (Courtesy of Andrea Baur, M.D., Klinikum Grosshadern, University of Munich.)

- Kawasaki's disease results in involved lymph nodes that are often hemorrhagic, demonstrating characteristic high signal intensity on T1W images
- Benign and malignant nodes enhance with overlap in appearance
- Central necrosis shown on gadolinium-enhanced fat-suppressed T1W GRE interstitial phase is relatively specific but not sensitive for malignant disease
  - *Retroperitoneal hematomas* are frequently spontaneous and associated with anticoagulation therapy, underlying coagulation disorders, or invasive procedures
    - Appears as a focal collection of fluid with a high-signal peripheral rim on noncontrast T1W images accentuated with fat suppression (fig. 9.19)
  - *Extramedullary hematopoiesis* is associated with hereditary hemolytic anemias, particularly thalassemia major, chronic leukemias, polycythemia vera, and diseases with extensive bone marrow infiltration
    - Commonly occurs in the retrocrural and presacral spaces
    - May develop an aggressive appearance and result in bone destruction
    - Intermediate in signal intensity on T1W images, intermediate to moderately high in signal intensity on T2W images, and enhances moderately after gadolinium administration (fig. 9.20)
  - *Neurilemoma* may have a characteristic high signal intensity on T2W images
  - *Retroperitoneal plexiform neurofibromas* are usually bilateral, slightly higher in signal intensity than muscles on T1W images, and high in signal intensity on T2W (fig. 9.17). Demonstration of tissue heterogeneity and increasing heterogeneity and lesion size on follow-up imaging studies are features worrisome for malignant disease
  - *Lipomas* show characteristic uniform fat signal on all images

Malignant Masses
Malignant Retroperitoneal Fibrosis (RPF)
- Background
  - Malignant retroperitoneal fibrosis is most commonly associated with cervical, bowel, breast, prostate, lung, and kidney cancers
  - The tumor consists of malignant cell infiltration of the retroperitoneum with associated desmoplastic reaction that often encases the aorta, IVC, and ureters
  - The contour of the mass is not lobular, distinguishing malignant retroperitoneal fibrosis from adenopathy, and may be infiltrative and irregular
- Imaging
  - Typically shows moderately high signal intensity on T2W images, exhibiting moderately intense enhancement with gadolinium (fig. 9.21), which may have an overlap in appearance with acute benign RPF
  - Infiltrative growth into neighboring structures favors malignant over benign RPF
  - Ureteral obstruction with bilateral hydronephrosis is common
  - Tissue sampling for pathological assessment may be indicated, but is challenging and should be obtained from multiple sites

Lymphoma
- Background
  - Lymphoma is the most common retroperitoneal malignancy, and both Hodgkin's and non-Hodgkin's lymphomas may involve the retroperitoneum
  - Non-Hodgkin's lymphoma more commonly involves a variety of nodal groups (in particular, mesenteric nodes are involved in more than 50% of cases) and extranodal sites
  - Intra-abdominal Hodgkin's lymphoma tends to be limited to the spleen and retroperitoneum and has a contiguous pattern of spread from node to node
- Imaging
  - Combined fat-suppressed T2W images and fat-suppressed gadolinium-enhanced T1W images is essential.
  - MRI performs well in the demonstration of enlarged lymph nodes (figs. 9.22 and 9.23), which typically appear relatively uniform in

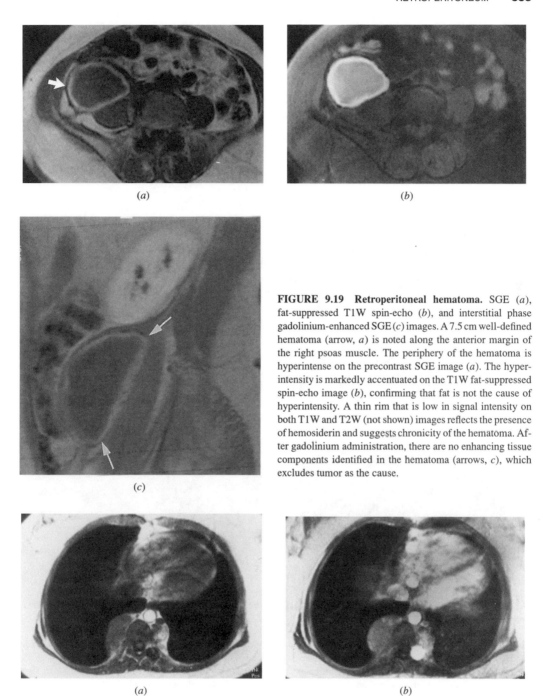

FIGURE 9.19 Retroperitoneal hematoma. SGE (*a*), fat-suppressed T1W spin-echo (*b*), and interstitial phase gadolinium-enhanced SGE (*c*) images. A 7.5 cm well-defined hematoma (arrow, *a*) is noted along the anterior margin of the right psoas muscle. The periphery of the hematoma is hyperintense on the precontrast SGE image (*a*). The hyperintensity is markedly accentuated on the T1W fat-suppressed spin-echo image (*b*), confirming that fat is not the cause of hyperintensity. A thin rim that is low in signal intensity on both T1W and T2W (not shown) images reflects the presence of hemosiderin and suggests chronicity of the hematoma. After gadolinium administration, there are no enhancing tissue components identified in the hematoma (arrows, *c*), which excludes tumor as the cause.

FIGURE 9.20 Extramedullary hematopoiesis in thalassemia major. SGE (*a*) and immediate postgadolinium SGE (*b*) images. Soft-tissue paravertebral masses in the lower thorax and abdomen are demonstrated. The hematopoietic masses are low in signal intensity on the SGE image (*a*) and demonstrate moderate enhancement on the immediate postgadolinium SGE image (*b*). (Reproduced with permission from Semelka RC, Shoenut JP, Kroeker MA: The retroperitoneum and the abdominal wall. In Semelka RC, Shoenut JP [eds.], *MRI of the Abdomen with CT Correlation*. New York: Raven Press, pp. 13–41, 1993.)

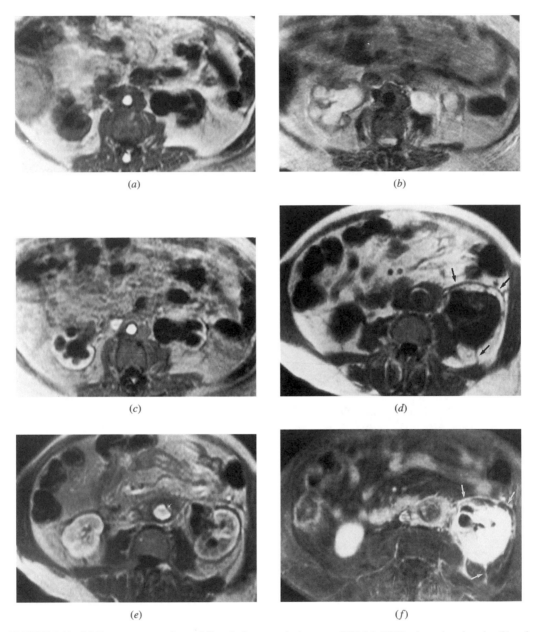

(a)   (b)

(c)   (d)

(e)   (f)

FIGURE 9.21   Malignant retroperitoneal fibrosis from cervical cancer. SGE (*a*), T2W echo-train spin-echo (*b*) and immediate postgadolinium SGE (*c*) images. The aorta is encased by abnormal soft tissue, which has slightly ill-defined margins. The soft tissue is low in signal intensity on the SGE image (*a*) and heterogeneous and moderate in signal intensity on the T2W echo-train spin-echo image (*b*) and demonstrates diffuse heterogeneous enhancement after gadolinium administration (*c*). This appearance is compatible with active malignant rather than chronic benign retroperitoneal fibrosis. Note bilateral hydronephrosis resulting from ureteral obstruction at a lower level.

SGE (*d*), immediate postgadolinium SGE (*e*), and postgadolinium T1W fat-suppressed spin-echo (*f*) images in a second patient with malignant retroperitoneal fibrosis. An oval-shaped mass encases the aorta. The mass is low in signal intensity on the SGE image (*d*), and demonstrates moderate heterogeneous enhancement on the immediate postgadolinium image (*e*) that progresses on the postgadolinium T1W fat-suppressed spin-echo image (*f*). The mass has aggressive infiltrating margins (arrows, *f*). The left perirenal fascia and perirenal septae are thickened (arrows, *d*) and demonstrate enhancement (arrows, *f*) on the gadolinium-enhanced T1W fat-suppressed spin-echo (*f*) image. Also noted is a dissection involving the abdominal aorta with good demonstration of the intimal flap (small arrow, *e*).

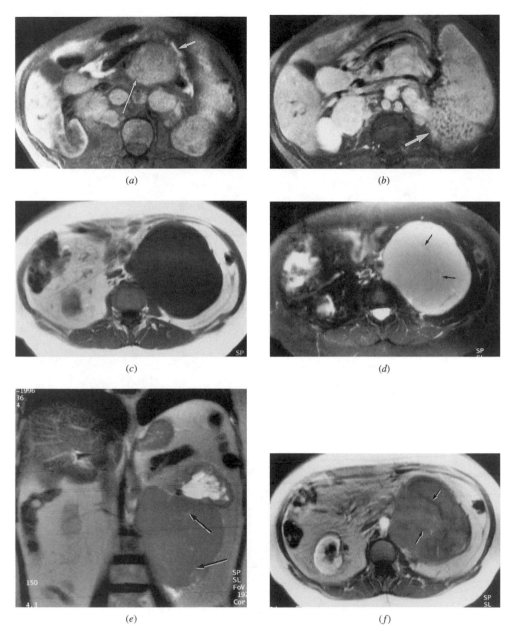

(a)

(b)

(c)

(d)

(e)

(f)

FIGURE 9.22   Non-Hodgkin's lymphoma. Precontrast (*a*) and gadolinium-enhanced (*b*) T1W fat-suppressed spin-echo images in a patient with retroperitoneal lymphadenopathy from non-Hodgkin's lymphoma. Extensive retroperitoneal and mesenteric lymphadenopathy is noted. The precontrast T1W fat-suppressed spin-echo image (*a*) permits distinction of the normal high-signal-intensity pancreas (short white arrow, *a*) from the retropancreatic nodal mass (long white arrow, *a*) and documents the extrapancreatic location of the mass. The nodal masses show moderate to intense enhancement on the gadolinium-enhanced image (*b*), whereas abnormal enhancement of the spleen (arrow, *b*) reflects lymphomatous infiltration. (Reproduced with permission from Semelka RC, Shoenut JP, Kroeker MA: The retroperitoneum and the abdominal wall. In Semelka RC, Shoenut JP [eds.], *MRI of the Abdomen with CT Correlation.* New York: Raven Press, pp. 13–41, 1993.) SGE (*c*), T2W fat-suppressed echo-train spin-echo (*d*), coronal T2W SS-ETSE (*e*), immediate postgadolinium SGE (*f*), and transverse (*g*) and sagittal (*h*) interstitial phase gadolinium-enhanced fat-suppressed SGE images in a patient with lymphoma presenting as a solitary retroperitoneal mass. A large, well-defined retroperitoneal mass is present. The mass is mildly heterogeneous and low in signal intensity on the T1W image (*c*) and moderately high signal intensity on the T2W image (*d*). Thin septations (arrows, *d, e*) are present in the mass. The coronal T2W SS-ETSE image demonstrates superior displacement and hydronephrosis of the left kidney secondary to ureteral compression caused by the mass.

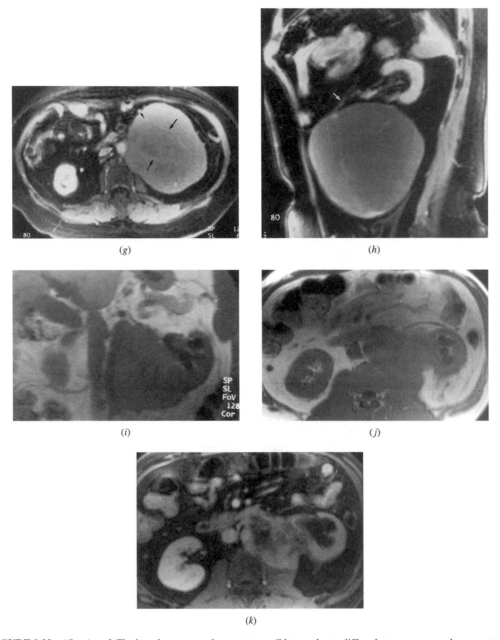

(g)   *(h)*

(i)   *(j)*

(k)

FIGURE 9.22   *(Continued)* The lymphoma mass demonstrates mild to moderate diffuse heterogeneous enhancement on the immediate postgadolinium SGE image (*f*), which becomes more homogeneous over time on the interstitial phase fat-suppressed SGE image (*g*). Note that the internal septations (arrows, *f, g*) show minimal enhancement on the immediate postgadolinium SGE image (*f*) and show progressive enhancement on the more delayed fat-suppressed SGE images (*g, h*), consistent with fibrous tissue. The anteriorly displaced ureter is identified at the anterior margin of the mass on the interstitial phase fat-suppressed SGE image (small arrow, *g*). Note that the sagittal image clearly demonstrates the fat plane between the kidney and the mass and depicts a segment of the anterosuperiorly displaced ureter (small arrow, *h*). A solitary mass lesion with no evidence of other sites of nodal or organ disease is a rare appearance for lymphoma. Coronal (*i*) and transverse (*j*) SGE and 90 s gadolinium-enhanced fat-suppressed SGE (*k*) images. There is a large heterogeneous mass originating in the retroperitoneum on the left that extends from the celiac axis inferiorly to the aortic bifurcation. This mass is isointense on noncontrast T1W images (*i, j*) and enhances heterogeneously (*k*). The mass encases the left renal artery and vein, as well as the ureter, resulting in hydronephrosis. This pattern is the most common form of kidney involvement by lymphoma. The psoas muscle is also compressed. This lesion represented large-cell lymphoma at histopathology.

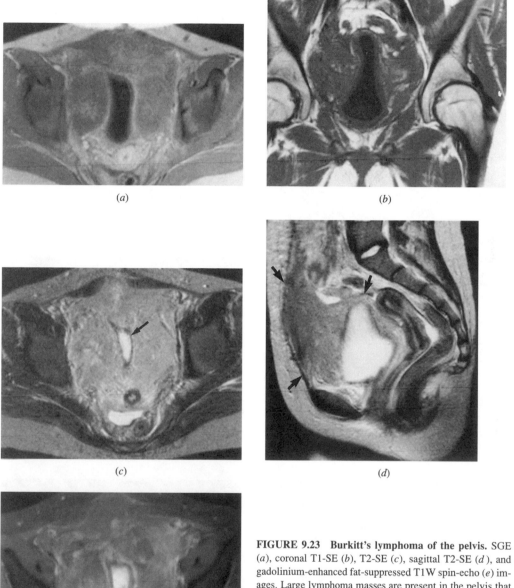

(a)

(b)

(c)

(d)

(e)

FIGURE 9.23 Burkitt's lymphoma of the pelvis. SGE
(*a*), coronal T1-SE (*b*), T2-SE (*c*), sagittal T2-SE (*d*), and
gadolinium-enhanced fat-suppressed T1W spin-echo (*e*) images. Large lymphoma masses are present in the pelvis that
cause compression of the urinary bladder (arrow, *c*), which
has an hourglass configuration, well shown on the coronal
T1-SE image (*b*). The sagittal T2-SE image depicts the large
lymphomatous mass (arrows, *d*) that extends along the dome
of the bladder into the uterovesicular space. The masses are
heterogeneous on both T1W and T2W images and show minimal enhancement after gadolinium administration (*e*).

signal and enhancement with only mild heterogeneity even in large masses (fig. 9.23), but can show heterogeneous enhancement in a subset of cases (fig. 9.22)
◦ MRI can outperform CT imaging in the evaluation of the upper abdominal paraaortic region and in patients who are thin

Metastatic Lymphadenopathy
• Background
  ◦ Carcinomas associated with retroperitoneal lymphadenopathy include kidney, colon, pancreas, lung, breast, testes, prostate, cervix, and melanoma

◦ MRI may be particularly helpful in thin patients, as the considerably greater soft-tissue contrast resolution than CT allows successful demonstration of nodes in the setting of minimal retroperitoneal fat
• Imaging
  ◦ Combined fat-suppressed. T2W images and fat-suppressed, gadolinium-enhanced images are essential
  ◦ Enlarged lymph nodes are usually moderate in signal intensity on T2W images and higher signal than adjacent psoas muscle (figs. 9.24 and 9.25)

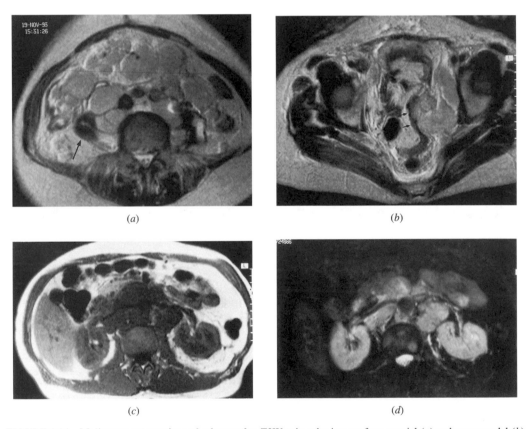

(a)   (b)

(c)   (d)

FIGURE 9.24   Malignant retroperitoneal adenopathy. T2W spin-echo images from cranial (*a*) and more caudal (*b*) levels. Enlarged retroperitoneal lymph nodes are demonstrated as rounded, well-defined masses of moderate signal intensity on both images. Note lateral displacement of the right psoas muscle (arrow, *a*) by enlarged paracaval lymph nodes, and medial displacement of the sigmoid colon (arrows, b) by enlarged left obturator lymph nodes.

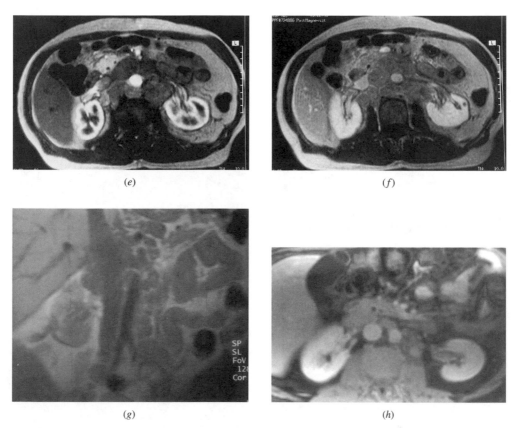

(e)   *(f)*

(g)   *(h)*

FIGURE 9.24   (*Continued*) SGE (*c*), T2W fat-suppressed spin-echo (*d*), and immediate (*e*) and 90 s (*f*) postgadolinium SGE images in a second patient who has prostate cancer. Multiple enlarged lymph nodes are present in the retroperitoneum displacing the aorta and the IVC anteriorly. The lymph nodes are low in signal intensity on the SGE image (*c*) and high in signal intensity on the T2W fat-suppressed spin-echo image (*d*). Fat suppression removes the competing high signal intensity of fat and renders the lymph nodes particularly conspicuous on the T2W image. The lymph nodes enhance minimally on the immediate postgadolinium SGE image (*e*) and show progressive enhancement on the 90 s postgadolinium SGE image (*f*).

Coronal SGE (*g*) and interstitial phase gadolinium-enhanced fat-suppressed SGE (*h*) images in a third patient, who has chronic lymphocytic leukemia. Diffuse abdominal adenopathy is appreciate in portocaval, periaortic, and iliac chains.

○ Benign and malignant enlarged lymph nodes demonstrate overlapping enhancement patterns

MR lymphography using iron oxide particles is currently under investigation. This technique has been shown in early patient experience to distinguish contrast-enhanced, low-signal-intensity benign lymph nodes from nonenhanced, intermediate, heterogeneous-signal-intensity malignant nodes on T2W images. Greater clinical experience is necessary to determine its accuracy.

Primary Retroperitoneal Neoplasms
• Background
  ○ The majority of primary retroperitoneal tumors (70–90%) are malignant
  ○ The most common histological types are malignant fibrous histiocytoma, liposarcoma, and leiomyosarcoma

• Imaging
  ○ On MR images, tumors are generally mixed low and intermediate in signal intensity on T1W images, and mixed medium and high in signal intensity on T2W images, and

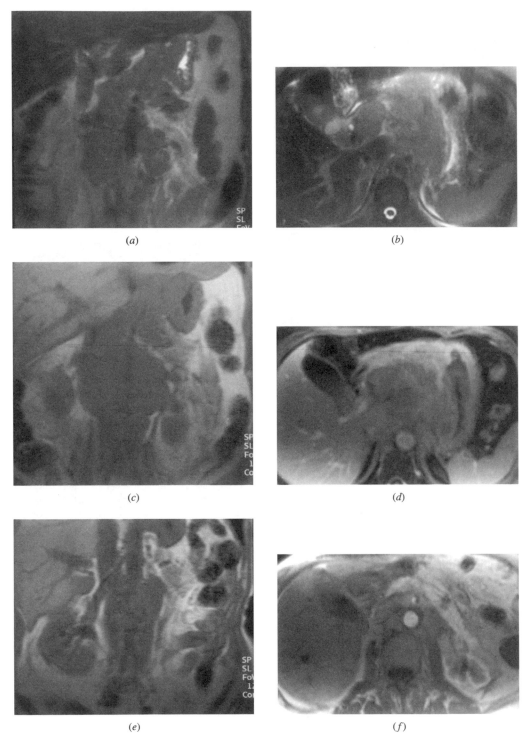

(a)

(b)

(c)

(d)

(e)

(f)

FIGURE 9.25 Malignant retroperitoneal lymphadenopathy. Coronal T2W SS-ETSE (*a*), transverse fat-suppressed T2W SS-ETSE (*b*), coronal SGE (*c*), and interstitial phase gadolinium-enhanced fat-suppressed SGE (*d*) images in a patient with gastric adenocarcinoma.

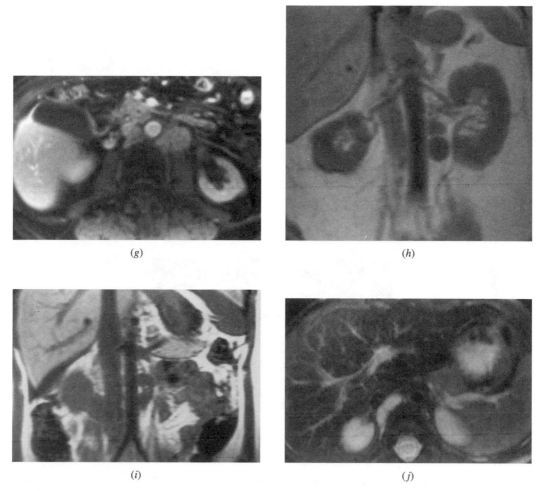

(g)

(h)

(i)

(j)

FIGURE 9.25 (*Continued*) There is a large, mildly heterogeneous lobulated mass involving the lesser curvature and extending into the gastrohepatic ligament (*d*). Extensive retroperitoneal lymph nodes are also appreciated.

Coronal SGE (*e*), immediate postgadolinium SGE (*f*), and interstitial phase gadolinium-enhanced fat-suppressed SGE (*g*) images in a second patient with recurrent colon cancer demonstrate the presence of aortocaval and left para-aortic bulky lymphadenopathy that extend superiorly to the level of the kidneys.

Coronal SGE image (*h*) in a third patient, who has carcinoma of the uterus, shows enlarged left para-aortic lymph nodes consistent with metastatic lymphadenopathy.

Coronal SGE image (*i*) in a fourth patient, who has endometrial stromal sarcoma, also demonstrates left para-aortic retroperitoneal adenopathy.

Transverse T2W fat-suppressed SS-ETSE image (*j*) in a fifth patient with neuroblastoma shows the presence of retrocrural lymph nodes that represent recurrent disease.

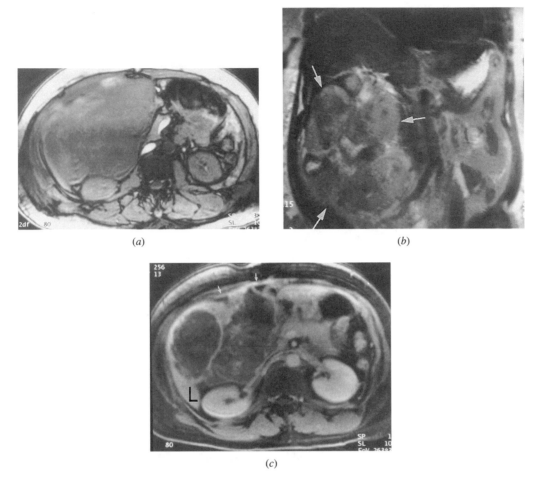

(a)   *(b)*

(c)

FIGURE 9.26 Retroperitoneal carcinoma. Out-of-phase SGE (*a*), coronal T2W SS-ETSE (*b*), and interstitial phase gadolinium-enhanced fat-suppressed SGE (*c*) images. A large, lobulated, heterogeneous mass is located in the right abdomen. The mass is heterogenous on both T1W (*a*) and T2W (arrows, *b*) images, displacing the aorta and IVC medially and the right kidney posteriorly. Areas of high signal intensity on the T2W image (*b*) represent necrotic areas. The mass demonstrates peripheral and patchy heterogeneous enhancement on the interstitial phase gadolinium-enhanced fat-suppressed SGE image (*c*). Invasion of the right lobe of the liver (L, *c*) is clearly demonstrated. The mass abuts the anterior abdominal wall, and enhancement of the anterior peritoneum (small arrows, *c*) is evident secondary to recent laparotomy attempt, which was aborted because of the large size of the mass.

enhance in a heterogeneous fashion (figs. 9.26–9.29)

◦ Leiomyosarcomas have a characteristic appearance, demonstrating hypervascularity with intense enhancement (fig. 9.27) with nonenhancing foci of necrosis

◦ Liposarcomas may show varying content of fat and soft tissue, with well-differentiated liposarcomas overlapping in appearance with benign lipoma

▪ Pathology is challenging, requiring removal of the entire mass for total evaluation

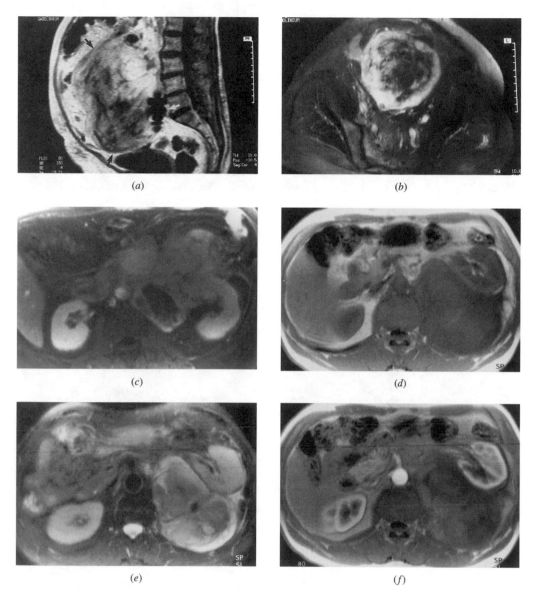

FIGURE 9.27   Retroperitoneal sarcoma. Sagittal T1-SE (*a*) and postgadolinium T1W fat-suppressed spin-echo (*b*) images in a patient with recurrent retroperitoneal leiomyosarcoma. A large, markedly heterogeneous mass (arrows, *a*) arises in the retroperitoneum immediately anterior to the lumbar spine and extends inferiorly to the pelvis. The mass demonstrates intense heterogeneous enhancement on interstitial phase gadolinium-enhanced images. Magnetic susceptibility artifacts are present that are caused by surgical clips (white arrow, *a*).

Transverse interstitial phase gadolinium-enhanced fat-suppressed SGE image (*c*) in a second patient, who has retroperitoneal leiomyosarcoma, demonstrates a large left-sided retroperitoneal mass that is heterogeneous in appearance and invades the lower and medial aspect of the left kidney.

SGE (*d*), T2W fat-suppressed echo-train spin-echo (*e*), immediate postgadolinium SGE (*f*), and transverse (*g*) and sagittal (*h*) interstitial phase gadolinium-enhanced fat-suppressed SGE images in a third patient, who has pleomorphic rhabdomyosarcoma. A large, left-sided retroperitoneal rhabdomyosarcoma mass is present. The mass displaces the left kidney anterolaterally, consistent with the retroperitoneal origin of the mass. The mass is heterogeneous and low in signal intensity on the precontrast SGE image (*d*) and heterogeneous and mixed high signal intensity on the T2W image (*e*). The mass demonstrates moderate and heterogeneous enhancement on the immediate postgadolinium SGE image (*f*) with progressive enhancement on the interstitial phase fat-suppressed SGE images (*g, h*).

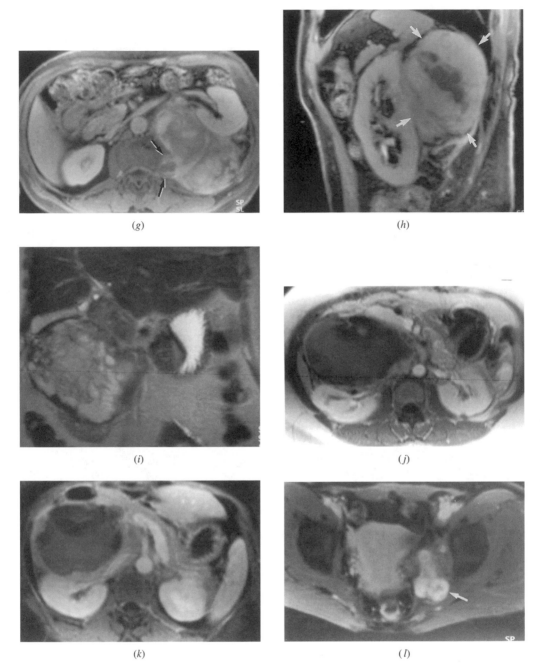

(g)

(h)

(i)

(j)

(k)

(l)

FIGURE 9.27 (*Continued*) Invasion of the left psoas muscle (arrows, *g*) is well shown on the interstitial phase fat-suppressed SGE image (*g*) as an enhancing area with irregular margins within the muscle. The sagittal image demonstrates the longitudinal extent of the mass (arrows, *h*) and anterior displacement of the kidney. Central necrosis is present that appears as a central area of lack of enhancement within the mass.

Coronal SS-ETSE (*i*), immediate postgadolinium SGE (*j*), and interstitial phase gadolinium-enhanced fat-suppressed SGE (*k*) in a fourth patient, who has retroperitoneal sarcoma. A large and heterogeneously enhancing tumor with septations and necrosis is seen in the right abdomen, abutting the head of the pancreas, porta hepatis, the right kidney, and the inferior vena cava.

interstitial phase gadolinium-enhanced fat-suppressed SGE (*l*) image in a fifth patient, who has retroperitoneal sarcoma. A heterogeneous, moderately intense mass (arrow, *l*) is present in the left pelvis. Involvement of the obturator internus and pyriformis muscles is apparent.

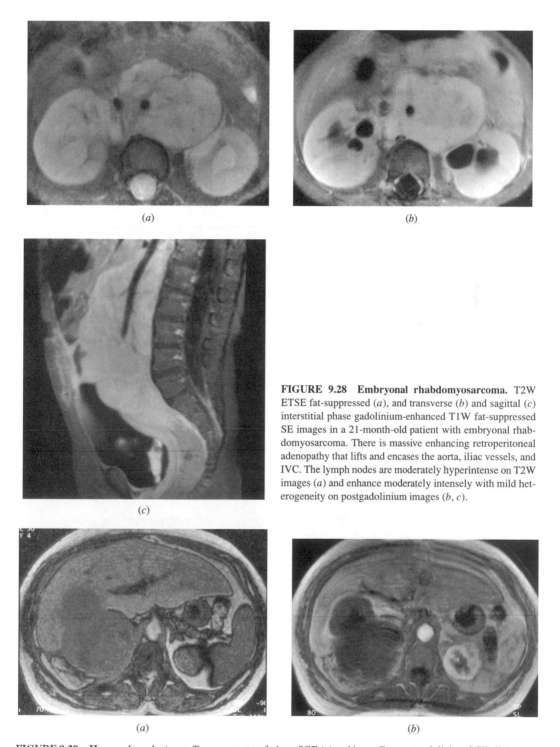

(a)

(b)

FIGURE 9.28 Embryonal rhabdomyosarcoma. T2W ETSE fat-suppressed (*a*), and transverse (*b*) and sagittal (*c*) interstitial phase gadolinium-enhanced T1W fat-suppressed SE images in a 21-month-old patient with embryonal rhabdomyosarcoma. There is massive enhancing retroperitoneal adenopathy that lifts and encases the aorta, iliac vessels, and IVC. The lymph nodes are moderately hyperintense on T2W images (*a*) and enhance moderately intensely with mild heterogeneity on postgadolinium images (*b*, *c*).

(c)

(a)

(b)

FIGURE 9.29   Hemangiopericytoma. Transverse out-of-phase SGE (*a*) and immediate postgadolinium SGE (*b*) images show a large lobulated necrotic mass in the right abdomen that invades the right kidney and the liver. Histopathologic examination established the diagnosis of hemangiopericytoma.

CHAPTER 10

PERITONEUM

Hernias

Abdominal Wall Hernias
- Background
  - Three main classifications
    - Inguinal
      - Congenital = indirect
        - A persistent processus vaginalis represents an opening from the peritoneal cavity through the inguinal ring into the scrotum that fails to close in infancy
      - Acquired = direct
        - Results from a disruption of the inguinal peritoneal lining, as may occur during stress of heavy lifting and increased intraperitoneal pressure
      - Represents a potential space into which omentum and bowel loops may invaginate (fig. 10.1)
    - Paraumbilical
      - May represent a congenital or acquired process (fig. 10.2)
      - Results from a peritoneal protrusion through the linea alba (fig. 10.3)
      - Risks include
        - Obesity
        - Recti abdomini diastasis
        - Multiparous female

- Spigelian
  - Peritoneal herniation through a defect in the aponeurosis between the transversus abdomini and rectus abdominis muscle into the lateral abdominal wall

Diaphragmatic Hernias
- Background
  - Three main classifications
    - Hiatal
      - Typically an acquired defect involving superior migration of the gastroesophageal junction (GEJ) into the posterior mediastinum (fig. 10.4)
      - Subclassifications
        - Sliding/fixed
        - Degree in terms of amount of stomach involved
        - Complications including rotation or incarceration of the stomach
        - Paraesophageal, involving the cardia or fundus of the stomach herniating superiorly through the hiatus while the GEJ remains in normal position
          - Considered at highest risk for complications

Primer on MR Imaging of the Abdomen and Pelvis, edited by Diego R. Martin, Michele A. Brown, and Richard C. Semelka ISBN 0-471-37340-0 Copyright © 2005 Wiley-Liss, Inc.

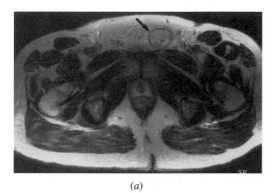
(a)

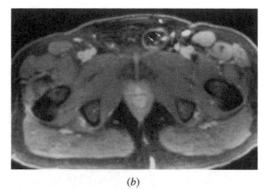
(b)

FIGURE 10.1 Inguinal hernia. Transverse 512-resolution T2W echo-train spin-echo (a) and interstitial phase gadolinium-enhanced fat-suppressed SGE (b) images in a patient with inguinal hernia. Expansion of the left inguinal canal (arrow, a) is well shown on the T2W image (a), which contains high-signal-intensity tissue with an appearance identical to surrounding fat. Fat within the expanded inguinal canal diminishes in signal intensity on the fat-suppressed image, and enhancing testicular vessels are well seen (arrows, b).

- Bochdalek
  - Results from congenital incomplete closure of the diaphragm, usually at the posterior and medial aspect of the left hemidiaphragm (fig. 10.5)
- Morgagni
  - Congenital defect typically involving the right hemidiaphragm anteriorly and medially

- Imaging
  - Peritoneal herniations are generally easily visualized by MRI, taking advantage of intrinsic multiplanar capabilities and a variety of sequences
- T2W single-shot spin-echo train
  - Motion insensitive to respiratory and bowel peristalsis, and insensitive to magnetic susceptibility effects of gastrointestinal gas
  - Obtain at least one acquisition with fat suppression in order to use fat as an endogenous contrast agent by varying signal of fat
  - Combination of nonfat-suppressed T1W images and fat suppressed T2W

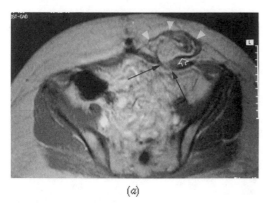
(a)

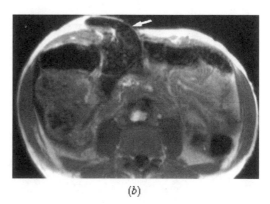
(b)

FIGURE 10.2 Spigelian hernia. Gadolinium-enhanced T1W SGE image (a) in a patient with spigelian hernia. A bowel-containing hernia sac (arrowheads, a) protrudes through a defect in the aponeurosis between the transversus and rectus muscles (solid arrows, a). The lateral margin of the hernia sac is the intact external oblique muscle and fascia (open arrow, a).

Transverse immediate postgadolinium T1W SGE image (b) in a second patient. A spigelian hernia with protrusion of bowel contents (arrow, b) is noted in the right anterior abdomen.

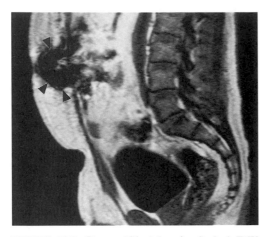

FIGURE 10.3 Paraumbilical hernia. Sagittal T1W SGE image shows signal-void air-containing bowel (arrowheads) in the subcutaneous tissues in a patient with a paraumbilical hernia.

images improves visualization of abnormal intraperitoneal or hernia fluid accumulation

- 3D GRE postgadolinium
  - To identify complications of bowel incarceration, including abnormal enhancement related to peritoneal or bowel inflammation or infection or bowel ischemia or infarction.

Intraperitoneal Fluid

- Background

Ascites

  ○ Causes: cirrhosis, malignancy, trauma, pancreatitis, hypoalbuminemic conditions, inflammation/infection, obstruction (venous or lymphatic), and inflammation

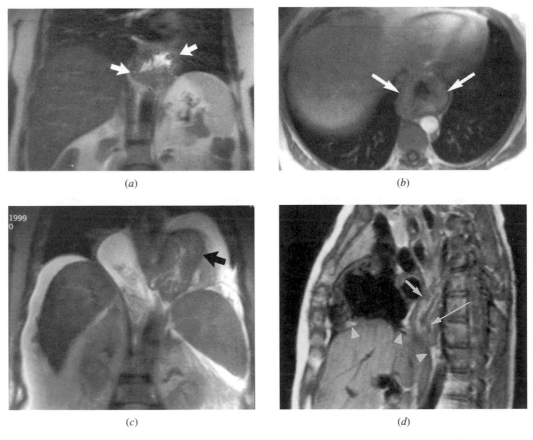

(a)

(b)

(c)

(d)

FIGURE 10.4 Hiatus hernia. Coronal T2W SS-ETSE (*a*) and transverse immediate postgadolinium SGE (*b*) images.

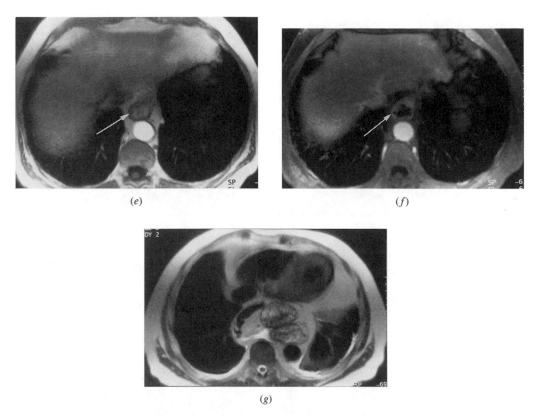

(e)   (f)

(g)

FIGURE 10.4 (*Continued*) The coronal T2W image demonstrates extension of the stomach (arrows, *a*) above the diaphragm. On the transverse postgadolinium image, the extent of gastric wall enhancement of the herniated part of the stomach (arrows, *b*) is comparable to the remainder of the stomach. Coronal T2W single-shot echo-train spin-echo (*c*) image in a second patient. There is a large hiatus hernia (arrow, *c*) in a patient with cirrhosis. Note that stomach, omentum, and ascites protrude through the hernia.

Sagittal T1W SGE image (*d*) in a third patient with a history of heartburn. The gastroesophageal junction (long arrow, *d*) is above the diaphragm (arrowheads, *d*), which is diagnostic of a hiatal hernia. Thickening of the esophageal wall (short arrow, *d*) is consistent with reflux esophagitis.

Immediate postgadolinium SGE (*e*) and 90 s postgadolinium SGE imaging (*f*) in a fourth patient demonstrate stomach in the lower mediastinum (arrows, *e*, *f*). Gastric rugae are well shown on the gadolinium-enhanced fat-suppressed image (*f*).

T2W SS-ETSE image (*g*) in a fifth patient shows a large hiatal hernia with surrounding herniated fat.

○ Simple transudates are low in signal intensity on T1W images and very high in signal intensity on T2W images (fig. 10.6)

○ Complex exudates, blood, enteric contents, and infected ascites will have higher signal intensity on T1W images and more variable signal intensity on T2W images (figs. 10.7 and 10.8)

○ Isolated greater sac fluid tends to have benign nonneoplastic etiology

○ Malignant fluid tends to involve the greater and lesser sac (fig. 10.9)

○ With inflammation or malignancy, bowel may appear tethered at multiple sites

Intraperitoneal Blood

○ Commonly associated with trauma, or spontaneous hemorrhage in a patient with a bleeding dyscrasia or who is anticoagulated

○ Blood produces age-dependent signal changes, but typically shows a mixture of T1W and T2W signals, with irregular areas of high to low signal intensity throughout the fluid, and may show a fluid-debris

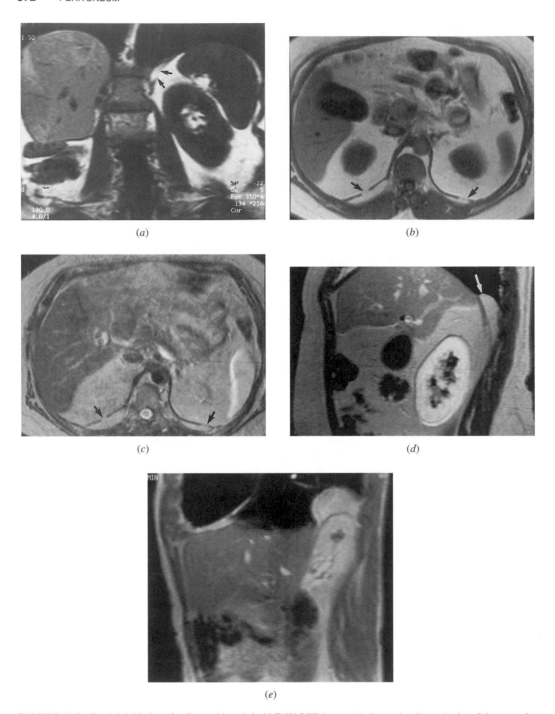

(a)

(b)

(c)

(d)

(e)

FIGURE 10.5 Bochdalek's hernia. Coronal breath-hold T1W SGE image (*a*) shows the discontinuity of the posterior diaphragm (arrows). The rent in the diaphragm allows fat and/or viscera to migrate superiorly into the chest. SGE (*b*), T2W spin-echo (T2-SE) (*c*), and sagittal 90 s postgadolinium SGE (*d*) images demonstrate rents in the diaphragm bilaterally (arrows, *b*, *c*) and herniation of fat into the pleural space (arrow, *d*).

Sagittal-plane gadolinium-enhanced T1W SGE (*e*) image in a third patient shows the herniation of kidney and fat into the thorax.

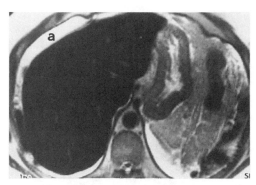

FIGURE 10.6   Ascites. T2W SS-ETSE image in a patient with simple transudative ascites. High-signal-intensity ascites (a) surrounds the abdominal viscera. The liver is low in signal intensity secondary to iron overload from multiple transfusions.

layer with dependent layering of blood products (fig. 10.10). Peripheral rim of high signal on T1W images is characteristic of hematomas due to peripheral accumulation of extracellular methemoglobin.

Intraperitoneal Bile
- ○ Most commonly related to recent surgery
- ○ Bile salts are very irritating to the peritoneum and can lead to chemical peritonitis
- ○ Bilomas result from adhesions walling off a bile fluid collection, usually in the perihepatic spaces
- ○ Typically seen as high signal on T2W, and demonstrates uniform abnormal peritoneal

enhancement of smoothly thickened peritoneum on fat-suppressed T1W post-gadolinium interstitial phase images (fig. 10.11)

Intraperitoneal Urine
- ○ Most commonly results from bladder leak
- ○ Classification of bladder rupture
  - ▪ Intraperitoneal
    - • Secondary to bladder dome rupture
    - • Associated with lap belt compression injury in motor vehicle accidents
  - ▪ Extraperitoneal
    - • Secondary to bladder base injury
    - • Associated with pelvic bone fractures
- • Imaging
  - ○ Single-shot echo-train T2W sequences provide motion-insensitive imaging with the ability to determine if the ascites is simple (uniform high signal) or complex (irregular or diminished signal)
  - ○ Gadolinium-enhanced T1W GE images can assess peritoneal thickening, nodularity, or masses
    - ▪ Differential for enhancing uniform peritoneal thickening
      - • Peritonitis
        - ○ T2W images show complex fluid
          - ▪ Pelvic sagittal images can show fluid-debris layering of debris and bacteria, which appears as dependent low signal material

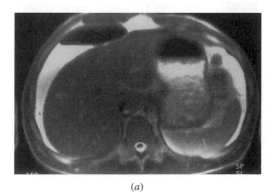

(a)

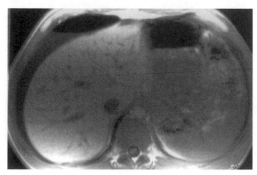

(b)

FIGURE 10.7   Postsurgical intraperitoneal air and fluid. Transverse T2W SS-ETSE (*a*) and SGE (*b*) images in a patient with a recent history of surgery demonstrate the presence of pneumoperitoneum and ascites. Note that air is invariably located along the nondependent surface in structures.

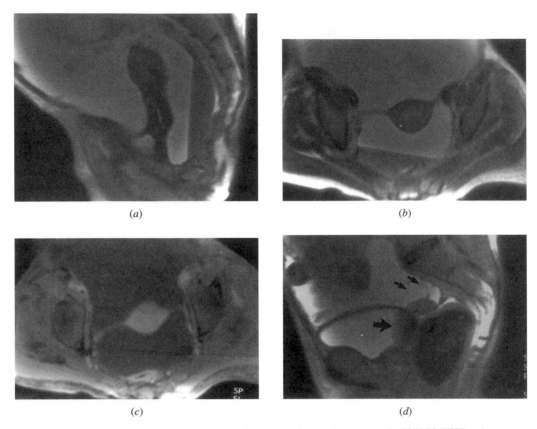

(a) (b)

(c) (d)

FIGURE 10.8 High-protein-content ascites, adhesions. Sagittal (a) and transverse (b) T2W SS-ETSE and transverse interstitial phase gadolinium-enhanced fat-suppressed SGE (c) images. A large volume of ascites is seen within the pelvis. In the posterior cul de sac, a fluid-fluid level is seen on the T2W image with the dependent fluid layer being low in signal, which is consistent with high protein content.

Sagittal T2W SS-ETSE image (d) in a second patient demonstrates a large volume of ascites in the pelvis with multiple thin septations (arrows, d) and a focal collection of proteinaceous material in the vesicorectal space. Low signal in the dependent portion of the bladder (large arrow, d) represents gadolinium.

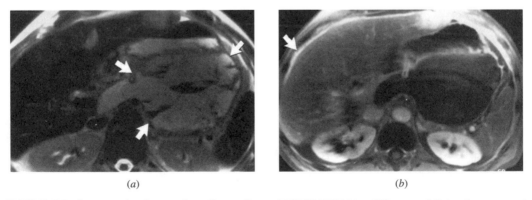

(a) (b)

FIGURE 10.9 Lesser sac involvement in malignant disease. T2W SS-ETSE (a) and 90 s postgadolinium fat-suppressed SGE (b) images. There is a dominant fluid collection in the lesser sac (arrows, a), which contains multiple septations and multiple fluid-fluid levels from proteinaceous debris as shown on the T2W image (a). The gadolinium-enhanced fat-suppressed image (b) obtained at the same anatomical level shows the lesser sac collection but not the internal septations. A thin layer of enhancing peritoneal disease (arrow, b) is appreciated on the gadolinium-enhanced fat-suppressed image that is not apparent on the T2W image.

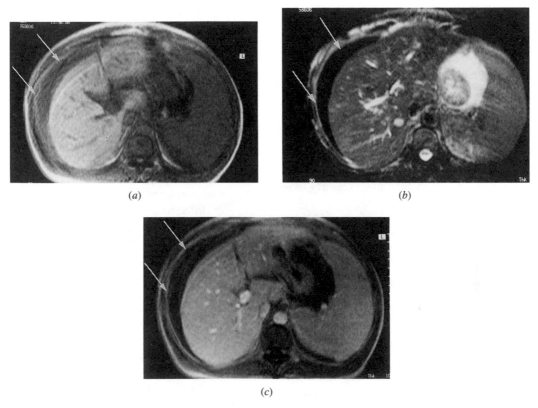

(a)   *(b)*

(c)

FIGURE 10.10   Intraperitoneal acute blood. SGE (*a*), T2W fat-suppressed spin-echo (*b*), and 1 min postgadolinium SGE (*c*) images in a patient status postpercutaneous liver biopsy. Fluid (arrows, *a–c*) surrounding the liver exhibits the signal characteristics of acute blood (deoxyhemoglobin): isointense or low signal intensity on T1W images and very low signal intensity on T2W images.

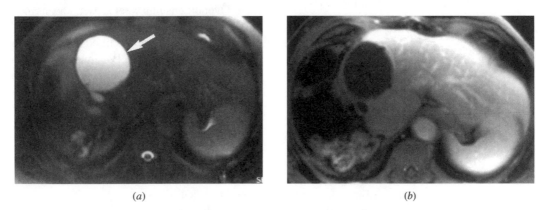

(a)   *(b)*

FIGURE 10.11   Biloma. T2W fat-suppressed SS-ETSE (*a*) and 90 s postgadolinium fat-suppressed SGE (*b*) images in a patient after right hepatectomy demonstrate a cystic mass along the resected surface of the left lobe (arrow, *a*) consistent with biloma.

- Portal hypertension and cirrhosis
  - T2W images show simple fluid
- Malignant ascites
  - Most common associated carcinomas
    - Ovary
    - Pancreas
    - Stomach
    - Colon
  - Ovary is the most common cause in females
- In bladder rupture
  - Fat-suppressed T2W images clearly show free intraperitoneal fluid
    - High-resolution (e.g., 512 × 512 matrix) T2W echo-train spin-echo images of the pelvis with 2.5–5 min acquisition time provide excellent anatomic delineation of the bladder, ureters, and urethra
  - Delayed gadolinium-enhanced images acquired at 10 min postinjection allow sufficient time to fill bladder and may demonstrate leakage from the lower urinary tract
    - If Foley catheter in place, it should be clamped to promote bladder filling and leakage during the exam
    - MR cystography can be performed by infusing 300 ml saline to which 1.25 ml gadolinium is added
      - Abdominal pelvic imaging can be obtained in a breath-hold acquisition using T1W 3D GRE
  - Mimickers of complex fluid
    - Large simple fluid pockets may develop focal areas of flow, resulting in flow-void artifacts that appear as a swirling pattern of low signal, most often shown adjacent to the liver in cirrhotic patients where respiratory induced flow is greatest. This arises because water proton excited by image acquisition flow out of the plane of imaging, leading to loss of signal during the readout phase. Dramatic variation in signal intensities from one slice to the next helps correctly identify this phenomenon.

Inflammation and Infection

Peritonitis
- Background
  - Etiologies
    - Sterile
      - Bile leak, pancreatitis
    - Infectious
      - Bowel perforation
        - Diverticulitis, peptic ulcer disease, Crohn's disease, traumatic bowel rupture
      - Bacterial peritonitis related to
        - Infected ascites with underlying
          - Cirrhosis and portal hypertension
          - Peritoneal dialysis
          - Hemorrhagic ascites
          - Pancreatitis
- Imaging
  - Seen as diffuse increased enhancement and increased thickness of the parietal and visceral peritoneum and mesentery
  - Demonstrated on gadolinium-enhanced fat-suppressed T1W GE images in the delayed equilibrium or interstitial phase (figs. 10.12 and 10.13)
  - In pancreatitis the fluid is complex, often collects preferentially in the lesser sac, and diffuse stranding pattern of enhancement is identified within the mesenteric and retroperitoneal fat spaces.
    - Over the ensuing weeks, pseudocysts may develop
      - If simple, these are filled with uniform high signal on T2W imaging with a thin wall that enhances, shown on post-gadolinium T1W fat-suppressed interstitial phase images

Abscess
- Background
  - Etiologies
    - Postsurgical complication
    - Diverticulitis
    - Crohn's disease
    - Following traumatic bowel rupture
- Imaging
  - Combination of motion-insensitive single-shot T2W, including fat-suppressed T2W,

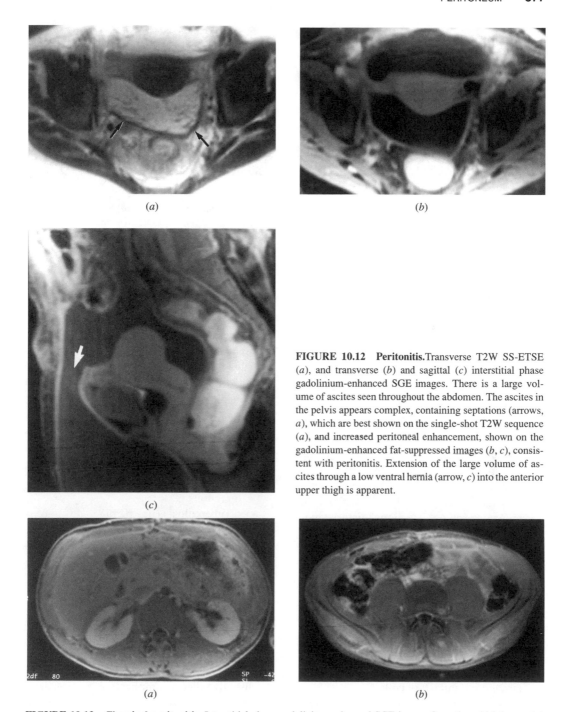

(a)

(b)

(c)

FIGURE 10.12   Peritonitis. Transverse T2W SS-ETSE (*a*), and transverse (*b*) and sagittal (*c*) interstitial phase gadolinium-enhanced SGE images. There is a large volume of ascites seen throughout the abdomen. The ascites in the pelvis appears complex, containing septations (arrows, *a*), which are best shown on the single-shot T2W sequence (*a*), and increased peritoneal enhancement, shown on the gadolinium-enhanced fat-suppressed images (*b*, *c*), consistent with peritonitis. Extension of the large volume of ascites through a low ventral hernia (arrow, *c*) into the anterior upper thigh is apparent.

(a)

(b)

FIGURE 10.13   Chemical peritonitis. Interstitial phase gadolinium-enhanced SGE images from the midabdomen (*a*) and pelvis (*b*) in a patient with chemical peritonitis, secondary to intraperitoneal administration of chemotherapeutic agents. Diffuse increased enhancement is present of peritoneal, mesenteric, and serosal surfaces, which has resulted in adherence of bowel loops to each other and linear enhancing strands in the mesentery. Bowel loops and mesenteric planes are ill-defined because of the generalized inflammatory process.

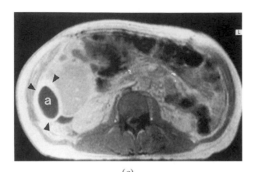
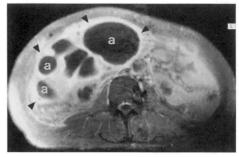

(a)   (b)

FIGURE 10.14 Intra-abdominal abscess. Interstitial-phase gadolinium-enhanced T1W SGE (a) and interstitial phase gadolinium-enhanced T1W fat-suppressed spin-echo (b) images in a patient with clinical suspicion of an abscess. Multiple loculated abscess collections are present along the liver capsule and in the right midabdomen (a, a, b). The thick enhancing rims (arrowheads, a, b) are characteristic of the inflammatory capsules associated with abscesses.

and fat-suppressed gadolinium-enhanced T1W GRE interstitial phase images are essential

○ Abscesses have a range of appearances depending on degree of maturation, but all show the following to varying extents:

▪ Thick enhancing wall surrounded by enhancing stranding in the adjacent soft tissues and/or fat

▪ A rounded abnormal structure with central nonenhancing low to intermediate T1W, and mixed intermediate to high T2W signal, shown as oval shaped and distinct from bowel by employing multiplanar imaging (fig. 10.14), with dependent layering of low-signal material most often present on T2W (fig. 10.15)

Mesenteric Panniculitis
• Background
  ○ Other terms include retractile mesenteritis and sclerosing mesenteritis
  ○ Represents nodular fibro-fatty thickening of the mesentery, localized or multifocal
  ○ Histologically identify fat necrosis, fibrosis, and inflammatory cells
  ○ Idiopathic or nonspecific in etiology with a variety of possible associated disorders including prior surgery, infection, trauma, and ischemia
    ▪ Diagnosis depends on excluding concomitant pancreatitis, Crohn's disease,

active infections, neoplasms, or arterial-vascular disease

• Imaging
  ○ T1W GRE breath-hold non-fat-suppressed images show stranding in the mesentery (fig. 10.16). Varying degrees of delayed gadolinium enhancement best shown with concomitant fat-suppression.

• Mimickers
  ○ Other causes of mesenteric inflammation and/or fibrotic reaction, including
    ▪ Neoplastic
      • Carcinoid, lymphoma, carcinomatosis
    ▪ Infectious
      • Tuberculosis (fig. 10.17)

Peritoneal Masses

Benign Masses
Cysts
• Background
  ○ Mesenteric cysts most commonly occur in the small-bowel mesentery
  ○ Uncertain etiology
  ○ Rarely symptomatic, and if symptomatic, usually reflects complication, such as hemorrhage, rupture, torsion, and bowel obstruction
  ○ Histologically a true cyst with endothelial, mesothelial, or epithelium of fallopian tube type, filled with serous or chylous fluid, and may contain protein or blood products

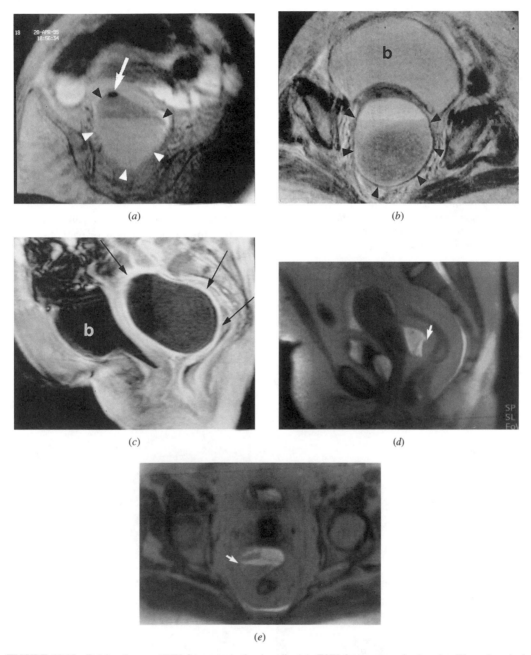

(a)

(b)

(c)

(d)

(e)

FIGURE 10.15   Pelvic abscess. T1W fat-suppressed spin-echo (*a*), T2W fat-suppressed spin-echo (*b*), and sagittal gadolinium-enhanced T1W fat-suppressed SGE (*c*) images in a patient with fever and an elevated white blood cell count. A complex fluid collection (arrowheads, *a*, *b*) is demonstrated in the pelvis. The variable signal intensity on the T1W images reflects a high protein content (*a*, *c*). On the T2W image (*b*), low-signal-intensity debris layers in the dependent portion of the abscess. A focus of signal–void air is present (arrow, *a*), which is not uncommonly observed in abscesses. The wall of the abscess (arrows, *c*) enhances substantially after gadolinium administration (bladder = b, *b*, *c*). Sagittal (*d*) and transverse (*e*) T2W SS-ETSE images in a second patient show a fluid collection in the cul de sac that exhibits layering of low–signal material on T2W images (arrow, *d*, *e*), consistent with abscess. A lesser volume of nonloculated fluid is also observed around the uterus.

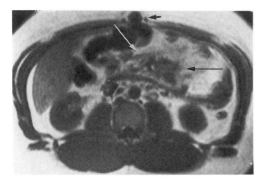

FIGURE 10.16 Mesenteric lipodystrophy and tuberculous peritonitis. SGE image (a) demonstrates low-signal-intensity stranding in the fat of the mesentery (long arrows), consistent with mesenteric lipodystrophy. A small ventral hernia is also present (short arrow).

- Imaging
  - Typically uniform simple fluid characteristics with high signal on T2W, low on T1W images, and a thin uniform wall (fig. 10.18)
  - Occasional complicated cyst will have decreased signal on T2W and elevated signal

on T1W images (fig. 10.18), with enhancement of the cyst wall and internal septations, if present

Pseudocysts
- Background
  - Cystic lesions with noncellular walls
  - Etiologies include pancreatitis or other causes of inflammation
- Imaging
  - Appear as simple or complicated cysts
  - Evaluate for abnormal tissue associations to determine cause, such as anatomic relationship to the pancreas or pancreatic duct in the setting of findings that indicate abnormal pancreatic parenchyma

Intraperitoneal Lipomas and Lipomatosis
- Background
  - Soft mobile masses
  - Simple lipomas are solitary smoothly marginated benign masses comprised of

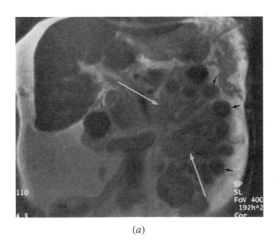

(a)

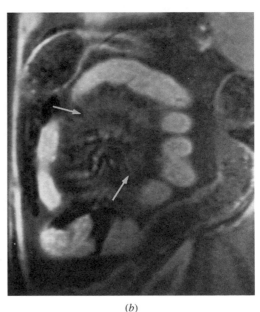

(b)

FIGURE 10.17 Coronal T2W SS-ETSE (a) and sagittal (b) interstitial phase fat-suppressed SGE images in a second patient, who has tuberculous peritonitis. A large volume of ascites is present. Multiple loops of thickened small bowel are appreciated (short arrows, a). The mesentery is infiltrated and intermediate in signal intensity (long arrows, a) on the T2W image (a). Terminal branches of the mesenteric vessels (arrows, b) fan out to the thickened loops of small bowel, creating a spoke-wheel-type pattern on the sagittal image. This appearance is that of retractile mesenteritis, which can be caused by a number of etiologies including tuberculosis.

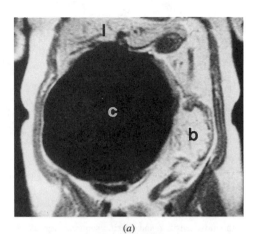

(a)

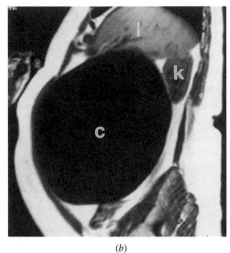

(b)

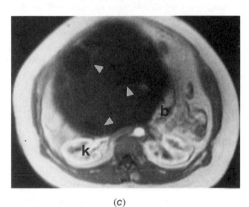

(c)

FIGURE 10.18 Mesenteric cyst. Coronal T1W magnetization-prepared single-shot gradient-echo (*a*), sagittal T1W SGE (*b*), and immediate postgadolinium fat-suppressed SGE (*c*) images. A large septated cystic mass (c, *a*, *b*) arising from the small-bowel mesentery causes mass effect upon the adjacent bowel (b, *a*, *c*), left kidney (k, *b*, *c*), and liver (l, *a*, *b*). Cysts that are low in signal intensity on T1W images (*a*, *b*) and high in signal intensity on T2W images (not shown) are consistent with serous fluid. Immediately after intravenous gadolinium administration (capillary phase) the septae traversing the cyst enhance (arrowheads, *c*). These imaging characteristics are consistent with an uncomplicated mesenteric cyst.

adipocytes and minimal stromal tissue, but can have various degrees of vascularized stromal tissue
- Lipomatosis represents benign proliferation of regional mesenteric fat, producing a mildly compressive but noninfiltrating mass effect on adjacent tissues
  - Associations include Cushing's syndrome or long-term steroid therapy
- Imaging
  - Diagnosis established by demonstration of a focal mass or mass effect by a fatty structure
    - T2W or T1W imaging shows the mass to be bright, with drop in signal on fat suppression, with negligible or no enhancing elements on T1W fat-suppressed gadolinium-enhanced images
- Mimickers

- Liposarcoma
  - Generally, as the extent of soft-tissue component increases, the likelihood that the mass is a liposarcoma is increased, with extensive enhancing soft-tissue elements and infiltration of surrounding structures making liposarcoma the most likely consideration
  - Overlap with lipoma exists, and histopathological assessment requires removal of the entire fatty mass

Endometriosis
- Background
  - Endometriosis is defined as the presence of endometrial glands or stroma in abnormal locations outside of the uterus
  - The three imaging hallmarks of endometriosis are

- Pelvic peritoneal endometrial implants
- Ovarian endometriomas (endometriotic cysts)
- Adhesions
  - The most common peritoneal sites of involvement are, in decreasing order of frequency,
    - Ovaries
    - Uterine ligaments
    - Cul-de-sac and pelvic peritoneum reflected over the uterus
    - Fallopian tubes
    - Rectosigmoid region
    - Bladder
  - Rare extraperitoneal sites include the lungs and the central nervous system
- Imaging
  - Endometriomas have variable signal intensity, but are commonly high in signal intensity on T1W images and heterogeneously high in signal intensity on T2W images
    - Protein and blood breakdown products tend to demonstrate a gradation of signal intensity on T2W images, which has been termed shading
  - Noncontrast T1W fat-suppressed image is the most sensitive MRI technique for identifying endometriomas (fig. 10.19)
  - Contrast-enhanced T1W may also be useful
  - Limitations
    - MR imaging of ovarian endometriomas is considered sensitive and moderate to high in specificity
    - However, imaging of extraovarian endometriosis in considered insensitive, and if imaging is negative, laparoscopic evaluation may be required for direct visualization

Desmoid Tumor
- Background
  - A rare gastrointestinal mesenchymal tumor
  - Desmoid tumors vary in histologic features from fibroproliferative disease to low-grade sarcoma
  - Commonly arises as a reactive response to prior surgery or accidental trauma, and tend to recur if resected

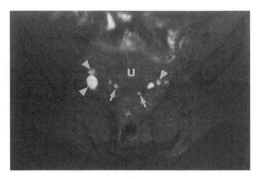

FIGURE 10.19 Endometriosis. T1W fat-suppressed spin-echo image demonstrates high-signal-intensity foci of ovarian endometriomas (arrowheads) and smaller endometriosis implants adherent to the uterine serosa (arrows). T1W fat-suppressed spin-echo or SGE technique is the most sensitive and specific sequence for detecting the blood product–laden deposits of endometriosis. (Reprinted with permission from Ascher SM, Agrawal R, Bis KG, Brown E, et al: Endometriosis: Appearance and detection with conventional, fat-suppressed, and contrast-enhanced fat-suppressed spin-echo techniques. *J Magn Reson Imaging* 5:251–257, 1995.)

  - Associations with polyposis syndromes
    - Gardner's and familial adenomatous polyposis syndromes
- Imaging
  - Varying appearance including diffuse, focal discrete, and multifocal disease (fig. 10.20)
  - Generally low signal on both T1W and T2W imaging
  - Enhances minimally on postgadolinium capillary and interstitial phase T1W imaging

Malignant Masses
Mesothelioma
- Background
  - Although similar in histology to pleural malignant mesothelioma, the incidence of peritoneal origin of this tumor is significantly lower
  - Risk factors are identical to pleural form, and predominantly associated with prior exposure to certain forms of asbestos
- Imaging
  - Best sequence for visualization is fat-suppressed gadolinium-enhanced T1W 2D or 3D GRE in the delayed interstitial phase

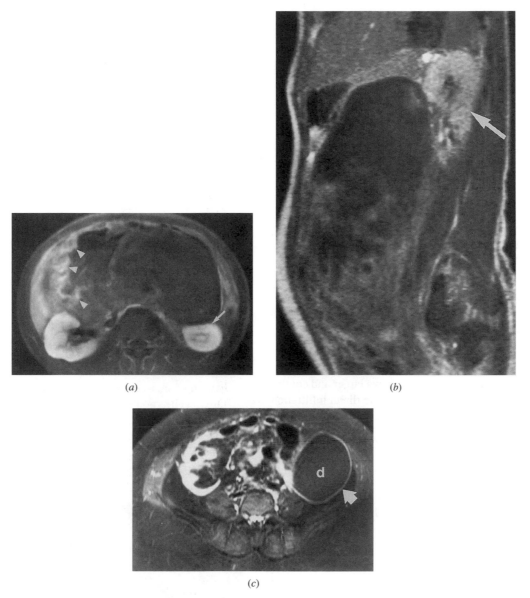

(a)   (b)

(c)

FIGURE 10.20   Desmoid tumor. Transverse 90 s postgadolinium T1W fat-suppressed spin-echo (a) and sagittal 10 min postgadolinium SGE (b) images in a woman with Gardner syndrome and intra-abdominal desmoid tumor. The right aspect of the mass enhances (arrowheads) more than the left aspect. The greater enhancement on the right reflects active disease. This large desmoid produces a mass effect on the kidneys (arrows, a, b). Imaging in the sagittal plane helps define the craniocaudad extent of the tumor.

Transverse interstitial phase gadolinium-enhanced T1W fat-suppressed spin-echo image (c) in a second woman with Gardner syndrome and intra-abdominal desmoid tumor. The desmoid tumor (d, c) exhibits minimal enhancement, confirming its fibrous nature. Thin mural enhancement is apparent (arrow, c). On the basis of this image alone, the tumor could be mistaken for a cyst. T2W images distinguish the two: a desmoid tumor remains low in signal intensity, whereas a cyst is high signal intensity.

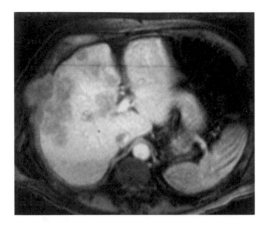

FIGURE 10.21 Mesothelioma. Transverse interstitial phase gadolinium-enhanced fat-suppressed SGE image in a patient with peritoneal mesothelioma demonstrates a large, lobulated hypointense mass in the right upper abdomen with invasion of the liver and abdominal wall. Note also the presence of extensive liver metastases. (Courtesy of Gregory Sica, M.D., Brigham and Women's Hospital, Boston, MA.)

- ○ Early disease appears as small nodular foci arising from the peritoneum
- ○ Advanced disease shows larger and confluent nodules with possible direct infiltration into intra-abdominal and abdominal wall soft tissues (fig. 10.21)

Metastases
- • Background
  - ○ Most common tumors include ovary, pancreas, stomach, and colon
    - ▪ These are the same tumors associated with malignant ascites
  - ○ Patterns of spread
    - ▪ Local
      - • Direct extension
        - ○ Also can extend along peritoneal ligaments and folds
          - ▪ For example, pancreatic cancer infiltration
            - • Along the transverse mesocolon to the transverse colon, obstructing the colon
            - • Along the hepatoduodenal ligament into the porta hepatis
            - • To contiguous tissue of the lesser curvature of the stomach, then to

liver along the gastrohepatic ligament
  - ▪ Draining lymph nodes
  - ▪ Intraperitoneal seeding
  - ▪ Hematogenous
  - ▪ Tumor patterns
    - • Ovary
      - ○ Metastases most often present initially with intraperitoneal seeding
    - • Colon, stomach, and pancreas
      - ○ Metastases most often present initially with local lymph node and/or liver metastases
      - ○ Pancreas almost invariably develops peritoneal seeding with advanced disease

- • Imaging
  - ○ Fat-suppressed gadolinium-enhanced T1W GRE interstitial phase images are superior for diagnostic assessment of local extension, metastatic nodes, or peritoneal deposits (i.e., suppression of high fat signal intensity greatly facilitates visualization of small enhancing abnormal structures, such as nodes surrounded by fat) (figs. 10.22 and 10.23)
  - ○ Liver metastases are best evaluated on optimally timed arterial-capillary phase T1W GRE enhanced images (see chap. 2)

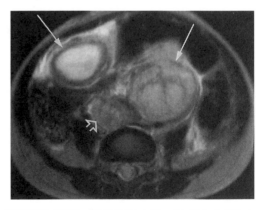

FIGURE 10.22 Metastatic yolk sac tumor. Transverse 512-resolution T2W echo-train spin-echo image in a patient with metastatic yolk sac tumor. Ovarian yolk sac tumors spread to the peritoneum (solid arrows), omentum, and retroperitoneal lymph nodes (open arrow).

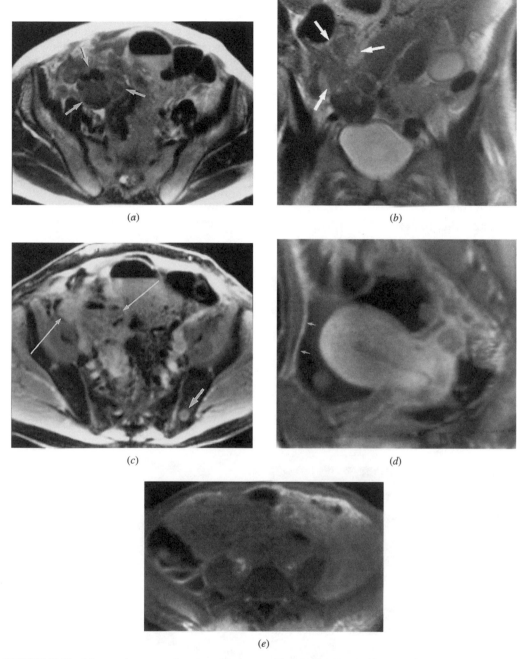

(a)

(b)

(c)

(d)

(e)

FIGURE 10.23 Metastatic pancreatic cancer. Transverse (*a*) and coronal (*b*) T2W single-shot echo-train spin-echo and interstitial phase gadolinium-enhanced T1W fat-suppressed SGE (*c*) images in a patient with metastatic pancreatic adenocarcinoma. The T2W images show a mass in the right lower quadrant (arrows, *a*, *b*). After intravenous contrast, the serosal and peritoneal metastases enhance (long arrows, *c*). Incidental note is made of an enhancing bone metastasis in the left ilium (short arrow, *c*). Sagittal (*d*) and transverse (*e*) interstitial phase gadolinium-enhanced fat-suppressed SGE images in a second patient, who has a neuroendocrine pancreatic tumor. There are multiple peritoneum-based nodular metastases throughout the pelvis. Diffuse peritoneal and serosal enhancement is present throughout the peritoneal cavity, consistent with large-volume peritoneal metastases. Virtually no uninvolved intraperitoneal or mesenteric fat is present because the entire contents of the peritoneal cavity at this level enhance substantially. The sagittal projection is effective at showing metastases along the lower anterior peritoneum (arrows, *d*).

385

Miscellaneous Metastatic Tumors Involving the Peritoneum

Carcinoid Tumors

- Background
  - Intestinal carcinoid tumor may involve the mesentery
  - Not uncommonly the primary intestinal site is not visible on imaging studies
  - These tumors commonly, but not always, induce an intense fibrotic reaction that leads to a stellate pattern of fibrous bands and retraction
- Imaging (fig. 10.24)

  - Non-fat-suppressed noncontrast T1W images show these tumors as low-signal-intensity stellate masses against the high-signal-intensity mesenteric fat. Fat-suppressed gadolinium-enhanced T1W interstitial phase shows these masses as mildly enhancing in a dark fat-suppressed background
  - T2W single-shot echo-train spin-echo sequences demonstrate low-signal-intensity tissue in a background of high signal intensity
  - These tumors generally enhance minimally

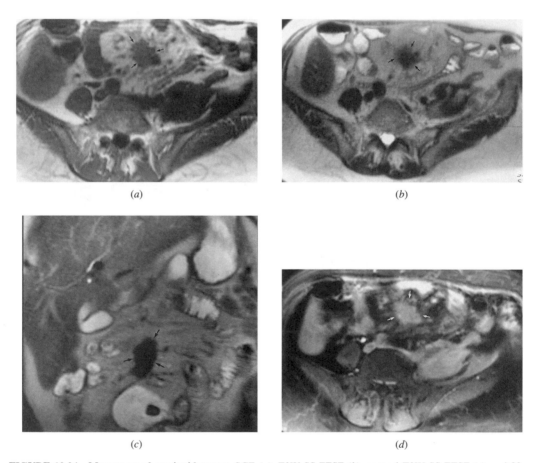

(a) (b)

(c) (d)

FIGURE 10.24 Metastases of carcinoid tumor. SGE (*a*), T2W SS-ETSE (*b*), coronal T2W SS-ETSE (*c*), and 90 s postgadolinium fat-suppressed SGE (*d*) images in a patient with a carcinoid tumor of the small bowel. Breath-hold T1W SGE images are well suited for imaging the low-signal-intensity metastasis in the root of the small-bowel mesentery (arrows, *a*); the radiating strands are highlighted by the surrounding high signal intensity of the intra-abdominal fat. The desmoplastic nature of these tumors is emphasized by its low signal intensity on T2W images (arrows, *b*, *c*) and only modest enhancement after intravenous contrast (arrows, *d*).

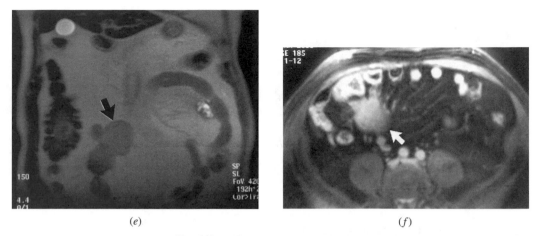

(e) (f)

FIGURE 10.24   (*Continued*) Coronal T2W SS-ETSE (e) and interstitial phase gadolinium-enhanced fat-suppressed SGE (f) images in a second patient with mesenteric metastasis from carcinoid tumor demonstrate a spiculated mass (arrow, e, f) with thin radiating linear strands that extend into the mesentery, caused by a desmoplastic fibrous reaction in the surrounding tissue.

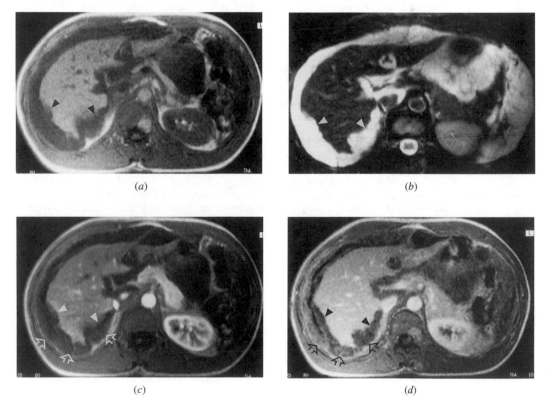

(a) (b)

(c) (d)

FIGURE 10.25   Pseudomyxoma peritonei. SGE (a), T2W fat-suppressed echo-train spin-echo (b), immediate (c) and interstitial phase (d) postgadolinium SGE, and coronal precontrast SGE (e) and 5 min postgadolinium SGE (f) images in a patient with pseudomyxoma peritonei secondary to rupture of an appendiceal mucinous cystadenocarcinoma.

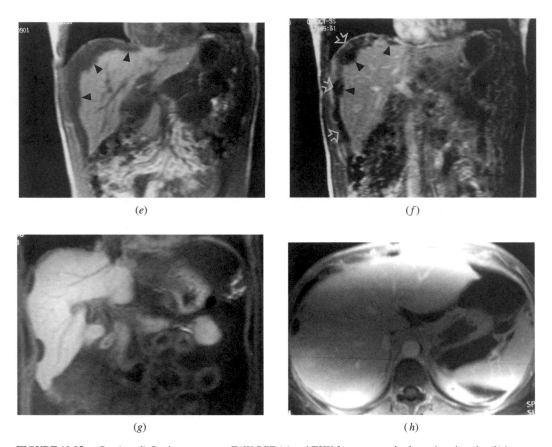

(e) (f)

(g) (h)

FIGURE 10.25   (*Continued*) On the precontrast T1W SGE (*a*) and T2W fat-suppressed echo-train spin-echo (*b*) images the gelatinous material surrounding the liver has regions in which the signal intensity resembles that of simple ascites. However, the characteristic scalloping of the liver margin (arrowheads, *a–f*), coupled with the enhancement of the material (open arrows, *c*, *d*, *f*) filling the abdomen, establishes the correct diagnosis. Free fluid within the abdomen does not enhance. Coronal images (*e*, *f*) provide a global view of the disease extent and demonstrate subdiaphragmatic disease well.

Coronal (*g*) and transverse (*h*) interstitial phase gadolinium-enhanced fat-suppressed SGE images in a second patient, who also has appendiceal mucinous cystadenocarcinoma. A large volume of ascites with extensive peritoneal enhancement is observed, associated with scalloping of the liver surface, features that are characteristic of pseudomyxoma peritonei.

Pseudomyxoma Peritonei
- Background
  - A mucinous tumor, most commonly originating from appendix, ovary, or pancreas
  - Can fill the peritoneal spaces with gelatinous mucin that is extremely difficult to remove surgically, and recurrence after debulking procedures is common
- Imaging
  - Characterized by scalloping tumor deposits along the surface capsule of liver and spleen (fig. 10.25)
  - Signal characteristics of the intraperitoneal mucinous material is
    - Mildly low signal on T1W
    - Mildly heterogeneous and moderately high signal on T2W
    - Mild early and late enhancement along peritoneum and organ margins

CHAPTER 11

BLADDER

OVERVIEW

For MR imaging of the bladder, it is useful to combine sequences that demonstrate high-signal-intensity urine (i.e., T2W imaging and delayed post gadolinium imaging) with techniques that demonstrate low-intensity urine (noncontrast T1W imaging with or without fat suppression and immediate postgadolinium dynamic SGE imaging). Half Fourier single-shot turbo spin-echo (HASTE) technique has the additional advantage of being breathing independent. Moderate bladder distention is important. If the bladder is not distended, it may be difficult to recognize small tumors. If the bladder is too distended, the patient becomes uncomfortable, and flat tumors can be missed. The patient should void 2 hours prior to the exam, and not again until after the exam to standardize bladder distension. Chemical-shift artifact can mimic or mask an invasive bladder cancer. To correct for this, chemically selective fat suppression can be performed, or the frequency-encoding gradient can be rotated. Routine use of a phased-array multicoil improves image quality.

Normal

- Bladder wall is 2–8 mm thick
- Low signal on T2W images
- Low signal on T1W images
- Mild enhancement which progresses slightly on late postcontrast images

Normal Variants and Congenital Disease
Congenital Anomalies
- Background
  - Agenesis and hypoplasia are rare
  - Duplication is slightly more common
  - Exstrophy is a clinical diagnosis; however, MR may contribute important information about associated skeletal, muscular, and peritoneal anomalies and position of the sex organs
- Imaging
  - In duplication, the septum is low signal on T1W and T2W images, and the walls of both cavities are equal in thickness and signal intensity, unlike diverticula

Primer on MR Imaging of the Abdomen and Pelvis, edited by Diego R. Martin, Michele A. Brown, and Richard C. Semelka ISBN 0-471-37340-0 Copyright © 2005 Wiley-Liss, Inc.

Congenital Diverticula
- Background
  ○ Herniations of bladder mucosa through focal weakness in the detrusor muscle
  ○ Most occur in males
  ○ Most occur at bladder base
  ○ At the ureteral meatus (Hutch diverticulum), may be associated with ureteral obstruction
  ○ Associated with urinary stasis, chronic infection, inflammation, dysplasia, leukoplakia, and squamous metaplasia, which may precede malignant tumor
  ○ Tumors originating within diverticula are rare, occurring in 2–7%, and are most commonly transitional cell carcinoma (78%), squamous cell carcinoma (17%), combined transitional and squamous cell (2%), and adenocarcinoma (2%)
- Imaging
  ○ Outpouchings from the native bladder
  ○ Wall of the diverticulum is thin and hypointense on T2W images
  ○ On T1W images with gadolinium, the diverticulum fills with contrast-enhanced urine

Mass Lesions

Benign Masses
Papilloma
- Background
  ○ 2–3% of all primary bladder tumors
  ○ Histologically benign, but may recur or become malignant
  ○ Axial fibrovascular core covered by well-differentiated urothelial layers
- Imaging (fig. 11.1)
  ▪ Best seen on immediate postgadolinium MR images (15–45 seconds)
  ▪ Small enhancing masses arising from lesser enhancing wall

Leiomyoma

- Background
  ○ Most common of the rare benign bladder tumors
  ○ Affects women 30–55 years of age

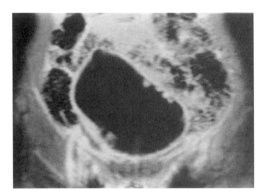

FIGURE 11.1 Multiple papillary tumors. Coronal T1W gadolinium-enhanced fat-suppressed spin-echo image. The enhancing papillomas are well shown as enhancing mass lesions in a background of low signal intensity of nongadolinium-containing urine.

  ○ Most commonly arises at the trigone, less commonly lateral and posterior walls
  ○ Intravesicular location (60%) may present with hematuria
  ○ Extravesicular (30%) and intramural (10%) are asymptomatic
- Imaging
  ○ On T2W images
    ▪ High signal intensity, in contrast to intermediate low-signal-intensity muscle in the bladder wall
    ▪ May have heterogeneous mixed signal intensity if degenerating
  ○ On T1W images
    ▪ Intermediate in signal intensity
    ▪ May have medium to high signal intensity if degenerating
- Mimickers
  ○ Leiomyomas and leiomyosarcomas cannot be consistently distinguished, although large size, heterogeneity, and irregular margins suggest malignancy

Pheochromocytoma
- Background
  ○ Catecholamine-producing tumors arising from chromaffin cells
  ○ Occur along the sympathetic nervous system

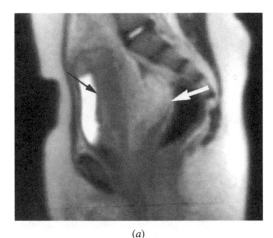

(a)

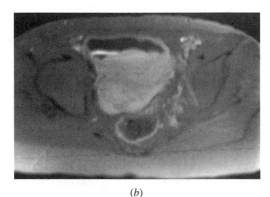

(b)

FIGURE 11.2   Neurofibroma. Sagittal T2W single-shot echo-train spin-echo (*a*) and T1W gadolinium-enhanced fat-suppressed spin-echo (*b*) images in a patient with a history of neurofibromatosis. There is a mildly heterogeneous and hypointense mass (black arrows, *a*) on the T2W image that involves the posterior aspect of the bladder wall and uterus (white arrow, *a*) and displaces the rectum posteriorly. Following gadolinium administration, there is moderately intense and slightly heterogeneous enhancement of the tumor (*b*). Histopathology demonstrated a plexiform neurofibroma in the bladder wall.

- 10–15% extra-adrenal
- 1% located in the bladder with predilection for the trigone
- 7% bladder pheochromocytomas are malignant
- Males and females have an equal incidence, with mean age of 41 years
- Half present with clinical triad of hypertension, gross intermittent hematuria, and attacks of sweating, headache, palpitations induced by micturition
- Characteristic features help distinguish from other tumors, including carcinoma
- Imaging
  - On T2W images: typically markedly increased, homogeneous signal intensity, but signal can be heterogeneously increased
  - On T1W images: hypointense or isointense signal intensity

Neurofibromas
- Background
  - Associated with neurofibromatosis
  - Genitourinary tract neurofibromas are rare, but bladder is most commonly affected

- Obstructive hydronephrosis is a common complication, presumably due to neurofibromas involving the trigone
- Imaging (fig. 11.2)
  - T1W signal intensity slightly greater than that of skeletal muscle
  - Markedly increased signal intensity relative to the surrounding tissues on T2W images
  - Larger tumors may be inhomogeneous with markedly increased signal intensity and well-defined central areas of decreased signal intensity
  - Most demonstrate enhancement with gadolinium administration

Ganglioneuromas
- Background
  - Rare
  - Similar appearance to neurofibromas
- Imaging (fig. 11.3)
  - On T2W images: hyperintense
  - On T1W images: isointense, enhance substantially

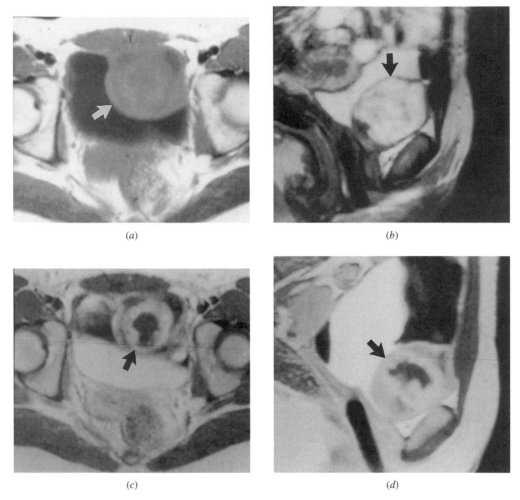

(a)   *(b)*

(c)   *(d)*

FIGURE 11.3   Ganglioneuroma. T1W spin-echo (*a*), sagittal T2W spin-echo (*b*), transverse (*c*), and sagittal (*d*) gadolinium-enhanced T1W spin-echo images. A 4 cm ganglioneuroma arises from the anteroinferior bladder wall. The tumor is intermediate in signal intensity on the T1W image (arrow, *a*), moderately hyperintense on the T2W image (arrow, *b*), and shows substantial enhancement on interstitial phase gadolinium-enhanced images (arrow, *c, d*) with central necrosis. (Courtesy of Hedvig Hricak, M.D., Ph.D.)

Hemangiomas
- Background
  ◦ Rare mesenchymal benign tumor of the bladder
  ◦ Most common presenting symptom is gross, painless hematuria
- Imaging
  ◦ On T2W images: very high signal intensity
  ◦ On T1W images: low signal with a multilocular pattern

Calcifications
- Background
  ◦ Bladder calculi
    ▪ Due to foreign body nidus, stasis, migration of upper tract stone, idiopathic
  ◦ Bladder wall calcification
    ▪ Seen in bilharziasis, usually caused by *Schistosoma haematobium*
    ▪ Symptoms include frequency, urgency, dysuria, flank pain, and hematuria

- Imaging
  - T2W images or late postgadolinium T1W images show considerable signal difference between high-signal-intensity urine and signal-void calculi within the bladder
  - Wall calcification is characteristically linear and continuous along the bladder wall, signal void on all MRI sequences

Malignant Masses

Overview

- Bladder cancer is the most common cancer of the urinary tract
- Incidence increases with age, most commonly seen in the sixth and seventh decades
- Incidence rising due to increased exposure to carcinogens such as tobacco, artificial sweeteners, coffee, cyclophosphamides, and various aromatic amines
- Classification based on three criteria
  - Cell type (urothelial, squamous, or glandular)
  - Pattern of growth (papillary, nonpapillary, noninfiltrating, or infiltrating)
  - Grading (degree of cellular differentiation)
- Nonpapillary urothelial tumors include
  - Invasive transitional cell carcinoma
  - Squamous cell carcinoma
  - Adenocarcinoma
  - Spindle cell carcinoma

Staging of Bladder Neoplasms

T0	No evidence of primary tumor
Ta	Noninvasive papillary carcinoma
Tis	Carcinoma in situ: "flat tumor"
T1	Tumor invades subepithelial connective tissue
T2	Tumor invades superficial muscle
T3	Tumor invades deep muscle or perivesical fat
T3a	Tumor invades deep muscle (outer half)
T3b	Tumor invades perivesical fat

T4	Tumor invades any of the following: prostate, uterus, vagina, pelvic wall, or abdominal wall
T4a	Tumor invades the prostate, uterus, or vagina
T4b	Tumor invades the pelvic or abdominal wall
N0	No regional lymph node metastases
N1	One homolateral solitary regional node (internal or external iliac)
N2–3	Contralateral or bilateral or multiple lymph node metastases
N4	Juxtaregional (common iliac, inguinal, or aortic) lymph node metastases
M0	No distant metastases
M1	Distant metastases or nodes above aortic bifurcation

Transitional Cell Carcinoma

- Background
  - Most common primary bladder malignancy, 85% of all bladder malignancies
  - Spread of invasive urothelial cancer:
    Radially through the wall of the bladder → circumferentially through the muscular layer → perivesical fat → prostate, seminal vesicles, or obturator internus muscles
  - Invasion of ureters or urethra common if tumor originates nearby
  - In women, rarely invades the uterus or cervix
  - 70–80% of bladder cancers diagnosed early stage with a 5-year survival rate of 81%
  - Overall 5-year mortality rate is almost 50%
  - Selection of appropriate treatment for bladder cancer depends on accurate diagnosis and staging
    - Superficial neoplasm: treated with transurethral resection and instillation of chemotherapeutic agents, BCG therapy, or both
    - Involvement of the superficial muscle layer: segmental cystectomy

- Invasive neoplasm/limited perivesical fat involvement: radical cystectomy
- Extension outside bladder into adjacent pelvic structures: presurgical chemotherapy or palliative radiation therapy
- MR useful to differentiate between muscular invasion (stage T3a) and invasion into the perivesical fat (stage T3b)
- Most common staging error in MRI (and CT) is overstaging
- Prior cystoscopic biopsy common cause of overstaging; MR should be performed at least 3 weeks after bladder biopsy
- Imaging
  - On T2W images
    - May differentiate superficial (stage T1) (fig. 11.4) and deep invasion of the muscular layer of the bladder wall (stage T3a) (fig. 11.5)
    - Intact dark bladder wall on T2W images: stage Tis, T1, or T2
- Bladder wall breached: stage T3a or higher
  - On T1W images
    - Invasion appears as low signal in the perivesical fat
    - Lymph nodes are low signal relative to surrounding fat
    - Metastases are low signal relative to bone marrow
    - Tumors typically show substantial enhancement with gadolinium
    - Well seen approximately 5–15 s after arterial enhancement, carcinomas enhance more than the surrounding bladder wall early after injection of contrast
    - Fast dynamic MR imaging differentiates between tumor and postbiopsy change, as tumor enhances earlier than postbiopsy tissue (6.5 s versus 13.6 s)
    - 2–5 min postcontrast fat-suppressed SGE images show lymph nodes and bone marrow metastases

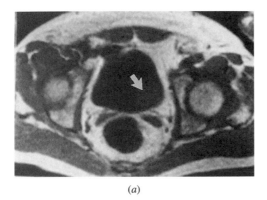

(a)

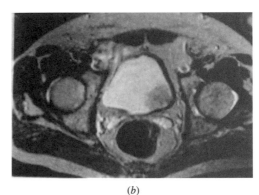

(b)

FIGURE 11.4 Transitional cell cancer, superficial invasion. T1W SGE (a), T2W echo-train spin-echo (b), and immediate postgadolinium SGE (c) images in a patient with superficial T1 transitional cell bladder cancer. The tumor is intermediate in signal intensity on the T1W image (arrow, a) and moderately high in signal intensity on the T2W image (b). Moderately intense tumor enhancement is appreciated on the postgadolinium image (c), and lack of wall invasion is shown. Intact low-signal-intensity muscular wall deep to the tumor is appreciated on the T2W (b) and immediate postgadolinium SGE (c) images.

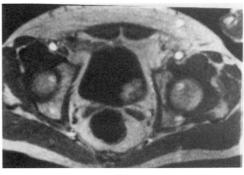

(c)

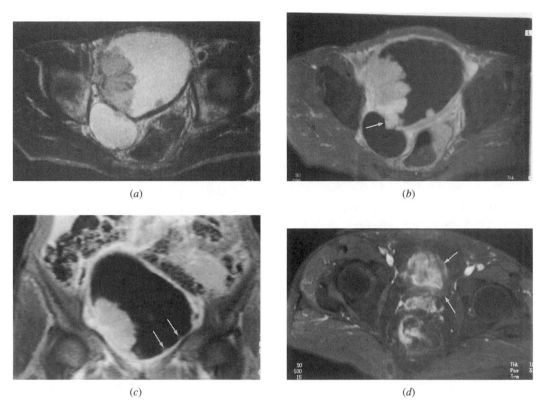

(a)   (b)

(c)   (d)

FIGURE 11.5   Invasive transitional cell carcinoma. T2W echo-train spin-echo (*a*), T1W gadolinium-enhanced fat-suppressed spin-echo (*b*), and coronal interstitial phase gadolinium-enhanced SGE (*c*) images. A frond-like, T3a papillary transitional cell cancer arises from the right lateral wall of the bladder. Note that the lesion extends into a diverticulum (arrow, *b*). On the T2W image, the low-signal-intensity muscular wall is not infiltrated by tumor (*a*). Multiple small papillomas are also identified (arrows, *c*).

▪ Enlarged hyperplastic lymph nodes and malignant nodes may look similar—another potential cause of overstaging (fig. 11.6)
- Mimickers
  ○ Other bladder tumors may have identical appearance
  ○ Fibrosis may be difficult to distinguish from tumor recurrence
    ▪ Following resolution of acute edema at 1 year, residual scar can be distinguished from recurrence of tumor using T2W images
    ▪ Fibrosis is low in signal intensity, whereas tumor recurrence is heterogeneous and moderate in signal intensity

▪ Prior to resolution of the edema, distinction between granulation tissue and recurrence is problematic

Squamous Cell Carcinoma
- Background
  ○ Most common form of neoplasia in chronic inflammation of the urinary bladder
  ○ Rare in Western countries, but is the most frequent form of bladder neoplasm (55%) in patients with schistosomiasis associated with squamous metaplasia
- Imaging
  ○ Intermediate in signal intensity on T1W images
  ○ Enhances with gadolinium
- Mimickers

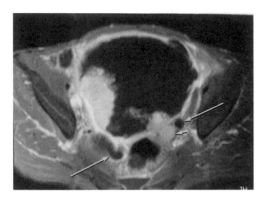

FIGURE 11.6 Transitional cell cancer and hyperplasic lymph node. T1W gadolinium-enhanced fat-suppressed spin-echo image. Multiple various-size papillary cancers are present with substantial enhancement of the mucosa following gadolinium administration. A 1.2 cm lymph node (small, arrow) is shown, which was considered consistent with nodal disease. At histopathology the enlarged nodes were benign and hyperplastic. Note also the dilated ureters (long arrows).

- Usually not distinguishable from transitional cell carcinoma

Adenocarcinoma
- Background
  - Rare
  - Found in patients with exstrophy of the bladder
  - Most commonly arises secondarily as extension from adjacent organs
  - As with squamous cell carcinoma, prognosis is poor
  - Most common tumor to arise at the vesicourachal remnant, but may arise in any location
- Imaging (fig. 11.7)
  - On T2W images: heterogeneous and moderately high signal
  - On T1W images: intermediate signal, enhances with gadolinium

Spindle Cell Carcinoma
- Background
  - Also known as carcinosarcoma
  - Contains spindle and giant cells
  - Epithelial component is most often transitional cell carcinoma
  - Prognosis is poor
- Imaging
  - Bulky tumors
  - Invariably deeply invade the bladder wall

Malignant Nonepithelial Neoplasms
- Background
  - Leiomyosarcoma, rhabdomyosarcoma, and lymphoma
  - Collectively account for less than 10% of all primary bladder tumors
- Imaging
  - On T2W images
    - High signal intensity
    - Intravesical disease may be obscured due to similar signal intensity of urine and tumor
  - On T1W images
    - Isointense to bladder wall
    - Early dynamic gadolinium-enhanced T1W images helpful for detecting bladder wall involvement
    - As on T2W images, intravesical tumor may be obscured on delayed post-gadolinium T1W images

Urachal Carcinoma
- Background
  - Urachus persists as a midline musculofibrous tube that can extend from the bladder dome to the umbilicus
  - Annual incidence of urachal carcinoma is estimated to be 1 in 5 million
  - Majority occur in men between the ages of 40 and 70
  - At presentation, the tumor is usually advanced. Overall 5-year survival is 10%.
  - Majority are adenocarcinomas
  - 75% mucin producing, may calicify
- Imaging
  - On T2W images: heterogeneous high signal
  - On T1W images: usually low signal, although signal characteristics vary due to differences in mucin content or necrosis

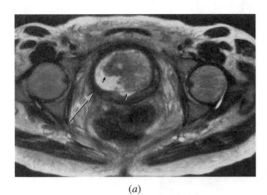

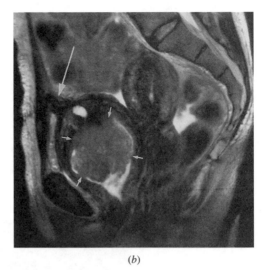

(a)   (b)

FIGURE 11.7   Adenocarcinoma. Transverse (*a*) and sagittal (*b*) T2W echo-train spin-echo images. A large pedunculated adenocarcinoma (short arrows, *a*, *b*) arises from the dome of the bladder. Diffuse bladder wall thickening is noted (long arrow, *a*). Heterogeneous signal of the bladder wall on the T2W image reflects deep bladder wall invasion. A urachal remnant is apparent on sagittal plane images (long arrow, *b*).

Metastatic Neoplasms
- Background
  - Direct invasion most common, may occur secondary to prostate, rectosigmoid, and uterine adenocarcinomas
  - Most common distant metastases: melanoma and gastric carcinoma
- Imaging (fig. 11.8)
  - Direct invasion obscures fat planes and may thicken bladder wall
  - Sagittal plane imaging is particularly effective for rectal and gynecological malignancies

Lymphoma
- Background
  - Bladder involvement more common in non-Hodgkin's lymphoma than Hodgkin's disease
  - Secondary bladder lymphoma more common than primary bladder lymphoma; occurs late in disease from direct invasion of pelvic masses
  - Primary bladder lymphoma has a relatively good prognosis, with the tumor remaining localized for a long period of time

- Imaging
  - Thickened bladder wall with intermediate signal intensity on T1W and T2W images
  - Mild gadolinium enhancement on early and late images
  - In secondary bladder lymphoma, tumor is of similar signal intensity to involved regional lymph nodes

Miscellaneous

Hypertrophy
- Background
  - Results from bladder outlet obstruction due to benign prostatic enlargement (the most common cause in males), prostate cancer, large pelvic tumors, bladder neck obstruction (functional or anatomic), and hydrocolpos
- Imaging
  - Thickened bladder wall, low in signal intensity on T2W images
  - Does not enhance substantially with gadolinium
  - Mucosal edema related to bladder outlet obstruction is usually located around the

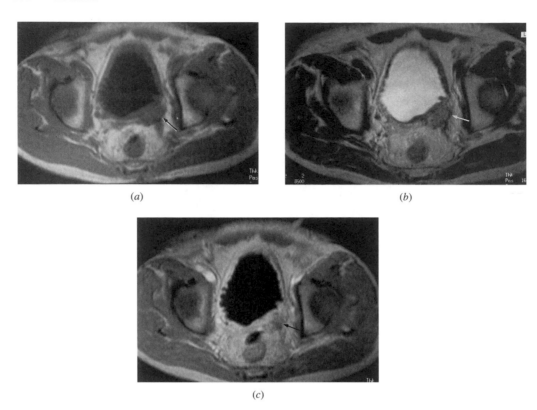

(a)   (b)

(c)

FIGURE 11.8   Bladder invasion by malignant disease–prostate cancer. T1W SGE (a), T2W single-shot echo-train spin-echo (b), and T1W postgadolinium SGE (c) images in a patient with recurrent prostate cancer invading the bladder. Tumor is intermediate in signal intensity on T1W (arrow, a) and T2W (arrow, b) images, and enhances minimally with gadolinium (arrow, c).

urethral orifice and is high signal intensity on T2W images
- Mimickers
  - Edema: thickened bladder wall, distinguished from bladder wall hypertrophy by its high signal intensity on T2W images

Cystitis
- Background
  - Due to infection, foreign bodies within the bladder, peritonitis, drug toxicity, or other causes
- Imaging (fig. 11.9)
  - Thickened bladder wall, may be focal or diffuse
  - On T2W images
    - Four layers can be appreciated within the inflamed bladder wall

- Innermost low-signal-intensity and inner high-signal-intensity bands represent the thickened epithelium and lamina propria, respectively
- Outer low-signal-intensity and outermost intermediate-signal-intensity represent the inner compact muscle layer and outer loose muscle layer, respectively
  - On T1W images
    - Increased enhancement after gadolinium administration
    - Extent of enhancement reflects the severity of the inflammatory process

Hemorrhagic Cystitis
- Background
  - Severe form of cystitis characterized by hematuria

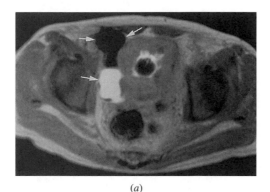
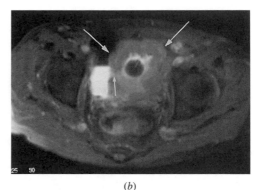

(*a*)   (*b*)

FIGURE 11.9   Bladder inflammation. 90 s postgadolinium SGE (*a*) and T1W postgadolinium fat-suppressed spin-echo (*b*) images in a patient with inflammation secondary to infection. Diffuse bladder wall thickening is present (arrows, *b*) and a large gadolinium-containing diverticulum (arrows, *a*) is identified arising from the right aspect of the bladder. A small high-signal-intensity tract represents the communication between the bladder and the diverticulum (short arrow, *b*).

- Due to radiation or infectious agents including *Escherichia coli* and viruses
- Imaging (fig. 11.10)
  - Thickened bladder wall
  - Complex signal based on the T1 and T2 characteristics of aging blood products

Granulomatous Disease
- Background
  - Bladder involvement common in genitourinary tuberculosis
  - Presents with dysuria and frequency
  - Earliest manifestations are mucosal edema and ulcerations, primarily surrounding the ureteral orifices, which can produce obstruction
- Imaging
  - Tuberculomas in the bladder wall can be large and simulate mass lesions
  - Focal granulomatous reactions are high signal intensity on T2W images
  - Epithelioid granulomatous lesions can occur with immunotherapy and may appear similar to malignant tumors

Pelvic Lipomatosis
- Background
  - Predominantly affects black males between the ages of 25 and 55
  - Can present with frequency, dysuria, perineal pain, or suprapubic discomfort

  - Benign process, but can cause renal failure and rectal compression
- Imaging
  - Extensive fat in pelvis, high signal on T1W images
  - Mass effect on bladder

Fistulas
- Background
  - May result from obstetrical procedures, surgery, trauma, radiation, infection, inflammatory bowel disease, or pelvic malignancies
  - Present with urinary or fecal incontinence, pneumaturia, fecaluria, or vaginal discharge
- Imaging
  - Sagittal plane effective at demonstrating vesicocervical fistulas because it displays these fistulas in profile
  - Typically insert low in the bladder, a region less well evaluated on transverse images due to volume averaging of the pelvic floor musculature
  - Gadolinium-enhanced T1W images with fat suppression best demonstrate bladder fistulas
    - On early postgadolinium images, the fistula wall is high signal and the tract is low signal

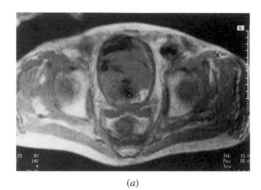

(a)

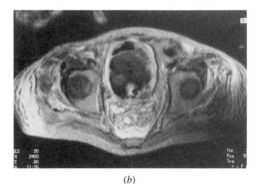

(b)

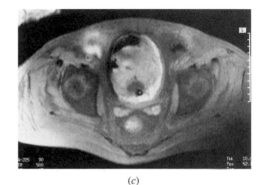

(c)

FIGURE 11.10 Hemorrhagic cystitis. T1W SGE (a), T2W spin-echo (b), and T1W fat-suppressed spin-echo (c) images in a patient with hemorrhagic cystitis. The bladder wall and intraluminal fluid show varying signal intensities, which represent the different phases of hemoglobin degradation.

- Late postgadolinium images may show high signal fluid within the fistula tract

Bladder Reconstruction
- Background
  - A variety of bladder surgical procedures are performed to alter the native bladder (e.g., bladder augmentation) or to create a neobladder (e.g., Indiana pouch)
- Imaging
  - MRI may be used to evaluate the reconstructed bladder and to examine for surgical complications or status of the kidneys
  - Delayed postgadolinium T1W images may be helpful to distinguish neobladder from bowel

Radiation Changes
- Background
  - Bullous edema may persist for months or years, and can progress to radiation cystitis with fibrosis and a contracted bladder

  - Bladder disease common when dose exceeds 4,500 cGy
  - Abnormalities on MRI may be present in the absence of symptoms
- Imaging
  - Mildest form
    - High signal intensity of the bladder mucosa on T2W images
    - Preservation of the bladder wall thickness
  - More severe injury
    - Wall thickening with uniformly high signal, or low signal in the inner layer with high signal at the periphery, on T2W images
    - Bladder wall shows increased enhancement, sometimes without other morphological changes on noncontrast images
    - Enhancement may occur up to 2.5 years after irradiation
  - Extreme radiation change
    - Fistula or sinus tracts
    - Other findings of radiation changes commonly present

CHAPTER 12

MALE PELVIS

BACKGROUND

MRI is an effective modality for the diagnosis, staging, and, follow-up of a variety of diseases affecting the male pelvis. Transverse and sagittal T2W echo-train spin-echo as well as postgadolinium transverse and sagittal fat-suppressed SGE sequences are used. The routine use of a phased-array multicoil results in reproducible high image quality. Endorectal coils may provide superior resolution for evaluation of prostate cancer. Supplemental T1W imaging through the abdomen and pelvis should be performed to assess for lymphadenopathy in cases of suspected malignancy.

Prostate and Posterior Urethra

Normal Anatomy
Prostate
- Background
  - Central zone
    - Periurethral
    - Surrounds verumontanum
  - Transitional zone
    - Surrounds central zone
    - Predominantly located within the base
    - Increases in size with age
  - Peripheral zone

- Greatest percentage of the gland
- Mostly in prostatic apex and midgland
- Posterior and posterolateral in location
- Imaging
  - T2W images: zonal anatomy well seen (fig. 12.1)
    - Peripheral zone: increased signal (abundant glandular material)
    - Central zone: decreased signal (more striated muscle and stroma)
    - Transitional zone: similar to central zone (large volume of stroma)
  - T1W images: prostate is homogeneous, intermediate signal, zonal anatomy not seen
  - Specific anatomic structures can be identified on high-resolution images
    - The anterior fibromuscular band
      - Surrounds anterolateral prostate
      - Low signal on T1W and T2W images
      - Divides prostate from preprostatic space
    - Prostatic capsule
      - Comprised of fibromuscular tissue, low signal on T2W images
    - Verumontanum
      - Central ovoid periurethral structure in midgland, high signal on T2W images
    - Neurovascular bundles

Primer on MR Imaging of the Abdomen and Pelvis, edited by Diego R. Martin, Michele A. Brown, and Richard C. Semelka ISBN 0-471-37340-0 Copyright © 2005 Wiley-Liss, Inc.

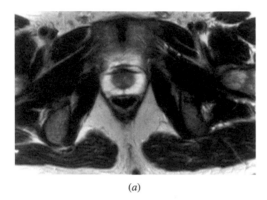
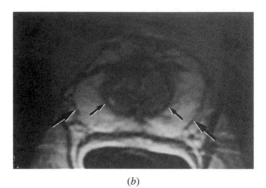

(a)   (b)

FIGURE 12.1   Normal prostate. Transverse T2W echo-train spin-echo image (*a*). The peripheral zone is high in signal intensity and surrounds the lower-signal transitional and central zones. T2W endorectal coil image (*b*) in a second patient demonstrates the central and transitional zones (short arrows, *b*) and the peripheral zone (long arrows, *b*).

- Posterolateral at 5 and 7 o'clock recto-prostatic angles

Posterior Urethra
- Background
  - Prostatic and membranous portions
- Imaging
  - Distal prostatic urethra: low-signal round structure in high-signal peripheral zone at apex on T2W images
  - Membranous urethra: extends from apex to bulb of penis; muscular wall forms external sphincter where Cowper's glands are located

Disease Entities

Congenital Abnormalities

Cyst
- Background
  - Most commonly encountered congenital anomalies of the prostate
  - Occur between prostatic urethra and bladder anteriorly or rectum posteriorly
  - Müllerian duct cysts may present with urinary retention, infection, or stone formation and are associated with increased incidence of squamous cell and adenocarcinomas
- Imaging
  - Generally high signal on T2W images
  - Variable signal on T1W images, depending on infection or hemorrhage
  - Characterized by location, which may be midline, paramedian, or lateral
    - Midline cysts
      - Utricular cysts (fig. 12.2)
        - Usually teardrop shaped, communicate with posterior urethra
        - Frequently associated with other genital anomalies
      - Müllerian duct cysts (fig. 12.3)
        - Do not communicate with posterior urethra
        - Connected by a stalk to verumontanum
        - Usually retrovesical in location
        - Rarely associated with renal agenesis
    - Paramedian cysts
      - Ejaculatory duct cysts
        - Congenital or postinflammatory
        - Generally result from obstruction along ductal system
      - Vas deferens cysts
        - Extremely rare
        - Most frequently involve the ampulla
- Mimickers
  - Large paramedian cysts may be identical to utricular or müllerian duct cysts
  - Aspirated cyst fluid contains spermatozoa, permitting differentiation from müllerian duct cysts

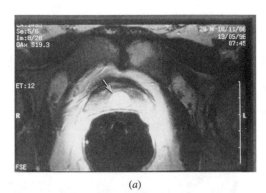

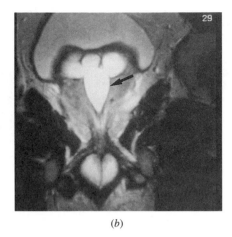

(a)   (b)

FIGURE 12.2   Utricular cyst. Transverse (*a*) and coronal (*b*) T2W spin-echo endorectal coil images. A rounded central structure is high signal and represents a utricular cyst.

Prostatic Agenesis and Hypoplasia
- Background
  ○ Much rarer anomalies
  ○ Often associated with other anomalies of genitourinary tract

Mass Lesions

Benign Masses
Benign Prostatic Hyperplasia (BPH)
- Background
  ○ Proliferation of glandular or interstitial elements of transitional zone
  ○ Observed in 50% of men over 45

- Imaging
  ○ T2W images (fig. 12.4)
    ▪ Usually medium to high signal, homogeneous or heterogeneous
    ▪ Compression of adjacent peripheral zone causes low-signal band called the surgical pseudocapsule
    ▪ Areas of infarction may be low signal
    ▪ Cystic ectasia (dilatation of glandular elements) is high signal
    ▪ Hyperplastic changes that predominantly involve the interstitium may cause heterogeneous low signal of enlarged gland

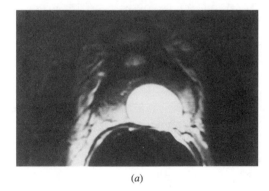

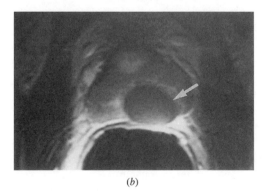

(a)   (b)

FIGURE 12.3   Müllerian cyst. Transverse T2W spin-echo (*a*) and immediate postgadolinium fat-suppressed T1 SGE (*b*) endorectal coil images. A large, ovoid müllerian cyst is seen in the dorsal aspect of the prostate near the midline, which is high in signal intensity on the T2W image (*a*) and intermediate in signal intensity on the postgadolinium image (white arrow, *b*).

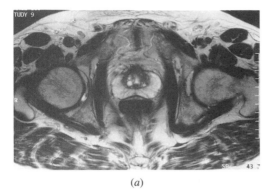

(a)

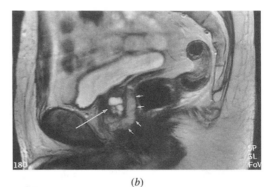

(b)

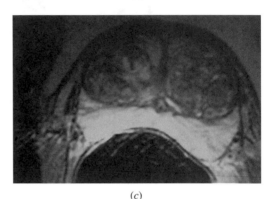

(c)

FIGURE 12.4 Benign prostatic hyperplasia. Transverse (*a*) and sagittal (*b*) T2W ETSE image. High-signal-intensity foci are present, representing cystic elements of interstitial BPH (long arrow, *b*). Normal signal intensity is seen within the surrounding peripheral zone (short arrows, *b*).

Transverse T2W ETSE endorectal coil image (*c*) in a second patient. Diffuse heterogeneous low signal intensity within an enlarged central gland is consistent with the predominantly glandular subtype of BPH.

- ▪ Focal alterations in signal may result from infarction or cystic changes within nodules of glandular BPH
  - ◦ T1W images
    - ▪ Low signal
    - ▪ Adenomatous changes may result in focal, nodular enlargement
- • Mimickers
  - ◦ Carcinoma: hyperplasia may occasionally infiltrate the peripheral zone, making distinction from carcinoma problematic

Postoperative Changes
- • Background
  - ◦ After surgical removal of periurethral tissue (transurethral, transvesical, or retropubic approach), prostatic urethra dilates to level of verumontanum
  - ◦ Widening of the prostatic urethra occurs following all forms of prostatectomies
  - ◦ Immediately following prostatectomy, the prostatic fossa is very wide and narrows over several weeks

- ◦ Residual prostatectomy defect is typically observed for years
- • Imaging
  - ◦ Configuration of the widening after cryocaustic prostate surgery is bottle shaped and different from that of transurethral resection (fig. 12.5)
  - ◦ Residual hyperplastic tissue may be low to medium signal on T2W images
  - ◦ Radical prostatectomy may result in periurethral scarring, also low signal on T2W images (fig. 12.6)
  - ◦ Fibrosis in the prostatic bed following total prostatectomy is low signal on T2W images and may mimic a small low-signal prostate and seminal vesicles

Malignant Masses
Rare Tumors
- • Background
  - ◦ Squamous cell cancer, transitional cell cancer, and sarcoma

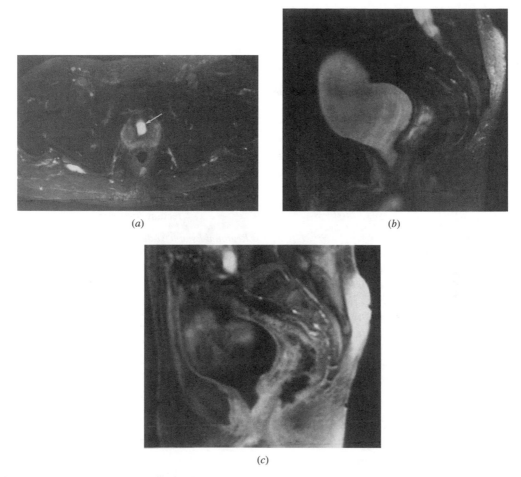

(a)   (b)

(c)

FIGURE 12.5   Defect from transurethral resection of the prostate (TRUP). Transverse (*a*) and sagittal (*b*) T2W fat-suppressed echo-train spin-echo and sagittal postgadolinium SGE (*c*) images. Dilatation of the prostatic urethra is observed after TURP.

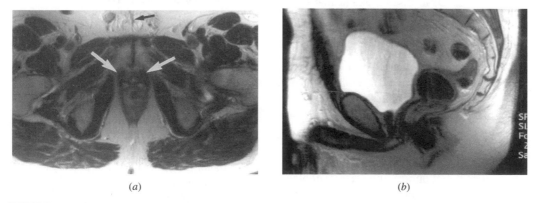

(a)   (b)

FIGURE 12.6   Postprostatectomy pelvis. Transversal (*a*) and sagittal (*b*) T2W ETSE images. Low-signal-intensity tissue surrounds the posterior urethra within the prostatic bed (white arrows, *a*) of this patient after prostatectomy. This appearance results from fibrosis and scarring at the operative site. Note the midline scar in the subcutaneous tissue (black arrow, *a*), which is a constant observation in postprostatectomy patients.

○ Uncommon, account for less than 5% of malignant prostatic tumors

Prostate Adenocarcinoma
• Background
  ○ Approximately 95% of malignant prostate lesions
  ○ Frequently latent, occurs in 80% of men over 80 and 50% of men over 50
  ○ Behavior depends on histological grade/stage and tumor volume
  ○ Approximately 70% arise in peripheral zone; remainder arise in transitional and central zones
  ○ Tumor spread
    Penetrates prostatic capsule → extends to the neurovascular bundles and seminal vesicles → invades bladder in advanced stage, may be extensive → infiltrates pelvic lymphatics, particularly obturator, external and internal iliac chains (precedes distant metastases to the bones and retroperitoneum) → metastasizes, most commonly to bone marrow and lymph nodes
  ○ Staging
    ▪ Table 12.1 outlines the American Joint Committee on Cancer's TNM staging classification of prostate carcinoma
    ▪ Table 12.2 briefly outlines the American Urological Association staging system developed by Whitmore and Jewett, which assigns alphabetical stages (A through D) to disease extent that corresponds roughly to the primary tumor staging (T1 through T4) of the TNM system
    ▪ Histologic grading may be by degree of anaplasia, DNA ploidy (diploid, tetraploid, or anaploid), or Gleason score, which sums the scores of the two most predominant glandular patterns of the tumor to predict aggressivity
  ○ Therapy
    ▪ Clinical assessment and treatment decisions based on imaging stage, pathological grade, prostate-specific antigen (PSA) levels, as well as patient age and general health

TABLE 12.1 American Joint Committee on Cancer Staging of Prostate

Carcinoma	

Primary Tumor

T0	No evidence of primary tumor
T1	Clinical inapparent, not visible by imaging
T2	Tumor confined to the prostate (may involve capsule)
T3	Tumor extends beyond capsule (may involve seminal vesicles)
T4	Invasion of adjacent structures other than seminal vesicles (bladder, rectum, levator m.)

Regional Lymph Nodes

N0	No regional lymph node metastasis
N1	Metastasis in a single node, 2 cm or smaller
N2	Metastasis in single node between 2 and 5 cm in size, or in multiple nodes each 5 cm or smaller
N3	Metastasis in a single node larger than 5 cm

Distant Metastasis

M0	No distant metastasis
M1	Distant metastasis (regional nodes, bone, other sites)

  ▪ Currently accepted therapies for stages A, B, and C disease are radical prostatectomy and radiation therapy with external beam irradiation or radioisotope implants
  ▪ Radical prostatectomy generally reserved for stage A or B disease
  ▪ Stage D disease treated palliatively with hormonal or radiation therapies

TABLE 12.2 American Urological Association Staging of Prostate Carcinoma

A	Clinical inapparent
B	Tumor cofined to the prostate
C	Tumor extends beond capsule (may involve seminal vesicles)
D	Metastatic disease to pelvic or distant nodes, bones, soft tissues, or organs

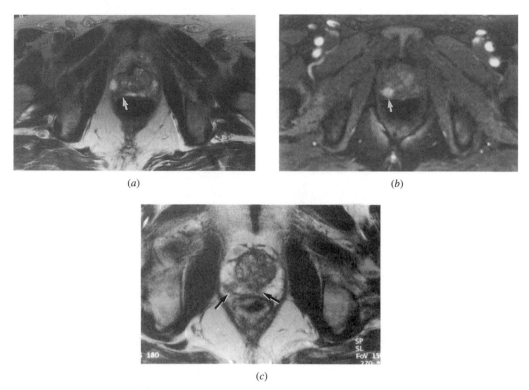

(a)   (b)

(c)

FIGURE 12.7   Prostate carcinoma. Transverse T2W ETSE (*a*) and transverse immediate postgadolinium fat-suppressed SGE (*b*) images. High-resolution T2W image (*a*) reveals a well-defined carcinoma within the peripheral zone of the right lobe of the prostate (arrow, *a*). Smaller tumor volume is present within the left lobe (*a*). Immediate postgadolinium image demonstrates enhancement of the tumor focus within the right lobe (arrow, *b*). More ill-defined enhancement is seen within the left lobe (*b*).

Transverse T2W ETSE (*c*) images in a second patient. There is a heterogeneous enlargement of the central aspect of the prostate consistent with prostatic hypertrophy. Several foci of low signal are noted at the 6 and 8 o'clock positions (arrow, *c*) within the gland consistent with prostate cancer.

- Detection of extracapsular extension precludes radical prostatectomy in younger patients
- Imaging (figs. 12.7, 12.8, and 12.9)
  - MRI detection limited primarily to tumors in peripheral zone
  - Increased staging accuracy can be achieved with T2W endorectal coil MRI and PSA values
  - Identifying invasion of neurovascular bundles is important because preservation of one or both bundles during radical prostatectomy significantly decreases incidence of impotency
  - On T2W images
    - Most tumors are hypointense, rarely isointense or hyperintense
    - When isolated to transitional zone, may appear heterogeneous, isointense, or hypointense, difficult to differentiate from BPH
    - Seminal vesicle invasion is seen as low signal
  - On T1W images
    - Generally isointense to peripheral zone
    - Tumors in peripheral zone demonstrate increased enhancement on immediate postgadolinium fat-suppressed SGE images

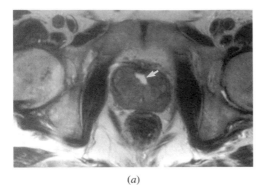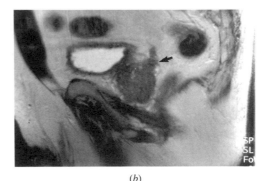

(a)   (b)

FIGURE 12.8 **Prostate carcinoma, diffuse involvement.** Transverse (a) and sagittal (b) SS-ETSE images. The prostate is enlarged with a transurethral prostatic resection defect in the superior aspect of the gland (arrow, a). The peripheral zone of the prostate is diffusely low signal on T2W images consistent with diffuse tumor infiltration. This is shown on both transverse and sagittal projection. Note seminal vesicle involvement on the sagittal projection (arrow, b).

- Bone metastases best seen on post-gadolinium fat-suppressed T1W images
  - Signs used to predict stage C disease by MRI
    - Focal contour abnormalities in prostatic capsule
    - Tumor volume
    - Apical location
    - Broad margins with the prostate capsule
    - Infiltration of the periprostatic fat
  - Neurovascular invasion may be seen as
    - Direct tumor extension posterolaterally into neurovascular bundles
    - Decreased signal obliterating the recto-prostatic angle
    - Focal contour abnormality in the posterolateral gland on transverse T2W images

  - Effect of therapy on MRI appearance
    - Hormonal and radiation therapies may cause low signal within the prostate
    - Cryosurgery may result in necrosis and loss of zonal anatomy
    - Postbiopsy hemorrhage may cause high signal in peripheral zone or seminal vesicles on T1W and T2W images; may conceal underlying tumor (fig. 12.10)
    - MRI should generally be delayed at least 3 weeks following intervention
- Mimickers
  - BPH involving the peripheral zone
  - Chronic prostatitis
  - Prostate metastasis (fig. 12.11)

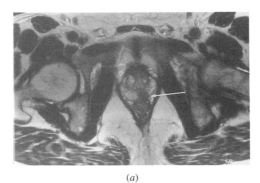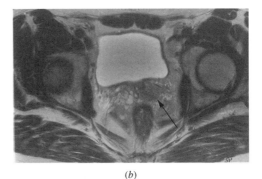

(a)   (b)

FIGURE 12.9 **Prostate cancer with seminal vesicle invasion.** Transverse T2W echo-train spin-echo images. A 1 cm tumor (white arrow, a) within the left aspect of the prostate at the midgland level is low signal. The left seminal vesicle (black arrow, b) is diffusely low in signal due to tumor involvement.

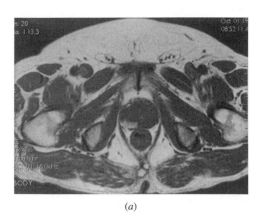

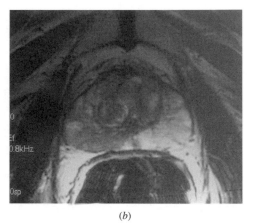

(a)   (b)

FIGURE 12.10   Postbiopsy hemorrhage within the prostate. Transverse T1W spin-echo (*a*) and endorectal coil T1W echo-train spin-echo (*b*) images demonstrate biopsy changes in the right aspect of the peripheral zone that appear high signal on T1 and low signal on T2. Biopsy changes may simulate or mask prostate cancer on T2W images. High signal on T1W images identifies hemorrhage.

Diffuse Disease

Prostatic Calcifications
- Background
  - Primary: form in ductal and acinar components

  - Acquired: arise in prostatic urethra or secondary to other etiologies, including infection, obstruction, necrosis, and radiation therapy
- Imaging
  - Signal-void focus on T1W and T2W images

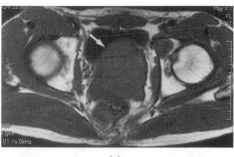

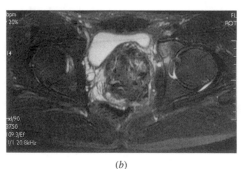

(a)   (b)

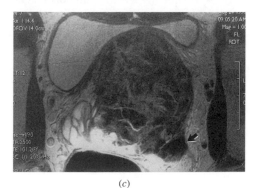

(c)

FIGURE 12.11   Prostate metastasis. T1W spin-echo (*a*), T2W echo-train spin echo (*b*), and endorectal coil transverse T2W echo-train spin-echo (*c*) images in a patient with colon cancer. A large metastasis is present in the prostate that is isointense on T1 (arrow, *a*) and heterogeneous and mildly hypointense on T2 (*b*, *c*). The left seminal vesicle is also extensively invaded (arrow, *c*).

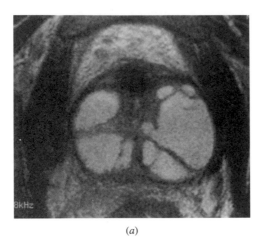
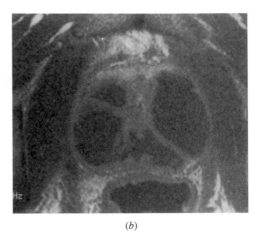

(a)   (b)

FIGURE 12.12   Prostate abscess. Endorectal T2W echo-train spin-echo (a) and gadolinium-enhanced T1W spin-echo (b) images. The prostate is enlarged and contains multiple fluid-filled spaces with intervening strands of prostate stroma. This appearance is consistent with extensive prostate abscess.

○ Primary are classically curvilinear
○ Acquired are generally larger and more irregular
○ Age-related changes are seen
  ▪ Peripheral zone enlarges 67% and central gland enlarges 175% between second and eighth decades
  ▪ Zonal anatomy becomes more clearly defined
  ▪ Periprostatic venous plexus and anterior fibromuscular stroma less easily distinguished

Inflammation and Infection

Prostatitis
• Background
  ○ Bacterial or nonbacterial in origin
  ○ 90–95% infectious prostatitis due to gram-negative organisms
    ▪ Approximately 80% *Escherichia coli*
    ▪ 10–15% klebsiella, serratia, proteus, pseudomonas, and enterobacter
  ○ 5–10% gram-positive organisms: enterococcus, streptococcus, staphylococcus
• Imaging
  ○ Acute prostatitis
    ▪ On T2W images
      • Enlarged gland with high signal in peripheral zone

    ▪ On T1W images
      • Low signal in peripheral zone
      • Areas of inflammation enhance avidly with gadolinium
      • May see extension of low signal into periprostatic fat
  ○ Chronic prostatitis
    ▪ Lesser inflammatory changes
    ▪ Focal low signal in peripheral zone may be seen in chronic granulomatous prostatitis and simulate prostate carcinoma
  ○ Abscesses (fig. 12.12)
    ▪ T2W images
      • Focal enlargement
      • Often very high signal
    ▪ T1W images
      • Frequently see inflammatory changes in the periprostatic fat
      • Enhancement of wall surrounding a signal-void center on gadolinium-enhanced images

Trauma

Posterior Urethral Trauma
• Background
  ○ Usually due to crush injuries or extensive pelvic fracturing

- May cause complete disruption of prostatomembranous urethra with erectile dysfunction and stricture formation
- Superior prostatic displacement seen on imaging may alter surgical approach
- Imaging
  - Disruption of the posterior urethra identified by urethral discontinuity and a low-signal-intensity band on T2W images
  - Stricture-associated fibrosis low signal on T1W and T2W images
  - Sagittal T2W images depicting elevation of prostatic apex above pubic symphysis may indicate suprapubic approach or pubectomy

Penis and Anterior Urethra
Normal Anatomy

Anatomy of the Penis and Anterior Urethra
- Background
  - Penis
    - Ventral compartment contains corpus spongiosum
    - Dorsal compartment contains the paired corpora cavernosa
    - Compartments separated by Buck's fascia, which encases the thin layer of tunica albuginea surrounding the ventral compartment and thicker layer surrounding the dorsal compartment
    - Posterior portion of the corpus spongiosum expands to form bulb of the penis, which is attached to the urogenital diaphragm
    - Inferior and lateral to bulb lies the bulbospongiosus muscle
    - Posterior aspects of corpora cavernosa form the crura, which are attached to the ischiopubic ramus and contiguous with the ischiocavernosus muscles inferomedially
  - Anterior urethra
    - Separated into bulbous and penile portions by the suspensory ligament
    - Surrounded by the corpus spongiosum
- Imaging (fig. 12.13)
  - Circular surface coil or a phased-array multicoil needed to achieve a good signal-to-noise ratio and spatial resolution
  - Greater delineation of anterior urethral and penile anatomy is achieved with fat saturation techniques
  - On T2W images
    - Corpus spongiosum is homogeneous high signal intensity
    - Corpora cavernosa may be homogeneously or heterogeneously increased

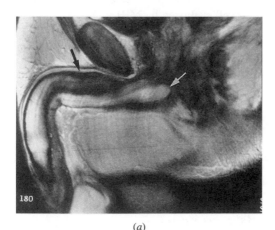

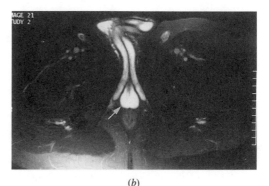

(*a*) (*b*)

FIGURE 12.13 Normal penis. Sagittal T2W ETSE image (*a*). The corpus cavernosum is high in signal intensity on the T2W image (black arrow, *a*). The high signal intensity of the bulb of the penis is seen posteriorly (white arrow, *a*).

A T2W fat-suppressed ETSE image (*b*) in a second patient. The bulb of the penis is well defined as a high-signal-intensity structure (white arrow, *b*).

signal, depending on perfusion distribution
- Fascial layers are low signal
- The bulb of the penis is high signal and may be a useful landmark
- The urethra and cavernous arteries are low-signal tubular structures within the centers of the corpus spongiosum and corpora cavernosa, respectively
  - On T1W images
    - Corpora spongiosa and cavernosa are homogeneous, medium signal intensity
    - Fascial layers are low signal
    - Gadolinium administration causes increased signal intensity of corpus spongiosum and corpora cavernosa, enabling improved differentiation from the surrounding muscle and fascial layers

Disease Entities

Congenital Abnormalities
Epispadias
- Background
  - Rare anomaly characterized by absence of the dorsal covering of distal urethra and ectopic placement of the proximal urethral aperture, which may be located anywhere along the length of the penis
  - Almost always associated with bladder exstrophy and accompanying pubic diastasis
- Imaging
  - Separation of the corpora cavernosa
  - Inversion of normal relationship of corpora cavernosa and corpus spongiosum at the level of the pubic symphysis
  - Urethra assumes a more cephalad position

Hypospadias
- Background
  - Frequently associated with a ventral fibrous band, resulting in a chordee deformity
- Imaging
  - Proximal, ventral location of meatus
  - There may be foreshortening of the urethra with either epispadias or hypospadias

Partial Aplasia of the Corpora Cavernosa
- Background
  - Rare, may lead to erectile dysfunction
  - Patients frequently have other associated genitourinary anomalies
- Imaging
  - Irregularity of length and caliber are well shown on T2W images

Diphallus
- Background
  - Rare anomaly resulting in partial or complete duplication of the erectile bodies and urethra
- Imaging
  - Frequently, there is associated shortening of the perineum or asymmetric development of the corpora cavernosa and ischiocavernosus muscles
  - MRI signal of supernumerary corpora identical to normal corpora

Mass Lesions

Benign Masses
Penile Prostheses
- Background
  - May develop postoperative complications such as infection and hematoma, which is well evaluated by MRI
- Imaging
  - Prostheses appear as tubular structures in central corpora cavernosa
  - Solid silicone prostheses appear signal void on all imaging sequences
  - Inflatable prostheses follow signal characteristics of the fluid they contain
  - Progressive decreased signal intensity on T2W images in the corpora cavernosa may reflect development of fibrosis

Malignant Masses
Cancer Involving the Urethra and Penis
- Background
  - Primary carcinomas extremely rare, <1% genitourinary cancers in males

- Penile carcinoma is squamous cell carcinoma in >95% of cases
- Urethral carcinoma is squamous cell in 78%, transitional cell in 15%, adenocarcinoma in 6%, and undifferentiated carcinomas in the rest
- Metastatic penile lesions may result from contiguous spread of prostatic, testicular, bladder, and osseous neoplasms, as well as disseminated leukemia and lymphoma

- Imaging
  - Primary neoplasms of the urethra and penis demonstrate isointense to low signal relative to corpus spongiosum on T1W and T2W images
  - Metastatic lesions are also low or intermediate signal on T1W images, but they may appear hypointense, isointense, or hyperintense to the corpus spongiosum on T2W images; heterogeneous enhancement is similar to rest of the malignant process

Diffuse Disease

Vascular Disorders
- Background
  - Impairment of arterial supply, intracorporeal sinusoids, or venous drainage networks
  - MRI can evaluate flow within the corpora spongiosum and cavernosa
  - Amyloid may also affect the anterior urethra

- Majority of cases are secondary to other disease states
- May result in stricture formation and calcified plaques in anterior urethra

- Imaging
  - Alteration in normal vascular flow (from central cavernosal arteries outward and distally) may provide evidence for erectile dysfunction
  - Focal low signal on T2W images may reflect amyloid deposition

Peyronie's Disease (induratio penis plastica)
- Background
  - Caused by focal inflammation of the tunica albuginea and corpora cavernosa
  - Resultant fibrosis and plaque formation lead to painful, deviated erections
  - Trauma, diabetes, gout, and hormonal dysfunction implicated as potential causes
  - Most common in patients 30–60 years of age
  - Rarely fibrosis may affect Buck's fascia: may indicate early Peyronie's disease or extension of fibrosis from other causes including trauma, sustained priapism, and collagen vascular disease
- Imaging (fig. 12.14)
  - On T2W images
    - Heterogeneity of the corpora cavernosa may be demonstrated

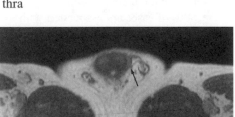
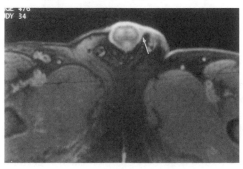

(*a*)   (*b*)

FIGURE 12.14   Fibrosis of Buck's fascia. Transverse T1W SGE (*a*) and 90 s postgadolinium fat-suppressed SGE (*b*) images. There is increased thickness of the left aspect of Buck's fascia (black arrow, *a*). Note the low-signal-intensity linear markings in the adjacent fat (*a*). The thickened fascia enhances diffusely after gadolinium administration (white arrow, *b*). These changes are compatible with early Peyronie's disease.

- Low-signal plaques may be visualized in the corpora cavernosa and tunica albuginea
  ○ On T1W images
    - Plaques are low signal
    - Plaque detection improved by gadolinium, with increased enhancement in areas of active inflammation

Urethritis
- Background
  ○ *Neisseria gonococcus, Chlamydia trachomatis, Condylomata acuminatum,* or *Mycobacterium tuberculosis*
- Imaging
  ○ Periurethral glands of Littre may become distended, may be seen on T2W images
  ○ Spread to periurethral tissues may lead to abscess
  ○ Aggressive infections may result in perineal/scrotal sinus formation

Trauma

Penile Trauma
- Background
  ○ Usually results from direct, blunt injury
- Imaging
  ○ On T2W images
    - Most common finding is a tear in the tunica albuginea seen as discontinuity of the low-signal ring
    - May see fracture or avulsion of corpora cavernosa from ischial attachments as focal low signal on T2W images
  ○ On T1W images
    - Signal characteristics of associated hematomas reflect acuity of trauma

Seminal Vesicles
Normal Anatomy

Anatomy of the Seminal Vesicles
- Background
  ○ Paired accessory glands located superior to the prostate
  ○ Each comprised of a single tube coiled upon itself
  ○ Surrounded by a fibromuscular sheet, narrows medially to form the excretory duct that joins the vas deferens to form the ejaculatory duct
  ○ Width and fluid content increase after puberty, peaking in fifth and sixth decades
- Imaging
  ○ On T2W images
    - Signal varies with fluid
    - In men younger than 60, seminal vesicles are high-signal "cluster of grapes" structures
    - Fluid content decreases after age 60; seminal vesicles appear progressively lower in signal
    - In normal aging, low signal is symmetric bilaterally and associated with decreased size
  ○ On T1W images
    - Seminal vesicles are homogeneous signal similar to muscle
    - After gadolinium, the convoluted walls of the vesicles enhance and can be more clearly defined with fat saturation

Disease Entities

Congenital Abnormalities
- Background
  ○ Ectopia, hypoplasia, and agenesis
  ○ Detection warrants evaluation of the entire genitourinary tract
  ○ Congenital seminal vesicle cysts are the most common abnormalities
    - 80% of cases are associated with ipsilateral renal dysgenesis
    - 8% of cases are associated with collecting system duplication
    - Frequently asymptomatic, but may become large enough to cause dysuria, perineal pain, increased frequency, or bladder outlet obstruction
- Imaging
  ○ Seminal vesical cysts are easily differentiated from müllerian or utricular cysts due to lack of connection to the prostate
  ○ Variable signal on T1W images (reflects hemorrhage or proteinacious content), high signal on T2W images

Mass Lesions

Benign Masses
- Background
  - Rare; leiomyomas are most common
  - More rarely lipomas, fibromas, cystadenomas, and angiomas may occur
- Imaging
  - Leiomyomas are usually well circumscribed, intermediate signal on T1W images and high signal on T2W images

Malignant Masses
- Background
  - Most due to local extension of prostatic, bladder, or rectal carcinomas
  - Primary malignancies are rare and are usually adenocarcinomas
  - Primary leiomyosarcomas and fibrosarcomas have also been reported
- Imaging
  - Invasion by prostate carcinoma causes loss of architecture and decreased signal on T2W images
- Mimickers
  - Postbiopsy change
    - Low signal on T2W images may be seen following prostatic biopsy
    - Postbiopsy change may be confused with tumor invasion and prevent radical prostatectomy in eligible patients
  - Senile amyloidosis
    - Common finding at autopsy
    - Appearing as low signal intensity on T2W images, it can also mimic malignancy (fig. 12.12)

Diffuse Disease

Calcifications
- Background
  - Most commonly associated with diabetes mellitus
  - Less often due to infectious etiologies such as tuberculosis and schistosomiasis
- Imaging
  - Low signal on T1W and T2W images

Infection of the Seminal Vesicles
- Background
  - Diagnosis is primarily clinical
  - Patients usually have associated prostatitis or epididymitis
  - Rare, isolated infection of the seminal vesicles classically results in hemospermia
- Imaging
  - Signal characteristics on MR images reflect presence or absence of blood products
  - The acutely inflamed gland may also appear enlarged and lower signal than the contralateral side
  - Chronic infection may cause fibrosis with decreased signal on T1W and T2W images

Testes, Epididymis, and Scrotum

Overview
- Phased-array surface coil or a circular surface coil overlying the testes
- Scrotum should be elevated by a folded towel placed between the thighs
- Small field-of-view T1W and T2W images obtained in axial, coronal, and sagittal planes
- Delayed gadolinium-enhanced images helpful in cases of tumor or inflammation

Normal Anatomy
Anatomy of the Testes, Epididymis, and Scrotum
- Background
  - The scrotum is comprised of internal cremasteric and external fascial layers, dartos muscle, and skin
  - The testes are encased by the tunica albuginea, a fibrous capsule that invaginates into the testis posteriorly to form the mediastinum testis
  - The processus vaginalis represents an extension of peritoneum, projecting between the tunica albuginea and dartos layers
  - The posterior testis and mediastinum testis are not covered by the tunica vaginalis, resulting in the bare area through which vascular structures and tubules pass

○ Approximately 400–600 seminiferous tubules are coiled within each testis
○ These converge to form the rete testis and ultimately the efferent ductules
○ The efferent ductules form the epididymal head posterior to the testis, then unify into a single coiled duct representing the epididymal body
○ The narrowed tail of the epididymis ultimately leads into the vas deferens
• Imaging
○ Testes are demarcated on T1W and T2W images by the low signal surrounding the tunica albuginea
○ Testes are homogeneous and isointense to muscle on T1W images and higher signal on T2W images
○ The mediastinum testis is a low-signal band in the posterior testis on T2W images
○ Low-signal fibrous projections from the mediastinum testis represent septulae, which divide the testis into lobules
○ The gubernaculum may be seen on T2W images as a low-signal curvilinear rim along the inferoposterior aspect of the testis
○ The signal intensity of the epididymis is slightly heterogeneous and hypo- to isointense to the testis on T1W images
○ The epididymis is more clearly differentiated from the testis on T2W images due to its low signal relative to the adjacent testis
○ Gadolinium causes hyperintensity of the epididymis relative to the testis

Disease Entities

Congenital Abnormalities
• Background
○ Hypoplasia and agenesis: unilateral or bilateral
○ Duplication
▪ Congenitally duplicated testes may be classified by their location within the scrotum, inguinal canal, or retroperitoneum
▪ There may be an associated ipsilateral inguinal hernia
▪ Polyorchia is associated with an increased incidence of testicular malignancy

○ Cryptorchidism
▪ The testes normally descend into the scrotum during the eighth month of gestation
▪ 80% of undescended testes are distal to the external inguinal ring
▪ Many cryptorchid testes will descend spontaneously during an infant's first year of life
▪ Fibrosis and impaired spermatogonia have been observed in undescended testes not surgically corrected by 2 years of age
▪ As a result of increased incidences of infertility and carcinoma, it is recommended that orchiopexy be performed between the first and second years of life
• Imaging
○ Undescended testes are low signal on T1W images and intermediate to high signal on T2W images, although low signal on T2W images may be seen in fibrotic or atrophic testes
○ Identification aided by the mediastinum testis, a low-signal-intensity structure on T2W images
○ Undescended testes often have a larger transverse than anteroposterior (AP) diameter while lymph nodes usually have a larger AP than transverse diameter
○ The low-signal gubernaculum testis remnant on coronal T2W images may be helpful, as the testis lies along its medial border

Mass Lesions

Benign Masses
Testicular Prostheses
• Background
○ Older prostheses contain silicone; newer prostheses contain solid elastomers
• Imaging
○ Recognized by the chemical shift artifact and the absence of spermatic cord
○ Silicone prostheses are low signal on T1W and T2W images
○ Solid elastomer prostheses are similar to native testes: intermediate signal on T1W images and high signal on T2W images

Cystic Lesions
- Background
  - Intratesticular cysts may be solitary or multiple
    - Occur in up to 10% of the male population
  - Seminiferous tubular ectasia in the rete testis
    - Ovoid lesions in continuity with the edge of the testis
    - Contain spermatozoa
    - Bilateral in 71% of cases
    - Ipsilateral spermatocele in 92% of cases
    - Centered at the mediastinum testis
    - Contiguous with the spermatocele along the bare area
  - Epididymal cysts
    - Occur anywhere in the epididymis
  - Spermatoceles (fig. 12.15)
    - Small cystic structures most commonly in the epididymal head
    - May be either solitary or multiloculated
- Imaging
  - Intratesticular cysts most commonly have simple fluid signal characteristics
  - Tubular ectasia in rete testis is typically lower in signal than testis on T1W images and nearly isointense to testis on T2W images
  - Epididymal cysts contain simple fluid; low signal on T1W images and high signal on T2W images
  - Spermatoceles are variable signal intensity, depending on presence of spermatozoa, fat, lymphocytes, and cellular debris

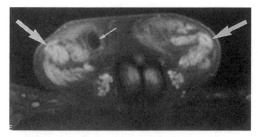

FIGURE 12.15 Spermatocele and bilateral varicoceles. Transverse gadolinium-enhanced T1W fat-suppressed spin-echo image demonstrates a nonenhancing ovoid structure within the right epididymal head consistent with a spermatocele (small arrow). There are also bilateral enhancing varicoceles (large arrows).

Benign Neoplasms

Testicular Neoplasms
- Background
  - Only 5% are benign
  - Of these, 90% are non-germ-cell tumors arising from Leydig cells, Sertoli cells, or connective tissue stroma

Extratesticular Neoplasms
Adenomatoid Tumor
- Background
  - Most common extratesticular neoplasm
  - Usually in the epididymis, can be in spermatic cord or tunica
- Imaging
  - Round and well defined, or occasionally plaque-like and less well defined

Lipomas
- Background
  - May arise in the spermatic cord
- Imaging
  - High signal on T1W images, follow fat on T2W images
  - Loss of signal on fat-suppressed images is diagnostic

Fibrous Pseudotumor
- Background
  - Benign, fibroproliferative tumor, etiology uncertain
  - Second most common extratesticular neoplasm
  - May occur in tunica albuginea or vaginalis, spermatic cord, or epididymis
  - Often associated with hydroceles or hematoceles
- Imaging
  - Frequently lobulated with frond-like projections, but may also cause circumferential thickening of the tunica albuginea
  - Low signal on T1W and T2W images, enhance negligibly with gadolinium

Other Benign Scrotal Lesions

Scrotal Fluid
- Background
  - Hydroceles, pyoceles, and hematoceles may occur with infection, tumor, or trauma

- Imaging
  - Hydroceles have signal characteristics typical of simple fluid
  - Pyoceles may have heterogeneous low signal on T1W images and heterogeneous high signal on T2W images
  - Hematoceles have varied signal depending on the chronicity of the blood products they contain

Varicoceles
- Background
  - More commonly left sided
- Imaging (fig. 12.15)
  - Multiple serpiginous structures in the pampiniform plexus, epididymal head, and spermatic cord
  - Signal intensity is dependent on flow velocity
  - Often intermediate signal on T1W images and higher signal on T2W images
  - Enhance with gadolinium

Scrotal Hernias
- Background
  - Usually diagnosed clinically; MRI may be helpful in equivocal cases
- Imaging
  - Complex mass within an enlarged inguinal canal. Mesenteric fat, loops of bowel, and intraluminal air may be visualized within the scrotal sac.
  - Imaging with HASTE and immediate post-gadolinium fat-suppressed SGE sequences may provide helpful information regarding entrapped bowel viability

Malignant Masses

Testicular Carcinomas
- Background
  - Primary
    - Less than 1% of tumors in males, but often occur in younger men, and 95% are malignant
    - Early detection and treatment are crucial, particularly for seminomas, which are chemotherapy and radiotherapy sensitive

- Testicular carcinomas may be divided into germ-cell and non-germ-cell subtype
- 95% of primary malignant neoplasms are of germ-cell origin
  - Seminomas (approximately 40%)
  - Nonseminomatous tumors
    - Embryonal carcinomas (~30%)
    - Teratocarcinomas (~25%)
    - Teratoma (10%)
    - Choriocarcinomas (1%)
    - Mixed histology (30%)
- Remainder are Sertoli, Leydig, or mesenchymal cell carcinomas
- Metastatic Spread
  - Lymphatics follow gonadal vessels to retroperitoneum
  - In cases of epididymis or spermatic cord invasion, may extend to pelvic nodes
  - Staged according to TNM criteria as outlined in Table 12.3
  - Secondary

TABLE 12.3   American Joint Committee on Cancer Staging of Testicular Carcinoma

Carcinoma	
Primary Tumor	
T0	No evidence of primary tumor
T1	Tumor limited to testis, including rete testis
T2	Tumor extends beyond tunica albuginea or into epididymis
T3	Tumor invades spermatic cord
T4	Tumor invades scrotum
Lymph Nodes	
N0	No lymph node metastasis
N1	Metastasis to a single lymph node 2 cm or smaller
N2	Metastasis to a single lymph node between 2 and 5 cm in size, or to multiple nodes each 5 cm or smaller
N3	Metastasis to a single lymph node larger than 5 cm
Distant Metastases	
M0	No distant metastases
M1	Distant metastases

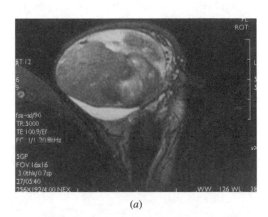
(a)

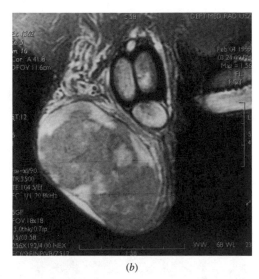
(b)

FIGURE 12.16   Testicular seminoma. Surface coil transverse (*a*) and coronal (*b*) T2W echo-train spin-echo images demonstrate a heterogeneous low-signal mass that exhibits extensive infiltration of the testicle. Remnants of uninvolved testicle appear high signal.

- Secondary involvement by leukemia, lymphoma
- Rarley, metastatic from lung, melanoma, genitourinary, or gastrointestinal malignancies
- Imaging
  - Tumors are low signal on T2W images
  - Lack of visualization of septulae found to be a sensitive indicator of malignant infiltration
  - Seminomas (fig. 12.16)
    - Isointense to normal tissue on T1W images and hypointense to normal tissue on T2W images
    - Most commonly homogeneously low signal on T2W images (fig. 12.16*a*, *b*)
    - May exhibit lobulation or occasionally central necrosis
    - Enhance to a lesser degree than normal testicular tissue; gadolinium may increase lesion conspicuity and aid detection of extension into surrounding tunica albuginea
  - Nonseminomatous tumors (fig. 12.17)
    - More heterogeneous on T2W images with more ill-defined margins (figs. 12.17*a*, *b* and 12.17*b*, *c*)

- Increased and decreased signals on T1W and T2W images correspond to foci of hemorrhage and necrosis, respectively, on histologic specimens
  - Lymphomatous infiltration may result in diffuse testicular enlargement, relative hypointensity on T2W images, and involvement of draining lymphatics (fig. 12.18)

Testicular Torsion

Acute Testicular Torsion
- Background
  - Arises when bare area is not sufficiently broad to anchor the testis, resulting in a "bell clapper" deformity.
  - <30% result in irreversible ischemia if diagnosis and surgery occur within 12 hours
  - Salvage rate then decreases rapidly with minimal surgical success after 24 hours of ischemia
- Imaging
  - MRI is not commonly used, as ultrasound and/or nuclear medicine examination enables timely diagnosis
  - Initial studies with P-31 MR spectroscopy in an animal model have revealed additional

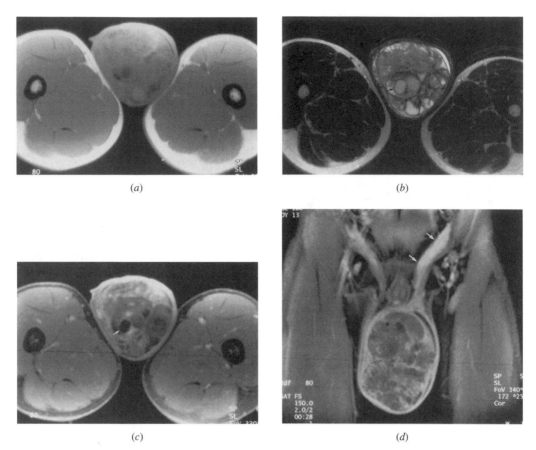

(a)   (b)

(c)   (d)

FIGURE 12.17   Nonseminomatous testicular neoplasma. Transverse SGE (a), T2W echo-train spin-echo (b), and transverse (c) and coronal (d) postgadolinium fat-suppressed SGE images. The left testicle is greatly enlarged. Tumor replaces the testicle and is mildly heterogeneous on the T1W image (a) and considerably heterogeneous on the T2W image (b). The tumor contains multiple cystic spaces that are well-defined, high-signal foci (arrow, b) on the T2W image and show lack of enhancement with gadolinium (arrows, c).

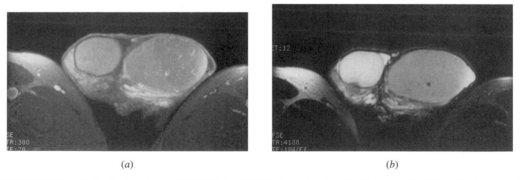

(a)   (b)

FIGURE 12.18   Testicular lymphoma. T1W SE (a) and T2W echo-train spin-echo (b) images. The left testicle is enlarged and exhibits diffuse infiltration with homogeneous tumor that is isointense on T1 and mildly hypointense on T2. Lymphoma is typically more homogeneous in appearance than other neoplasms.

promise for the evaluation of testicular torsion in the acute setting

Subacute Testicular Torsion

- Background
  - ◦ Bilateral orchiopexy is still indicated in the subacute period when ultrasound and nuclear medicine may be equivocal
  - ◦ MRI may provide assistance in differentiating from epididymo-orchitis
- Imaging
  - ◦ Common MRI findings include an enlarged spermatic cord with diminished flow, diffusely decreased signal intensity of the testis, decreased testicular size, and mild to moderate thickening of the tunica albuginea and epididymis
  - ◦ There may also be increased-signal-intensity foci on T1W images, reflecting hemorrhage, visualization of the pedicular

attachment of the testicle in a bellclapper deformity, or an associated hematocele
  - ◦ Identification of a whirling pattern within the spermatic cord and an associated low-signal-intensity knot at the point of maximal torsion on T2W images provides specific evidence for the diagnosis

Infection

Epididymal Orchitis

- Background
  - ◦ Vast majority of acute epididymitis cases are isolated; up to 20% may be associated with orchitis
  - ◦ Therapy is conservative and limited to antibiotics unless there is infarction from extensive edema or abscess formation
  - ◦ With the exception of mumps orchitis (fig. 12.19), isolated acute infection of the testes is rare
- Imaging

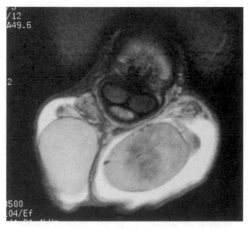

(a)

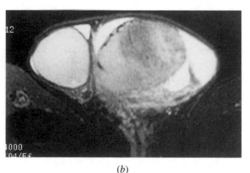

(b)

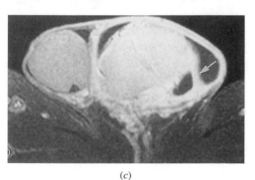

(c)

FIGURE 12.19 Mumps orchitis. Coronal T2W fat-suppressed echo-train spin-echo (*a*), transverse T2W fat-suppressed ETSE (*b*), and T1W postgadolinium fat-suppressed spin-echo (*c*) images. There is enlargement of the left testis relative to the contralateral side (*b*, *c*). The affected testis is heterogeneous and low in signal intensity on the T2W images (*a*, *b*) and enhances slightly more than unaffected testis on the postgadolinium image (*c*). Note the enhancing, thickened septations within the scrotal sac (arrow, *c*). There are accompanying hydroceles bilaterally.

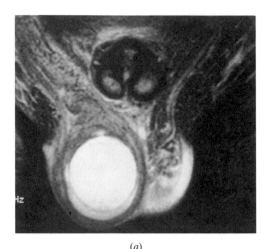
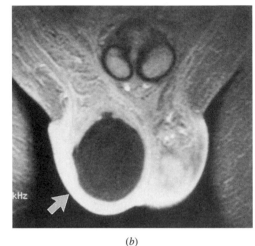

(a)   (b)

FIGURE 12.20   Testicular abscess. Coronal T2W ETSE (a) and gadolinium-enhanced T1W spin-echo (b) images. A complex fluid collecion within the right testis is heterogeneously high in signal intensity on the T2W image (a) and heterogeneously low in signal intensity on the postgadolinium T1W image, which is consistent with an abscess. There is extensive enhancement of the surrounding scrotal tissues secondary to adjacent inflammatory changes (arrow, b).

- ◦ Epididymal and/or testicular inflammation is most commonly manifested by generalized enlargement of the organ
- ◦ The epididymis may be hyperintense on T1W images and of variable signal relative to the contralateral side on T2W images
- ◦ There is frequently decreased signal intensity of the involved testis on T2W images
- ◦ The testicular septulae remain well defined but thickened, in contrast to the loss of normal architecture observed with malignancy
- ◦ Abscesses are high signal on T2W images, show wall enhancement with gadolinium (fig. 12.20), and are often accompanied by pyoceles
- ◦ There is marked gadolinium enhancement of the inflamed structure and surrounding tissues
- ◦ Acute inflammation often results in enlargement and edema of the spermatic cord. However, in contrast to avascularity in torsion, there is increased vascularity with infection.

- ◦ Identification of the bare area virtually excludes the possibility of a bell-clapper deformity, and thus of torsion

Trauma

Testicular Trauma
- • Background
  - ◦ MRI may provide important information for clinical management
- • Imaging
  - ◦ Intratesticular hematomas may appear high signal on T1W images and variable signal on T2W images
  - ◦ Contusion in the absence of hemorrhage may be detected as decreased signal of the involved testis on T2W images with relative decrease in gadolinium enhancement
  - ◦ Careful inspection of the low-signal tunica albuginea is necessary to evaluate for the possibility of acute testicular rupture, which ofter requires surgery; discontinuity on T2W images is suspicious for rupture

CHAPTER 13

FEMALE PELVIS

BACKGROUND

- Patient Preparation
  - Voiding prior to pelvic MRI improves patient comfort and minimizes artifacts of the distended urinary bladder induced by motion
  - Intrauterine contraceptive devices are safe, appear as signal void on T1W and T2W sequences, and do not significantly degrade images
  - Using faster sequences and compensation techniques, artifacts from peristalsis are usually not detrimental, but they can be reduced with glucagon if necessary
- Coils
  - Phased-array surface coil should be used routinely
  - In obese or pregnant patients, torso phased-array or body coil
  - Endoluminal coils can provide superior resolution when needed
- Routine Protocol (benign conditions)
  - Phased-array surface coil
  - Breath-hold imaging
    - Coronal single shot echo-train spin-echo (eg: HASTE or SSFSE)

- Sagittal T2W echo-train spin-echo (ETSE)
- Angled axial (to endometrium)
  - T2W ETSE
  - T1W GRE in- and out-of-phase (dual echo)
- Modifications
  - Cancer
    - Dynamic gadolinium-enhanced SGE
    - Delayed fat-suppressed T1W images
  - Urethral or vaginal imaging
    - Orthogonal transverse and coronal high-resolution small field-of-view T1W and T2W images oriented to urethra (transverse and sagittal for vagina)
  - Uterine anomalies
    - Angled coronal (to endometrium) T2W images
  - Fetal Imaging
    - Typically supine position, but decubitus position should be considered in advanced pregnancy
    - Primarily ultrafast T2W imaging, such as single-shot echo-train spin-echo
    - Images acquired according to fetal position in the axial, coronal, and sagittal planes

Primer on MR Imaging of the Abdomen and Pelvis, edited by Diego R. Martin, Michele A. Brown, and Richard C. Semelka ISBN 0-471-37340-0 Copyright © 2005 Wiley-Liss, Inc.

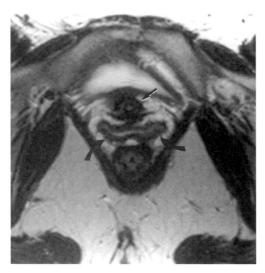

FIGURE 13.1   Normal anatomy of the female urethra and vagina. Tranverse pelvic coil FSE images show the normal urethral zonal anatomy (from central to peripheral), high-signal central spot, low-signal mucosa, moderately high-signal submucosa, and low-signal muscularis (arrow). The vagina is located posteriorly and reveals (from central to peripheral) high-signal mucosa/secretions, low SI muscular wall (curved arrow), and high-signal-intensity perivaginal venous plexus.

○ T1W information can be obtained with breath-hold spoiled gradient-echo sequences

Urethra

Normal (fig. 13.1)

- Transverse T2W images: "target" appearance
  ○ Dark outer ring: outer circular striated and inner longitudinal smooth-muscle layers
  ○ Middle high-signal-intensity ring: vascular submucosal layer
  ○ Dark central dot: mucosal layer
- A tiny dot of high-signal urine or mucus is sometimes seen inside the mucosal layer
- Zonal anatomy not always apparent in post-menopausal women
- On gadolinium-enhanced T1W images: marked enhancement of middle submucosal layer with little enhancement of remaining urethra

Mass Lesions

Benign Masses
Urethral Leiomyoma

- Background
  ○ Unusual benign tumors arising from smooth-muscle layer
  ○ Present with dysuria or palpable mass, mimicking urethral diverticulum
  ○ May grow during pregnancy, malignant degeneration not reported
- Imaging
  ○ Low to intermediate signal on T1W and T2W images due to smooth-muscle content

Malignant Masses
Primary Urethral Carcinomas

- Background
  ○ Uncommon, occur in middle age or later
  ○ Most are squamous cell, arise from distal (anterior) urethra
  ○ Transitional cell and adenocarcinomas originate from proximal (posterior) urethra
  ○ Spread contiguously, then lymphatically
    ▪ Anterior urethral tumors involve inguinal nodes first, then pelvic nodes
    ▪ Posterior urethral lesions drain to iliac, obturator, and para-aortic nodes
- Imaging
  ○ T2W and T1W images before and after contrast administration provide complementary information
  ○ Axial and sagittal T2W images useful for invasion of bladder, vagina, and pelvic floor
  ○ T1W images demonstrate extension into periurethral fat

Secondary Urethral Malignancies

- Background
  ○ Metastases from renal cell carcinoma or melanoma
  ○ Contiguous spread from bladder, uterus, cervix, and vagina

Miscellaneous

Urethral Diverticulum

- Background

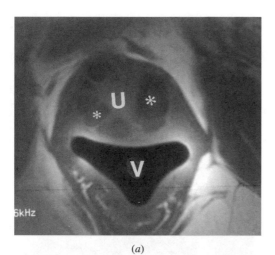

(a)

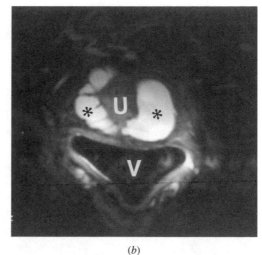

(b)

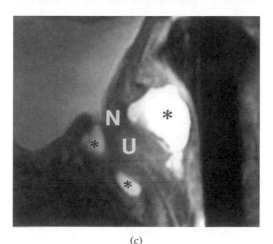

(c)

FIGURE 13.2   MR endovaginal coil demonstration of a saddlebag diverticulum. Axial T1W (a) and T2W (b) fast spin-echo images show the multiloculated diverticulum (*) that almost entirely surrounds the circumference of the urethra (U). The vaginal coil (V) is positioned posterior to the urethra. Sagittal T2W fast spin-echo image (c) reveals the superior extent of the diverticulum relative to the bladder neck (N) and also shows the portions of the diverticulum located anterior to the urethra (U).

- ◦ Due to recurrent infection and obstruction of periurethral glands, which rupture and drain into urethra
- ◦ Often asymptomatic, but can become infected, form stones or cause dyspareunia, dribbling, or a palpable mass
- Imaging (fig. 13.2)
  - ◦ MRI is current modality of choice; accuracy exceeds urethrography and urethroscopy
  - ◦ Low signal on T1W images and high signal on T2W images
  - ◦ Variety of configurations seen, commonly saddlebag appearance
  - ◦ May see connection to urethral lumen
  - ◦ Carcinomas rare; most often adenocarcinomas, reflecting ductal origin

Caruncle
- Background
  - ◦ Small benign, often asymptomatic inflammatory mass
  - ◦ Typically occurs in older postmenopausal women and arises on or near the external meatus
  - ◦ Occasionally causes pain or hematuria
  - ◦ Hyperplastic squamous epithelium with underlying submucosal vascularity, fibrosis, and inflammation

Stress Incontinence
- Background
  - ◦ Risk factors: advancing age, childbirth, smoking, and obesity

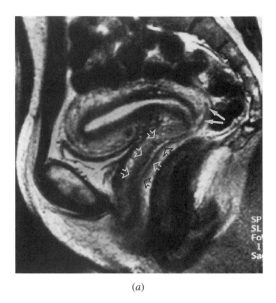
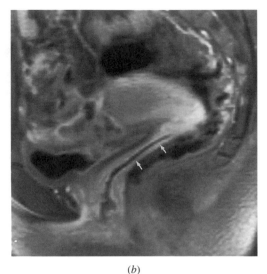

(*a*)   (*b*)

FIGURE 13.3   Normal Vagina. Sagittal T2W echo-train spin-echo (*a*) and immediate postgadolinium fat-suppressed SGE (*b*) images. On the T2W images the low-signal-intensity muscular wall and the central higher-signal-intensity mucosal layer of the vagina are apparent. The sagittal T2W image (*a*) shows vagina (open arrows, *a*) as well as the posterior vaginal fornix (closed arrows, *a*). Relationship with uterus and cervix is well seen. On the immediate postgadolinium fat-suppressed image (*b*), intense enhancement of vaginal mucosa (arrows, *b*) is present. (Courtesy of Susan M. Asher, M.D., Dept. of Radiology, Georgetown University Medical Center, Washington, D.C.).

- Imaging
  - Single-shot echo-train spin-echo and fast gradient-echo imaging used
  - Sagittal images obtained at rest and during straining
  - Urethral hypermobility depicted by a change in the normal vertical orientation of urethra to horizontal during straining
  - Periurethral collagen is well shown on T2W images and appears high in signal intensity
  - Complications of mechanical sphincters include fistula formation, periurethral abscess, and erosion
  - Sagittal single-shot echo-train spin-echo technique also valuable for enteroceles and cystoceles, which are also associated with pelvic floor relaxation

Vagina

Normal
- Inner mucosal layer and intraluminal fluid/mucus appear as central low signal on T1W images and high signal on T2W images (fig. 13.3)
- The middle layer of the vagina is low in signal intensity on both T1W and T2W images and consists of the submucosa and muscularis layers (inner longitudinal and outer circular smooth muscle layers)
- The vaginal venous plexus in the outer adventitial layer is high in signal intensity on T2W images due to slow venous flow
- After gadolinium administration, the vaginal wall enhances, and occasionally a low-signal-intensity line is present centrally, which may represent the lumen or inner epithelial layer

Normal Variants and Congenital Disease
Vaginal Agenesis and Partial Agenesis
- Background
  - May have associated abnormalities of the uterus, cervix, upper urinary tract, and skeleton
- Imaging
  - Thin-section T2W transverse images accurately demonstrate agenesis

Duplication and Partial Duplication
- Background
  - Typically seen with uterus didelphys
  - Associated with ipsilateral renal agenesis
- Imaging
  - Well seen on transverse T2W images
    - May have longitudinal vaginal septum (low signal on T2W images), which can cause dyspareunia or can obstruct a hemivagina and its associated uterine cavity
    - May have transverse vaginal septum, which presents like imperforate hymen with amenorrhea and cyclical abdominal pain (fig. 13.4)

Ambiguous Genitalia
- Background
  - Pseudohermaphrodites
    - Male pseudohermaphrodites: have testes and ambiguous internal/external genitalia
      - Phenotypically female, blind-ended vagina, no uterus or fallopian tubes

- Female pseudohermaphrodites: normal 46 XX
  - Normal ovaries, virilized external genitalia
  - No male internal genitalia
- Imaging
  - MRI helps identify internal genitalia
  - T2W imaging particularly helpful in preoperative location of the testes in male pseudohermaphrodites

Mass Lesions

Benign Masses
Bartholin's Cyst
- Background
  - Retention of secretions in Bartholin's glands due to trauma or chronic inflammation
  - Usually asymptomatic unless infected, most commonly with *Neisseria gonorrhoeae*

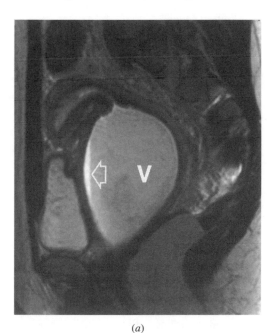

(a)

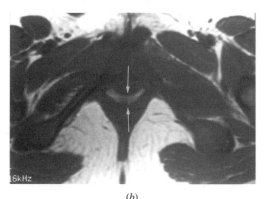

(b)

FIGURE 13.4   Hematocolpos secondary to a low transverse vaginal septum. Sagittal T2W fast spin-echo image (*a*) shows a distended vaginal canal (V) that is filled with complex fluid with a fluid-fluid level (arrow). Axial T1W image obtained through the lower vagina (*b*) shows that the vaginal canal (arrows) contains high signal intensity, representing the T1-shortening effects of protein and/or methemoglobin within subacute blood. A low transverse septum may have a similar appearance to an imperforate hymen on MR imaging. The treatment of the two conditions, however, is similar.

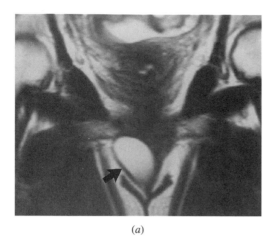
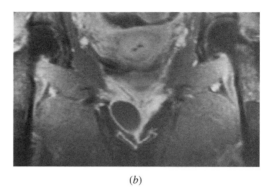

(a)   (b)

FIGURE 13.5   Asymptomatic Bartholin's gland cyst. Coronal T2W echo-train spin-echo image (a) obtained though the low pelvis shows a high-signal-intensity mass (arrow) within the lateral aspect of the distal vagina near the introitus. Coronal postgadolinium fat-suppressed T1W SGE image (b) shows a rim-enhancing cyst with low-signal contents.

- Imaging (fig. 13.5)
  - Small fluid-filled structures in lower third of vagina
  - High signal on T2W images
  - Medium to high signal on T1W images, depending on contents
  - Rim enhancement with gadolinium suggests infection

Gartner Duct Cyst
- Background
  - Usually asymptomatic, but large lesions can cause dyspareunia or difficult delivery
  - Can be associated with genitourinary abnormalities
- Imaging (fig. 13.6)
  - Fluid-filled structure in anterolateral aspect of upper vagina
  - High signal on T2W images
  - Low signal on T1W images, may be high depending on contents
  - Rim enhancement is not a typical feature

Cavernous Hemangioma
- Occurs mostly in infants, tends to stabilize or regress
- Symptoms unusual, can include bleeding, ulceration, or hemorrhage during vaginal delivery

- STIR and fat-suppressed T2W images demonstrate high-signal serpiginous vascular lakes

Malignant Masses
Primary Vaginal Malignancies
- Background
  - Up to 95% are squamous cell
  - Peak age incidence 60–70 years
  - Often asymptomatic, but can present with increased vaginal discharge or spotting
  - Typically arise from upper posterior vagina, can spread through wall to adjacent structures
  - Tumors in upper third spread to iliac nodes, in lower two-thirds spread to inguinal nodes
  - Clear-cell adenocarcinomas are rare
    - Associated with in utero diethylstilbestrol exposure
    - Often arise anteriorly in upper third of vagina
    - 5-year survival rate of 80% for vaginally confined disease, 20% for locally advanced or metastatic tumors
  - Other rare primary vaginal malignancies include leiomyosarcomas in adults, endodermal sinus tumors in infants, lymphoma, and melanoma

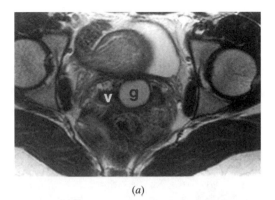

(a)

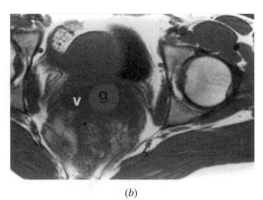

(b)

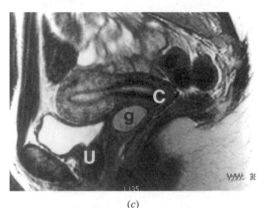

(c)

FIGURE 13.6   Gartner duct cyst. Axial T2W spin-echo image (*a*) shows a well-circumscribed high-signal-intensity mass (G) centered within the proximal vagina (V). Corresponding axial T1W fast spin-echo image (*b*) reveals high signal intensity within the cyst, representing intracystic protein. Sagittal T2W fast spin-echo image (*c*) reveals that the mass is located above the urethra (arrow) and below the cervix (curved arrow) within the proximal vagina. The normal zonal anatomy of the uterus is present.

- Imaging (fig. 13.7)
  - Intermediate signal intensity on T1W images, may be occult when small
  - Well seen on T2W images, moderately high signal
  - Variable gadolinium enhancement
  - Differentiation of inflammatory changes from tumor may sometimes be problematic
  - Differentiation of postoperative changes from recurrent tumor may be difficult
    - Recurrent tumor is generally irregular in contour and usually high signal on T2W images, whereas fibrosis and granulation tissue are low signal on T2W images
    - Recurrent tumor frequently enhances in a heterogeneous intense fashion on gadolinium-enhanced fat-suppressed images
    - Inflammatory changes within 9 months to 1 year following radiation therapy result in increased signal intensity on T2W images and may mimic tumor recurrence

Vaginal Metastases
- Background
  - 80% of all vaginal tumors
  - Majority due to local spread from cervical and endometrial carcinoma
- Imaging
  - Sagittal and transverse plane images useful for tumor extension to vagina
  - T2W echo-train spin-echo images and gadolinium-enhanced T1W fat-suppressed images can define tumor involvement

Vulvar and Perineal Carcinomas
- Background
  - Uncommon, occur in older patients, typically squamous cell
  - Symptoms include vulvar pruritus, pain, bleeding, and palpable mass
- Imaging (fig. 13.8)
  - May appear intermediate signal on T2W echo-train spin-echo images
  - Heterogeneous gadolinium enhancement

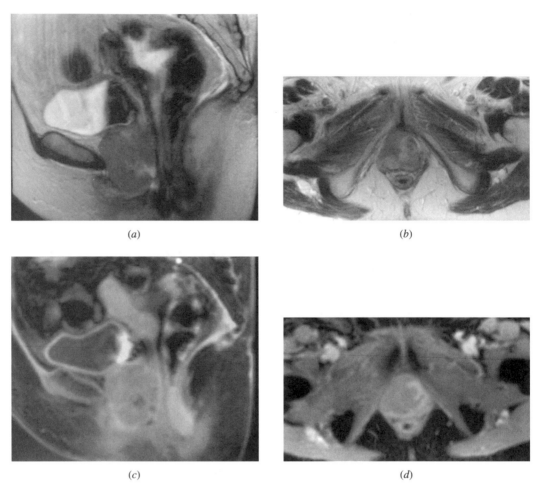

(a) (b)

(c) (d)

FIGURE 13.7 Vaginal carcinoma. Sagittal (*a*) and transverse (*b*) T2W ETSE and sagittal (*c*) and transverse (*d*) interstitial phase gadolinium-enhanced fat-suppressed SGE images. There is a large, irregular soft tissue mass arrising from the vagina and involving the urethra. The uterus is small and low signal secondary to prior radiation therapy.

Miscellaneous

Radiation Change

- Background
  - Acute radiation changes less than 1 year: interstitial edema and capillary leakage
  - Chronic changes after more than 1 year: fibrosis, diminished interstitial fluid, and diminished vascularity
- Imaging (fig. 13.9)
  - Acute: vaginal wall thickening, high signal on T2W images, gadolinium enhancement
  - Chronic: vaginal wall atrophy, low signal on T2W images, diminished gadolinium

enhancement, necrosis of vaginal wall with fistula can occur

Fistulas

- Background
  - Occur in setting of gynecological malignancy after radiation therapy, hysterectomy, or inflammatory bowel disease
  - MRI can evaluate soft tissue to determine if fistula is due to benign or malignant disease
- Imaging
  - Sagittal and transverse planes with T2W and postgadolinium fat-suppressed T1W images maximize detection

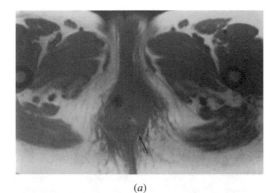

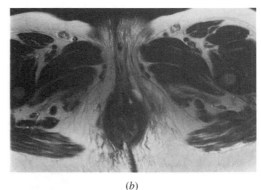

(a)   (b)

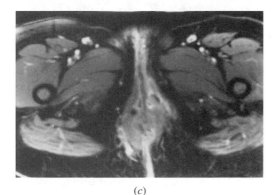

(c)

FIGURE 13.8   Vulvar carcinoma. Transverse SGE (*a*), 512-resolution T2W echo-train spin-echo (*b*), and 90 s post-gadolinium fat-suppressed SGE (*c*) images. The T1W image (*a*) shows an irregular low-signal-intensity mass arising from the vulva with posterior extension to involve the anus (arrow). On the T2W image (*b*), mass is intermidate in signal intensity. In part, this reflects the high signal intensity of fat on echo-train spin-echo sequences. Heterogeneous enhancement of tumor is seen on postgadolinium imaging (*c*).

Uterus and Cervix

Normal Anatomy and Changes with Menstrual Cycle/Menopause
Anatomy of the Uterus
- Corpus
  - Zonal anatomy best seen on T2W sagittal images (figs. 13.10 and 13.11)
  - Zonal anatomy not apparent on T1W images

- Three zones on T2W images; vary with hormonal status
  - Central high-signal stripe = endometrium and secretions
    - Thickness varies with menstrual cycle
    - 3–6 mm in follicular phase to 5–13 mm in secretory
  - Low signal band "junctional zone" = inner layer of myometrium

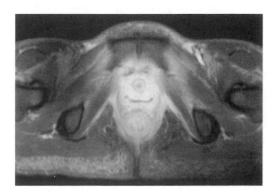

FIGURE 13.9   Radiation changes after treatment for vaginal carcinoma. Transverse gadolinium-enhanced T1W fat-suppressed spin-echo image. Enhancing tissue is seen involving the urethra, vagina, and anal canal. Diffuse thickening of the vaginal wall is appreciated. Enhancement from acute rediation changes cannot be easily distinguished from tumor, but symmetric changes favor benign disease.

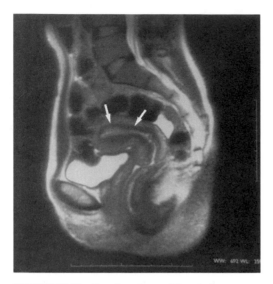

FIGURE 13.10 Zonal anatomy of the uterine corpus. Sagittal T2W fast spin-echo image. The central, high-signal-intensity stripe represents the endometrium. The band of low signal intensity subjacent to the endometrial stripe represents the inner myometrium, the so-called junctional zone (JZ) (arrows). The outer layer of the myometrium is of intermediate signal intensity.

- Immediately subjacent to the endometrial stripe
- Mean thickness 2–8 mm
- During the menstrual phase, intense early enhancement may be observed at dynamic imaging

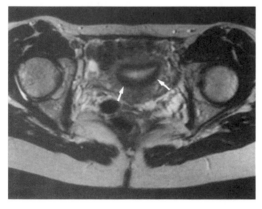

FIGURE 13.11 Short-axis view of the uterus. T2W fast spin-echo sequence. The zonal anatomy is well depicted: hyperintenss endometrium, junctional zone (arrows) representing the innermost part of the myometrium of low signal intensity and the myometrium of intermediate signal intensity.

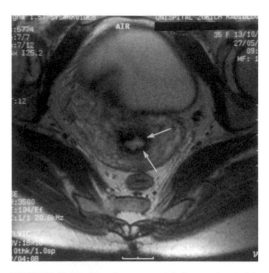

FIGURE 13.12 Zonal anatomy of the cervix. Axial-oblique T2W fast spin-echo image. A thin hypointense fibrous cervical stroma (arrows) is seen surrounding a high-signal-intensity central area representing the cervical mucosa and probably some cervical mucus. The wide peripheral zone is due to a large portion of muscle tissue extending from the uterus to the cervix.

- Intermediate signal band = outer layer of myometrium
  - Postmenopausal uterus
    - Small, zonal anatomy indistinct, junctional zone not always visualized
    - Endometrium 3 mm or less in women not receiving hormones, 6 mm or less in women receiving hormonal replacement therapy
- Cervix
  - Four zones on T2W imaging; do not vary with hormonal status (fig. 13.12)
    - Central hyperintense zone = mucus within the endocervical canal
    - Inner high-signal zone = endocervix columnar epithelium
    - Hyopintense zone = fibrous stroma, 3–8 mm thick
    - Medium-signal zone = smooth muscle continuous with the outer myometrium
  - Gadolinium enhancement
    - Endocervical mucosa enhances rapidly
    - Stroma shows more gradual enhancement
    - Fibrous stroma enhances more slowly than outer zone of smooth muscle

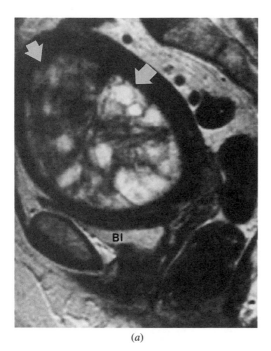
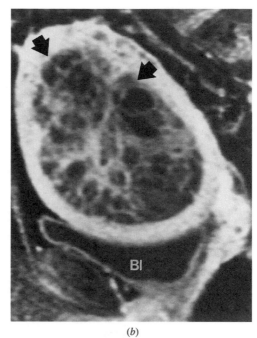

(a)   (b)

FIGURE 13.13 Tamoxifen-induced changes. Sagittal T2W ETSE (*a*) and gadolinium-enhanced fat-suppressed SGE (*b*) images. The endometrial complex is markedly enlarged (arrows, *a, b*) and shows heterogeneous signal intensity. A lattice-like pattern of enhancement is present. A benign polyp was found at histopathology. Bl, bladder.

Exogenous Hormone Therapy
- Prolonged use of oral contraceptives
  - Decrease in uterine size
  - Endometrium thin; junctional zone is less prominent
  - Signal intensity of the myometrium on T2W images is increased
- Tamoxifen
  - Spectrum of endometrial abnormalities reported
    - Proliferative changes
    - Hyperplasia
    - Polyps
    - Carcinoma
  - Two different MR imaging patterns described
    - T2W homogeneously hyperintense endometrium, mean thickness of 0.5 mm, enhancement of the endometrial-myometrial interface with signal void in the lumen on gadolinium-enhanced images
    - T2W: images: heterogeneous, widened endometrium (mean thickness 1.8 cm)

with enhancement of the endometrial-myometrial interface and a lattice-like enhancement circumscribing well-defined cystic spaces (fig. 13.13)

Congenital Uterine Anomalies
Müllerian Duct Anomalies
- Background
  - Nondevelopment or nonfusion of müllerian ducts
  - Frequently associated with urinary tract anomalies
  - Usually asymptomatic, but can be associated with
    - Primary amenorrhea
    - Menstrual disorders
    - Impaired fertility
  - HSG has several limitations
    - Only horns that communicate with the main endometrial cavity are opacified
    - External contour of the uterus cannot be evaluated, thereby limiting differentiation between bicornuate and septate uteri

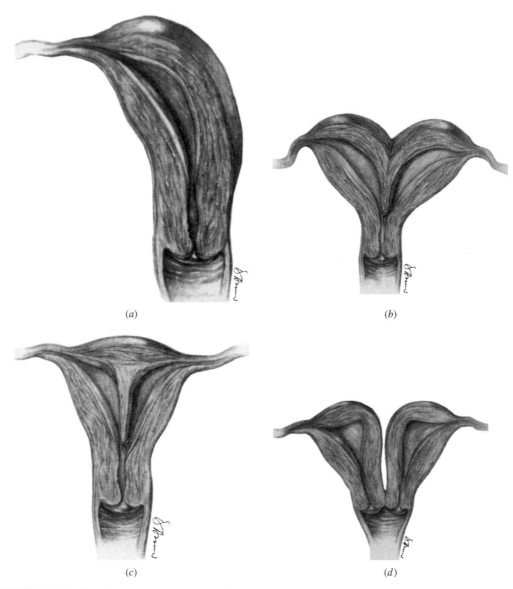

(a)   *(b)*

(c)   *(d)*

FIGURE 13.14   Classification of uterine anomalies. Unicornuate uterus (*a*), bicornuate uterus (*b*), septate uterus (*c*), and uterus didelphys (*d*).

- ○ Buttram and Gibbons classification (fig. 13.14)
  - ▪ Class I: segmental agenesis or hypoplasia
  - ▪ Class II: unicornuate uterus (with or without rudimentary horn)
  - ▪ Class III: uterus didelphys
  - ▪ Class IV: bicornuate uterus (complete division down to internal os, partial division, arcuate uterus)
  - ▪ Class V: septate uterus (complete or incomplete)
- • Imaging
  - ○ Class 1: vaginal agenesis or hypoplasia, intact ovaries and fallopian tubes, variable anomalies of the uterus, urinary tract, and skeletal system
  - ○ Class II (fig. 13.15): elongated, curved uterus, normal zonal anatomy on T2W

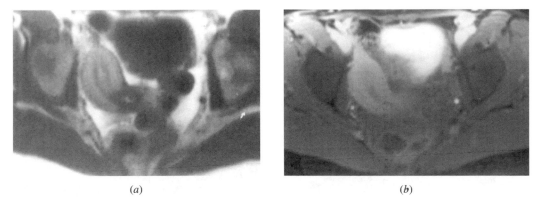

FIGURE 13.15   Unicornuate uterus. Transverse T2W SS-ETSE (*a*) and interstitial phase gadolinium-enhanced fat-suppressed SGE (*b*) images demonstrate a curved and elongated uterus that represents a unicornuate uterus. No rudimentary horn on the left is identified. Note that the zonal anatomy is normal.

images, a rudimentary horn may or may not contain endometrium
- Class III (fig. 13.16): two normal-sized uteri and cervices, possibly a septate vagina with

transverse or longitudinal septum; septate vagina can occur with any müllerian duct anomaly, but is most commonly associated with uterus didelphis; when transverse,

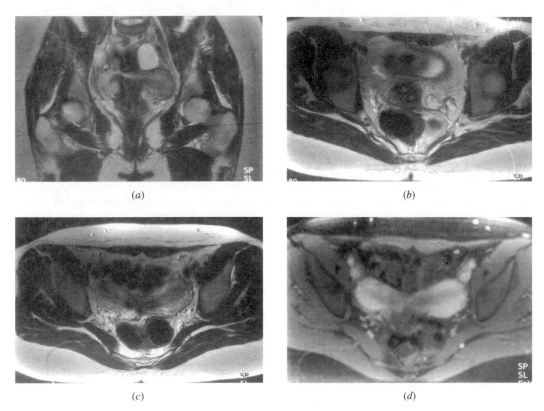

FIGURE 13.16   Uterus didelphys. Coronal (*a*) and transverse (*b, c*) T2W echo-train spin-echo and transverse post-gadolinium SGE (*d*). Two normal-sized uteri and cervices are identified. Note that normal zonal anatomy of the uteri is present.

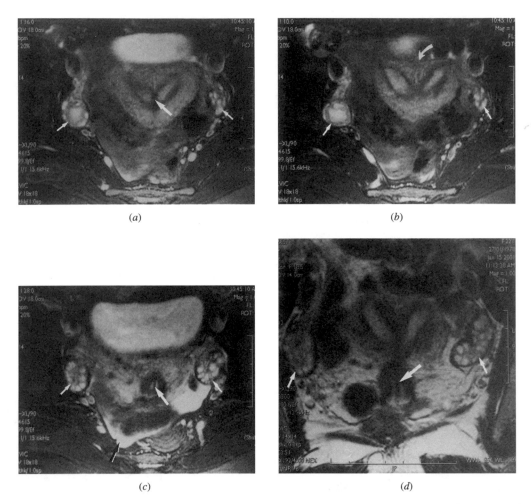

(a)   (b)

(c)   (d)

FIGURE 13.17   Septate uterus. Axial T2W fat-saturated fast spin-echo images at the level of the uterine corpus (*a, b*) and cervix (*c*). Axial-oblique T2W fast spin-echo image parallel to the cavum uteri (*d*) allows for better visualization of the hyperintense septum extending into the cervix (large white arrow, *a, c, d*). Note flat fundal contour (curved arrow, *b*) consistent with septate uterus. The ovaries present with hyperintense cysts (small arrows, *a–d*). Fluid is seen in the pouch of Douglas (black arrow, *c*).

the septum can obstruct the outflow of blood into the vagina and result in hematoculpometra, which is seen as a distended vagina and uterine horn with contents following the signal characteristics of blood on T1W and T2W sequences
○ Class IV: Divergent uterine horns with an intercornual distance exceeding 4 cm and indentation of the fundal contour more than 1 cm in depth; septum may terminate at internal os (unicollis) or extend to external os (bicollis)

○ Class V (fig. 13.17): convex, flat, or minimally indented fundal contour, normal intercornual distance (2–4 cm)

Diethylstilbestrol Exposure
• Background
○ Uterine anomalies include hypoplasia, T shape, constrictions, polypoid defects, and synechiae
○ Increased risk of clear-cell carcinoma of the vagina
○ No increased incidence of urinary tract anomalies

- Imaging
  - Areas of uterine cavity constriction with focal thickening of the junctional zone
  - Hypoplasia of the cervix and uterine cavity, with normal zonal anatomy

Benign Diseases of the Uterine Corpus

Endometrial Hyperplasia
- Background
  - Can result from conditions of prolonged estrogen excess
  - Can lead to metrorrhagia
- Imaging
  - Diffuse thickening of endometrial stripe on T2W images
  - Isointense or slightly hypointense compared to normal endometrium
  - MRI characteristics nonspecific, cannot distinguish from endometrial carcinoma

Polyps of the Endometrium
- Background
  - Seen in about 10% of all uteri, typically in postmenopausal patients
  - Mostly asymptomatic, but may cause irregular or persistent bleeding
  - Malignant transformation into endometrial cancer in less than 1%
- Imaging (fig. 13.18)
  - On T2W images, usually isointense or slightly hypointense to normal endometrium, but may be entirely isointense and present as diffuse or focal thickening
  - Pronounced gadolinium enhancement
  - MRI can distinguish polyps from submucosal leiomyomas
  - MRI can distinguish most polyps from endometrial carcinoma, but accuracy is not sufficient to obviate biopsy; carcinomas and polyps frequently coexist

Leiomyomas
- Background
  - Synonyms: fibroids, fibroleiomyomas
  - Benign neoplasm of smooth-muscle-cell origin
  - Classified according to location: submucosal, intramural, subserosal, or cervical
  - Occasionally seen in the broad ligament or other locations detached from uterus
  - If >8 cm in diameter, likely to degenerate
  - Most are asymptomatic, but may be associated with a variety of symptoms:
    - Bleeding disorders
    - Pressure effects
    - Infertility
    - Second-trimester abortions
    - Dystocia
    - Palpable pelvic-abdominal mass
    - Rarely: torsion, infection, and sarcomatous degeneration
    - Pain is usually the result of acute degeneration (e.g., hemorrhagic infarction during pregnancy), torsion (pedunculated subserosal), or prolapse (pedunculated submucosal)
  - Benign metastasizing leiomyoma is an unusual variant, with tumors in the lungs, lymph nodes, or abdomen thought to originate from a benign uterine leiomyoma not uncommonly removed many years earlier
  - Treatment options for symptomatic leiomyomas
    - Medical (gondatotropin-releasing hormone analogs)
    - Surgical (hysterectomy or myomectomy)
    - Percutaneous uterine artery embolization
  - MRI monitors change in size of leiomyomas, postprocedural complications such as hematoma, abscess, uterine rupture, and peritoneal inclusion cyst
  - In cases of uterine artery embolization, MRI is helpful
    - Preprocedure: helps select patients based on size and location of leiomyomas (e.g., embolization of a pedunculated subserosal tumor may lead to its detachment from the uterus), and extent of vascularity
    - Demonstration of change in size and loss of enhancement after therapy
- Imaging (fig. 13.19)
  - MRI indicated for
    - Localization prior to uterine-sparing surgery

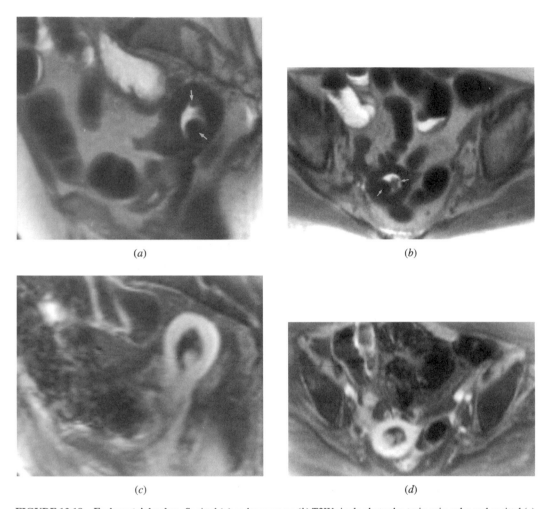

(a)

(b)

(c)

(d)

FIGURE 13.18   Endometrial polyp. Sagittal (a) and transverse (b) T2W single-shot echo-train spin-echo and sagittal (c) and transverse (d) postgadolinium fat-suppressed SGE images. The uterine cavity is mildly distended and contains multiple polypoid lesions (arrows, a, b) that enhance compable to myometrium on postgadolinium images (c, d).

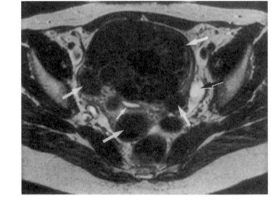

FIGURE 13.19   Multiple uterine leiomyomas. Axial T2W fat-saturated fast spin-echo image: multiple leiomyomas of different size are shown as sharply marginated masses of low signal intensity (white arrows). Endometrial cavity (small arrow). Left ovary (black arrow).

- May be resected hysteroscopically if submucosal
- Laparoscopic or transabdominal approach if intramural or subserosal
- Visualization of endometrium or ovaries in patients with large leiomyomas
- Distinguishing between pedunculated leiomyoma and solid ovarian mass
- Differentiating leiomyomas from other pathological conditions
  - Typically sharply marginated and low signal on T1W and T2W sequences
  - Dark signal on T2W images differentiates from malignant tumors
  - Small hyperintense rim may be seen on T2W images
  - Orthogonal planes oriented to the uterus are helpful for accurate localization
  - Contrast-enhanced T1W images are not usually needed for detection
  - Enhancement varies, usually less than surrounding myometrium
  - Extent of enhancement may indicate likely response to uterine artery embolization and allows evaluation of response postprocedure
  - A myomectomy site may contain high signal intensity on both T1W and T2W images, indicating subacute hematoma (fig. 13.20)
  - Degenerative change causes various MR appearances

- Inhomogeneous high signal intensity on T2W images
- Lack of enhancement on gadolinium-enhanced T1W images
- In hemorrhagic (red) degeneration as seen in pregnancy, hyperintense areas on T1W images are typically seen
- Secondary calcification in about 4%, more frequently in older women
  - MRI usually differentiates leiomyoma from polyp or carcinoma, but leiomyomas have variable signal characteristics that may overlap with those of other endometrial pathology
  - Malignant degeneration is uncommon, but may be suspected if MRI shows sudden enlargement (especially following menopause) or indistinct/irregular border
  - Lipoleiomyoma is a rare type of leiomyoma that contains fat

Adenomyosis
- Background
  - Aberrant endometrial stroma and glands within the myometrium
  - Affects women during menstrual years, higher incidence in multiparous women
  - Commonly associated with leiomyomas
  - Histologically demonstrated in up to 24% of all hysterectomy specimens

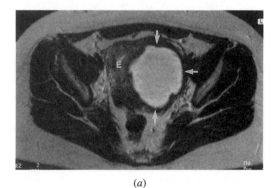

(a)

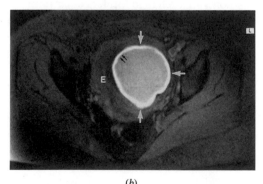

(b)

FIGURE 13.20   Postmyomectomy hematoma. T2W echo-train spin-echo sequence, (*a*). Fat-suppressed T1W SGE sequence (*b*). A well-delineated mass of moderately high signal intensity (arrows, *a*, *b*) consistent with a hematoma is present in the surgical bed. Note the peripheral rim of higher signal intensity (small arrows, *b*), which is typical of a subacute hematoma. E, endometrium.

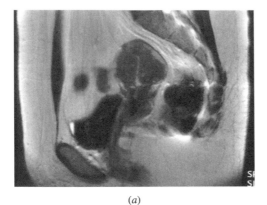

(a)

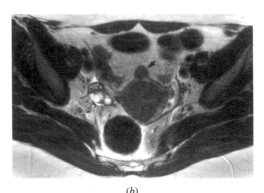

(b)

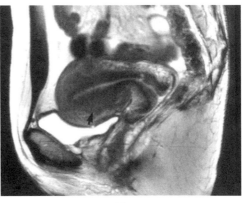

(c)

FIGURE 13.21 Diffuse adenomyosis. Sagittal (a) and transverse (b) T2W ETSE images. There is diffuse broadening of the junctional zone of the uterine body consistent with diffuse adenomyosis. Note also a small subserosal leiomyoma (arrow, b) located anteriorly. Sagittal T2W ETSE image (c) in a second patient with diffuse adenomyosis demonstrates a lesser degree of broadening of the junctional zone.

- ○ Does not contain functional endometrium, thus not affected by hormonal stimulation; does not contain hemorrhage (in contrast to endometriosis)
- ○ May be microscopic, focal, or diffuse; adenomyoma refers to focal, nodular form
- ○ May be asymptomatic, or present with pelvic pain, hypermenorrhea, and/or uterine enlargement (similar to leiomyoma), typically in the fourth to fifth decade
- ○ Diagnosis is important because uterine-conserving therapy is possible with leiomyomas, whereas hysterectomy is the definitive treatment for debilitating adenomyosis
- • Imaging (fig. 13.21)
  - ○ T2W images most important
    - ▪ Thickening of the junctional zone to 12 mm or more
    - ▪ Multiple spots of hyperintensity, most likely representing islands of ectopic endometrium, cystically dilated endometrial glands, or hemorrhagic fluid

- ○ T1W images
  - ▪ Typically unremarkable
  - ▪ Less frequently, foci of high signal seen corresponding to areas of hemorrhage (mechanism unclear)
  - ▪ When the degree of hemorrhage is extensive, cystic adenomyosis can result, presenting with well-circumscribed, cystic myometrial lesions with hemorrhage in different stages of organization at MR imaging
- ○ Diffuse form may result in uterine enlargement
- ○ Focal form characterized by circumscribed thickening of the junctional zone with blurring of its border toward the myometrium
- ○ Adenoma characterized by a low-signal myometrial mass with ill-defined borders
  - ▪ Differential diagnosis: leiomyoma
  - ▪ Features favoring adenomyosis include poorly defined borders, elliptical shape along endometrium, minimal mass effect

relative to size, internal punctate high signal foci, and linear striations extending from endometrium into myometrium
  ○ Contrast not needed for diagnosis; enhancement is variable

Benign Disease of the Cervix

Nabothian Cysts
- Mucous distention of endocervical glands or clefts, rarely symptomatic
- Medium to high signal on T1W images, hyperintense on T2W images
- No enhancement after contrast administration

Malignant Disease of the Uterine Corpus and Cervix

Endometrial Carcinoma
- Background
  ○ Most common malignancy of the female genital tract
  ○ Primarily occurs in postmenopausal women
  ○ Postmenopausal bleeding is the most common and often only symptom
  ○ Adenocarcinomas account for 80–90%
  ○ Frequently invades myometrium, but rarely extends through serosa
  ○ Lymphatic, hematogenous spread occurs later than in cervical carcinoma
  ○ The International Federation of Gynecology and Obstetrics (FIGO) classification is used for tumor staging (Table 13.1)
  ○ Myometrial invasion is an important prognostic factor, as there is close correlation between the depth of myometrial invasion and lymphatic spread
  ○ Para-aortic lymphadenopathy may occur without pelvic node involvement
  ○ Hematogenous metastases occur with disseminated disease and most frequently involve lungs
  ○ MR can identify invasion of cervix and/or extrauterine spread
- Imaging (figs. 13.22 and 13.23)
  ○ Indications for MRI
    ▪ Advanced disease suspected on clinical grounds
    ▪ Histologic subtypes that carry a worse prognosis

- Endovaginal ultrasound technically limited or indeterminate
- Coexisting myometrial pathology such as leiomyomas
  ○ Noninvasive endometrial carcinoma (FIGO stage IA) has nonspecific appearance
    ▪ Uterus may appear entirely normal
    ▪ Endometrial stripe may be widened
    ▪ Heterogeneous mass may distend endometrial cavity
  ○ These changes are also seen in endometrial hyperplasia, polyps, or coagulated blood; thus, histologic sampling is required to establish the diagnosis
  ○ T2W Imaging
    ▪ Signal similar to that of normal endometrium on T2W sequences
      • Limited ability to detect small tumors
      • Larger tumors result in widening of the endometrial cavity
      • In patients with FIGO stage IA disease, the junctional zone will remain intact
    ▪ Myometrial invasion (FIGO stages Ib and Ic)
      • Disruption of junctional zone by hyperintense tumor
        ○ Pitfall: junctional zone is not always visualized in postmenopausal women
      • Deep invasion suggested by hyperintense tumor in outer half of myometrium
    ▪ Cervical invasion
      • Superficial extension of endometrial carcinoma to the cervical mucosa (FIGO stage IIA) is demonstrated by direct tumor visualization and widening of the endocervical canal
      • Invasion of the cervical fibrous stroma (FIGO stage IIB) is diagnosed when hypointense cervical stroma is disrupted by the hyperintense tumor mass
  ○ T1W Imaging
    ▪ Tumor that is confined to uterus is not typically visualizable
    ▪ Lymph nodes are well shown
    ▪ Nodes exceeding 1.0 cm short axis diameter are considered pathologic
  ○ Gadolinium-enhanced T1W imaging

TABLE 13.1   Revised FIGO Staging of Endometrial Carcinoma with Corresponding MRI Findings

Revised FIGO Staging[1]

Stage 0	Carcinoma in situ	
Stage I	Tumor confined to corpus	
	IA	Tumor limited to endometrium
	IB	Invasion <50% of myometrium
	IC	Invasion >50% of myometrium
Stage II	Tumor invades cervix but does not extend beyond uterus	
	IIA	Invasion of endocervix
	IIB	Cervical stromal invasion
Stage III	Tumor extends beyond uterus but not outside true pelvis	
	IIIA	Invasion of serosa, adnexa, or positive peritoneal cytology
	IIIB	Invasion of vagina
	IIIC	Pelvic and/or para-aortic lymphadenopathy
Stage IV	Tumor extends outside of true pelvis of invades bladder or rectal mucosa	
	IVA	Invasion of bladder or rectal mcosa
	IVB	Distant metastases (includes intraabdominal or inguinal lymphadenopathy)

Corresponding MR Findings[2]

Stage 0		Normal or thickened endometrial stripe
Stage I	IA	Thickened endometrial stripe with diffuse or focal abnormal signal intensity. Endometrial stripe may be normal. Intact junctional zone with smooth endometrial-myometrial interface[3]
	IB	Signal intensity of tumor extends into myometrium <50% Partial or full-thickness disruption of junctional zone with irregular endometrial-myometrial interface
	IC	Signal intensity of tumor extends into myometrium >50% Full-thickness disruption of junctional zone[3] Intact stripe of normal outer myometrium
Stage II	IIA	Internal os and endocervical canal are widened Low signal intensity of fibrous stroma remains intact
	IIB	Disruption of fibrous stroma
Stage III	IIIA	Disruption of continuity of outer myometrium Irregular uterine configuration
	IIIB	Segmental loss of hypointense vaginal wall
	IIIC	Regional lymph nodes >1.0 cm in diameter
Stage IV	IVA	Tumor signal disrupts normal tissue planes with loss of low signal intensity of bladder or rectal wall
	IVB	Tumor masses in distant organs or anatomic sites

[1] All stages are further subdivided into three tumor grades (not shown).
[2] MRI findings seen on T2-weighted or contrast-enhanced T1-weighted images.
[3] For patients with adenomyosis, criteria may not apply.

- Typically enhances to a lesser extent than adjacent myometrium
- Gadolinium enhancement is of value to permit distinction between enhancing tumor and fluid distending the endometrial canal, a distinction that may not be feasible on T2W images

Uterine Sarcoma
- Rare
- Invades blood vessels, lymphatics, and contiguous pelvic structures
- Lung is the most common site of distant metastases

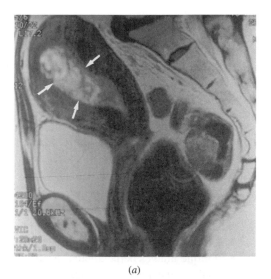
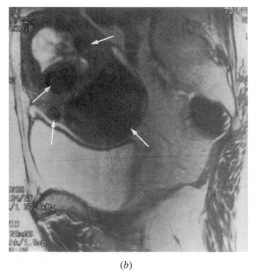

(a)   *(b)*

FIGURE 13.22   Endometrial carcinoma stage IA, multiple leiomyomas. Sagittal T2W fast spin-echo images (*a*, *b*). The patient was referred to MRI for staging of endometrial carcinoma proven by D&C. Clinically advanced tumor stage was suspected. MRI shows widening of the endometrial cavity due to inhomogeneously hyperintense tumor. The junctional zone (small arrows), however, was intact and thus a stage IA diagnosed. The large uterus found at clinical examination and prompting the suspicion of advanced tumor stage could be explained by multiple sharply delineated, hypointense leiomyomas (arrows, *b*).

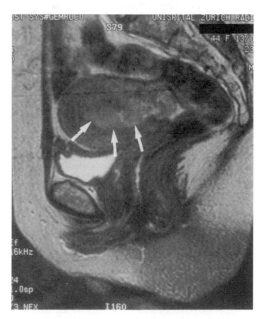

FIGURE 13.23   Endometrial carcinoma stage IC. Sagittal T2W fast spin-echo images. Endometrial carcinoma, isointense relative to endometrium, is seen, resulting in asymmetric widening of the endometrium. Whereas the junctional zone (arrows) can be delineated ventrally, the tumor invades the inner myometrium along the posterior aspect.

- MRI not reliable in differentiating sarcomas from other uterine neoplasms, but a large heterogeneous mass with indistinct or irregular borders should raise concern (fig. 13.24)

Cervical Carcinoma
- Background
  - Average age at diagnosis is 45
  - Intermenstrual bleeding is the most common symptom when invasive
  - Up to 90% are squamous cell
  - 10% are adenocarcinomas, adenosquamous carcinomas, and undifferentiated carcinomas
  - Adenocarcinomas tend to have a worse prognosis
  - Other indicators of a poor prognosis
    - Young age
    - Lymphadenopathy
    - Tumor diameter larger than 4 cm
    - Depth of stromal invasion greater than 5 mm
    - Advanced stage at presentation
  - Advances predominantly via direct extension and local spread

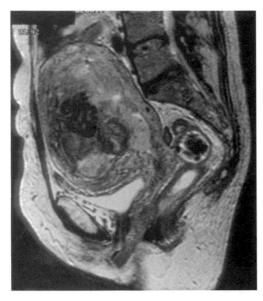

FIGURE 13.24 Endometrial sarcoma. Sagittal T2W fast spin-echo image. A large, heterogeneous uterine mass with indistinct borders is demonstrated.

- Lymph node involvement
  - External iliac > obturator > common and internal iliac
  - Para-aortic nodes in 45% of cases with pelvic side wall or lower vagina involvement
  - Inguinal nodes if lower vagina involved
- Hematogenous spread rare
  - Occurs only in advanced disease
  - Liver and lung are the most common sites
- Staged clinically according to the FIGO staging system (Table 13.2)
- Preoperative staging predicts prognosis and defines choice of treatment
  - FIGO stage Ia: simple hysterectomy or even fertility-preserving surgery
  - Invasive carcinoma (FIGO stage Ib) or tumor extending to the upper vagina (FIGO stage IIa): radical hysterectomy and pelvic lymph node dissection
  - Advanced disease (stage IIB or beyond): radiation therapy
- Lymphadenopathy, large tumor volume, and tumor extension to the uterine corpus affect prognosis, but are not evaluated in the FIGO staging system

- Imaging (figs. 13.25 to 13.28)
  - Not used for detection; however, MRI found superior to CT for local staging
  - MRI especially helpful in select circumstances
    - Tumors larger than 2 cm in size
    - Tumors located entirely within the endocervical canal
    - Concomitant pelvic masses
    - Pregnant patients
  - MRI technique
    - T2W sequence is most important for staging
    - Axial and sagittal sequences routinely performed
    - Oblique images perpendicular to the cervical canal can improve staging accuracy
    - Axial T1W sequences used to detect lymphadenopathy, both noncontrast T1W and gadolinium-enhanced fat-suppressed T1W GRE
  - T2W Imaging
    - Tumor is high signal intensity compared to the hypointense cervical stroma
      - FIGO stage Ib is restricted to the cervix: fully preserved hypointense rim of cervical stroma
      - Stage IIa invades the upper two-thirds of the vagina: disruption of the low-signal-intensity vaginal wall or thickened hyperintense vagina
      - Stage IIb extends to parametrium: complete disruption of the cervical stroma, irregularity or stranding within the parametrial fat
      - Stage IIIa extends to lower third of the vagina
      - Stage IIIb infiltrates pelvic wall or obstructs one or both ureters: dilated ureter can be well seen adjacent to the psoas muscle on axial fat-saturated T2W images. Pelvic side-wall invasion suggested when the normal low signal intensity of the levator ani, pyriformis, or obturator internus muscle is disrupted.
      - Stage IVa invades bladder or rectal wall: fat planes between organs

TABLE 13.2   FIGO Staging of Cervical Carcinoma with Corresponding MRI Findings

FIGO Staging [1]

Stage 0		Carcinoma in situ
Stage I		Tumor confined to cervix (extension to corpus should be disregarded)
	IA	Microinvasion
	IB	Clinically invasive. Invasive component >5 mm in depth and >7 mm in horizontal spread
Stage II		Tumor extends beyond cervix but not to pelvic side wall or lower third of vagina
	IIA	Vaginal invasion (no parametrial invasion)
	IIB	Parametrial invasion
Stage III		Tumor extends to lower third of vagina or pelvic side wall; ureter obstruction
	IIIA	Invasion of lower third of vagina (no pelvic side-wall extension)
	IIIB	Pelvic side wall extension or ureteral obstruction
Stage IV		Tumor extends outside true pelvis of invades bladder or rectal mucosa
	IVA	Invasion of bladder or rectal mucosa
	IVB	Distant metastases

Corresponding MRI findings [2]

Stage 0		No tumor mass present
Stage I	IA	No tumor mass or localized widening of the endocervical canal with a small tumor mass
		Fibrous stroma intact and symmetric
	IB	Partial or complete disruption of low-signal-intensity fibrous stroma
		Rim of intact cervical tissue surrounding tumor
Stage II	IIA	Segmental disruption of hypointense vaginal wall (upper two-thirds)
	IIB	Complete disruption of low signal intensity fibrous stroma with tumor signal extending into parametrium
Stage III	IIIA	Segmental disruption of hypointense vaginal wall (lower third)
	IIIB	Same findings as IIB with tumor signal, most frequently extending to involve obturator internus, piriformis, or levator ani muscles
		Dilated ureter
Stage IV	IVA	Tumor signal disrupts normal tissue planes with loss of low signal intensity of bladder or rectal wall
	IVB	Tumor masses in distant organs or anatomic sites

[1] The presence of metastatic lymph nodes is not included in the FIGO classification.
[2] MRI findings seen on T2-weighted or contrast-enhanced T1-weighted images.

obliterated, hyperintense disruption of the hypointense bladder or rectal wall, nodular wall thickening or intraluminal masses
- T1W Imaging
  - Tumor confined to cervix, vagina, or uterine corpus not visualizable
  - Lymph nodes well shown
  - Fat planes well demonstrated
- Cervical carcinoma may obstruct cervix, leading to hematometra or pyometra

- Uterine cavity distended with variable signal on T1W and T2W images, depending on content (e.g., retained secretions, blood, or tumor)
- Other causes of obstruction: benign stenosis, endometrial carcinoma

Recurrent Cervical Carcinoma
- Background
  - Typical manifestations include recurrent pelvic mass and lymphadenopathy

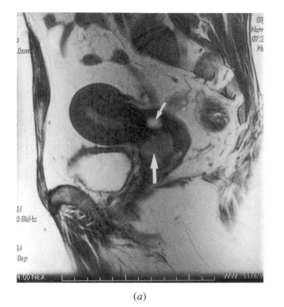

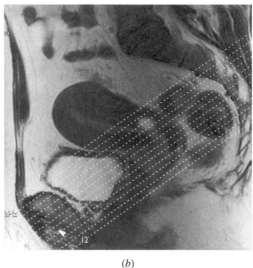

(a)

(b)

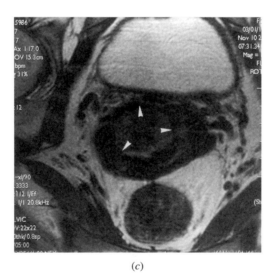

(c)

FIGURE 13.25 Cervical carcinoma stage IB. Sagittal T2W fast spin-echo images (*a, b*). On the sagittal image in (*b*), an oblique imaging plane perpendicular to the cervical canal is prescribed graphically. Resulting axial-oblique T2W fast spin-echo image (*c*). A tumor (arrow) of intermediate signal is shown within the cervix. The tumor is in the entire circumference surrounded by normal hypointense cervical stroma (arrowheads, *c*) and parametrial invasion could thus be excluded. Incidentally, Nabothian cysts (small arrow, *a*) are seen within the cervix.

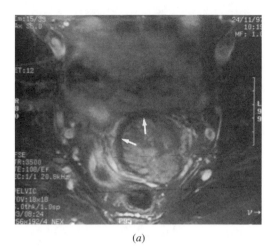

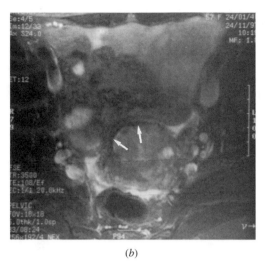

(*a*)   (*b*)

FIGURE 13.26   Cervical carcinoma stage IIB. Axial T2W fat-suppressed fast spin-echo images (*a*, *b*). A large inhomogeneously hyperintense cervical tumor is seen. Whereas the normal hypointense cervical stroma can be delineated at the ventral aspect (small arrows), it is disrupted dorsally. The diagnosis of parametrial invasion was histologically confirmed.

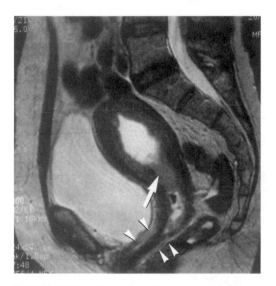

FIGURE 13.27   Cervical carcinoma with vaginal extension. Sagittal T2W fast spin-echo image. Hyperintense cervical carcinoma (arrow) with extension to the vagina. The tumor results in a cervical stenosis with fluid retention within the uterine cavum. Note that the fat planes between the cervix and the urinary bladder as well as the rectal wall can be well delineated (arrowheads); bladder or rectal wall infiltration can thus be excluded.

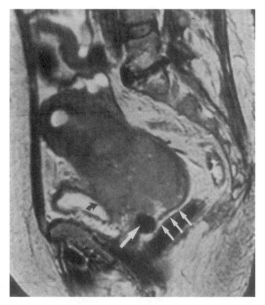

FIGURE 13.28   Cervical carcinoma with urinary bladder invasion (FIGO stage IV). Sagittal T2W fast spin-echo image. Hyperintense cervical carcinoma (arrow) with extension to the vagina (large arrow: tampon) and urinary bladder invasion. Note that the fat plane between the cervix and rectal wall can be well delineated (small arrows); rectal wall infiltration can thus be excluded.

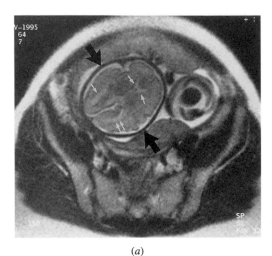
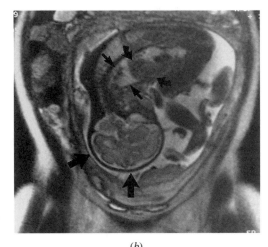

(a)   *(b)*

FIGURE 13.29   Normal fetus. Central nervous system (CNS) third trimester. Axial (*a*) and coronal HASTE (*b*) sequences through the maternal pelvis. The contour of the fetal head (large arrows *a*, *b*) and the cerebral hemispheres are well delineated. Cerebral ventricles (small arrows, *a*) are hyperintense relative to brain tissue. Fetal lungs (arrows, *b*) are of high signal intensity because of their water content. The liver (curved arrows, *b*) is of intermediate signal intensity and occupies most of the abdominal cavity. The lung-liver interface outlines the diaphragm.

- ○ Less common sites of recurrence are solid organs (e.g., liver or bones) or peritoneal carcinomatosis
- ○ MRI helpful to assess local recurrence and enlarged lymph nodes
- • Imaging
  - ○ Radiation therapy presents a diagnostic challenge because differentiation between radiation changes and residual or recurrent disease is frequently difficult
    - ▪ Irradiation in premenopausal patients results in decreased uterine size, endometrial thinning, decreased signal of the myometrium, and loss of zonal anatomy, resembling a postmenopausal uterus
    - ▪ Both tumor and radiation fibrosis are low signal on T1W images
    - ▪ On T2W images
      - • After 12 months, radiation fibrosis is distinct from tumor
        - ○ Tumor is hyperintense relative to adjacent muscle and fat
        - ○ Radiation fibrosis is hypointense
      - • During the initial 6–12 months, radiation change may be hyperintense; an identifiable mass favors recurrence

- ▪ Gadolinium-enhanced T1W images
  - • Enhancement of the cervix is nonspecific
  - • Helpful in demonstrating parametrial and pelvic side-wall recurrence

MRI and Pregnancy

Overview
- • MRI is considered safe for the developing fetus after the first trimester
- • Gadolinium-based contrast agents should generally be avoided, unless essential to show a life-threatening disease process
- • Gadolinium should be avoided in the first trimester

The Fetus
- • Background
  - ○ Ultrasonography remains the imaging technique of choice for assessment of the fetus
  - ○ The role of fetal MRI is increasing (figs. 13.29 to 13.34)
  - ○ MRI can demonstrate much fetal anatomy in detail, including the CNS, lungs, and major abdominal viscera beginning at the second trimester

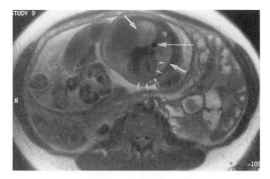

FIGURE 13.30   Normal fetus. Heart and vessels. Axial HASTE sequence through the maternal pelvis. Fetal lungs (arrows) are depicted on either side of the thorax. The heart is visible, and the contrast between the signal-void area generated by the circulating blood and the intermediate signal intensity of the myocardium (small arrows) allows assessment of ventricular wall thickness. The thoracic aorta (long, thin arrow) is depicted as a signal-void area in front of the thoracic spine.

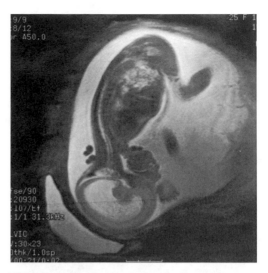

FIGURE 13.31   Hydrocephalus in a fetus of 22 weeks of gestation. Sagittal T2W single-shot fast spin-echo image shows marked dilatation of lateral ventricles.

- Imaging
  - Fetal brain maturation is reliably evaluated with fast T2W imaging (fig. 13.29)
    - 12–23 weeks: smooth surface except for the interhemispheric fissure; 2–3 layers in the cerebral cortex can be delineated; cerebral ventricles are large, gradually becoming smaller after 23 weeks
    - 24–26 weeks: a few shallow groves in central sulcus; 3 cortical layers seen (immature cortex, intermediate zone, germinal matrix)

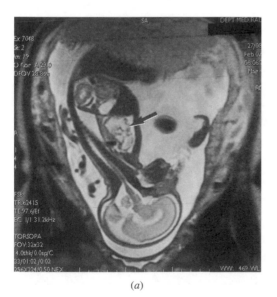

(a)

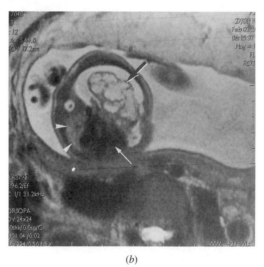

(b)

FIGURE 13.32   Fetus with adenomatoid cystic malformation at 28 weeks of gestation. Sagittal (*a*) and axial (*b*) T2W single-shot fast spin-echo images of the fetus. A mainly cystic, hyperintense lesion is seen within the left hemithorax (black arrows). The heart (white arrow) is pushed to the contralateral side. Hypoplasia of the right lung (arrowheads). Associated polyhydramnios was seen.

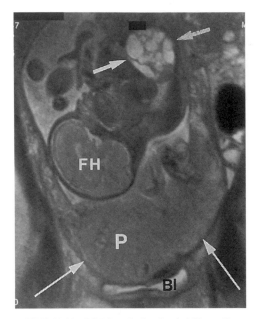

FIGURE 13.33 Multicystic dysplastic kidney disease. Coronal SS-ETSE sequence through the maternal pelvis. The fetal kidney (arrows) shows multiple high-signal-intensity cysts, which is consistent with multicystic dysplastic renal disease. In addition, a complete placenta previa is demonstrated (long, thin arrows). FH, fetal head; P, placenta; Bl, maternal bladder.

- 27–29 weeks: sulcus formation in various regions of the brain parenchyma
- 30 weeks: sulcation in the whole cerebal cortex
- 33 weeks: infolding of the cortex and opercular formation
- Subarachnoid space appears dilated at all gestational ages, most markedly at 21–26 weeks
  - Thorax (fig. 13.30)
    - Lung and tracheobronchial tree
      - Filled with amniotic fluid, hyperintense on T2W images
      - Sagittal and coronal images of the fetus delineate thorax and abdomen
      - MRI detects congenital diaphragmatic hernia, adenomatoid-cystic pulmonary malformation (fig. 13.33) or broncho-pulmonary sequestration
    - Heart, pulmonary vasculature, and great vessels are hypointense on T2W images
  - Abdomen
    - Stomach, esophagus, intestine, urinary collecting system, and bladder are high signal on T2W images

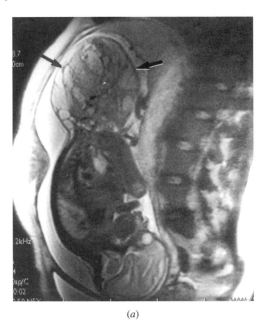

(a)

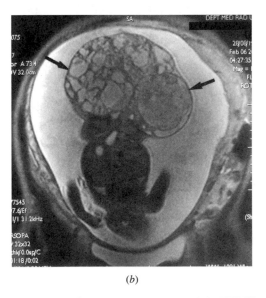

(b)

FIGURE 13.34 Fetus with sacrococcygeal teratoma at 28 weeks of gestation. Sagittal (a) and coronal (b) T2W SS-ETSE images of the fetus. A large, predominantly cystic, hyperintense lesion is delineated in the sacral region (arrows, a, b) consistent with a sacrococcygeal teratoma. Associated polyhydramnios is present.

- Liver, spleen, and kidneys appear hyperintense on T2W images
- On T1W imaging, the intestinal loops are relatively high signal due to meconium
  - Amniotic fluid
    - Hypointense on T1W sequences and hyperintense on T2W sequences
    - Volume measurements allow detection of oligohydramnios and polyhydramnios (fig. 13.34)

The Placenta
- Background
  - MRI can depict placental masses
  - MRI is highly accurate in the diagnosis of placenta previa (fig. 13.35), and invasive placenta can also be detected
- Imaging
  - Normal placenta is homogeneous intermediate signal on T1W
  - Homogeneous increased signal T2W images in the second trimester

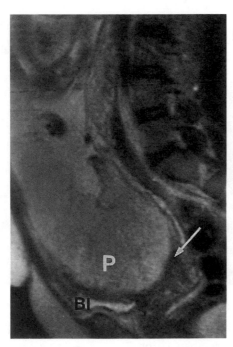

FIGURE 13.35   Complete placenta previa. Sagittal SS-ETSE image through the maternal pelvis shows that the placenta (P) completely covers the internal cervical os (arrow). Bl, maternal bladder.

- Becomes more heterogeneous on T2W images in third trimester, with visualization of internal architecture with cotyledon formation

Gestational Trophoblastic Disease
- Background
  - Complete or partial hydatidiform mole, invasive mole, choriocarcinoma
  - Clinically presents with hyperemesis gravidarum, severe preeclampsia before 24 weeks of gestation, a large-for-date uterus, or first-trimester bleeding
  - Markedly elevated human chorionic gonadotropin (β-hCG) diagnostic
- Imaging (fig. 13.36)
  - While the role of imaging is limited, MRI may help establish the degree of myometrial invasion in patients with invasive mole or choriocarcinoma
  - Complete hydatidiform moles are most common and have a typical MR appearance
    - Heterogeneous mass with multiple cystic spaces distending endometrial cavity
    - Rim of hypointense myometrium at the periphery
    - Uterine zones distorted with irregular boundary between tumor and myometrium
    - On T1W sequences, foci of high signal are apparent corresponding to hemorrhage
    - Intense enhancement with gadolinium

Pelvimetry
- Background
  - Performed in patients who desire a trial of labor with breech presentation, have a history of secondary cesarean section due to dystocia, or present with pelvic deformity
  - MRI accurately measures bony structures without ionizing radiation
- Imaging (fig. 13.37)
  - Gradient-echo sequences have been suggested due to short acquisition times and relatively low specific absorption rate

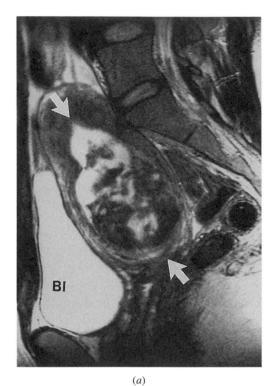

BI

(*a*)

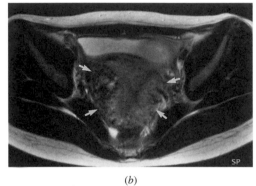

(*b*)

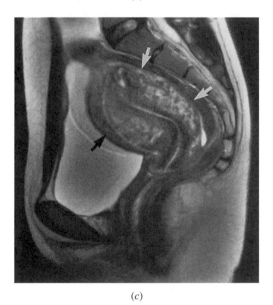

(*c*)

FIGURE 13.36   Hydatidiform mole and invasive mole.
Sagittal T2W ETSE image (*a*) in a patient with a partial hydatidiform mole. A large heterogeneous mass is seen within
the endometrial cavity (arrows) in a patient with elevated
serum β-HCG levels. Note that there is no definite evidence
of myometrial invasion. Transverse (*b*) and sagittal (*c*) T2W
ETSE images in a second patient who has an invasive mole.
Note that in distinction from the patient with the hydatid
mole there is diffuse heterogeneous high signal intensity of
the myometrium consistent with invasion (arrows *b*, *c*). Bl,
bladder.

The Maternal Side
Adnexal Masses
  ○ May become symptomatic during preg-
    nancy as a result of extrinsic compression,
    hemorrhage, or torsion

  ○ MRI differentiates simple cysts from more
    complex lesions
  ○ Relationship between the mass and the
    pregnant uterus can be established

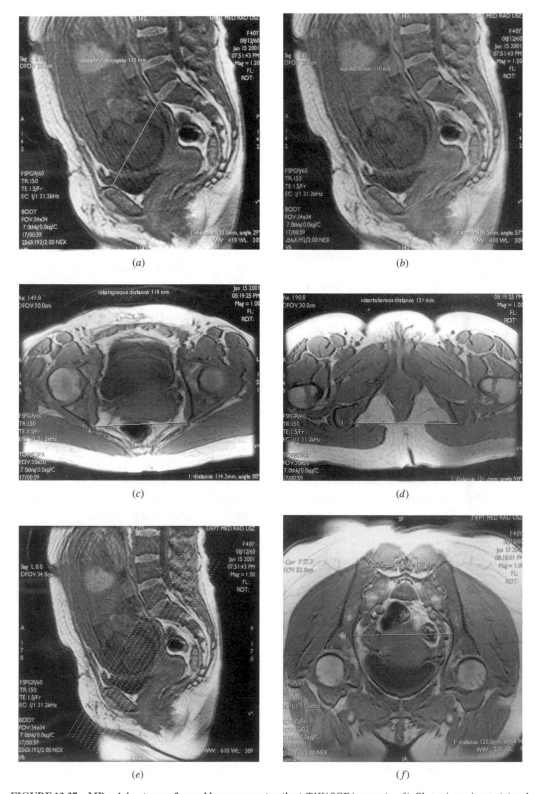

FIGURE 13.37 **MR pelvimetry performed in a pregnant patient.** T1W SGE images (*a–f*). Obstetric conjugate (*a*) and sagittal outlet (*b*) are measured on a midsagittal plane, interspinous distance (*c*) and intertuberous distance (*d*) on transverse planes. The transversal distance (*f*) is measured on an oblique plane acquired as shown on the localizing image (*e*).

Uterine Leiomyomas
- May outgrow their vascular supply, resulting in degeneration
- Most commonly hemorrhagic infarction and necrosis (red degeneration)
  - Peripheral or diffuse high signal on T1W images
  - Variable signal with or without low-signal rim on T2W images
- Presence in the lower uterine segment might influence route of delivery

Cervical Carcinoma
- Approximately 1 per 1,200 to 10,000 pregnancies
- MRI is currently the best imaging modality for evaluating pregnant patients with cervical carcinoma
- With close surveillance, deliberate delay of therapy to achieve fetal maturity is a reasonable option for patient with early-stage cancer, since tumor characteristics and maternal survival do not appear adversely affected by pregnancy

Urography
- MRI can be helpful in distinguishing physiologic hydronephrosis from other causes of urinary tract dilatation such as calculi

Postpartum Uterus
- Background
  - MR may be useful to evaluate postdelivery complications such as hemorrhage, ovarian vein thrombosis, and retained products of conception
- Imaging (fig. 13.38)
  - Returns to normal size by 6 months
  - Blood in the endometrial cavity is common and resolves usually within 1 week
  - The junctional zone is visualized again in 2 weeks
  - A small amount of free pelvic fluid is normal
  - Cesarean section incision typically seen as an area of moderately high signal intensity on both T1W and T2W sequences, suggesting subacute hematoma

- Ovarian vein thrombosis is seen as a low-signal filling defect in the ovarian vein on interstitial phase gadolinium-enhanced T1W images

Adnexa

Ovaries (fig. 13.39)
- Two patterns on T2W images
  - Lower signal cortex and stroma with higher signal in the medulla
    - More prevalent in premenopausal subjects
    - Small high-signal foci, largely peripherally located, representing follicles
  - More homogeneous low signal of the cortex and medulla
    - More common in postmenopausal women
- On T1W images
  - Homogeneously isointense to the myometrium
  - Gadolinium enhancement varies with hormonal status
    - Premenopausal enhancement tends to be less than myometrium
    - Postmenopausal enhancement is equivalent to myometrium
- Transposed ovaries have similar imaging features to normal ovaries

Mass Lesions

Benign Masses
Functional Cysts
- Background
  - Common regardless of age and hormonal status
  - Include follicular, corpus luteal, and corpus albicans cysts
- Imaging
  - Uncomplicated cysts are very high signal on T2W images, low to intermediate signal on T1W images
  - Cyst walls are usually low signal on T2W images; enhancement is variable
  - Corpus luteal cysts have thicker walls that enhance intensely

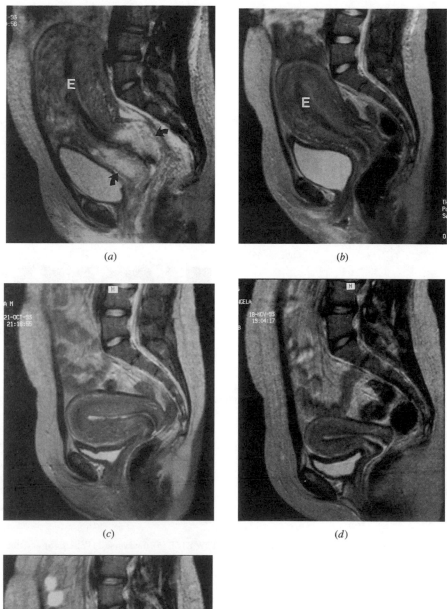

(a)

(b)

(c)

(d)

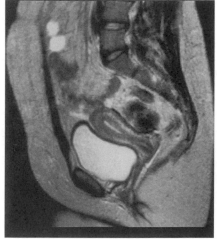

(e)

FIGURE 13.38   Postpartum uterus. Sagittal T2W ETSE
images at 24 h (*a*), 1 week (*b*), 1 month (*c*), 2 months (*d*),
and 6 months (*e*) after delivery. Acute and/or subacute blood
is shown within the endometrial cavity (E) in the first week
postpartum (*a, b*). The outer cervical stroma or smooth-
muscle layer is hyperintense (curved arrows, *a*) in the first
30 h after delivery. The inner fibrous stroma, however, remains hypointense throughout the postpartum period (*a–e*).
The myometrium is of intermediate and heterogeneous signal intensity during the early postpartum period (*a–c*). By
6 months, complete reconstitution of the junctional zone
(JZ) is evident (*e*). Note the gradual decreases in size of the
uterus from *a* to *e*.

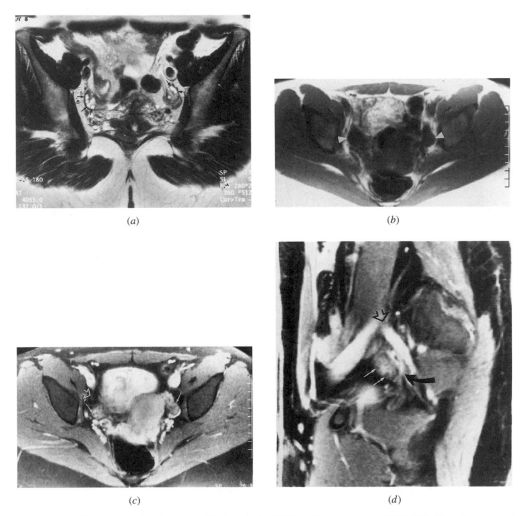

(a)

(b)

(c)

(d)

FIGURE 13.39   Normal ovaries. Paracoronal 512-resolution T2W ETSE (*a*), transverse T1W SGE (*b*), and transverse (*c*) and sagittal (*d*) gadolinium-enhanced T1W fat-suppressed SGE images of a woman with normal ovaries. The ovaries reside in the ovarian fossa and are intermediate in signal intensity on the unenhanced T1W image (arrowheads, *b*). On the T2W image (*a*), follicles are identified as high-signal-intensity structures (arrows, *a*). After contrast the ovarian parenchyma enhances, whereas the follicles (arrows, *c, d*) are signal-void foci. The enhanced images show some of the anatomic boundaries of the ovarian fossa: the bifurcation of the common iliac vessels superiorly (open arrow, *d*), obliterated umbilical artery anteriorly (open arrow, *c*), and the internal iliac vessels posteriorly (curved arrow, *d*). (Courtesy of Susan M. Ascher, M.D., Department of Radiology, Georgetown University.)

∘ Complicated cysts must be differentiated from endometriomas and neoplasm
  ▪ Follow-up showing resolution of the cyst easily classifies it as functional
  ▪ On any single study there are features that can aid in differentiation
    • Papillary projections are a feature of neoplasm not present in functional cysts

• Hemorrhagic cysts have high signal on T1W images and high or low signal on T2W images and can mimic endometriomas (fig. 13.40)

Mature Cystic Teratoma (Dermoid Cyst)
• Background
  ∘ Most common ovarian neoplasm, 90% unilateral

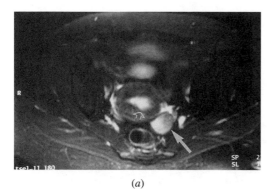
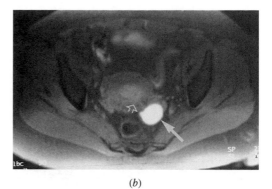

(a)   (b)

FIGURE 13.40   Left adnexal hemorrhagic cyst in patient with endometrial carcinoma. T2W fat-suppressed ETSE (a) and T1W fat-suppressed SGE (b) images. Hemorrhagic cysts can mimic endometriomas with high signal intensity on T1W images (arrow, b) and heterogeneous high signal intensity on T2W images (arrow, a). Note the focus of endometrial carcinoma that thins the junctional zone (open arrow, a, b). (Courtesy of Susan M. Ascher, M.D., Department of Radiology, Georgetown University.)

- ◦ Peak incidence during mid-reproductive years
- ◦ Symptoms can occur due to mass effect, torsion, infection, or rupture
- ◦ Malignant transformation in 1–3%, typically in postmenopausal women
  - ▪ Majority are squamous cell carcinoma while minority are adenocarcinoma, sarcoma, transitional cell carcinoma, or melanoma
  - ▪ Prognosis poor: most patients survive less than 1 year
- • Imaging (fig. 13.41)
  - ◦ Characteristic features: gross fat, fat-fluid or fluid-fluid levels, layering debris, calcification, and Rokitansky nodules (dermoid plugs on cyst wall)
  - ◦ Interfaces between fat and water/soft tissue cause chemical shift artifact
  - ◦ Fat suppressed or out-of-phase T1W images improve diagnosis, with fat suppression showing loss of signal of fatty components and out-of-phase T1W images showing development of phase cancellation artifact at fat-tissue boundaries
  - ◦ Struma ovarii (fig. 13.42)
    - ▪ Composed almost entirely of thyroid tissue
    - ▪ Multilocular masses with solid components

- ▪ The different locules have variable signal, often low to intermediate on T1W and very low on T2W images
- ▪ Solid components of thyroid tissue enhance intensely

Serous Cystadenomas
- • Background
  - ◦ Occur in women between 20 and 50 years of age
  - ◦ 20% of benign ovarian neoplasms
  - ◦ 20% are bilateral
  - ◦ Treated by resection or unilateral oophorectomy, they do not recur or spread
- • Imaging (fig. 13.43)
  - ◦ Most commonly a thin-walled unilocular cyst
  - ◦ Papillary projections occasionally seen
    - ▪ Hallmark of epithelial neoplasms
    - ▪ May be a predictor of malignancy
    - ▪ Benign tumors have fewer and smaller projections
  - ◦ Dark on T1W and bright on T2W sequences, if uncomplicated
  - ◦ When complicated by hemorrhage, T1 and T2 signal altered
  - ◦ Unilocular thin-walled lesions can be mistaken for functional cysts
  - ◦ Multilocular lesions may be mistaken for malignant tumors or hydrosalpinx

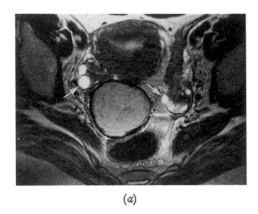

(a)

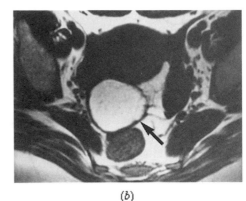

(b)

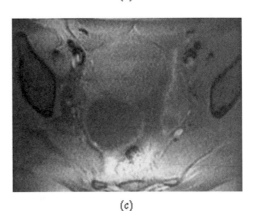

(c)

FIGURE 13.41 Dermoid. Transverse 512-resolution T2W ETSE (*a*), T1W SE (*b*), and T1W fat-suppressed SE (*c*) images in a second patient. An exophytic right ovarian dermoid is present that is uniformly high in signal intensity on the T1W image (arrow, *b*) and suppresses uniformly on the fat-suppressed image (*c*). Follicles are well shown in both ovaries (arrows, *a*) on the high-resolution image, and the exophytic nature of the dermoid is clearly demonstrated. (Courtesy of Susan M. Ascher, M.D., Department of Radiology, Georgetown University).

- ○ Papillary projections should be carefully sought; gadolinium aids detection

Mucinous Cystadenomas
- • Background
  - ○ More common after age 40
  - ○ 20% of benign ovarian neoplasms
  - ○ 5% bilateral
  - ○ Treatment same as serous cystadenoma
- • Imaging (fig. 13.44)
  - ○ Tend to be multilocular, helps distinguish them from serous type
  - ○ Multiple locules, varying signal due to protein content
  - ○ Hemorrhage may be seen in one or more locules
  - ○ Papillary projections suggest malignancy

Endometriosis
- • Background
  - ○ Benign entity affecting women in their reproductive years
  - ○ May be incidental or present with pain or infertility
  - ○ <1% undergo malignant transformation
  - ○ Enlargement during pregnancy does not indicate malignant transformation
  - ○ Most common sites of involvement: ovaries, cul-de-sac, posterior uterine wall, uterosacral ligaments, anterior uterine wall, and bladder dome
  - ○ Other sites: sigmoid colon, fallopian tubes, and distal ureters
- • Imaging (fig. 13.45)
  - ○ Endometriomas
    - ▪ Thick-walled cysts with extensive surrounding fibrosis and adhesions
    - ▪ High signal on T1W images, best seen with fat suppression
    - ▪ Gradient of low signal (shading) seen on T2W images uncommon in functional or hemorrhagic cysts
    - ▪ Variable mural enhancement

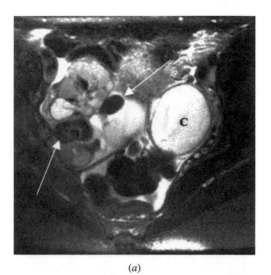

(a)

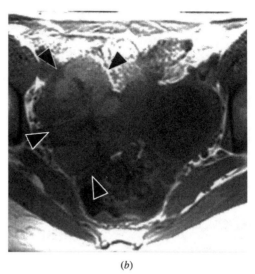

(b)

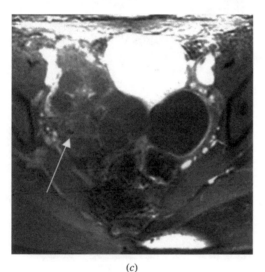

(c)

FIGURE 13.42   Struma ovarii. T2W FSE (*a*), T1W SE (*b*), and gadolinium-enhanced T1W fat-suppressed SGE (*c*) images in a patient with struma ovarii. Note a multiloculated mass in the right ovary (arrowheads, *b*), which shows lace-like enhancement on postgadolinium images. Some cysts show low signal intensity on T2W images (arrows, *a*, *b*). Struma ovarii is a monodermal teratoma in which the tumor may produce thyroid hormones.

- ○ Endometrial implants
  - ▪ Small implants may be difficult to visualize
  - ▪ High-resolution fat-suppressed T1W sequences most sensitive
  - ▪ Some implants enhance
  - ▪ Usually low signal on T2W images
  - ▪ Laparoscopic or surgical diagnosis, staging and treatment often needed
- ○ Solid endometrioma
  - ▪ May invade adjacent organs and tissue
  - ▪ Characteristic low-signal poorly marginated mass on T2W images

Polycystic Ovary Disease
- • Background
  - ○ Hormone imbalance causing ovarian stimulation without maturation of dominant follicle, always affecting both ovaries
  - ○ Numerous follicles, increased stromal tissue, capsular hypertrophy
  - ○ Stein-Levanthal syndrome (hirsutism, amenorrhea, infertility) present in minority
- • Imaging (fig. 13.46)
  - ○ Multiple peripheral small follicles of similar size

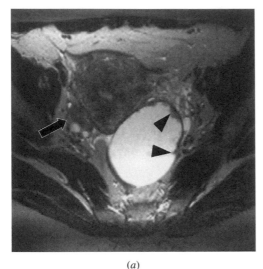

(a)

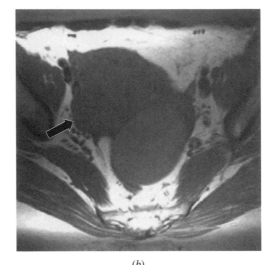

(b)

FIGURE 13.43 Normal right ovary and left ovarian serous cystadenocarcinoma. T2W ETSE (*a*), T1W SE (*b*), gadolinium-enhanced T1W fat-suppressed SGE (*c*) images in a 40-year-old woman with a left adnexal mass. The normal right ovary (arrow, *a–c*) contains several follicles that have enhancing rims following contrast. Note that the ovarian stroma enhances less than adjacent myometrium. Apparent thickening of the wall of the cyst (arrowheads, *a*) is confirmed on the postgadolinium image, which demonstrates enhancing papillary projections (arrowheads, *c*). (Reprinted with permission from Outwater EK, Mitchell DG: Normal ovaries and functional cysts: MR appearance. *Radiology* 198:397–402, 1996.)

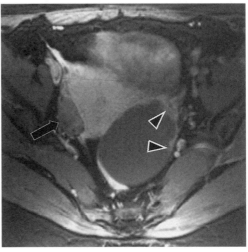

(c)

- Universally high signal of cysts on T2W images (hemorrhage not seen)
- Thickened fibrotic capsule may be evident
- Hypointense central stroma on T2W images

Theca-Lutein Cysts
- Background
  - May be large and multiple with elevated human chorionic gonadotropin (β-hCG), observed in gestational trophoblastic disease, fertility medications, twin pregnancy

- Usually asymptomatic, may present with pain (cyst rupture/hemorrhage, ovarian torsion)
- Imaging (fig. 13.47)
  - Numerous cysts, often multilocular, measuring up to 4 cm
  - Ovaries generally between 6 and 12 cm, can reach 20 cm
  - Cysts are low to high signal on T1W, high signal on T2W sequences
  - An associated hypervascular endometrial mass is seen in gestational trophoblastic disease

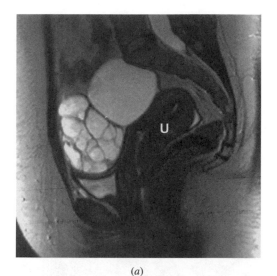

(a)

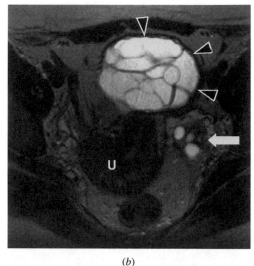

(b)

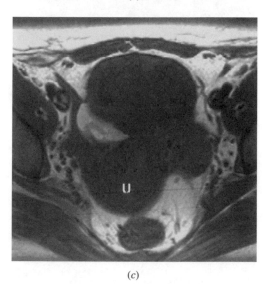

(c)

FIGURE 13.44 Mucinous cystadenoma. Sagittal (a) and transverse (b) T2W ETSE and transverse T1W SE (c) images. Multiple internal cysts and septations are typical findings in mucinous cystadenoma. The low-signal-intensity fibrotic wall of the mass (arrowheads, b) and the adjacent normal left ovary (arrow, b) are noted. The sagittal image (a) demonstrates displacement of the uterus (uterus = U, a–c) posteriorly by the mass. (Courtesy of Susan M. Ascher, M.D., Department of Radiology, Georgetown University.)

○ Ascites may indicate ovarian hyperstimulation syndrome in women undergoing fertility treatment

○ In these cases, an intrauterine or ectopic gestation may also be evident

Paraovarian and Peritoneal Cysts
• Background
  ○ Paraovarian cysts account for 10–20% of adnexal masses
  ○ Peritoneal inclusion cysts occur in women with functioning ovaries and adhesions due to prior surgery or endometriosis

• Imaging
  ○ Paraovarian cysts are round, low signal on T1W and high signal on T2W images
  ○ Peritoneal inclusion cysts have similar signal, but may be irregular in shape

Benign Solid Tumors
• Background
  ○ Most commonly composed of fibrous cells (fibroma), thecal cells (thecoma), or a combination of the two (fibrothecoma)
  ○ Pure thecomas arise most often in menopausal women

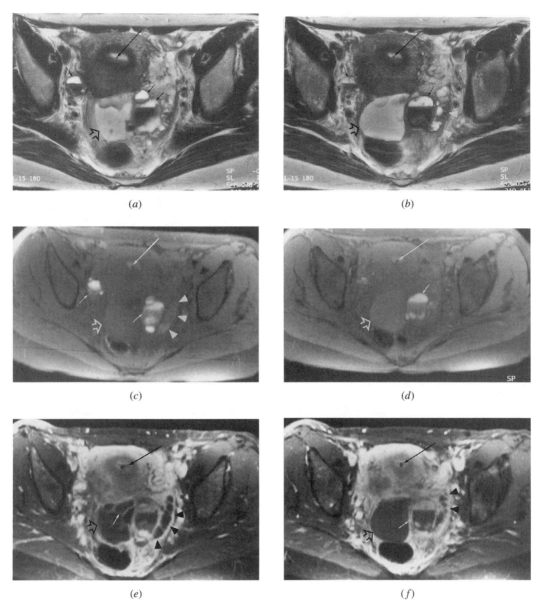

(a)   *(b)*

(c)   *(d)*

(e)   *(f)*

FIGURE 13.45   Endometriosis. Transverse 512-resolution T2W ETSE (*a*, *b*), T1W fat-suppressed SE (*c*, *d*), and gadolinium-enhanced T1W fat-suppressed SE (*e*, *f*) images in a 42-year-old woman with a 2 month history of pelvic pain, elevated CA-125, and complex adnexal masses on transvaginal sonography. Bilateral adnexal masses have high-signal-intensity components on T1W images, which demonstrate shading with fluid-fluid levels on T2W images consistent with endometriomas (short solid arrows, *a–d*). Note the serpentine left hydro/hematosalpinx (arrowheads, *b*, *c*, *e*, *f*). Posterior to the uterus is a polygonal fluid collection (open arrow, *a–f*). Following contrast, both the rims and septations of the masses (short solid arrows, *e*, *f*) enhance, as do the walls of the dilated left fallopian tube (arrowheads, *e*, *f*). The polygonal fluid collection has similar enhancement characteristics. Orthogonal views confirm the findings. Note the IUD within the endometrium (long, solid arrow *a–f*). At laparoscopy, bilateral endometriomas, endometriosis implants, left hydro/hematosalpinx, adhesions, and a peritoneal pseudocyst behind the uterus were found. MRI can add specificity to the finding of an elevated CA-125.

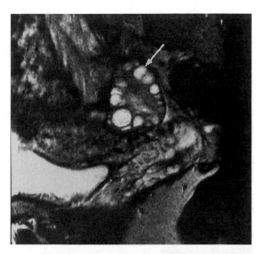

FIGURE 13.46   Polycystic ovary disease. Sagittal 512-resolution T2W ETSE image demonstrates a mildly enlarged ovary that contains multiple, similar-sized cysts (arrow). Central ovarian tissue is low in signal intensity, reflecting increased medullary cellular stroma.

- 15% have endometrial hyperplasia
- 29% have endometrial carcinoma
- Many are discovered during workup for abnormal bleeding
  - Pure fibromas are diagnosed more frequently in younger women
    - Usually asymptomatic
    - With ascites and right pleural effusion = Meig's syndrome
- Imaging (fig. 13.48)
  - The MR characteristics of fibromas and thecomas are similar: hypointense on T1W and T2W images
  - May be difficult to distinguish from pedunculated subserosal leiomyomata
    - Exophytic leiomyoma may have bridging vascular sign = curvilinear tortuous vascular structures will be seen crossing between uterus and mass
    - Exophytic leiomyoma may exhibit definable attachment to uterus
    - Compressed ovarian tissue surrounding an ovarian tumor is a helpful observation
  - Variable enhancement

Brenner Tumor
  - Less common, arises from surface epithelium of ovary

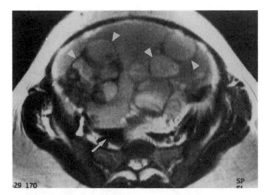

FIGURE 13.47   Theca-lutein cysts. Transverse T2W ETSE image in a patient on ovulation induction medicine who presented with acute pain and hypotension. Bilateral multilocular ovarian cysts (arrowheads) are identified in association with a gravid uterus (not shown) and marked free abdominopelvic fluid. Some of the cysts are complicated by hemorrhage. There is also evidence of hemoperitoneum. Note that the dependent fluid is decreased in signal intensity on T2W images, which is consistent with blood products (arrow). The hyperstimulation syndrome is a well-recognized, life-threatening complication of ovulation induction therapy for infertility. (Courtesy of Susan M. Ascher, M.D., Department of Radiology, Georgetown University.)

  - Majority benign
  - Associated with other ovarian tumors in 30%, usually in ipsilateral ovary
  - Signal similar to fibroma with homogeneous low signal on T2W images

Ovarian Torsion
- Background
  - Most common in prepubertal girls and during pregnancy
  - Underlying ovarian mass predisposes to torsion
  - Typically present with acute pain, sometimes episodic
  - Venous flow restricted first, causing enlargement, edema, interstitial hemorrhage
  - Arterial flow restricted later, causing necrosis
  - In chronic intermittent torsion, massive ovarian edema may occur
- Imaging (fig. 13.49)
  - Acute torsion

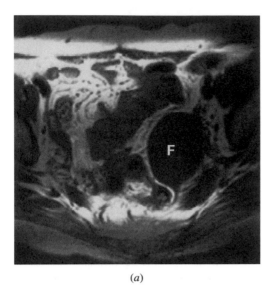

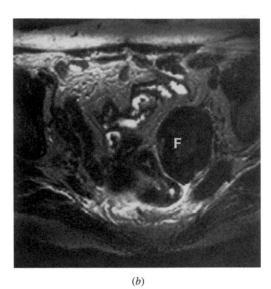

(a)   (b)

FIGURE 13.48   Fibroma/thecoma. Transverse T1W SE (*a*) and T2W ETSE (*b*) images in a patient with a left ovarian fibroma (F, *a*, *b*). The tumor is well defined and low in signal intensity on T1W and T2W images. (Courtesy of Susan M. Ascher, M.D., Department of Radiology, Georgetown University.)

- Adnexal protrusion continuous with uterus, to which engorged blood vessels converge
  - Generally low signal on T1W and T2W images
  - High-signal foci reflect hemorrhage/congestion

- Thick, straight vessels draping around the lesion
  - Vessels on the surface of the ovary and/or lesion distal to the torsion
- Complete absence of enhancement
  - Indicates significant arterial compromise

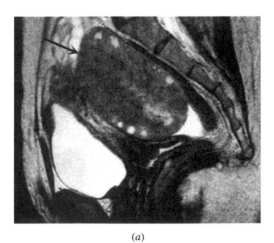

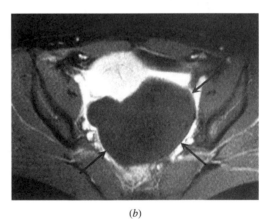

(a)   (b)

FIGURE 13.49   Ovarian torsion. Sagittal T2W ETSE image (*a*) in a patient with pelvic pain, low-grade fever, and mild leukocytosis shows a large, solid pelvic mass (arrow, *a*) posterior to the uterus. Peripheral follicles are noted, indicating that the mass is a markedly enlarged ovary. Gadolinium-enhanced T1W images (*b*) show no enhancement of the pelvic mass consistent with infarction (arrows, *b*). Surgery confirmed ovarian torsion with an infarcted ovary. Histopathologic evaluation showed an infarcted ovary with hemorrhagic necrosis. (Courtesy of Russell Low, M.D., Sharp Clinic, San Diego.)

- If torsion incomplete, some enhancement will be seen, may be better appreciated with subtraction imaging
- High-signal rim of hemorrhage may be seen on T1W images; however, this is nonspecific
  ◦ Chronic intermittent torsion
    ▪ Marked enlargement of the ovary
    ▪ Increased T2 signal

Malignant Masses

Primary Ovarian Carcinoma
- Background
  ◦ Second most common reproductive tract malignancy
  ◦ Primarily middle age and older women
- Imaging
  ◦ Five criteria of malignancy described: (1) size >4 cm; (2) solid mass or a large solid component; (3) wall thickness >3 mm; (4) septa thickness >3 mm or the presence of nodularity or vegetations; and (5) necrosis
  ◦ Four additional findings also indicative of malignancy: (1) involvement of adjacent organs or the pelvic side wall; (2) peritoneal, mesenteric, or omental disease; (3) ascites; and (4) adenopathy

Epithelial Origin
- Background
  ◦ 75–85% of patients with epithelial neoplasms present with peritoneal disease
  ◦ May spread lymphatically to para-aortic nodes and along the broad ligament to pelvic nodes
  ◦ Traditionally surgical staging
  ◦ Prognosis depends on tumor stage, residual disease after initial surgery, and tumor grade
  ◦ Four major cell types: mucinous, serous, endometrioid, and clear cell
    ▪ Serous cell type
      - 50% of ovarian malignancies
      - 30% contain psammoma bodies
    ▪ Mucinous cell type
      - More aggressive than serous
      - Generally very large, higher stage

- Endometrioid cell type
  - 15% of ovarian malignancies
  - Invasive, 25% bilateral
  - Arise de novo or from endometriosis
  - Up to one-third associated with endometrial hyperplasia or carcinoma
  - Typically a mixture of cystic and solid elements, rarely purely solid, papillary projections uncommon
- Clear cell type
  - 5% of ovarian malignancies
  - 13% bilateral
  - Invasive, but more often local disease, better prognosis
  - Typically unilocular with mural nodules, may mimic serous tumors
- Undifferentiated epithelial neoplasm
  - Do not fit into a category based on the four cell types
  - Poorest prognosis, often widespread at diagnosis
- Imaging
  ◦ MR appearance variable with cystic and solid components
  ◦ Gadolinium enhancement with fat suppression essential for detection of solid components and peritoneal implants
  ◦ Papillae suggest serous origin (fig. 13.50)
    ▪ Bilateral in 50%
    ▪ Predominantly unilocular cysts
    ▪ Intermediate-signal papillary projections within a cystic lesion
    ▪ Projections enhance with gadolinium
  ◦ Mucinous tumors are generally multiloculated (fig. 13.51)
    ▪ More often bilateral
    ▪ Different signal in various locules
    ▪ Septae between locules enhance with gadolinium
    ▪ Hemorrhage, necrosis, solid elements may be seen
  ◦ Clear-cell carcinomas tend to be large unilocular masses with solid mural elements

Sex Cord Stromal Origin
- Background
  ◦ 5% of all ovarian neoplasms

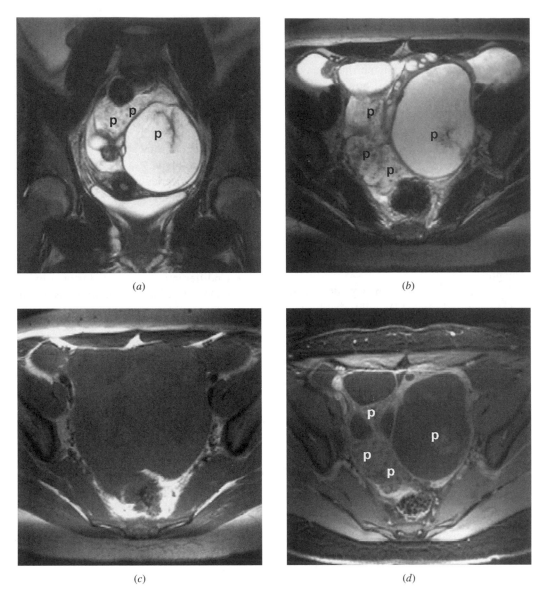

FIGURE 13.50 **Serous cystadenocarcinoma.** Coronal (*a*) and transverse (*b*) T2W ETSE, T1W SGE (*c*), and gadolinium-enhanced T1W SE (*d*) images in a 19-year-old woman with a low-malignant-potential serous tumor. Complex bilateral adnexal masses are noted. The T2W images demonstrate papillary projections (p, *a*, *b*). After gadolinium administration, the papillary projections show marked enhancement (p, *d*). Contrast administration helps to differentiate between vascularized solid elements and debris within cystic masses. (Courtesy of Susan M. Ascher, M.D., Department of Radiology, Georgetown University.)

- ○ Classified according to differentiation: ovarian follicles, testicular tubules, Leydig cells or adrenal cortical cells
- ○ Granulosa cell tumors are most common
- ○ 50% in postmenopausal women; 5% in prepubertal girls

- • Imaging
  - ○ Appearance varies ranging from solid to unilocular to multicystic
  - ○ Granulosa cell tumors are generally solid, with variable amounts of cystic change and intratumoral hemorrhage (fig. 13.52)

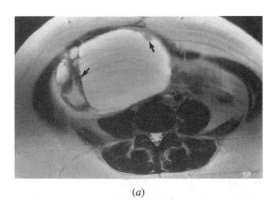

(a)

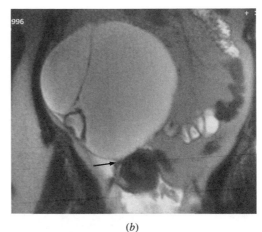

(b)

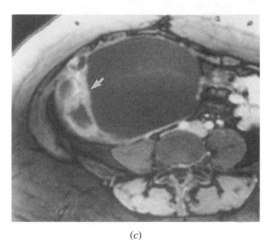

(c)

FIGURE 13.51   Mucinous cystadenocarcinoma. Transverse 512-resolution T2W ETSE (*a*), coronal T2W SS-ETSE (*b*), and transverse gadolinium-enhanced T1W fat-suppressed SGE (*c*) images in a patient with advanced mucinous ovarian cancer. A large cystic mass with septations and nodules (arrows, *a*) abuts the uterus (arrow, *b*). Following contrast, the enhancing tumor excrescences are well shown (arrow, *c*).

- ○ On T2W images the tumors are of heterogeneous high signal
- ○ On T1W images the tumors are of intermediate signal intensity
- ○ After gadolinium, solid areas enhance while cystic change or hemorrhage will not
- ○ Local invasion, especially into the sacrum, is well seen with sagittal imaging
- ○ Associated uterine changes due to hormone elaboration are seen in most patients and include uterine enlargement and thickening of the endometrium, also well demonstrated on sagittal images

Germ Cell Origin
- • Background
  - ○ Dysgerminomas most common

  - ▪ Occur in adolescents and young women
  - ▪ Bilateral in up to 15%
  - ▪ Lymphatic spread is more common than peritoneal seeding
  - ▪ Very radiosensitive
  - ▪ Generally solid
  - ○ Endodermal sinus tumors second most common
    - ▪ Similar age distribution to other germ cell tumors
    - ▪ Very malignant, but most are confined to one ovary
    - ▪ Rupture and ascites are not uncommon
    - ▪ Prognosis is poor without surgery and aggressive chemotherapy regimens
  - ○ Immature teratomas comprise about 20% of germ cell tumors

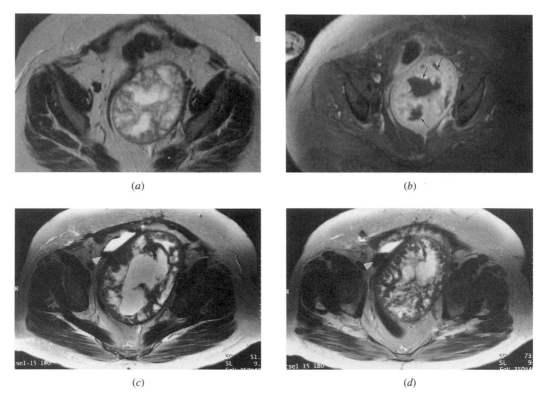

(a)　　　　　　　　　　　　　　(b)

(c)　　　　　　　　　　　　　　(d)

FIGURE 13.52　Granulosa cell tumor. T2W ETSE (*a*) and gadolinium-enhanced T1W fat-suppressed SGE (*b*) images in a woman with a granulosa cell ovarian tumor. The tumor is heterogeneous on the T2W image, and following contrast the solid elements enhance. Necrotic foci interspersed in an otherwise solid mass is a common feature of granulosa cell tumors (arrows, *b*). Transverse 512-resolution T2W ETSE (*c, d*) images 9 months later show interval growth of tumor and increasing necrosis. Note that the bladder is displaced anterolaterally by the mass. Low signal intensity in the dependent portion of the bladder reflects excreted concentrated gadolinium (arrowhead, *c, d*).

- Occur in children and young adults
- Usually large at presentation but unilateral
- Tend to spread by seeding the peritoneum
- Imaging
  - MR appearance of germ cell tumors is nonspecific
  - May be quite large at presentation
  - Immature teratomas may contain foci of fat

Other Primary Tumors
- Of mesenchymal tumors, smooth muscle are most common
  - Benign leiomyoma most common
  - Malignant transformation reported
  - Leiomyosarcomas are rare
- Also reported are lipoleiomyoma, hemangioma, myxoma, fibrosarcoma, rhabdomyosarcoma, schwannoma, osteosarcoma, chondrosarcoma, fibrosarcoma, and endometrial stromal sarcoma
- MR appearance of these tumors is similar to their appearance elsewhere

Lymphoma
- Background
  - Rare cases of primary ovarian lymphoma reported
  - Generally part of a disseminated disease presentation
  - Most commonly non-Hodgkin's in children and large cell in adults

- Imaging
  - Usually bilateral masses (secondary lymphoma)
  - Homogeneous slight hyperintensity on T2W images
  - Homogeneous hypointensity on T1W images
  - Contrast enhancement is mild to moderate with mild heterogeneity
  - Cystic change and necrosis are rare, even in large tumors
  - Physiologic follicles may be retained

Metastases
- Background
  - Most common sites of origin: colon, stomach, breast, and hematopoietic tissues
  - Spread by one of several routes: direct extension, hematogenous, lymphatic, or peritoneal
  - Krukenberg's tumor (mucin-filled signet-ring cells found) classically associated with gastric origin, but may arise from breast, colon, and appendix primaries
- Imaging
  - Krukenberg's tumors generally have both cystic and solid components
  - Cystic components
    - Generally high signal on T2W, may be variable
    - Variable signal on T1W images, reflecting content
  - Solid components
    - May be hypointense on T1W and T2W images corresponding to dense collagenous stroma
    - May show intense enhancement
  - Although rare, metastatic melanoma may be distinguished by peripheral high T1 signal within the mass

Inflammation
Pelvic Inflammatory Disease (PID)/Tubo-Ovarian Abscess (TOA)
- Background
  - Condition of women of reproductive age

  - Ascending spread; women after hysterectomy are not at risk
  - Women with an intrauterine device are at increased risk. Actinomyces is especially common in these women.
  - Uncomplicated PID (myometritis, endometritis, and oophoritis) generally managed with antibiotics
  - TOA or pyosalpinx may require percutaneous or surgical drainage
  - Long-term sequelae of PID include infertility, chronic pelvic pain, and an increased risk of ectopic pregnancy
- Imaging (fig. 13.53)
  - Inflammation seen as ill-defined hyperintensity on fat-suppressed T2W images that enhance markedly on postgadolinium fat-suppressed T1W images
  - TOA has variable MR appearance, but is generally a round or tubular thick-walled, fluid-filled mass in the adnexal region
    - Generally hypointense on T1W images and hyperintense or heterogeneous on T2W images
    - Intense rim enhancement, corresponding to granulation tissue
    - Increased enhancement of surrounding tissues
    - Differential diagnosis of TOA: endometrioma, ovarian neoplasm, infected ovarian cyst, and an abscess from another source such as Crohn's disease, appendicitis, or diverticulitis
  - Chronic PID/TOA results in similar but less severe changes

Fallopian Tubes

Mass Lesions
Benign Masses
- Entities described above (endometriosis, leiomyomata, adenomatoid tumors, and teratoma) can affect the fallopian tubes with the same MR characteristics
- Endometriosis generally affects the surface of the tube

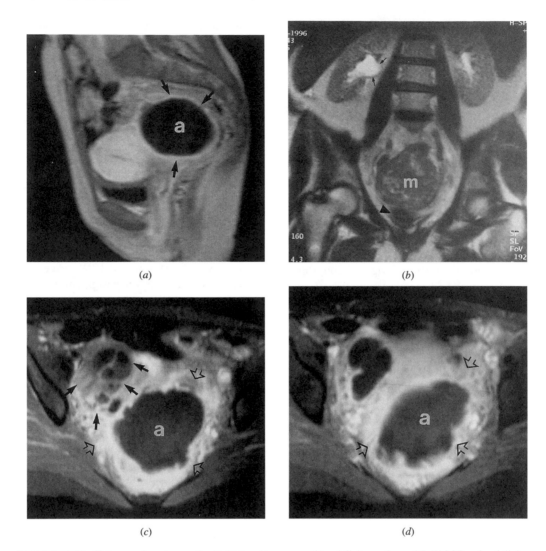

(a)   (b)

(c)   (d)

FIGURE 13.53   Tubo-ovarian abscess. Sagittal (*a*) and transverse (*b*) gadolinium-enhanced T1W SGE and gadolinium-enhanced T1W fat-suppressed SE (*c, d*) images in a woman with fever and a fluctuant adnexal mass on bimanual exam. A large loculated abscess occupies the posterior pelvis (a, *a–d*). The right ovary is enlarged and is invested with an abscess (solid arrows, *b, c*). The well-formed abscess capsule (arrows, *a*) and septations enhance markedly, as does the inflammation in the surrounding fat (open arrows, *b–d*). The associated inflammatory changes are more conspicuous on the fat-suppressed images. Tubo-ovarian abscess is a well-recognized complication of PID. Whereas most cases of PID can be managed conservatively, the presence of an abscess usually necessitates surgical intervention.

- Leiomyomata are exceedingly rare and discovered incidentally

Hydrosalpinx
- Background
  - Occlusion of the fimbriated end of the tube, resulting in dilatation

- If complicated by hemorrhage, the term *hematosalpinx* may be applied
- If complicated by infection, the term *pyosalpinx* is used
- Causes of tubal obstruction include PID, endometriosis, adjacent tumors, and adhesions from prior surgery

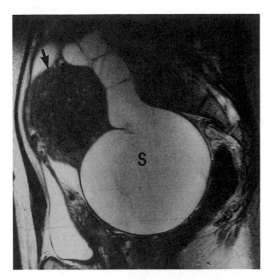

FIGURE 13.54   Hydrosalpinx. Sagittal 512-resolution T2W ETSE image demonstrates a large hydrosalpinx (S). Adenomyosis of the uterus (arrow) is also present.

- Imaging (fig. 13.54)
  - Tubular fluid-filled structure folded on itself
  - Multiplanar imaging especially useful for recognizing that a multicystic structure represents a dilated tube
  - Signal varies with tubal contents

Ectopic Pregnancy
- Background
  - Most common sites are fallopian tubes and ovaries
  - Incidence rising due to increased use of treatments for infertility
- Imaging
  - Fallopian tube hematoma: intermediate to high signal on T1W images
  - Bloody ascites: increased signal intensity on fat-suppressed T1W images
  - Enhancement of fallopian tube wall
  - Gestational sac-like structure
  - Heterogeneous adnexal mass

Malignant Masses
Primary Fallopian Tube Carcinoma
- Background
  - Rare; 0.5% of all gynecologic tumors

- Most commonly adenocarcinoma; sarcoma (leiomyosarcoma, carcinosarcoma, and mixed müllerian tumor) and choriocarcinoma are even more rare
  - Average age 55
  - Poor prognosis due to late stage at diagnosis
- Imaging
  - Typically a small adnexal mass with low T1 signal and high T2 signal
  - Enhancement is seen
  - Associated findings include hydrosalpinx, peritumoral ascites, and intrauterine fluid

Metastases
- More common than primary carcinoma
- Generally the result of direct extension from the ovary, endometrium, or cervix
- Tumors arising outside of the genital system include breast and gastrointestinal cancers
- Lymphatic spread accounts for the majority of tubal involvement

Inflammation
Salpingitis
- Background
  - Seen in the setting of PID/TOA
- Imaging
  - Tubal enlargement due to obstruction of fimbriated end
  - Serpentine adnexal lesion; central signal varies with the tube contents
  - Purulent material is of variable signal on T1W and T2W images, may show a fluid-debris level
  - Tube wall enhances

Pelvic Varices
- Background
  - Associated with pelvic pain syndrome, chronic pelvic pain without obvious cause
  - Generally affects multiparous women of reproductive age
  - Patients complain of a deep, dull pelvic ache made worse by activity or actions that increase intra-abdominal pressure

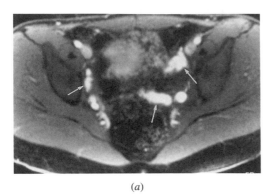 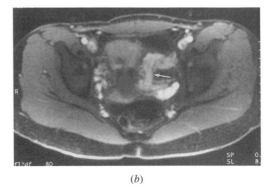

(a)   (b)

FIGURE 13.55   Pelvic varices. Transverse 45 s postgadolinium fat-suppressed SGE images (*a, b*) in a patient with chronic pelvic pain. Pelvic varices, left greater than right, show marked enhancement after intravenous gadolinium administration (arrows, *a, b*). The concurrent use of fat suppression increases the conspicuity of the dilated vessels by removing the competing high signal intensity of fat. Pelvic varices are a common, though rarely recognized, cause of chronic pelvic pain. In imaging a patient with pelvic pain of unknown etiology, the presence or absence of varices should be noted.

- In contrast, secondary pelvic varices are not generally associated with pain but do herald a potentially serious underlying abnormality such as inferior vena caval obstruction, portal hypertension, increased pelvic blood flow, or vascular malformations

- Imaging (fig. 13.55)
  - On T1W and T2W images, serpentine parauterine and paraovarian structures
  - Enhances significantly with gadolinium, especially if an appropriate delay is employed (2 min)

BIBLIOGRAPHY

CHAPTER 1

Brown MA, Semelka RC: *MRI: Basic Principles and Applications,* 2nd ed. New York: Wiley-Liss, 1999.

de Gonzalez AB, Darby S: Risk of cancer from diagnostic x-rays: Estimates for the UK and 14 other countries. *The Lancet* 363:345–351, 2004.

Gaa J, Hutabu H, Jenkins RL, Finn JP, Edelman RR: Liver masses: Replacement of conventional T2-weighted spin echo MR imaging with breath-hold MR imaging. *Radiology* 200:459–464, 1996.

Lee VS, Lavelle MT, Rofsky NM, Laub G, Thomasson DM, Krinsky GA, Weinreb JC. Hepatic MR imaging with a dynamic contrast-enhanced isotropic volumetric interpolated breath-hold examination: Feasibility, reproducibility, and technical quality. *Radiology* 215:365–372, 2000.

Low RN, Semelka RC, Worawattanakul S, Alzate GD. Extrahepatic abdominal imaging in patients with malignancy: Comparison of MR imaging and helical CT in 164 patients. *J Magn Reson Imag* 12:269–277, 2001.

Low RN, Semelka RC, Worawwattanakul S, Alzate GD, Sigeti JS. Extrahepatic abdominal imaging in patients with malignancy: Comparison of MR imaging and helical CT, with subsequent surgical correlation. *Radiology* 210:625–632, 1999.

Noone TC, Semelka RC, Chaney DM, Reinhold C: Abdominal imaging studies: Comparison of diagnostic accuracies resulting from ultrasound, computed tomography, and magnetic resonance imaging in the same individual. *J Magn Reson Imag* 22:19–24, 2004

Rofsky NM, Lee VS, Laub G, Pollack MA, Krinsky GA, Thomasson D, Ambrosino MM, Weinreb JC. Abdominal MR imaging with a volumetric interpolated breath-hold examination. *Radiology* 212:876–884, 1999.

Semelka RC, Balci NC, Op de Beeck B, Reinhold C. Evaluation of a 10-minute comprehensive MR imaging examination of the upper abdomen. *Radiology* 211:189–195, 1999.

Semelka RC, Kelekis NL, Thomasson D, Brown MA, Laub GA: HASTE MR imaging: Description of technique and preliminary results in the abdomen. *J Magn Reson Imag* 6:698–699, 1996.

Semelka RC, Willms AB, Brown MA, Brown ED, Finn JP: Comparison of breath-hold T1-weighted MR sequences for imaging of the liver. *J Magn Reson Imag* 4:759–765, 1994

CHAPTER 2

Bader TR, Beavers KL, Semelka RC: MR imaging features of primary sclerosing cholangitis: Patterns of cirrhosis in relationship to clinical severity of disease. *Radiology* 226:675–685, 2003.

Balci NC, Semelka RC, Noone TC, Ascher SM. Acute and subacute liver-related hemorrhage: MRI findings. *J Magn Reson Imag* 17(2):207–211, 1999.

Bassignani M, Fulcher AS, Szucs RA, Chong WK, Prasad UR, Marcos A. Use of imaging for living donor liver transplantation. *Radiographics* 21:39–52, 2001.

Brandhagen DJ, Fairbanks VF, Batts KP, Thebodeau SN. Update on hereditary hemochromatosis and the HFE gene. *Mayo Clin Proc* 74:917–921, 1999.

Brown JJ, Borrello JA, Raza HS, Balfe DM, Baer AB, Pilgram TK, Atilla S: Dynamic contrast-enhanced MR imaging of the liver: Parenchymal enhancement patterns. *J Magn Reson Imag* 13:1–8, 1995.

Bruneton JN, Raffaelli C, Maestro C, Padovani B: Benign liver lesions: Implications of detection in cancer patients. *Eur Radiol* 5:387–390, 1995.

Buetow PC, Buck JL, Pantongrag-Brown L, Ros PR, Devaney K, Goodman ZD, Cruess DF: Biliary cystadenoma and cystadenocarcinoma: Clinical-imaging-pathologic correlations with emphasis on the importance of ovarian stroma. *Radiology* 196:805–810, 1995.

Buetow PC, Buck JL, Ros PR, Goodman ZDLC: Malignant vascular tumors of the liver: Radiologic-pathologic correlation. *Radiographics* 14:153–166, 1994.

Buetow PC, Rao P, Marshall H: Imaging of pediatric liver tumors. *MRI Clin N Am* 5(2):397–413, 1997.

Burdeny DA, Semelka RC, Kelekis NL, Kettritz U, Woosley JT, Cance WG, Lee JKT: Chemotherapy treated liver metastases mimicking hemangiomas on MR images. *Abdom Imag* 24:378–382, 1999.

Caudana R, Morana G, Pirovano GP, Nicoli N, Portuese A, Spinazzi A, Di Rito R, Pistolesi GF: Focal malignant hepatic lesions: MR imaging enhanced with gadolinium benzoxypropionictetra-acetate(BOPTA)—preliminary results of phase II clinical application. *Radiology* 199:513–520, 1996.

Corrigan K, Semelka RC: Dynamic contrast-enhanced MR imaging of fibrolamellar hepatocellular carcinoma. *Abdom Imaging* 20:122–125, 1995.

Danet IM, Semelka RC, Leonardou P, Braga L, Vaidean G, Woosley JT, Kanematsu M: Spectrum of MRI appearances of untreated metastases of the liver. *Am J Roentgenol* 181:809–817, 2003.

Danet IM, Semelka RC, Nagase LL, Woosely JT, Leonardou P, Armao D: Liver metastases from pancreatic adenocarcinoma: MR imaging characteristics. *J Magn Reson Imag* 18:181–188, 2003.

de Sousa JM, Portmann B, Williams R: Nodular regenerative hyperplasia of the liver and the Budd-Chiari syndrome. Case report, review of the literature and reappraisal of pathogenesis. *J Hepatol* 12:28–35, 1991.

Fauerholdt L, Schlichting P, Christensen E, et al.: Conversion of micronodular cirrhosis into macronodular cirrhosis. *Hepatology* 3:928–931, 1983.

Gore RM: Diffuse liver disease. In: Gore RM, Levine NS, Laufer I (eds.), *Textbook of Gastrointestinal Radiology*. Philadelphia, PA: Saunders, 1994, pp. 1968–2017.

Hagspiel KD, Neidl KF, Eichenberger AC, Weder W, Marincek B: Detection of liver metastases: Comparison of superparamagnetic iron oxide–enhanced and unenhanced MR imaging at 1.5 T with dynamic CT, intraoperative US, and percutaneous US. *Radiology* 196:471–478, 1995.

Hamm B, Thoeni RF, Gould RG, Bernardino ME, Luning M, Saini S, Mahfouz AE, Taupitz M, Wolf KJ: Focal liver lesions: Characterization with nonenhanced and dynamic contrast material-enhanced MR imaging. *Radiology* 190:417–423, 1994.

Hamrick-Turner J, Abbitt PL, Ros PR: Intrahepatic cholangiocarcinoma: MR appearance. *Am J Roentgenol* 158:77–79, 1992.

Ito K, Siegelman ES, Stolpen AH, Mitchell DG: MR imaging of complications after liver transplantation. *Am J Roentgenology* 175:1145–1149, 2000.

Jeong MG, Yu JS, Kim KW: Hepatic cavernous hemangioma: Temporal peritumoral enhancement during multiphase dynamic MR imaging. *Radiology* 216:692–697, 2000.

Kanematsu M, Semelka RC, Leonardou P, Mastropasqua M, Lee JKT: Hepatocellular carcinoma of diffuse type: MR imaging findings and clinical manifestations. *J Magn Reson Imag* 18:189–195, 2003.

Kelekis NL, Semelka RC, Siegelman ES, Ascher SM, Outwater EK, Woosley TJ, Reinhold C, Mitchell DG: Focal hepatic lymphoma: MR demonstration using current techniques including gadolinium enhancement. *J Magn Reson Imag* 15(6):625–636, 1997.

Kelekis NL, Semelka RC, Worawattanakul S, et al.: Hepatocellular carcinoma in North America: A multiinstitutional study of appearance on T1-weighted, T2- weighted, and serial gadolinium-enhanced gradient-echo images. *Am J Roentgenol* 170:1005–1013, 1998.

Kelekis NL, Warshauer DM, Semelka RC, Eisenberg LB, Woosley JT: Inflammatory pseudotumor of the liver: Appearance on contrast enhanced helical CT and dynamic MR images. *J Magn Reson Imag* 5:551–553, 1995.

Klatskin G, Conn HO: *Histopathology of the Liver*, pp. 368, 371. New York: Oxford University Press, 1993.

Krinsky GA, Lee VS: MR imaging of cirrhotic nodules. *Abdom Imag* 25:471–482, 2000.

Lebovics E, Thung SN, Schaffner F: The liver in the acquired immunodeficiency syndrome: A clinical and histologic study. *Hepatology* 5:293–298, 1995.

Liou J, Lee JK, Borrello JA, Brown JJ: Differentiation of hepatomas from nonhepatomatous masses: Use of MnDPDP-enhanced MR images. *J Magn Reson Imag* 12:71–79, 1994.

Low RN, Sigeti JS, Francis IR, Weinman D, Bower B, Shimakawa A, Foo TK: Evaluation of malignant biliary obstruction: Efficacy of fast multiplanar spoiled gradient-recalled MR imaging vs. spin-echo MR imaging, CT, and cholangiography. *Am J Roentgenol* 162:315–323, 1994.

MacSween RNM, Anthony PP, Scheuer PJ, Burt AD, Portamann BC. *Pathology of the Liver*, p. 10, 3rd ed. London: Churchill Livingstone, 1994.

Marti-Bonmati L, Talens A, del Olmo J, de Val A, Serra MA, Rodrigo JM, Ferrandez A, Torres V, Rayon M, Vilar JS: Chronic hepatitis and cirrhosis: Evaluation by means of MR imaging with histologic correlation. *Radiology* 188:37–43, 1993.

Martin DR: MR imaging of diffuse liver disease. *Topics in MRI* 13:151–164, 2002.

Martin DR, Semelka RC: Imaging of benign and malignant focal liver lesions. *MRI Clin N Am* 9:785–802, 2001.

Martin DR, Semelka RC, Chung JJ, Balci NC, Wilber K: Sequential use of gadolinium chelate and mangafodipir trisodium for the assessment of focal liver lesions: Initial observations. *J Magn Reson Imag* 18:955–963, 2000.

Meissner K: Hemorrhage caused by ruptured liver cell adenoma following long-term oral contraceptives: A case report. *Hepato-gastroenterology* 45(19):224–225, 1998.

Mitchell DG: Focal manifestations of diffuse liver disease at MR imaging. *Radiology* 185:1–11, 1992.

Mitchell DG. Liver I: Currently available gadolinium chelates. MRI Clin N Am 4:37–51, 1996.

Mortelé KJ, Praet M, Vlierberghe HV, Kunnen M, Ros PR: CT and MR imaging findings in focal nodular hyperplasia of the liver: Radiologic-pathologic correlation. *Am J Roentgenol* 175:687–692, 2000.

Nagel HS, Bernardino MELC: Contrast-enhanced MR imaging of hepatic lesions treated with percutaneous ethanol ablation therapy. *Radiology* 189:265–270, 1993.

Noone TC, Semelka RC, Balci NC, Graham ML: Common occurrence of benign liver lesions in patients with newly diagnosed breast cancer investigated by MRI for suspected liver metastases. *J Magn Reson Imag* 10:165–169, 1999.

Noone TC, Semelka RC, Siegelman ES, Balci NC, Hussain SM, et al.: Budd-Chiari syndrome: Spectrum of appearances of acute, subacute, and chronic disease with magnetic resonance imaging. *J Magn Reson Imag* 11:44–50, 2000.

Ohtomo K, Itai Y, Ohtomo Y, Shiga J, Iio M: Regenerating nodules of liver cirrhosis: MR imaging with pathologic correlation. *Am J Roentgenol* 154:505–507, 1990.

Oi H, Murakami T, Kim T, Matsushita M, Kishimoto H, Nakamura H: Dynamic MR imaging and early-phase helical CT for detecting small intrahepatic metastases of hepatocellular carcinoma. *Am J Roentgenol* 166:369–374, 1996.

Paulson EK, McClellan JS, Washington K, Spritzer CE, Meyers WC, Baker ME: Hepatic adenoma: MR characteristics and correlation with pathologic findings. *Am J Roentgenol* 163:113–116, 1994.

Pollard JJ, Nebesar RA: Altered hemodynamics in the Budd-Chiari syndrome demonstrated by selective hepatic and selective splenic angiography. *Radiology* 89:236–243, 1967.

Ralls PW, Henley DS, Colletti PM, Benson R, Raval JK, Radin DR, Boswell WD Jr., Halls JM: Amebic liver abscess: MR imaging. *Radiology* 165:801–804, 1987.

Rooholamini SA, Au AH, Hansen GC, Kioumehr F, Dadsetan MR, Chow PP, Kurzel RB, Mikhail G: Imaging of pregnancy-related complications. *Radiographics* 13:753–770, 1993.

Ros PR, Freeny PC, Marms SE, et al: Hepatic MR imaging with ferumoxides: A multicenter clinical trial of the safety and efficacy in the detection of focal hepatic lesions. *Radiology* 196:481–488, 1995.

Sallah Sabah, Semelka RC, Kelekis N, Worawattanakul S, Sallah W: Diagnosis and monitoring response of treatment of hepatosplenic candidiasis in patients with acute leukemia using magnetic resonance imaging. *Acta Haematol* 100:77–81, 1998.

Semelka RC, Chung JJ, Hussain SM, Marcos HB, Woosley JT: Chronic hepatitis: Correlation of early patchy and late linear enhancement patterns on gadolinium-enhanced MR images with histopathology-initial experience. *J Magn Reson Imag* 13:385–391, 2001.

Semelka RC, Heimberger TKG: Contrast agents for MR imaging of the liver. *Radiology* 218:227–238, 2001.

Semelka RC, Hussain SM, Marcos HB, Woosley JT: Biliary hamartomas: Solitary and multiple lesions shown on current MR techniques including gadolinium enhancement. *J Magn Reson Imag* 10:196–201, 1999.

Semelka RC, Hussain SM, Marcos HB, Woosley JT: Perilesional enhancement of hepatic metastases: Correlation between MR imaging and histopathologic findings—initial observations. *Radiology* 215:89–94, 2000.

Semelka RC, Kelekis NL, Sallah S, Worawattanakul S, Ascher SM: Hepatosplenic fungal disease: Diagnostic accuracy and spectrum of appearance on MR imaging. *Am J Roentgenology* 169(5):1311–1316, 1997.

Semelka RC, Lee JKT, Worawattanakul S, Noone TC, Patt RH, Asher SM: Sequential use of ferumoxide particles and gadolinium chelate for the evaluation of focal liver lesions on MRI. *J Magn Reson Imag* 8:670–674, 1998.

Semelka RC, Martin DR, Balci Cem, Lance T: Focal liver lesions: Comparison of dual phase CT and multisequence multiplanar MR imaging including dynamic gadolinium enhancement. *J Magn Reson Imag* 13:397–401, 2001.

Semelka RC, Martin DR, Balci NC, Trang L: Focal liver lesions: Comparison of dual-phase CT and multisequence multiplanar MR imaging including dynamic gadolinium enhancement. *JMRI* 13:397–401, 2001.

Semelka RC, Shoenut JP, Ascher SM, Kroeker MA, Greenberg HM, Yaffe CS, Micflikier AB: Solitary hepatic metastasis: Comparison of dynamic contrast-enhanced CT and MR imaging with fat-suppressed T2-weighted, breath-hold T1-weighted FLASH, and dynamic gadolinium-enhanced FLASH sequences. *J Magn Reson Imag* 4:319–323, 1994.

Semelka RC, Shoenut JP, Kroeker MA, Greenberg HM, Simm FC, Minuk GY, Kroeker RM, Micflikier AB: Focal liver disease: Comparison of dynamic contrast-enhanced CT and T2-weighted fat-suppressed, FLASH, and dynamic gadolinium-enhanced MR imaging at 1.5 T. *Radiology* 184:687–694, 1992.

Shoenut JP, Semelka RC, Levi C, Greenberg H: Ciliated hepatic foregut cysts: US, CT, and contrast-enhanced MR imaging. *Abdom Imag* 19:150–152, 1994.

Shortell CK, Schwartz SI: Hepatic adenoma and focal nodular hyperplasia. *Surg Gynecol Obstet* 173:426–431, 1991.

Siegelman ES, Outwater E, Hanau CA, Ballas SK, Steiner RM, Rao VM, Mitchell DG: Abdominal iron distribution in sickle cell disease: MR findings in transfusion and nontransfusion dependent patients. *J Comput Assist Tomogr* 18:63–67, 1994.

Soyer P, Lacheheb D, Caudron C, Levesque M: MRI of adenomatous hyperplastic nodules of the liver in Budd-Chiari syndrome. *J Comput Assist Tomogr* 17:86–89, 1993.

Stark DD, Goldberg HI, Moss AA, Bass NM: Chronic liver disease: Evaluation by magnetic resonance. *Radiology* 150:149–151, 1984.

Stark DD, Wittenberg J, Butch RJ, Ferrucci JT Jr: Hepatic metastases: Randomized, controlled comparison of detection with MR imaging and CT. *Radiology* 165:399–406, 1987.

Vassiliades VG, Foley WD, Alarcon J, Lawson T, Erickson S, Kneeland JB, Steinberg HV, Bernardino ME: Hepatic metastases: CT versus MR imaging at 1.5 T. *Gastrointest Radiol* 16:159–163, 1991.

Venkataraman S, Semelka RC, Braga L, Danet IM, Woosley JT: Inflammatory myofibroblastic tumor of the hepatobiliary system: Report of MR imaging appearance in four patients. *Radiology* 227:758–763, 2003.

Vogl TJ, Kummel S, Hammerstingl R, Schellenbeck M, Schumacher G, Balzer T, Schwarz W, Muller PK, Bechstein WO, Mack MG, Sollner O, Felix R: Liver tumors: Comparison of MR imaging with Gd-EOB-DTPA and Gd-DTPA. *Radiology* 200:59–67, 1996.

Wanless IR, Mawdsley C, Adams R: On the pathogenesis of focal nodular hyperplasia of the liver. *Hepatology* 5(6):1194–1200, 1985.

Yamashita Y, Mitsuzaki K, Yi T, et al.: Small heptacellular carcinoma in patients with chronic liver damage: Prospective comparison of detection with dynamic MR imaging and helical CT of the whole liver. *Radiology* 200:79–84, 1996.

Yates CK, Streight RA: Focal fatty infiltration of the liver simulating metastatic disease. *Radiology* 159:83–84, 1986.

CHAPTER 3

Ernst O, Asselah T, Sergent G, et al.: MR cholangiography in primary sclerosing cholangitis. *Am J Roentgenol* 171:1027–1030, 1998.

Fulcher AS, Turner MA, Capps GW, Zfass AM, Baker KM: Half-Fourier RARE MR cholangiopancreatography: Experience in 300 subjects. *Radiology* 207(1):21–32, 1998.

Furuta A, Ishibashi T, Takahashi S, Sakamoto K: MR imaging of xanthogranulomatous cholecystitis. *Radiat Med* 14(6):315–319, 1996.

Hirao K, Miyazaki A, Fujimoto T, Isomoto I, Hayashi K: Evaluation of aberrant bile ducts before laparoscopic cholecystectomy: Helical CT cholangiography versus MR cholangiography. *Am J Roentgenol* 175(3):713–720, 2000.

Irie H, Honda H, Kuroiwa T, Yoshimitsu K, Aibe H, Shinozaki K, Masuda K: Pitfalls in MR cholangiopancreatographic interpretation. *RadioGraphics* 21:23–37, 2001.

Ito K, Mitchell DG, Outwater EK, Blasbalg R: Primary sclerosing cholangitis: MR imaging features. *Am J Roentgenol* 172(6):1527–1533, 1999.

Kiefer B, Grassner J, Hausmann R: Image acquisition in a second with half-Fourier acquisition single shot turbo spin echo. *J Magn Reson Imag* 4(P):86–87; 1994.

Kim MJ, Cha SW, Mitchell DG, Chung JJ, Park S, Chung JB: MR imaging findings in recurrent pyogenic cholangitis. *Am J Roentgenol* 173(6): 1545–1549, 1999.

Lee YM, Kaplan MM: Primary sclerosing cholangitis. *N Engl J Med* 332:924–932, 1995.

Loud PA, Semelka RC, Kettritz U, Brown JJ, Reinhold C: MRI of acute cholecystitis: Comparison with the normal gallbladder and other entities. *J Magn Reson Imag* 14(4):349–355, 1996.

Miller FH, Gore RM, Nemcek AA Jr, Fitzgerald SW: Pancreaticobiliary manifestations of AIDS. *Am J Roentgenol* 166(6):1269–1274, 1996.

Pavone P, Laghi A, Catalano C, Materia A, Basso N, Passariello R: Caroli's disease: Evaluation with MR cholangiopancreatography (MRCP). *Abdom Imag* 21:117–119, 1996.

Regan F, Fradin J, Khazan R, Bohlmann M, Magnuson T: Choledocholithiasis: Evaluation with MR cholangiography. *Am J Roentgenol* 167:1441–1445, 1996.

Rooholamini SA, Tehrani NS, Razavi MK, Au AH, Hansen GC, Ostrzega N, Verma RC: Imaging of gallbladder carcinoma. *Radiographics* 14:291–306, 1994.

Semelka RC, Kelekis NL, John G, Ascher SM, Burdeny DA, Siegelman ES: Ampullary carcinoma: Demonstration by current MR techniques. *J Magn Reson Imag* 7:153–156, 1997.

Semelka RC, Shoenut JP, Kroeker MA, Hricak H, Minuk GY, Yaffe CS, Micflikier AB: Bile duct disease: Prospective comparison of ERCP, CT, and fat suppression MRI. *Gastrointest Radiol* 17:347–352, 1992.

Soto JA, Alvarez O, Munera F, Velez SM, Valencia J, Ramirez N: Diagnosing bile duct stones: Comparison of unenhanced helical CT, oral contrast-enhanced CT cholangiography, and MR cholangiography. *Am J Roentgenol* 175(4):1127–1134, 2000.

Soyer P, Bluemke DA, Reichle R, Calhoun PS, Bliss DF, Scherrer A, Fishman EK: Imaging of intrahepatic cholangiocarcinoma: 1. Peripheral cholangiocarcinoma. *Am J Roentgenol* 165:1427–1431, 1995.

Soyer P, Bluemke DA, Reichle R, Calhoun PS, Bliss DF, Scherrer A, Fishman EK: Imaging of intrahepatic cholangiocarcinoma: 2. Hilar cholangiocarcinoma. *Am J Roentgenol* 165:1433–1436, 1995.

Taourel P, Reinhold C, Bret PM, Barkun AN, Atri M: Biliary and pancreatic ductal anatomy: Normal findings and variants demonstrated with MR cholangiopancreatography (abstract). *RSNA,*

Radiological Society of North America 197(P):502, 1995.

Todani T, Watanabe Y, Narusue M, Tabuchi K, Okajima K: Congenital bile duct cysts: Classification, operative procedures, and review of thirty-seven cases including cancer arising from choledochal cyst. *Am J Surg* 134(2):263–269, 1977.

Yoshimitsu K, Honda H, Jimi M, Kuroiwa T, Hanada K, Irie H, Tajima T, Takashima M, Chijiiwa K, Shimada M, Masuda K: MR diagnosis of adenomyomatosis of the gallbladder and differentiation from gallbladder carcinoma: Importance of showing Rokitansky-Aschoff sinuses. *Am J Roentgenol* 172(6):1535–1540, 1999.

CHAPTER 4

Buetou PC, Rao P, Thompson LDR: From the archives of the AFIP. Mucinous cystic neoplasm of the pancreas: Radiologic-pathologic correlation. *Radiographics* 18:433–449, 1998.

Carlson B, Johnson CD, Stephens DH, Ward EM, Kvois LK: MRI of pancreatic islet cell carcinoma. *J Comput Assist Tomogr* 17:735–740, 1993.

Catalano C, Pavone P, Laghi A, Panebianco V, Scipioni A: Pancreatic adenocarcinoma: Combination of MR imaging, MR angiography and MR cholangiopancreatography for the diagnosis and assessment of respectability. *Eur Radiol* 8:428–434, 1998.

Delhaye M, Engelholm, Cremer M: Pancreas divisum: Congenital anatomic variant or anomaly? Contribution of endoscopic retrograde dorsal pancreatography. *Gastroenterology* 89:951–958, 1985.

del Pilar Fernandez M, Bernardino ME, Neylan JF, Olson RA: Diagnosis of pancreatic transplant dysfunction: Value of gadopentatate dimeglumine-enhanced MR imaging. *Am J Roentgenol* 156:1171–1176, 1991.

Fulcher AS, Turner MA: MR pancreatography: A useful tool for evaluationg pancreatic disorders. *Radiographics* 19:5–24, 1999.

Gabata T, Matsui O, Kadoya M, et al: Small pancreatic adenocarcinomas: Efficacy of MR imaging with fat suppression and gadolinium enhancement. *Radiology* 193:683–688, 1994.

Hough DM, Stephens DH, Johnson CD, Binkovitz LA: Pancreatic lesions in von Hippel–Lindau disease: Prevalence, clinical significance, and CT findings. *Am J Roentgenol* 162:1091–1094, 1994.

Irie H, Honda H, Aibe H, Kuroiwa T, Yoshimizu K: MR cholangiopancreatography differentiation of benign and malignant intraductal mucin-producing tumors of the pancreas. *Am J Roentgenol* 174:1403–1408, 2000.

King LF, Scurr ED, Murugan N: Hepatobiliary and pancreatic manifestation of cystic fibrosis: MR imaging appearances. *RadioGraphics* 20:767–777, 2000.

Krebs TL, Daly B, Cheong JJWY, Carroll K, Barlett ST: Acute pancreatic transplant rejection: Evaluation with dynamic contrast-enhanced MR imaging compared with histopathologic analysis. *Radiology* 210:437–442, 1999.

Low RN, Semelka RC, Worawattanakul S, Alzate GD: Extrahepatic abdominal imaging in patients with malignancy: Comparison of MR imaging and helical CT in 164 patients. *J Magn Reson Imag* 12:269–277, 2000.

Martin DR, Karabulut N, Yang M, Chang WL, MacFadden DW: Peripancreatic signal changes identified on fat suppressed gradient echo imaging associated with fat necrosis and poor clinical outcome. *J Magn Reson Imag* 1:49–58, 2003.

Martin DR, Semelka RC: MR imaging of pancreatic masses. *MRI Clin N Am* 8(4):787–811, 2000.

McFarland EG, Kaufman JA, Saini S, et al: Preoperative staging of cancer of the pancreas: Value of MR angiography versus conventional angiography in detecting portal venous invasion. *Am J Roentgenol* 166:37–43, 1996.

Mitchell DG, Winston CB, Outwater EK, Ehrlich SM: Delineation of pancreas with MR imaging: Multiobserver comparison of five pulse sequences. *J Magn Reson Imag* 5:193–199, 1995.

Mozell E, Stenzel P, Woltering EA, Rosch J, O'Dorisio TM: Functional endocrine tumors of the pancreas: Clinical presentation, diagnosis, and treatment. *Curr Probl Surg* 27:304–385, 1990.

Ohtomo K, Furai S, Oneone M, Okada Y, Kusano S, Uchiyama G: Solid and papillary epithelial neoplasm of the pancreas: MR imaging and pathologic correlation. *Radiology* 184:567–570, 1992.

Procacci C, Megibow AJ, Carbognin G, Guarise A, Spoto E: Intraductal papillary mucinous tumor of the pancreas: A pictorial essay. *Radiographics* 19:1447–1463, 1999.

Semelka RC, Ascher SM: MRI of the pancreas—state of the art. *Radiology* 188:593–602, 1993.

Semelka RC, Custodio CM, Balci C, Woosley JT: Neuroendocrine tumors of the pancreas: Spectrum of appearances on MRI. *J Magn Res Imag* 11:141–148, 2000.

Semelka RC, Kelekis NL, Molina PL, Scharp T, Calvo B: Pancreatic masses with inconclusive findings on spiral CR. Is there a role for MRI? *J Magn Reson Imag* 6:585–588, 1996.

Semelka RC, Shoenut JP, Kroeker MA, Micflikier AB: Chronic pancreatitis: MR imaging features before and after administration of gadopentetate dimeglumine. *J Magn Reson Imag* 3:79–82, 1993.

Semelka RC, Simm FC, Recht M, Deimling M, Lenz G, Laub GA: MRI of the pancreas at high field strength—a comparison of six sequences. *J Comput Assist Tomogr* 15(6):966–971, 1991.

Steer ML, Waxman I, Freedman S: Chronic pancreatitis. *N Engl J Med* 332:1482–1490, 1995.

Thompson NW, Eckhauser FE, Vinik AI, Lloyd RV, Fiddian-Green RD, Strodel WE: Cystic neuroendocrine neoplasms of the pancreas and liver. *Ann Surg* 199:158–164, 1984.

Winston CB, Mitchell DG, Outwater EK, Ehrlich SM: Pancreatic signal intensity on T1-weighted fat saturation MR images: Clinical correlation. *J Magn Reson Imag* 5:267–271, 1995.

CHAPTER 5

Applegate KE, Goske MJ, Pierce G, Murphy D: Situs revisited: Imaging of the heterotaxy syndrome. *Radiographics* 19:837–852, 1999.

Disler DG, Chew FS: Splenic hemangioma. *Am J Roentgenol* 157:44, 1991.

Hill SC, Damaska BM, Ling A, Patterson K, et al.: Gaucher disease: Abdominal MR imaging findings in 46 patients. *Radiology* 184:561–566, 1992.

Ito K, Mitchell DG, Honjo K, Fujita T, et al.: MR imaging of acquired abnormalities of the spleen. *Am J Roentgenol* 168:697–702, 1997.

Kelekis N, Semelka RC, Burdeny DA: Dark ring sign: Finding in patients with fungal liver lesions undergoing treatment with antifungal antibiotics. *J Magn Reson Imag* 14:615–618, 1996.

Mirowitz SA, Brown JJ, Lee JKT, Heiken JP: Dynamic gadolinium-enhanced MR imaging of the normal spleen: Normal enhancement patterns and evaluation of splenic lesions. *Radiology* 179:681–686, 1991.

Mirowitz SA, Gutierrez E, Lee JKT, Brown JJ, et al.: Normal abdominal enhancement patterns with dynamic gadolinium-enhanced MR imaging. *Radiology* 180:637–640, 1991.

Ohtomo K, Fukuda H, Mori K, Minami M, et al.: CT and MR appearances of splenic hamartoma. *J Comput Assist Tomogr* 16:425–428, 1992.

Ramani M, Reinhold C, Semelka RC, Siegelman ES, Liang L, Ascher SM, Brown JJ, Eisen RN, Bret PM: Splenic hemangiomas and hamartomas: MR imaging characteristics of 28 lesions. *Radiology* 202:166–172, 1997.

Sagoh T, Hoh K, Togashi K, et al.: Gamna-Gandy bodies of the spleen: Evaluation with MR imaging. *Radiology* 172:685–687, 1989.

Semelka RC, Shoenut JP, Greenberg HM, Bow EJ: Detection of acute and treated lesions of hepatosplenic candidiasis: Comparison of dynamic contrast-enhanced CT and MR imaging. *J Magn Reson Imag* 2:341–345, 1992.

Semelka RC, Shoenut JP, Lawrence PH, Greenberg HM, Madden TP, Kroeker MA: Spleen: Dynamic enhancement patterns on gradient-echo MR images enhanced with gadopentetate dimeglumine. *Radiology* 185:479–482, 1992.

Siegelman ES, Mitchel DG, Semelka RC: Abdominal iron deposition: Metabolism, MR findings, and clinical importance. *Radiology* 199:13–22, 1996.

Urrutia M, Mergo PJ, Ros LH, Torres GM, Ros PR: Cystic masses of the spleen: Radiologic-pathologic correlation. *Radiographics* 16:107–129, 1996.

Warshauer DM, Semelka RC, Ascher SM: Nodular sarcoidosis of the liver and spleen: Appearance on MR images. *J Magn Reson Imaging* 4:553–557, 1994.

Weissleder R, Elizondo G, Stark DD, Hahn PF, et al.: The diagnosis of splenic lymphoma by MR imaging: Value of superparamagnetic iron oxide. *Am J Roentgenol* 152:175–180, 1989.

Weissleder R, Hahn PF, Stark DD, Elizondo G, et al.: Superparamagnetic iron oxide: Enhanced detection of focal splenic tumors with MR imaging. *Radiology* 169:399–403, 1988.

CHAPTER 6

Bakker J, Beek FJA, Beutler JJ, Hené RJ, Kort GAP, Lange EE, et al.: Renal artery stenosis and accessory renal arteries: Accuracy of detection and visualization with gadolinium-enhanced breath-hold MR angiography. *Radiology* 207:497–504, 1998.

Balci NC, Semelka RC, Patt RH, Dubois D, Freeman JA, Gomez-Caminero A, Woosley JT: Complex renal cysts: Findings on MR imaging. *AM J Roentgenol* 172:1485–1500, 1999.

Bard RH, Lord B, Fromowitz: Papillary adenocarcinoma of kidney. *Urology* 19:16–20,1982.

Bosniak MA: The small (<3.0 cm) renal parenchymal tumor: Detection, diagnosis, and controversies. *Radiology* 179:307–317, 1991.

Brown ED, Semelka RC: Renal abscesses: Appearance on gadolinium-enhanced magnetic resonance images. *Abdom Imaging* 21:172–176, 1996.

Burdeny DA, Semelka RC, Kelekis NL, Reinhold C, Ascher SM: Small (<1.5 cm) angiomyolipomas of the kidney: Characterization by combined use of in-phase and fat attenuated MR techniques. *J Magn Reson Imag* 15(2):141–145, 1997.

Choyke PL, Frank JA, Girton ME, et al.: Dynamic Gd-DTPA-enhanced MR imaging of the kidney: Experimental results. *Radiology* 170:713–720, 1989.

Choyke PL, Glenn GM, Wlather MM, Patronas NJ, Linehan WM, Zbar B: von Hippel–Lindau disease: Genetic, clinical, and imaging features. *Radiology* 194:629–642, 1995.

Chung JJ, Semelka RC, Martin DR. Acute renal failure: Common occurrence of preservation of corticomedullary differentiation on MR images. (Submitted)

Davidson AJ, Hayews WS, Hartman DS, McCarthy WF, Davis CJ: Renal oncocytoma and carcinoma: Failure of differentiation with CT. *Radiology* 186:693–696, 1993.

Debatin JF, Ting RH, Wegmuller H, et al.: Renal artery blood flow: Quantification with phase-contrast MR imaging with and without breath holding. *Radiology* 190:371–378, 1994.

Esparza AR, McKay DB, Cronan JJ, Chazan JA: Renal parenchymal malakoplakia. Histologic spectrum and its relationship to megalocytic interstitial nephritis and xanthogranulomatous pyelonephritis. *Am J Surg Pathol* 13(3):225–236, 1989.

Gabow PA: Autosomal dominant polycystic kidney disease. Review article. *N Engl J Med* 329:332–342, 1993.

Gylys-Morin V, Hoffer FA, Kozakewich H, Shamberger RC: Wilms' tumor and nephroblastomatosis: Imaging characteristics at gadolinium-enhanced MR imaging. *Radiology* 188:517–521, 1993.

Haustein J, Niendorf HP, Krestin G, et al.: Renal tolerance of gadolinium-DTPA/dimeglumine in patients with chronic renal failure. *Invest Radiol* 27:153–156, 1992.

Ishikawa I: Uremic acquired cystic disease of kidney. *Urology* 26:101–107, 1985.

John G, Semelka RC, Burdeny DA, Kelekis NL, Kettritz U, Freeman JA: Renal cell cancer: Incidence of hemorrhage on MR images in patients with renal insufficiency. *J Magn Reson Imag* 7:157–160, 1997.

Kettritz U, Semelka RC, Brown ED, Sharp TJ, Lawing WL, Colindres RE: MR findings in diffuse renal parenchymal disease. *J Magn Reson Imag* 6:136–144, 1996.

Kettritz U, Semelka RC, Siegelman ES, Shoenut JP, Mithell DG: Multilocular cystic nephroma: MR imaging appearance with current techniques, including gadolinium enhancement. *J Magn Reson Imag* 1:145–148, 1996.

Kikinis R, von Schulthess GK, Jager P, et al.: Normal and hydronephrotic kidney: Evaluation of renal function with contrast-enhanced MR imaging. *Radiology* 165:837–842, 1987.

Leo ME, Petrou SP, Barrett DM: Transitional cell carcinoma of the kidney with vena caval involvement: Report of 3 cases and a review of the literature. *J Urol* 148:398–400, 1992.

Liou JTS, Lee JKT, Heiken JP, Totty WG, Molina PL, Flye WM: Renal transplants: Can acute rejection and acute tubular necrosis be differentiated with MR imaging. *Radiology* 179:61–65, 1991.

Low RN, Martinz AG, Steinberg SM, Alzate GD, et al.: Potencial renal transplant donors: Evaluation with gadolinium-enhanced MR angiography and MR urography. *Radiology* 207:165–172, 1998.

Mitnick JS, Bosniak MA, Mitton S, Raghavendra BN, Subramanyan BR, Genieser NB: Cystic renal disease in tuberous sclerosis. *Radiology* 147:85–87, 1983.

Mosetti MA, Leonardou P, Motohara T, Kanematsu M, Armao D, Semelka RC: Autosomal dominant polycystic kidney disease: MR imaging evaluation using current techniques. *J Magn Reson Imag* 18:210–215, 2003.

Muller MR, Prasad PV, Bimmler D, Kaiser A, Edelman RR: Functional imaging of the kidney by means of measurement of the apparent diffusion coefficient. *Radiology* 193:711–715, 1994.

Mulopulos GP, Patel SK, Pessis D: MR imaging of xanthogranulomatous pyelonephritis. *J Comput Assist Tomogr* 10:154–156, 1986.

Murad T, Komako W, Oyesu R, Bauer K: Multilocular cystic renal cell carcinoma. *Am J Clin Pathol* 95(5):633–637, 1991.

Neimatallah MA, Dong Q, Schoenberg SO, Cho KJ, Prince MR: Magnetic resonance imaging in renal transplantation. *J Magn Reson Imag* 10:357–368, 1999.

Newhouse JH, Wagner BJ: Renal oncocytomas. *Abdom Imag* 23:249–255, 1998.

Osterling JE, Fishman EK, Goldman SM, Marshall FF: The management of renal angiomyolipoma. *J Urol* 135:1121–1124, 1986.

Oto A, Herts BR, Remer EM, Novick AC: Inferior vena cava tumor thrombus in renal cell carcinoma: Staging by MR imaging and impact on surgical treatment. *Am J Roentgenol* 171:1619–1624, 1998.

Press GA, McClennan BL, Melson GL, Weyman PJ, Mauro MA, Lee JKT: Papillary renal cell carcinoma: CT and sonographic evaluation. *Am J Roentgenol* 143:1005–1010, 1984.

Prince MR, Narasimham DL, Stanley JC, Chenevert TL, Williams DM, Marx MV, Cho KJ: Breathhold gadolinium-enhanced MR angiography of the abdominal aorta and its major branches. *Radiology* 197:785–792, 1995.

Quinn MJ, Hartman DS, Friedman AC, et al: Renal oncocytoma: New observations. *Radiology* 153:49–53, 1984.

Regan F, Bohlman ME, Khazan R, Rodriguez R, Schultze-Haakh H. MR urography using HASTE imaging in the assessment of ureteric obstruction. *Am J Roentgenol* 167:1115–1120, 1996.

Reichard EAP, Roubidoux MA, Dunnick NR: Renal neoplasms in patients with renal cystic diseases. *Abdom Imag* 23:237–248,1998.

Ros PR, Gauger J, Stoupis C, Burton SS, Mao J, Wilcox C, Rosenber EB, Briggs RW: Diagnosis of renal artery stenosis: Feasibility of combining MR angiography, MR renography, and gadopentetate-based measurements of glomerular filtration rate. *Am J Roentgenol* 165:1447–1457, 1995.

Rothpearl A, Frager D, Subramanian A, Bashist B, Baer J, Kay C, Cooke K, Raia C: MR urography: Technique and application. *Radiology* 194:125–130, 1995.

Semelka RC, Corrigan K, Ascher SM, Brown JJ, Colindres RE: Renal corticomedullary differentiation: Observation in patient with differing serum creatinine levels. *Radiology* 190:149–152, 1994.

Semelka RC, Hricak H, Tomei E, Floth A, Stoller M: Obstructive nephropathy: Evaluation with dynamic Gd-DTPA-enhanced MR imaging. *Radiology* 175:797–803, 1990.

Semelka RC, Kelekis NL, Burdeny DA, Mitchell DG, Brown JJ, Siegelman ES: Renal lymphoma: Demonstration by MR imaging. *Am J Roentgenol* 166:823–827, 1996.

Semelka RC, Shoenut JP, Greenberg HM, Bow EJ: Detection of acute and treated lesions of hepatosplenic candidiasis: Comparison of dynamic contrast-enhanced CT and MR imaging. *J Magn Reson Imag* 2:414–420, 1992.

Strotzer M, Lehner KB, Becker K: Detection of fat in a renal cell carcinoma mimicking angiomyolipoma. *Radiology* 188:427–428, 1993.

Tempany CMC, Morton RA, Marshall FF: MRI of the renal veins: Assessment of nonneoplastic venous thrombosis. *J Comput Assist Tomogr* 16(6):929–934, 1992.

Van Ball JG, Smits NJ, Keeman JN, et al.: The evolution of renal angiomylipomas in patients with tuberous sclerosis. *J Urol* 152:35–38, 1994.

Weeks SM, Brown ED, Brown JJ, Adamis MK, Eisenberg LB, Semelka RC: Transitional cell carcinoma of the upper urinary tract staging by MRI. *Abdom Imag* 20:365–367, 1995.

Winalski CS, Lipman JC, Tumeh SS: Ureteral neoplasms. *Radiographics* 10:271–283, 1990.

Wise SW, Hartman DS, Hardesty LA, Mosher TJ: Renal medullary cystic disease: Assessment by MRI. *Abdom Imag* 23(6):649–651, 1998.

Wolf GL, Hoop B, Cannillo JA, Rogowska JA, Halpern EF: Measurement of renal transit of gadopentetate dimeglumine with echo-planar MR imaging. *J Magn Reson Imag* 4:365–372, 1994.

Wolf RL, King BF, Torres VE, Wilson DM, Ehman RL: Measurement of normal renal arterial blood flow: Cine phase-contrast MR imaging vs. clearance of p-aminohippurate. *Am J Roentgenol* 161:995–1002, 1993.

Yoshimitsu K, Honda H, Kuroiwa T, Irie H, Tajima T, Jimi M, Kuroiwa K, et al.: Fat detection in granular-cell renal cell carcinoma using chemical-shift gradient-echo MR imaging: another renal tumor that contains fat. *Abdom Imag* 25:100–102, 2000.

CHAPTER 7

Aisen AM, Ohl DA, Chenevert TL, Perkins P, Mikesell W: MR of an adrenal pseudocyst. *Magn Reson Imag* 10:997–1000, 1992.

Baker ME, Blinder R, Spritzer C, Leight GS, Herfkens RJ, Dunnick NR: MR evaluation of adrenal masses at 1.5 T. *Am J Roentgenol* 153:307–312, 1989.

Belden CJ, Powers C, Ros PR: MR demonstration of a cystic pheochromocytoma. *J Magn Reson Imag* 5:778–780, 1995.

Bush WH, Elder JS, Crane RE, Wales LR: Cystic pheochromocytoma. *Urology* 25:332–334, 1985.

Chung JJ, Semelka RC, Martin DR: Adrenal adenomas: Characteristic post-gadolinium capillary blush dynamic MR imaging. *J Magn Reson Imag* 13:242–248, 2001.

Crecelius SA, Bellah R: Pheochromocytoma of the bladder in an adolescent: Sonographic and MR imaging findings. *Am J Roentgenol* 165:101–103, 1995.

Custodio CM, Semelka RC, Balci NC, Mitchell KM, Freeman JA: Adrenal neuroblastoma in an adult with tumor thrombus in the inferior vena cava. *J Magn Reson Imag* 9:621–623, 1999.

Feinstein RS, Gatewood OMB, Fishman EK, Goldman SM, Siegelman SS: Computed tomography of adult neuroblastoma. *J Comput Assist Tomogr* 8:720–726, 1984.

Hamrick-Turner JE, Cranston PE, Shipkey FH: Cavernous hemangiomas of the adrenal gland: MR findings. *Magn Reson Imag* 12(8):1263–1267, 1994.

Hauser H, Gurret JP: Miliary tuberculosis associated with adrenal enlargement CT appearance. *J Comput Assist Tomogr* 10:254–256, 1986.

Ichikawa T, Ohtomo K, Uchiyama G, Koizumi K, Monzawa S, Oba H, et al.: Adrenal adenomas: Characteristic hyperintense rim sign on fat-saturated spin-echo MR images. *Radiology* 193:247–250, 1994.

Korobkin M, Giordano TJ, Brodeur FJ, et al.: Adrenal adenomas: Relationship between histologic lipid and CT and MR findings. *Radiology* 200:743–747, 1996.

Krestin GP, Steinbrich W, Friedmann G: Adrenal masses: Evaluation with fast gradient-echo MR imaging Gd-DTPA-enhanced dynamic studies. *Radiology* 171:675–680, 1989.

Mayo-Smith WW, Lee MJ, McNicholas MMJ, Hahn PF, Boland GW, Saini S: Characterization of adrenal masses (<5 cm) by use of chemical shift MR imaging: Observer performance versus quantitative measures. *Am J Roentgenol* 165:91–95, 1995.

McLoughlin RF, Bilbey JH: Tumors of the adrenal gland: Findings on CT and MR imaging. *Am J Roentgenol* 163:1413–1418, 1994.

McMurry JF Jr, Long D, McClure R, Kotchen TA: Addison's disease with adrenal enlargement on computed tomographic scanning. *Am J Med* 77:365–368, 1984.

McNicholas MMJ, Lee MJ, Mayo-Smith WW, Hahn PF, Boland GW, Mueller PR: An imaging algorithm for the differential diagnosis of adrenal adenomas and metastases. *Am J Roentgenol* 165:1453–1459, 1995.

Mitchell DG, Grovello M, Matteucci T, Peterson RO, Miettinen MM: Benign adenocortical masses: Diagnosis with chemical shift MR imaging. *Radiology* 185:345–351, 1992.

Musante F, Derchi LE, Bazzochi M, et al.: MR imaging of adrenal myelolipomas. Journal of Computer Assisted Tomography (JCAT) 15:111–114, 1991.

Outwater EK, Siegelman ES, Huang AB, Birnbaum BA: Adrenal masses: Correlation between CT attenuation value and chemical shift ratio at MR imaging with in-phase and opposed-phase sequences. *Radiology* 200:749–752, 1996.

Outwater EK, Siegelman ES, Radecki PD, Piccoli CW, Mitchell DG: Distinction between benign and malignant adrenal masses: Value of T1-weighted chemical-shift MR imaging. *Am J Roentgenol* 165:579–583, 1995.

Paling MR, Williamson BRJ: Adrenal involvement in non-Hodgkin lymphoma. *Am J Roentgenol* 141:303–305, 1983.

Provenzale JM, Ortel TL, Nelson RC: Adrenal hemorrhage in patients with primary antiphospholipid syndrome: Imaging findings. *Am J Roentgenol* 165:361–364, 1995.

Reinig JW, Doppman JL, Dwyer AJ, Frank J: MRI of indeterminate adrenal masses. *Am J Roentgenol* 147:493–496, 1986.

Reining JW, Doppman JL, Dwyer AJ, Johnson AR, Knop RH: Adrenal masses differentiated by MR. *Radiology* 158:81–84, 1986.

Reinig JW, Stutley JE, Leonhardt CM, Spicer KM, Margolis M, Caldwell CB: Differentiation of adrenal masses with MR imaging: Comparison of techniques. *Radiology* 192:41–46, 1994.

Sato N, Watanabe Y, Saga T, Mitsudo K, Dohke M, Minami K: Adrenocortical adenoma containing a fat component CT and MR image evaluation. *Abdom Imag* 20:489–490, 1995.

Schwartz LH, Panicek DM, Koutcher JA, Brown KT, Getrajdman GI, Heelan RT, et al.: Adrenal masses in patients with malignancy: Prospective comparsion of echo-planar, fast spin-echo, and chemical shift MR imaging. *Radiology* 197:421–425, 1995.

Semelka RC, Shoenut JP, Lawrence PH, Greenberg HM, Maycher B, Madden TP, Kroeker MA: Evaluation of adrenal masses with gadolinium enhancement and fat suppressed MR imaging. *J Magn Reson Imag* 3:337–343, 1993.

Silverman SG, Mueller PR, Pinkney LP, Koenker RM, Seltzer SE: Predictive value of image-guided adrenal biopsy: Analysis of results of 101 biopsies. *Radiology* 187:715–718, 1993.

Small WC, Bernardino ME: Gd-DTPA adrenal gland enhancement at 1.5 T. *J Magn Reson Imag* 9:309–312, 1991.

Smith SM, Patel SK, Turner DA, et al: Magnetic resonance imaging of adrenal cortical carcinoma. *Urol Radiol* 11:1–6, 1989.

Tsushima Y, Ishizaka H, Matsumoto M: Adrenal masses: Differentiation with chemical shift, fast low-angle shot MR imaging. *Radiology* 186:705–709, 1993.

Westra SJ, Zaninovic AC, Hall TR, Kangarloo H, Boechat MI: Imaging of the adrenal gland in children. *Radiographics* 14:1323–1340, 1994.

CHAPTER 8

Acheson ED: The distribution of ulcerative colitis and regional enteritis in United States veterans with particular reference to the Jewish religion. *Gut* 1:291–293, 1960.

Blot WJ et al.: Continuing climb in rates of esophageal adenocarcinoma: An update. *JAMA* 270 (11):1320, 1993.

Brown JJ, Duncan JR, Heiken JP, et al.: Perflurocetylbromide as a gastrointestinal contrast agent for MR imaging: Use with and without glucagon. *Radiology* 181:455–460, 1991.

Chou CK, Chen LT, Sheu RS, Wang ML, et al.: MRI manifestations of gastrointestinal wall thickening. *Abdom Imag* 19:389–394, 1994.

Chou CK, Chen LT, Sheu RS, Yang CW, et al.: MRI manifestations of gastrointestinal lymphoma. *Abdom Imag* 19:495–500, 1994.

Chung JJ, Semelka RC, Martin DR, Marcos HB: Colon diseases: MR evaluation using combined T2-weighted single-shot echo train spin-echo and gadolinium-enhanced spoiled gradient-echo sequences. *J Magn Reson Imag* 12:297–305, 2000.

Coggon D, Acheson ED: The geography of cancer of the stomach. *Br Med Bull* 40:335–341, 1984.

Dragosics B, Bauer P, Radaasziewicz T: Primary gastrointestinal non-Hodgkin's lymphomas. *Cancer* 55:1060–1073, 1985.

Gomberg JS, Friedman AC, Radecki PD, Grumbach K, Caroline DF: MRI differentiation of recurrent colorectal carcinoma from postoperative fibrosis. *Gastrointest Radiol* 11:361–363, 1986.

Haenszel W, Kurihara M: Studies of Japanese migrants: 1. Mortality from cancer and other disease among Japanese in the United States. *J Natl Cancer Inst* 40:43–68, 1968.

Hamed MM, Hamm B, Ibrahim ME, Taupitz M, Mahfouz AE: Dynamic MR imaging of the abdomen with gadopentetate dimeglumine: Normal enhancement pattern of liver, spleen, stomach, and pancreas. *Am J Roentgenol* 158:303–307, 1992.

Ito K, Kato T, Tadokoro M, et al.: Recurrent rectal cancer and scar: Differentiation with PET and MR imaging. *Radiology* 182:549–552, 1992.

Jetmore AB, Ray JE, Gathright BJ, McMullen KM, et al.: Rectal carcinoids: The most frequent carcinoid tumor. *Dis Colon Rectum* 35:717–725, 1992.

Kahrihas PJ, Kishk SM, Helm JF, Dodds WJ, et al.: Comparison of pseudoachalasia and achalasia. *Am J Med* 82:439–446, 1987.

Kaminsky S, Laniado M, Gogoll M, et al.: Gadopentetate dimeglumine as a bowel contrast agent: Safety and efficacy. *Radiology* 178:503–508, 1991.

Kee F, Wilson RH, Gilliland R, Sloan JM, et al.: Changing site distribution of colorectal cancer. *Br Med J* 305:158, 1992.

Kettritz U, Isaacs K, Warshauer DM, Semelka RC: Crohn's disease: Pilot study comparing MRI of the abdomen with clinical evaluation. *J Clin Gastroenterol* 21:249–253, 1995.

Lee JK, Marcos HB, Semelka RC: MR imaging of the small bowel using the HASTE sequence. *Am J Roentgenol* 170:1457–1463, 1998.

Low RN, Barone RM, Lacey C, Sigeti JS, Alzate GD, Sebrechts CP: Peritoneal tumor: MR imaging with dilute oral barium and intravenous gadolinium-containing contrast agents compared with unenhanced MR imaging and CT. *Radiology* 204:513–520, 1997.

Low RN, Francis IR: MR imaging of the gastrointestinal tract with IV gadolinium and diluted barium oral contrast media compared with unenhanced MR imaging and CT. *Am J Roentgenol* 169:1051–1059, 1997.

Macpherson RI: Gastrointestinal tract duplications: Clinical, pathologic, etiologic and radiologic considerations. *Radiographics* 13:1063–1080, 1993.

Marcos H, Semelka RC: Stomach diseases: MR evaluation using combined T2-weighted single-shot echo train spin echo and gadolinium–enhanced spoiled gradient-echo sequences. *J Mag Reson Imag* 10:950–960, 1999.

Marcos HB, Semelka RC: Evaluation of Crohn's disease using half-Fourier RARE and gadolinium-enhanced SGE sequences initial results. *J Mag Reson Imag* 18:263–268, 2000.

Martin, DR, Yang M, Thomasson D, Acheson C: MR colonography: Development of optimized methodology using ex vivo and in vivo systems. *Radiology* 225:597–602, 2002.

Outwater E, Schiebler ML: Pelvic fistulas: Findings on MR images. *Am J Roentgenol* 160:327–330, 1993.

Perzin KH, Bridge MY: Adenomas of the small intestine: A clinicopathologic review of 51 cases and a study of their relationship to carcinoma. *Cancer* 48(3):799–819, 1981.

Rafal RB, Markisz JA: Magnetic resonance imaging of an esophageal duplication cyst. *Am J Gastroenterol* 86:1809–1811, 1991.

Rubesin SE, Gilchrist AM, Bronner M, Saul SH, et al.: Non-Hodgkin lymphoma of the small intestine. *Radiographics* 10:985–998, 1990.

Rubin DL, Muller HH, Sidhu MK, Young SW, et al.: Liquid oral magnetic particles as a gastrointestinal contrast agent for MR imaging: Efficacy in vivo. *J Magn Reson Imag* 3:113–118, 1993.

Schnall MD, Furth EE, Rosato F: Rectal tumor stage: Correlation of endorectal MR imaging and pathologic findings. *Radiology* 190:709–714, 1994.

Semelka RC, Hricak H, Kim B, et al.: Pelvic fistulas: Appearances on MR images. *Abdom Imag* 22:91–95, 1997.

Semelka RC, John G, Kelekis NL, Burdeny DA, Ascher SM: Bowel related abscesses: Demonstration by current MR techniques. *J Magn Reson Imag* 16:855–861, 1998.

Semelka RC, Marcos HB: Polyposis syndromes of the gastrointestinal tract: MR findings. *J Mag Reson Imag* 11:51–55, 2000.

Semelka RC, Shoenut JP, Silverman R, Kroeker MA, Yaffe CS, Micflikier AB: Bowel disease: Prospective comparison of CT and 1.5 T pre- and postcontrast MR imaging with T1-weighted fat-suppressed and breath-hold FLASH sequences. *J Magn Reson Imag* 1:625–632, 1991.

Shoenut JP, Semelka RC, Magro CM, Silverman R, Yaffe CS, Mickflikier AB: Comparison of magnetic resonance imaging and endoscopy in distinguishing the type and severity of inflammatory bowel diseases. *J Clin Gastroenterol* 19:31–35, 1994.

Shoenut JP, Semelka RC, Silverman R, Yaffe CS, Mickflikier AB: Magnetic resonance imaging in inflammatory bowel disease. *J Clin Gastroenterol* 17:73–78, 1993.

Shoenut JP, Semelka RC, Silverman R, Yaffe CS, Mickflikier AB: Magnetic resonance imaging evaluation of the local extent of colorectal mass lesions. *J Clin Gastroenterol* 17:248–253, 1993.

Stoker J, Hussain SM, van Kempen D, Elevelt AJ, Laneris JS: Endoanal coil MR imaging in anal fistulas. *Am J Roentgenol* 166:360–362, 1996.

Wesbey GE, Brasch RC, Goldberg HI, Engelstad BL: Dilute oral iron solutions as gastrointestinal contrast agents for magnetic resonance imaging: Initial clinical experience. *J Magn Reson Imag* 3:57–66, 1985.

CHAPTER 9

Arrive L, Hricak H, Tavares NJ, Miller TR: Malignant versus nonmalignant retroperitoneal fibrosis: Differentiation with MR imaging. *Radiology* 172:139–143, 1989; 955–956, 1983.

Auffermann W, Olofsson PA, Rabahie GN, Tavares NJ, Stoney RJ, Higgins CB: Incorporation versus infection of retroperitoneal aortic grafts: MR imaging features. *Radiology* 172:359–362, 1989.

Bretan PN Jr., Williams RD, Hricak H: Preoperative assessment of retroperitoneal pathology by magnetic resonance imaging. Primary leiomyosarcoma of inferior vena cava. *Urology* 28:251–255, 1986.

Connolly J, Eisner D, Goldman S, Stutzman R, Steiner M: Benign retroperitoneal fibrosis and renal cell carcinoma. *J Urol* 149:1535–1537, 1993.

Douek PC, Revel D, Chazel S, Falise B, Villard J, Amiel M: Fast MR angiography of the aortoiliac arteries and arteries of the lower extremity: Value of bolus-enhanced, whole-volume subtraction technique. *Am J Roentgenol* 165:431–437, 1995.

Ecklund K, Hartnell GG, Hughes LA, Stokes KR, Finn JP: MR angiography as the sole method in evaluating abdominal aortic aneurysms: Correlation with conventional techniques and surgery [see comments]. *Radiology* 192:345–350, 1994.

Ellis JH, Bies JR, Kopecky KK, Klatte EC, Rowland RG, Donohue JP: Comparison of NMR and CT imaging in the evaluation of metastatic retroperitoneal lymphadenopathy from testicular carcinoma. *J Comput Assist Tomogr* 8:709–719, 1984.

Gatanaga H, Ohnishi S, Miura H, Kita H, Matsuhashi N, Kodama T, Minami M, Okudaira T, Imawari M, Yazaki YRC: Retroperitoneal fibrosis leading to extrahepatic portal vein obstruction. *Intern Med* 33:346–350, 1994.

Glazer HS, Lee JK, Levitt RG, Heiken JP, Ling D, Totty WG, Balfe DM, Emani B, Wasserman TH, Murphy WA: Radiation fibrosis: Differentiation from recurrent tumor by MR imaging. *Radiology* 156:721–726, 1985.

Hahn PF, Saini S, Stark DD, Papanicolaou N, Ferrucci JT, Jr.: Intraabdominal hematoma: The concentric-ring sign in MR imaging. *Am J Roentgenol* 148:115–119, 1987.

Hartman DS, Hayes WS, Choyke PL, Tibbetts GP: From the archives of the AFIP. Leiomyosarcoma of the retroperitoneum and inferior vena cava: Radiologic-pathologic correlation. *Radiographics* 12:1203–1220, 1992.

Ichikawa T, Koyama A, Fujimoto H, Honma M, Saiga T, Matsubara N, Ozeki Y, Uchiyama G, Ohtomo K: Abdominal wall desmoid mimicking intra-abdominal mass: MR features. *J Magn Reson Imag* 12:541–544, 1994.

Johnson WK, Ros PR, Powers C, Stoupis C, Segel KH: Castleman disease mimicking an aggressive retroperitoneal neoplasm. *Abdom Imag* 19:342–344, 1994.

Justich E, Amparo EG, Hricak H, Higgins CB: Infected aortoiliofemoral grafts: Magnetic resonance imaging. *Radiology* 154:133–136, 1985.

Kelekis NL, Semelka RC, Hill ML, Meyers DC, Molina PL: Malignant fibrous histiocytoma of the inferior vena cava: Appearances on contrast-enhanced spiral CT and MRI. *Abdom Imag* 21:461–463, 1996.

Koep L, Zuidema GD: The clinical significance of retroperitoneal fibrosis. *Surgery* 81:250–257, 1977.

Lane RH, Stephens DH, Reiman HM: Primary retroperitoneal neoplasms: CT findings in 90 cases with clinical and pathologic correlation. *Am J Roentgenol* 152:83–89, 1989.

Lepor H, Walsh PC: Idiopathic retroperitoneal fibrosis. *J Urol* 122:1–6, 1979.

Lindell OI, Sariola HV, Lehtonen TA: The occurrence of vasculitis in perianeurysmal fibrosis. *J Urol* 138:727–729, 1987; 155:407–412, 1985.

Prince MR, Narasimham DL, Jacoby WT, Williams DM, Cho KJ, Marx MV, Deeb GM: Three-dimensional gadolinium enhanced MR angiography of the thoracic aorta. *Am J Roentgenol* 166:1387–1397, 1996.

Vlahos L, Trakadas S, Gouliamos A, Plataniotis G, Papavasiliou C: Retrocrural masses of extramedullary hemopoiesis in beta-thalassemia. *Magn Reson Imag* 11:1227–1229, 1993.

Williams DM, Joshi A, Dake MD, Deeb GM, Miller DC, Abrams GD: Aortic cobwebs: An anatomic marker identifying the false lumen in aortic dissection—imaging and pathologic correlation [see comments]. *Radiology* 190:167–174, 1994.

Williams WM, Kosovsky PA, Rafal RB, Markisz JA: Retroperitoneal germ cell neoplasm: MR and CT. *Magn Reson Imag* 10:325–331, 1992.

Wolff KA, Herold CJ, Tempany CM, Parravano JG, Zerhouni EA: Aortic dissection: Atypical patterns seen at MR imaging. *Radiology* 181:489–495, 1991.

CHAPTER 10

Berger PE: Hernias of the abdominal wall and peritoneal cavity. In Franken EA Jr, Smith WL (eds.), *Gastrointestinal Imaging in Pediatrics*. Philadelphia: Harper & Row, pp. 446–456, 1982.

Dooms GC, Fisher MR, Hricak H, Higgins CB: MR of intramuscular hemorrhage. *J Comput Assist Tomogr* 9:908–913, 1985.

Gougoutas CA, Siegelman ES, Hunt J, Outwater EK: Pelvic endometriosis: Various manifestations and MR imaging findings. *Am J Roentgenol* 175:353–358, 2000.

Hahn PF, Saini S, Stark DD, Papanicolauo N, et al.: Intra-abdominal hematoma: The concentric-ring sign in MR imaging. *Am J Roentgenol* 148:115–119, 1987.

Haynes JW, Brewer WH, Walsh JW: Focal fat necrosis presenting as a palpable abdominal mass: CT evaluation. *J Comput Assist Tomogr* 9:568–569, 1985.

Katz ME, Heiken JP, Glazer HS, Lee JKT: Intra-abdominal panniculitis: Clinical, radiographic, and CT features. *Am J Roentgenol* 145:293–296, 1985.

Kurachi H, Murakami T, Nakamura H, et al.: Imaging of peritoneal pseudocysts: Value of MR imaging compared with sonography and CT. *Am J Roentgenol* 160:589–591, 1993.

Low RN, Semelka RC, Worawattanakul S, Altaze GD, Sigeti JS: Extrahepatic abdominal imaging in patients with malignancy: Comparison of MR imaging and helical CT, with subsequent surgical correlation. *Radiology* 210:625–632, 1999.

Meyers MA, Oliphant M, Berne AS, Feldberg MAM: The peritoneal ligaments and mesenteries: Pathways of intra-abdominal spread of disease. *Radiology* 163:593–604, 1987.

Noone TC, Semelka RC, Worawattanakul S, Marcos HB: Intraperitoneal abscesses: Diagnostic accuracy of and appearances at MR imaging. *Radiology* 208:525–528, 1998.

Novetsky GJ, Berlin L, Epstein AJ, Lobo N, et al.: Pseudomyxoma peritonei. *J Comput Assist Tomogr* 6:398–399, 1982.

Picus D, Glazer HS, Levitt RG, Husband JE: Computed tomography of abdominal carcinoid tumors. *Am J Roentgenol* 143:581–584, 1984.

Reitamo JJ, Hayry P, Nykyri E, Saxen E: The desmoid tumor. I. Incidence, sex, age, and anatomical distribution in the Finnish population. *Am J Clin Pathol* 77(6):665–673, 1982.

Sabate JM, Torrubia S, Maideu J, Franquet T, Monill JM, Perez C: Sclerosing mesenteritis: Imaging findings in 17 patients. *Am J Roentgenol* 172:625–629, 1999.

Semelka RC, John G, Kelekis NL, Burdeny DA, Ascher SM: Bowel related abscesses: MR demonstration preliminary results. Magnetic Resonance Imaging. 16:855–61, 1998.

Semelka RC, Lawrence PH, Shoenut JP, Heywood M, et al.: Primary malignant ovarian disease: Prospective comparison of contrast enhanced CT and pre- and post-intravenous Gd-DTPA enhanced fat suppressed and breath hold MRI with histological correlation. *J Magn Reson Imag* 3:99–106, 1993.

Smith TR: Malignant peritoneal mesothelioma: Marked variability of CT findings. *Abdom Imag* 19:27–29, 1994.

Unger EC, Glazer HS, Lee JKT, Ling D: MRI of extracranial hematomas: Preliminary observations. *Am J Roentgenol* 146:403–407, 1986.

Walls SD, Hricak H, Baily GD, Kerlan RK Jr., et al.: MR of pathologic abdominal fluid collections. *J Comput Assist Tomogr* 10:746–750, 1986.

Young RH, Gilks CB, Scully RE: Mucinous tumors of the appendix associated with mucinous tumors of the ovary and pseudomyxoma peritonei. A clinico-pathological analysis of 22 cases supporting an origin in the appendix. *Am J Surg Pathol* 15: 415–429, 1991.

CHAPTER 11

Barentsz JO, Engelbrecht M, Jager GJ, Witjes JA, de Larossete J: Fast dynamic gadolinium-enhanced MR imaging of urinary bladder and prostate cancer. *J Magn Reson Imag* 10(3):295–304, 1999.

Barentsz JO, Ruijs SHJ, Strijk SP: The role of MR imaging in carcinoma of the urinary bladder. *Am J Roentgenol* 160:937–947, 1993.

Cheng D, Tempany CMC: Mr imaging of the prostate and bladder. *Semin Ultrasound, CT, and MRI* 19:67–89, 1998.

Ebner F, Kressel HY, Mints MC, et al.: Tumor recurrence versus fibrosis in the female pelvis: Differentiation with MR imaging at 1.5 T. *Radiology* 166:333–340, 1988.

Hahn D: Neoplasms of the urinary bladder. In Pollack HM (ed.), *Clinical Urography*, vol. 2. Philadelphia: WB Saunders, 1990, pp. 1355–1377.

Heiken JP, Forman HP, Brown JJ: Neoplasm of the bladder, prostate, and testis. *Radiol Clin N Am* 32:81–98, 1994.

Hricak H: The bladder and female urethra. In Hricak H, Carrington BM (eds.), *MRI of the Pelvis : A Text Atlas*. London: Martin Dunitz, 1991, pp. 417–461.

Hricak H: Magnetic resonance imaging evaluation of the irradiated female pelvis. *Semin Roentgenol* 29:70–80, 1994.

Kim B, Semelka RC, Ascher SM, Chalpin D, Carroll P, Hricak H: Bladder tumor staging: Comparison of contrast enhanced CT, T1- and T2-weighted MR imaging, dynamic gadolinium-enhanced imaging, and late gadolinium-enhanced imaging. *Radiology* 193:239–245, 1994.

Menahem MM, Slywotzky C: Urinary bladder leiomyoma: Magnetic resonance imaging findings. *Urol Radiol* 14:197–199, 1992.

Narumi Y, Kadota T, Inoue E, et al.: Bladder tumors: Staging with gadolinium-enhanced oblique MR imaging. *Radiology* 187:145–150, 1993.

Narumi Y, Kadota T, Inoue E, et al.: Bladder wall morphology: In vitro MR imaging—histopathologic correlation. *Radiology* 187:151–155, 1993.

Persad R, Kabala J, Gillatt D, Penry B, Gingell JC, Smith JB: Magnetic resonance imaging in the staging of bladder cancer. *Br J Urol* 71:566–573, 1993.

Semelka RC, Hricak H, Kim B, Forstner R, Bis KG, Ascher SM, Reinhold C: Pelvic fistulas: Appearances on MR images. *Abdom Imag* 22:91–95, 1997.

Siegelman ES, Schnall MD: Contrast-enhanced MR imaging of the bladder and prostate. *MRI Clin N Am* 4:153–169, 1996.

Warshawsky R, Bow SN, Waldbaum RS, Cintron J: Bladder pheochromocytoma with MR correlation. *J Comput Assist Tomogr* 13:714–716, 1989.

CHAPTER 12

Cramer BM, Schiegel E, Thuroff J: MR imaging in the differential diagnosis of scrotal and testicular disease. *Radiographics* 11:9–21, 1991.

Di Santis D: Urethral inflammation. In Pollack H (ed.), *Clinical Urography*. Philadelphia: WB Saunders, 1990, pp. 925–939.

Harris R, Schned A, Heaney J: Staging of prostate cancer with endorectal MR imaging: Lessons from a learning curve. *Radiographics* 15:813–829, 1995.

Helweg G, Judmaier W, Buchberger W, Wicke K, Oberhauser H, Knapp R, Ennemoser O, Zur Nedden D: Peyronie's disease: MR findings in 28 patients. *Am J Roentgenol* 158:1261–1264, 1992.

Hricak H: The testis. In Hricak H, Carrington BM (eds.), *MRI of the Pelvis*. Norwalk: Appleton & Lange, 1991, pp. 343–382.

Hricak H: The penis and male urethra. In Hricak H, Carrington BM (eds.), *MRI of the Pelvis*. Norwalk: Appleton & Lange, 1991, pp. 383–416.

Hricak H: The prostate gland. In Hricak H, Carrington BM (eds.), *MRI of the Pelvis*. Norwalk: Appleton & Lange, 1991, pp. 249–312.

Hricak H, White S, Vigneron D, et al.: Carcinoma of the prostate gland: MR imaging with pelvic phased-array coils versus integrated endorectal-pelvic phased-array coils. *Radiology* 193:703–709, 1994.

Huch Boni R, Boner J, Debatin J, Trinkler F, Knonagel H, Von Hochstetter A, Helfenstein U, Krestin G: Optimization of prostate carcinoma staging: Comparison of imaging and clinical methods. *Clin Radiol* 50:593–600, 1995.

Huch Boni R, Boner J, Lutolf U, Trinkler F, Pestalozzi D, Krestin G: Contrast-enhanced endorectal coil MRI in local staging of prostate carcinoma. *J Comput Assist Tomogr* 19(2):232–237, 1995.

Kalbhen CL, Hricak H, Shinohara K, et al.: Prostate carcinoma: MR imaging findings after cryosurgery. *Radiology* 198:807–811, 1996.

King BF, Hattery RR, Lieber MM, Berquist TH, Williamson B Jr., Hartman GW: Congenital cystic disease of the seminal vesicle. *Radiology* 178:207–211, 1991.

King BF, Hattery RR, Lieber MM, Williamson B Jr., Hartman GW, Berquist TH: Seminal vesicle imaging. *Radiographics* 9:653–676, 1989.

Lovett K, Rifkin MD, McCue PA, Choi H: MR imaging characteristics of noncancerous lesions of the prostate. *J Magn Reson Imag* 2:35–39, 1992.

McDermott VG, Meakem III TJ, Stolpen AH, Schnall MD: Prostatic and periprostatic cysts: Findings on MR imaging. *Am J Roentgenol* 164:123–127, 1995.

Nunes LW, Scheibler MS, Rauschning W, Schnall MD, Tomaszewski JE, Pollack H, Kressel H: The normal prostate and periprostatic structures: Correlation between MR images made with an endorectal coil and cadaveric microtome sections. *Am J Roentgenol* 164:923–927, 1995.

Outwater E, Schiebler M, Tomaszewski J, Schnall M, Kressell H: Mucinous carcinomas involving the prostate: Atypical findings at MRI. *J Magn Reson Imag* 2:597–600, 1992.

Quinn S, Franzini D, Demlow T, Rosencrantz D, Kim J, Hanna R, Szumowski J: MR imaging of prostate cancer with an endorectal surface coil technique: Correlation with whole mount-specimens. *Radiology* 190:323–327, 1994.

Semelka R, Anderson M, Hricak H: Prosthetic testicle: Appearance at MR imaging. *Radiology* 173:561–562, 1989.

Sommer FG, Nghiem HV, Herfkens R, McNeal J: Gadolinium-enhanced MRI of the abnormal prostate. Magn Reson Imaging 11:941–948, 1993.

Tempany C, Rahmouni A, Epstein J, Walsh P, Zerhouni E: Invasion of the neurovascular bundle by prostate cancer: Evaluation with MR imaging. *Radiology* 181:107–112, 1991.

Yu KK, Hricak H: Imaging prostate cancer. *Radiol Clin North Am* 38:59–85, 2000.

CHAPTER 13

Amin RS, Nikolaidis P, et al.: Normal anatomy of the fetus at MR imaging. *Radiographics* 19:201–214, 1999.

Buttram VC Jr., Gibbons WE: Müllerian anomalies: A proposed classification (an analysis of 144 cases). *Fertil Steril* 32:40–46, 1979.

Carrington BM, Hricak H, et al.: Müllerian duct anomalies: MR imaging evaluation. *Radiology* 176:715–720, 1990.

Hamm B, Kubik Huch RA, et al.: MR imaging and CT of the female pelvis: Radiologic-pathologic correlation. *Eur Radiol* 9:3–15, 1999.

Hricak H, Secaf E, Buckley DW, Brown JJ, Tanagho EA, McAninch JW. Female urethra: MR imaging. *Radiology* 178:527–535, 1991.

Kim B, Hricak H, Tanagho EA. Diagnosis of urethral diverticula in women: Value of MR imaging. *Am J Roentgenol* 161:809–815, 1993.

Levine D, Barnes PD: Cortical maturation in normal and abnormal fetuses as assessed with prenatal MR imaging. *Radiology* 210:751–758, 1999.

Morrow CP, Curtin JP. Tumors of the ovary: Sex cord stromal tumors and germ cell tumors. In Morrow CP, Curtin JP (eds.), *Synopsis of Gynecologic Oncology*. New York: Churchill Livingstone, 1998, pp. 281–306.

Murase E, Seigelman ES, et al.: Uterine leiomyomas: Histopathologic features, MR imaging findings, differential diagnosis, and treatment. *Radiographics* 19:1179–1197, 1999.

Outwater EK, Dunton CJ. Imaging of the ovary and adnexa: Clinical issues and applications of MR imaging. *Radiology* 194:1–18, 1995.

Outwater EK, Huang AB, Dunton CJ, et al.: Papillary projections in ovarian neoplasms: Appearance on MRI. *Journal of Magnetic Resonance Imaging* 7:689–695, 1997.

Outwater EK, Schiebler ML, Owens RS, et al.: MRI characterization of hemorrhagic adnexal masses: A blinded reader study. *Radiology* 186:489–494, 1993.

Pannu HK, Kaufman HS, Cundiff GW, Genadry R, Bluemke DA, Fishman EK. Dynamic MR imaging of pelvic organ prolapse: Spectrum of abnormalities. *Radiographics* 20:1567–1582, 2000.

Reinhold C, Tafazoli F, et al.: Uterine adenomyosis: Endovaginal US and MR features with histopatholigic correlation. *Radiographics* 19:147–160, 1999.

Romanzi LJ, Groutz A, Blaivas JG. Urethral diverticulum in women: Diverse presentations resulting in diagnostic delay and mismanagement. *J Urol* 164:428–433, 2000.

Siegelman ES, Outwater EK: Tissue characterization in the female pelvis by means of MR imaging. *Radiology* 212:5–18, 1999.

Siegelman ES, Outwater EK, Banner MP, Ramchandani P, Anderson TL, Schnall MD: High-resolution MR imaging of the vagina. *Radiographics* 17:1183–1203, 1997.

Sironi S, De Cobelli F, et al.: Carcinoma of the cervix: Value of plain and gadolinium-enhanced MR imaging in assessing degree of invasiveness. *Radiology* 188:780–797, 1993.

Stevens SK, Hricak H, Campos Z: Teratomas versus cystic hemorrhagic adnexal lesions: Differentiation with proton-selection fat saturation MR imaging. *Radiology* 186:481–488, 1993.

Sugimura K, Okizuka H, Iamaoka I, et al.: Pelvic endometriosis: Detection and diagnosis with chemical shift MR imaging. *Radiology* 188:435–438, 1993.

Togashi K, Nishimura K, Kimura I, et al.: Endometrial cyst: Diagnosis with MR imaging. *Radiology* 180:73–78, 1991.

Woo GM, Twickler DM, et al.: The pelvis after cesarean section and vaginal delivery. Normal MR findings. *Am J Roentgenol* 161:1249–1252, 1993.

Yamashita Y, Torashima M, Hatanaka Y, et al.: Adnexal masses: Accuracy of characterization with transvaginal US and precontrast and postcontrast MR imaging. *Radiology* 194:557–565, 1995.

Young RH, Scully RE: Metastatic tumors in the ovary. In Blaustein A (ed.), *Pathology of the Female Genital Tract*. New York: Springer-Verlag, 1994, pp. 939–974.

Zaloudek C: The Ovary. In Gompel C and Silverberg SG (eds.), *Pathology in Gynecology and Obstetrics*. Philadelphia: Lippincott, 1994, pp. 313–413.

INDEX

A

Abdominal wall hernia, peritoneal imaging, 368–370

Abdominoperineal resection (APR), large bowel imaging, 325–326

Abscesses:
  diverticular, large bowel imaging, 318—320
  gastrointestinal tract imaging, 257–259
  kidney imaging, 193, 195, 198
  liver imaging:
    amoebic abscess, 24, 26
    fungal abscess, 27–30
    nonpyogenic, 24, 26
    pyogenic, 23–25
  peritoneal imaging, 376, 378—381
  prostate imaging, 410
  retroperitoneum imaging, postoperative graft evaluation, 340, 343–344
  splenic imaging, cryptococcal abscess, 144–146
  testicular, 422
  tubal ovarian abscess, 469–470

Accesory spleen, imaging study, 125

Acromegaly, adrenal gland hyperplasia, 225

Acute Budd-Chiari syndrome, 52–53

Acute pancreatitis:
  imaging studies, 92–93, 95
  pseudocyst formations, 95–100

Acute pyelonephritis, imaging studies, 188, 193, 196–197

Acute tubular necrosis, kidney imaging, 205, 209

Addison's disease, adrenal gland imaging, 256

Adenocarcinomas:
  bladder imaging, 396–397
  cervical, 443–444
  esophageal masses, 261
  gallbladder, 66–69
  large bowel imaging, 304–311
  prostate, imaging and staging, 406–409
  small bowel imaging, 276–277
  stomach imaging, 265–266
  vaginal malignancies, 428–429

Adenomas:
  adrenal gland imaging, 225–236
    bilateral, 226–227, 229
    mild capillary blush, 226
    signal drop-no capillary blush, 226–227
  focal nodular hyperplasia, differential diagnosis, 20–22
  kidney imaging, 171, 174
  large bowel imaging, 297, 299–302
  small bowel imaging, 273–274

Adenomatoid tumor:
  extratesticular region, 417
  fetal cystic malformations, 448–450

Adenomyomatosis, gallbladder imaging, 63–64

Adenomyosis, uterine corpus, 439–441

Adnexal masses. *See also* Ovaries
  ovarian cysts, 454, 456–461
  in pregnancy, 452

Adrenal cortical carcinoma, imaging studies, 238, 242, 248–250

Primer on MR Imaging of the Abdomen and Pelvis, edited by Diego R. Martin, Michele A. Brown, and Richard C. Semelka ISBN 0-471-37340-0 Copyright © 2005 Wiley-Liss, Inc.

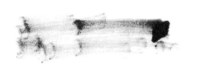